THE JOHNS HOPKINS WHIT[E PAPERS]

2 0 0 8

JOHNS HOPKINS

MEDICINE

Arthritis

Back Pain and Osteoporosis

Colon Cancer

Coronary Heart Disease

Depression and Anxiety

Diabetes

Digestive Disorders

VOLUME 1

Prepared by the Editors of
The Johns Hopkins White Papers
Published by Medletter Associates, LLC

JOHNS HOPKINS MEDICINE
BALTIMORE, MARYLAND

THE JOHNS HOPKINS MEDICAL LETTER
HEALTH AFTER 50

THE JOHNS HOPKINS WHITE PAPERS *are published in association with* THE JOHNS HOPKINS MEDICAL LETTER: HEALTH AFTER 50. *This monthly eight-page newsletter provides practical, timely information for anyone concerned with taking control of his or her own health care. The newsletter is written in clear, non-technical, easy-to-understand language and comes from the century-old tradition of Johns Hopkins excellence. For information on how to subscribe to this newsletter, please write to Health After 50, P.O. Box 420179, Palm Coast, FL 32142.*

Get subscription information—along with the latest perspectives from our experts—at our website:

www.JohnsHopkinsHealthAlerts.com/library

Please visit

www.JohnsHopkinsHealthAlerts.com/library

for articles, updates, special reports, information on our other products, including the Heart, Memory, Depression, Prostate, and Arthritis quarterly bulletins, and more.

Published in the United States in 2008 by Medletter Associates, LLC,
6 Trowbridge Drive, Bethel CT 06801

ISBN: 978-1-933087-72-6 Johns Hopkins White Papers, Volume One

Printed in the United States.

Note:
This book is not intended as an alternative to personal medical advice. The reader should consult a physician in all matters relating to health and particularly in respect of any symptoms that may require diagnosis or medical attention. While the advice and information are believed to be accurate and true at the time of going to press, neither the authors nor the publisher can accept any legal responsibility or liability for any errors or omissions that may have occurred.

ARTHRITIS

John A. Flynn, M.D.,

and

Timothy Johnson, M.D.

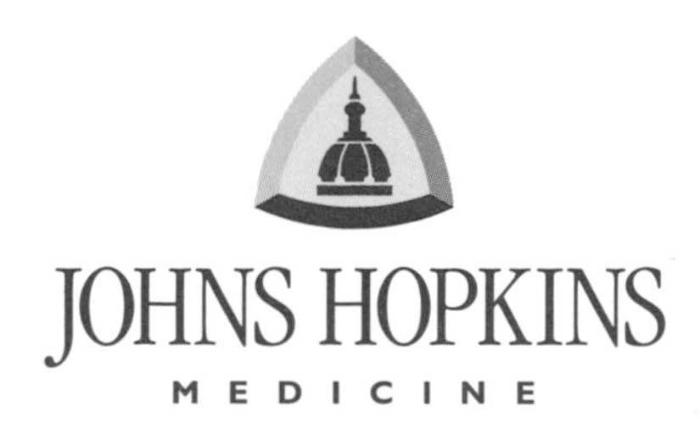

Dear Reader:

Welcome to the 2008 *Arthritis White Paper*—your Johns Hopkins guide to the prevention, diagnosis, and management of arthritis problems, ranging from osteoarthritis, rheumatoid arthritis, gout, and bursitis to lupus, ankylosing spondylitis, fibromyalgia, and Lyme disease.

This year's highlights include:

- Why **smoking** is bad for your knees. (page 7)
- How to find a **qualified fitness trainer** to keep you fit *and* comfortable. (page 8)
- **New NSAID guidelines** focus on safer forms of pain relief. (page 14)
- **Exercise after joint replacement:** How much? What kind? (page 27)
- Obesity: Who is too heavy for **joint replacement surgery**? (page 28)
- Alternatives that work, including an ancient Chinese **exercise that helps relieve knee pain**. (page 35)
- **The sleep–inflammation link**: How a restful night can improve arthritis symptoms. (page 38)
- A **new blood test** that may identify rheumatoid arthritis before symptoms appear. (page 44)
- The importance of **early aggressive treatment** of rheumatoid arthritis in preventing permanent disability. (page 49)
- How rheumatoid arthritis raises your **risk of osteoporosis**. (page 50)
- Why experts think **chronic Lyme disease** doesn't exist. (page 66)

You'll also find a new "Ask the Doctor" column on pages 25, 31, 43, 61, and 63. This year's questions came from my patients, but next year I'd like to answer a few of yours. If you have any arthritis-related queries you want answered in the White Papers or comments about the White Papers in general, please e-mail the editors at whitepapers@johnshopkinshealthalerts.com.

Wishing you the best of health in 2008,

John A. Flynn, M.D.
Associate Professor of Rheumatology
Department of Medicine
Johns Hopkins University School of Medicine

P. S. Don't forget to visit www.HopkinsArthritis.com for the latest news on arthritis and other information that will complement your Johns Hopkins White Paper.

THE AUTHORS

John A. Flynn, M.D., M.B.A., F.A.C.P., F.A.C.R., is a graduate of the University of Missouri-Columbia School of Medicine, where the University of Missouri Medical Alumni Organization selected him as a recipient of the "Outstanding Young Physician Award." He completed his internship and residency in Internal Medicine at the Johns Hopkins University School of Medicine, followed by a fellowship in Clinical Rheumatology.

Dr. Flynn is an Associate Professor in the Divisions of General Internal Medicine and Rheumatology in the Department of Medicine at the Johns Hopkins University School of Medicine. He holds the D. William Schlott, M.D., Professorship of Clinical Medicine and serves as the Clinical Director of the Division of General Internal Medicine and as the Medical Director of the Spondyloarthritis Program. Dr. Flynn has joint appointments in the Department of Psychiatry and Behavioral Sciences as well as at the School of Nursing at Johns Hopkins University. He also serves as an advisor to the Colleges Advisory/Clinical Skills Program at the Johns Hopkins University School of Medicine. His clinical interests include spondyloarthritis. His research interests include ambulatory education and the delivery of primary care in an academic setting.

Dr. Flynn is a recipient of the Clinician Scholar Educator Award from the American College of Rheumatology; the award is designed to recognize and support rheumatologists dedicated to providing exemplary educational experiences for medical trainees. He was also awarded the Alumni Association Award for Excellence in Teaching from the Johns Hopkins University School of Medicine. This award recognizes those whose investment in teaching students at both the pre- and postdoctoral levels is of the highest order.

Dr. Flynn has published in journals such as *Arthritis & Rheumatism*, *Arthritis Care & Research*, *The New England Journal of Medicine*, and the *Journal of General Internal Medicine*. He is Co-Editor of the textbook *Cutaneous Medicine* and Editor of the *Oxford American Handbook of Clinical Medicine*.

■ ■ ■

Timothy Johnson, M.D., received his medical degree from Yale University, followed by a residency and fellowship in sports medicine and shoulder surgery at Weill Medical College of Cornell University–Hospital for Special Surgery. Now an Assistant Professor of Orthopedic Surgery at the Johns Hopkins University School of Medicine, he is a member of the American Board of Orthopedic Surgery. With special interests in arthroscopic surgery of the elbow, knee, shoulder, and hip, as well as sports injuries, Dr. Johnson is currently a team physician for the Baltimore Orioles.

CONTENTS

ARTHRITIS

If you suffer from joint pain and stiffness, you are not alone. By age 50, almost every man and woman has occasionally experienced these symptoms. But if joint pain and stiffness persist, it could mean that you have arthritis.

Fortunately, having arthritis does not have to prevent you from engaging in many of the activities you enjoy. You can take a number of measures to keep your joints pain free and mobile, and if these don't relieve your pain, many medications are also available. If these strategies fail to keep you comfortable and active, surgery may be able to help.

This White Paper will help you discover the best ways to relieve pain and live well with arthritis. The paper begins with a discussion of osteoarthritis, the most common form of arthritis, then addresses rheumatoid arthritis, which is much less common but far more severe. The White Paper concludes with sections on other rheumatoid disorders: ankylosing spondylitis, bursitis, fibromyalgia, gout, lupus, and the arthritis that may arise as a late complication of Lyme disease. Although less prevalent than osteoarthritis and rheumatoid arthritis, together these rheumatic conditions affect nearly 5% of the American population.

What Is Arthritis?

The word "arthritis" means joint inflammation (derived from "arth," which in Greek means joint, and "itis," meaning inflammation). To date, scientists have identified more than 100 types of arthritis, many of which affect the skin, muscles, bones, and internal organs as well as the joints. Together, these conditions are known as rheumatic diseases. Physicians who specialize in treating these diseases are called rheumatologists.

Prevalence

Arthritis is one of the most common chronic health problems in the United States. It is also the number one cause of disability. About one of every three adults—approximately 70 million Americans in all—has been diagnosed with arthritis or has chronic joint symptoms such as pain and stiffness. Women are particularly at risk. According to the Arthritis Foundation, arthritis in general affects about twice as many women as men.

The economic cost of arthritis in the United States for medical care and lost wages is almost $175 billion annually. Of course, the most important cost is the pain, suffering, and disability that can significantly affect a person's quality of life.

Prognosis

Arthritis is a chronic condition—a disease that persists for a long time, often for a lifetime. At present, there is no cure. That may seem discouraging, but fortunately, there's much reason for optimism. New research has led to early diagnosis and better control of many forms of arthritis. It is now clear, for example, that regular exercise is not a hazard to people with arthritis but is instead essential for preventing pain and disability.

Thanks to new drugs and new surgical procedures, fewer people with arthritis now develop severe joint deformities and permanent disabilities. With proper care from their doctors—and active participation in managing their own treatment plan—most people who have arthritis continue to lead active lives, even in their later years.

If you or someone you care about has arthritis, obtaining accurate information is an important part of the treatment plan. Contrary to ads for miracle cures and instant pain relievers that you may hear on the radio or see in newspapers or magazines, arthritis treatment often involves trial and error to find the best combination of therapies and medications to relieve your symptoms. The more you know about arthritis, the more you will understand the rationale behind the treatment, and the better prepared you will be to participate in your own arthritis management.

Anatomy of the Joints

Before you can understand the causes and treatments of arthritis, you need to know more about your joints. A joint is the place where two or more movable bones come together (articulate). Think of your knees, hips, and the many joints in your hands and feet.

Healthy joints move smoothly, thanks to a complex system of lubrication and shock absorption. The components that make this system work include:

- **Cartilage:** a tough, slippery material that coats the ends of the

How Different Forms of Arthritis Affect the Joints

Normal Joint

The entire joint is enclosed in a capsule. The synovial membrane, or inner lining, of this capsule produces a slippery fluid that lubricates the space between the bones. The end of each bone is covered with resilient cartilage, which acts as a natural shock absorber. Outside the joint capsule, tendons connect bones to muscles, while the bursae produce a lubricant that eases movement between muscles and bones.

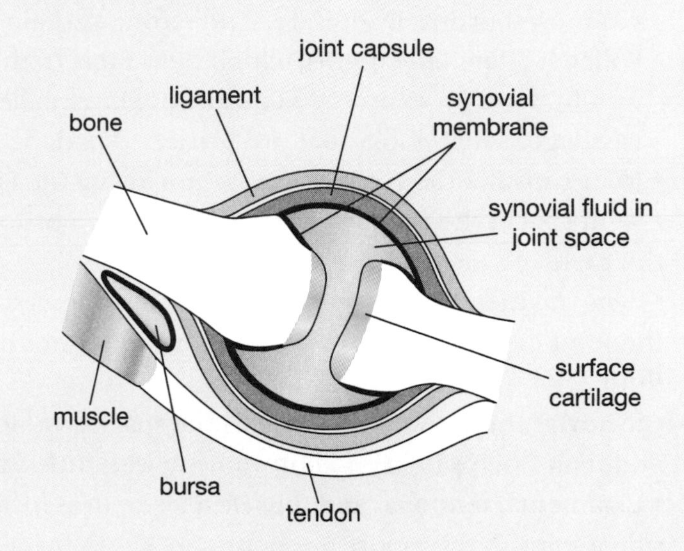

Joint With Osteoarthritis

In a joint affected by osteoarthritis (the most common type of arthritis, prevalent in people over age 50), the cartilage progressively breaks down so that bone surfaces are not protected from rubbing together. The joint gradually loses its shape and alignment. The ends of the bones thicken and develop uneven bony growths, known as spurs or osteophytes. Fragments of loose cartilage or bone may float around within the joint space. All of this damage can cause pain and limit the joint's range of motion.

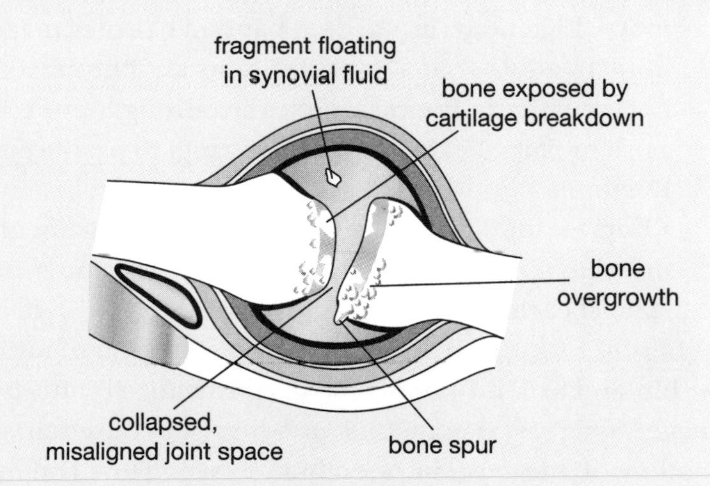

Joint With Rheumatoid Arthritis

Rheumatoid arthritis results when—for reasons unknown—the body's immune system erroneously begins to attack tissue in the joint as if the tissue were a foreign or infectious invader. This attack results in inflammation of the synovial membrane. Inflammatory cells release enzymes that eat away at the tissues inside the joint capsule, including bone and cartilage. As with osteoarthritis, the joint loses its shape and alignment—sometimes severely so. Pain, loss of movement, and eventual destruction of the joint may ensue.

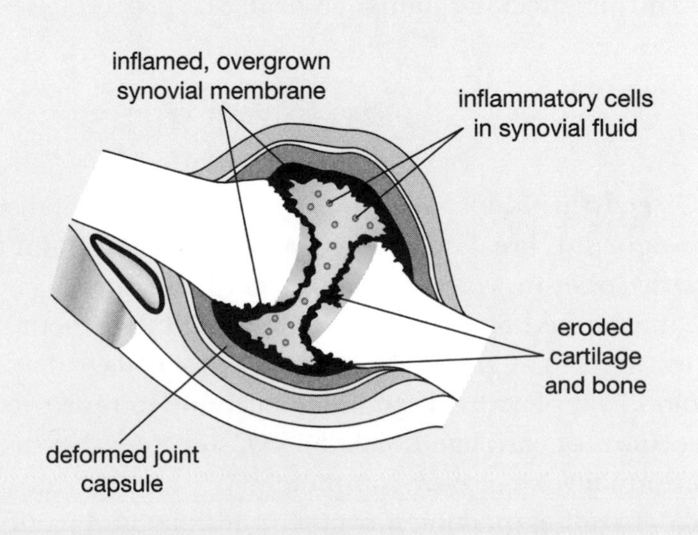

bones and provides a shock-absorbing cushion to prevent the bones from rubbing together. Joint (articular) cartilage is composed primarily of water and strong protein fibers called collagen. The knee joints, which bear most of the body's weight, have an extra shock-absorbing layer called meniscal cartilage, which looks like two C-shaped pads.

- **Joint capsule:** the membrane sac enclosing the entire joint.
- **Joint space:** the narrow, open area between two bones, where the cartilage meets.
- **Synovial membrane (synovium):** the inner membrane lining the joint capsule. It secretes a slippery substance called synovial fluid.
- **Synovial fluid:** the fluid that fills the space around and between bones and helps to keep joints moving with little friction.
- **Ligaments, tendons, and muscles:** structures located just outside a joint that support the bones and help the joint bend and move. Ligaments are strong, band-like tissues that connect one bone to another at a joint. Tendons are fibrous cords that connect muscles to bones. Muscles are strong, fibrous tissues that work in pairs, flexing and contracting, to produce movement in the joints.
- **Bursae:** fluid-filled sacs located between ligaments, tendons, muscles, and bones. Bursae help these structures move smoothly against each other.

Different forms of arthritis cause inflammation of various structures within and around joints. Osteoarthritis mostly affects the joint cartilage, whereas rheumatoid arthritis generally starts with inflammation of the synovial membrane (see "How Different Forms of Arthritis Affect the Joints" on page 3).

OSTEOARTHRITIS

Osteoarthritis, also known as degenerative joint disease, involves a progressive breakdown of cartilage and other joint tissues. It starts with softening of the smooth cartilage surface, which then becomes pitted and frayed. Unlike most of the body's tissues, which are able to regrow when damaged, cartilage has a very limited blood supply, which hampers its ability to repair itself. Over time, sections of cartilage break down faster than they are repaired and, eventually, wear away completely. Without this cushion, the bones rub together, making movement difficult and painful. The friction can also cause bony outgrowths called osteophytes or "spurs," which can add to the discomfort.

Osteoarthritis is the most common form of arthritis and one of the most common causes of physical disability in adults. An estimated 21 million people in the United States have the condition. By age 40, approximately 90% of us have at least some signs of osteoarthritis that can be seen on x-rays of the weight-bearing joints (the hips and knees, for example), but symptoms of pain and stiffness usually don't start until later in life. Before age 55, osteoarthritis is more common in men; after age 55, it is more common in women.

As cartilage continues to break down, the joints lose their normal shape, and bony growths (called spurs) may form. Bits of bone or cartilage often break off into the joint space, causing more pain and joint damage. The cartilage breakdown may cause inflammation of the synovial membrane, which in turn leads to production of enzymes and cytokines (inflammatory proteins) that cause further cartilage damage. The quality of a substance called hyaluronic acid in the synovial fluid also may change, and this can reduce its protective effects.

Osteoarthritis occurs most often in the knees, hips, spine, small joints of the fingers, and base of the thumb and big toe, although it can affect any joint. When severe osteoarthritis affects the knees, hips, and spine, it may significantly limit activity and diminish a person's quality of life. The good news: Osteoarthritis generally has little or no effect on longevity—in other words, it won't shorten your life.

Causes of Osteoarthritis

Osteoarthritis is often called a wear-and-tear disease because it develops in joints after many years of use. Aging increases the risk of developing osteoarthritis, but it's not the sole cause. Scientists are not sure exactly what causes the condition, but several factors play a role: genetic predisposition, obesity, prior joint injuries, wear and tear on the joints due to chronic overuse or sports-related activities, muscle weakness, and nerve injury. Osteoarthritis is classified as primary or secondary, depending on the presence of underlying conditions and the number of affected joints.

Primary osteoarthritis. The most common type, it results from the gradual breakdown of cartilage that occurs with age. Why the cartilage starts to break down is not clear. Individuals who have primary osteoarthritis have no inflammation in their joints and no indication that an injury or repetitive activities could have caused their joint problems. But in some people with a family history of osteoarthritis, genetics seems to play a role. In a study of female twins, heredity contributed to 39–65% of the hand and knee osteoarthritis that developed. Research also suggests that middle-aged women with low levels of estrogen are more likely to develop osteoarthritis than those with normal levels.

Primary osteoarthritis typically affects the joints of the lower back, hips, knees, big toe, fingers, and base of the thumb. It can be present in only one of these joints or in all of them.

Secondary osteoarthritis. This type results from specific conditions that damage joint cartilage, including a prior injury (a fracture or torn ligament), chronic joint inflammation due to another type of arthritis (such as rheumatoid arthritis), or repetitive overuse of the joint from activities such as heavy lifting, kneeling, or operating certain types of equipment. One study found that people whose jobs required at least one hour a day of kneeling or squatting were almost twice as likely to have osteoarthritis in the knees as people who didn't perform such activities. Because trauma or overuse hastens the degeneration of joint cartilage, symptoms of secondary osteoarthritis often appear at a much younger age than symptoms of primary osteoarthritis.

Stress on a joint—from obesity, for example—is probably the most common risk factor for secondary osteoarthritis. Obesity is especially hard on the knees and the other major weight-bearing joints such as the hips and spine. Studies show that osteoarthritis of the knee is nearly four times more common in obese women than in normal-weight women and nearly five times more common in obese men than in normal-weight men.

Secondary osteoarthritis may also be due to a prior infection in a joint, inherited metabolic conditions such as excess body iron (hemochromatosis), overproduction of certain hormones, or bone disorders that affect the joints. With some of these conditions, osteoarthritis is limited to one or just a few joints. With disorders that affect the entire body, osteoarthritis may develop in numerous joints.

Prevention of Osteoarthritis

Fortunately, taking a few steps can reduce your risk of developing osteoarthritis in the first place or prevent osteoarthritis from getting worse if you already have it. Although none of these methods is guaranteed to work, they are nonetheless good for your overall health.

Weight Control

Losing weight could be your best strategy to prevent osteoarthritis in your weight-bearing joints. A team of Johns Hopkins rheumatologists found a significant association between body mass index (the best indicator of overweight) and significant knee, hip, and back pain.

What's more, it does not take very much weight loss to decrease your risk of osteoarthritis. Studies show that overweight or obese women who lose as little as 11 lbs cut their risk of knee osteoarthritis in half.

Exercise

Although arthritis is a wear-and-tear condition, mild to moderate exercise will not damage your joints. In fact, a careful, regular exercise program can dramatically lower the risk of osteoarthritis by strengthening the muscles that support weight-bearing joints. Exercise will also help with weight loss, which also reduces your risk. To help ensure that your exercise program is not doing more harm than good, try working with a physical therapist or a fitness trainer (see "How To Find a Qualified Fitness Trainer" on pages 8–9).

What about vigorous exercise and sports activities? Studies show that even distance runners don't have an increased risk of osteoarthritis. But the risk is increased in athletes who sustain joint injuries, especially in collision sports like football. If you do suffer a joint injury, proper bracing, physical therapy, and, if necessary, surgical repair can reduce your risk of developing osteoarthritis.

Injury Prevention

For someone who already has signs of osteoarthritis, the best way to minimize the risk of secondary osteoarthritis is to prevent joint injuries. If your daily activities require frequent kneeling, squatting, or repetitive hand motions (at the computer keyboard, for example), you may want to ask your doctor about braces or other supportive devices to protect your joints.

Symptoms of Osteoarthritis

Because primary osteoarthritis develops slowly, people rarely notice any symptoms before their 40s or 50s. When symptoms first appear, they are usually mild. For example, your joints may ache after doing physical work or exercise, or you may feel stiff for a few minutes when you get out of bed in the morning.

NEW RESEARCH

Smoking May Lead to Knee Cartilage Loss

If you smoke and one of your parents has knee osteoarthritis, you may be upping your own chances of developing the condition, according to a recent study.

Researchers measured knee cartilage in 325 middle-aged people, 163 of whom had at least one parent with severe knee osteoarthritis, and they repeated the measurements two years later. The participants reported on their smoking habits and knee pain through questionnaires.

The researchers found that people who smoked and who had a parent with knee osteoarthritis were much more likely to lose cartilage on the end of the tibia, or shin bone, and to have defects in the cartilage itself than nonsmokers with no family history of osteoarthritis. And heavy smokers had nearly 10 times the risk of having cartilage defects than nonsmokers.

In people with or without a family history of osteoarthritis, current smokers were more likely to have knee pain than former smokers or nonsmokers; 41% vs. 33%, respectively. Current smokers also lost cartilage faster and had more cartilage defects than nonsmokers.

These results are the first to suggest that smoking may interact with certain genes in a way that increases the risk of knee osteoarthritis—another reason to chuck your smokes into the nearest trash can.

ARTHRITIS & RHEUMATISM
Volume 56, page 1521
May 2007

How To Find a Qualified Fitness Trainer

Asking the right questions is key to a successful partnership

Has your rheumatologist recommended exercise to improve your osteoarthritis or rheumatoid arthritis symptoms, but you're not quite sure what to do or how to do it? Working with a good fitness trainer can ensure that your exercise regimen meets your needs and that you learn to do the exercises properly, minimizing the risk of overuse or injury.

But beware—the qualifications of fitness trainers vary widely: Some are nearly as qualified as physical therapists, while others have merely passed a week-long course. And don't expect your doctor to oversee the trainer; most doctors are just too busy to be more than minimally involved in this aspect of your care.

So how can you find a good trainer who has worked with arthritis patients? And what's the best way to open and maintain the lines of communication between your doctor and your trainer?

The Right Credentials

The first step is to ask your rheumatologist or physical therapist to refer you to a qualified trainer. You can also check with your local chapter of the Arthritis Foundation (see page 77 for contact information), which may have a list of trainers experienced in working with people who have arthritis. Another option is to ask friends, family, or reputable local health clubs for referrals.

Although no laws require trainers to be certified or even to have particular training, certification by a reputable agency ensures that you are working with someone who understands the mechanics of exercise. Reputable certifying associations include the American College of Sports Medicine (www.acsm.org), the National Strength and Conditioning Association (www.nsca-lift.org), and the American Council on Exercise (www.acefitness.org). All of these organizations have locators on their websites that list the names of certified trainers. To find other reputable certifying groups, check with the National Commission for Certifying Agencies (www.noca.org), which sets the standards for credentialing agencies.

Ask Questions

Once you've selected several trainers and determined their certification, you'll need to interview them, asking the following:

• ***Have you worked with someone who has my kind of arthritis?*** The answer should, of course, be yes. Ask for and contact one or two references from the trainers.

• ***Are you willing to coordinate my program with my rheumatologist or physical therapist?*** You want someone who has worked with physicians and physical therapists and knows how to

Pain and Swelling

As osteoarthritis advances, you may hear cracking or creaking sounds or feel mild pain when moving joints in your hands, knees, hips, and spine. Increased activity makes the pain worse and rest relieves it. Some swelling and joint deformity may occur as the disease progresses. If you develop inflammation (hot, red, or tender joints), you may have rheumatoid arthritis, not osteoarthritis.

Knobby Nodes

Enlargement of the finger joints is common in the later stages of osteoarthritis. Knobby overgrowths of the joints nearest to the fingertips (Heberden's nodes) occur more often in women and tend to run in families. Similar enlargements located on the middle joints of the fingers are known as Bouchard's nodes.

communicate with them about your condition.

• ***How will you decide what program to put me on?*** The trainer's answer should be that his or her plan will depend on your goals, your fitness level, and the input of your doctor or physical therapist about your limitations and medications.

• ***What would you do if someone has this kind of limitation (name one of yours)? If someone has a flare-up?*** If he or she has no suggestions or doesn't know what a flare-up is, that should be a red flag.

Meeting with a trainer is not a one-way street. A good trainer will ask you questions as well, such as:

- What kind of arthritis do you have? What are your goals?
- What are your limitations?
- Have you ever had a joint replacement?
- What medications do you take?
- Have you exercised before?
- What kind of activities do you like?
- Do you prefer individual or group exercise?

Doctor-Trainer Coordination

As noted previously, your rheumatologist should be able to refer you to a reputable physical therapist or, perhaps, even to a personal trainer, but providing extensive advice about exercise is generally beyond his or her realm of expertise. And, in reality, with multiple demands, most doctors are simply too pressed for time. Nevertheless, that does not mean that you should not try to coordinate your work with a personal trainer and your doctor's recommendations.

You can begin by giving your trainer your doctor's contact information and asking him or her to send the doctor a note, explaining your exercise program and inquiring if any of the activities are ones you shouldn't be doing. Many doctors prefer notes to phone calls since their time is so limited. Be sure to give the doctor permission to discuss your case with your trainer.

If your doctor has nixed a certain exercise that your trainer feels might help you, ask your trainer to send any scientific evidence to your doctor. The doctor may give the okay, or he or she may tell the trainer something about your limitations that, regardless of the studies, should keep you from the particular exercise.

If your trainer's advice collides with your doctor's, you can also do some sleuthing on your own and then let both professionals know what you have found.

Your health and fitness are the top priority. And anything you can do to nurture efficient, effective communication among you, your doctor, and your fitness trainer only enhances your chances of staying well. ■

Disease Progression

In many people, osteoarthritis symptoms progress very little; in others, pain and stiffness gradually worsen until they limit daily activities, such as walking, climbing stairs, or preparing meals. But discomfort and loss of function are not inevitable.

In fact, research shows that the prognosis of osteoarthritis is generally good. For example, one study followed 63 people with osteoarthritis of the hand or knee. Knee x-rays and reports of pain over an average of 11 years, showed that the disease made little progression among people whose initial symptoms were mild or moderate—which is the case for most people with osteoarthritis.

Researchers are also looking into new drugs and procedures that may halt disease progression. One example under investigation is the osteoporosis medication risedronate (Actonel), which may help preserve bone beneath cartilage. And research suggests that the antibiotic, doxycycline, appears to slow joint space narrowing. Investigators are also studying the use of adult stem cells to regenerate cartilage, muscle, and bone (see "Stem Cells for Cartilage Implants" on page 33).

Diagnosis of Osteoarthritis

If you develop joint pain and stiffness, your doctor will take your medical history and do a physical examination to determine which type of arthritis you have.

Important Questions

The first step in obtaining a diagnosis is answering a detailed set of questions about where, when, and how your symptoms first occurred. Because no lab test can confirm osteoarthritis, these questions are used to eliminate other possibilities.

Here are some questions your doctor is likely to ask:

- Which joints are involved?
- What triggers your pain?
- When is the pain at its worst?
- Does anything provide relief?
- Have your joints been red and swollen?
- Do you have morning stiffness, and how long does it last?
- Have you had fever, chills, or unexplained weight loss?
- What are some of your current and past work and recreational activities?
- What other medical conditions do you have?
- What medications are you taking?

Physical Examination

During the physical exam, the doctor will ask you to walk, bend, and move the joints of your hands, arms, legs, feet, and spine. This will show how many joints are affected and whether the arthritis occurs symmetrically (in matching joints on both sides of the body). The doctor may also need to check your skin, heart, lungs, eyes, and digestion, because they can be affected by certain rheumatic diseases.

X-rays

X-rays are not essential to confirm a diagnosis of osteoarthritis. In most instances, your doctor will be able to make the diagnosis based solely on the results of your medical history and physical examination. But x-rays may be taken to determine the extent of cartilage loss, bone damage, bone spurs, and narrowing of the joint spaces.

The severity of osteoarthritis indicated on an x-ray and in a physical exam may be quite different, however. Some people whose x-rays show joint changes have no symptoms. In other cases, x-rays of people who have many sore and stiff joints may show little joint damage.

Joint Aspiration

When the diagnosis is unclear, your doctor may use a procedure called joint aspiration to obtain a sample of synovial fluid from the affected joint. The aspiration is performed by injecting a local anesthetic into the joint and then inserting a syringe and withdrawing a small amount of fluid. Examination of the fluid for the number and type of white blood cells can help determine whether osteoarthritis is causing your joint symptoms.

Other Tests

If the doctor suspects that your joint symptoms may be due to rheumatoid arthritis or another type of rheumatic disease (such as gout or lupus), he or she may also order blood and urine tests.

Treatment of Osteoarthritis

Your doctor cannot predict how quickly your joint symptoms will worsen or how severe the symptoms will become. In addition, no current treatment can stop or reverse the progression of osteoarthritis. But your doctor can recommend a combination of therapies that will decrease joint pain and stiffness, improve joint movement, and increase your ability to perform routine activities. By following your doctor's treatment recommendations, you will see improvements in your quality of life.

Your doctor will base your treatment on your age, occupation, and everyday activities. He or she will also take into consideration the severity of your osteoarthritis, which of your joints are affected, what symptoms are present, and whether you have other medical problems.

Osteoarthritis treatment usually requires several or all of the following approaches:

- Weight loss to decrease stress on your weight-bearing joints
- Exercise to improve mobility

NEW RESEARCH

Being Overweight Raises the Risk of Knee—Not Hip—Osteoarthritis

Obesity is a well-known risk factor for developing osteoarthritis. But one study offers a surprising new insight: a high body-mass index (BMI), a measure of body fat, is associated with the development and progression of osteoarthritis of the knee but not the hip.

Researchers drew 3,585 participants from the Rotterdam Study, a study of chronic diseases of the elderly begun in 1990. They included only those with knees and hips that showed some signs of osteoarthritis in x-rays taken at the start of the study. They divided the participants into three groups: people who had a healthy BMI of 25 or lower; those with a BMI of 25–27.5 (overweight), and those with a BMI greater than 27.5 (obesity).

When they compared baseline x-rays with those taken 6.5 years later, the people with BMIs over 27.5 had more than three times the risk of developing knee osteoarthritis than the group with a BMI of 25 or lower. But they found no significant relationship between a high BMI and hip osteoarthritis.

The extra weight may cause a misalignment in the knee, a hinge joint, that it would not cause in the hip, a ball-and-socket joint, say the researchers. The weight on a misaligned joint may result in a force that's double or triple the force on a normal joint.

This study suggests that even if you have osteoarthritis in your knees, maintaining a healthy weight might help slow its progression.

ANNALS OF THE RHEUMATIC DISEASES
Volume 66, page 158
February 2007

- Rest and joint self-care
- Drugs for pain management
- Physical and occupational therapy to maintain flexibility and strengthen the muscles around your joints
- Assistive devices such as braces, canes, crutches, and walkers
- Alternative therapies such as supplements or acupuncture
- Surgery, as a last resort, if the above treatments do not provide sufficient pain relief.

Self-Management Techniques

You are the most important partner in the treatment plan for your arthritis. The plan will have two complementary goals: improving your physical function and managing your pain. The former involves a balance between mobility and rest. Being fit and flexible will reduce your pain, but many individuals with osteoarthritis need medications to help them feel well enough to remain active. If all goes well, you may find yourself in a positive cycle, in which medication helps you exercise, and exercise helps you lose weight, so that you have less joint damage, less pain, and less need for drugs.

Weight loss

Because being overweight puts extra stress on the joints, losing as many extra pounds as you can is important. In one study, researchers randomly assigned 21 obese people who had knee osteoarthritis to either an exercise program or a combination of exercise and diet. After six months, people in the exercise group lost an average of 4 lbs while people in the exercise and diet group lost an average of 19 lbs. Both groups had a significant reduction in knee pain, but improvements were greater in those who had lost more weight.

The Arthritis, Diet, and Activity Promotion Trial (ADAPT), which focused on overweight osteoarthritis patients over age 60, also found that modest weight loss plus moderate exercise provided the greatest improvement in knee pain and mobility. In a Johns Hopkins study of overweight or obese osteoarthritis patients, a 15-lb weight loss improved their symptoms more than common pain relievers did.

Other research shows that people who have osteoarthritis in one knee can reduce the likelihood that it will develop in the other knee if they lose weight. If you are overweight and haven't been successful in your weight loss efforts, consult a dietitian for help in improving your eating habits.

Exercise

When you are experiencing significant joint pain, resting your joints is important. But when your pain improves, exercise is equally essential to maintain joint motion, muscle strength, and fitness.

Appropriate exercise won't "wear out" your damaged joints. In fact, research shows that it's one of the best treatments for osteoarthritis. Regular exercise also improves mood, increases flexibility, and promotes heart health. In addition, it can improve balance, which is often impaired in people with knee osteoarthritis. Without exercise, you will lose muscle strength, and your osteoarthritis may progress faster.

Ideally, you should exercise every day. Studies show that people who exercise daily achieve the greatest improvement in pain and function, compared with those who exercise less often.

But how do you know which exercises are right for you? That's where a physical therapist comes in. With your doctor's approval, a physical therapist can develop an exercise program for you, based on your age, physical condition, and the severity of your symptoms. At first, you may have to visit the therapist's office to learn the exercises. But once you know how to do them correctly, you can continue the exercises at home or at a fitness center, with only periodic visits to the physical therapist to monitor your progress. Improvement takes time, and patience is crucial to your success.

The physical therapist is likely to recommend three types of exercises—range of motion, muscle strengthening, and aerobic—and a schedule for doing these exercises.

Range-of-motion exercises. These exercises involve gently moving a joint as far as possible in every direction, without causing pain. The purpose of range-of-motion exercises is to maintain flexibility, reduce pain and stiffness, and improve joint function. These stretching exercises are also recommended as a warm-up before a workout. Here's an example of a range-of-motion exercise: Try standing with your arms at your side. Then raise one arm straight up close to your ear, stretching it gently while keeping your elbow straight. Return your arm slowly to your side, and then repeat the exercise with your other arm.

Muscle-strengthening exercises. These exercises increase structural support for the joints, lessening the load placed on them. For example, lifting light hand weights is a good way to strengthen arm muscles. Or lie on your back, raise one leg, hold it up for several seconds, and then lower it slowly, feeling the pull in the thigh muscles that help to support your knee. Repeat the exercise with your other leg.

NEW RESEARCH

Walking and Jogging: Do They Raise Knee Osteoarthritis Risk?

If worry about osteoarthritis is keeping you off the walking trail, relax. A nine-year study finds that walking and jogging won't raise or lower your risk of knee osteoarthritis, even if you're overweight.

The researchers reviewed the records of 1,705 adults, ages 26 to 81, who were overweight or obese but who did not have knee osteoarthritis. The participants answered questions about their physical activities and knee symptoms, such as pain or stiffness, and had x-rays taken of their knees. Of the initial group, 1,279 repeated the same process nine years later. Researchers examined x-rays for changes in the knee joints and for a reduction in the space between the joints, which signals a loss of cartilage.

The researchers divided participants into three groups: those who didn't exercise; those who walked six or more miles per week, and those who walked six miles or less weekly. Nine years later, there was little difference in the number of people from each group who developed knee osteoarthritis. Of those who did no exercise, 7.5% got knee arthritis, as did about 6% of people who walked more than six miles weekly and nearly 5% who logged less than six miles.

People who are overweight or obese do have a higher risk of knee osteoarthritis, but it's not exercise that's boosting—or lowering—the risk. So, go ahead and hit the trails. If your knees are healthy, they aren't likely to complain.

ARTHRITIS & RHEUMATISM
Volume 57, page 6
February 15, 2007

Pain Relief Without NSAIDs

New guidelines recommend NSAIDs as a last resort for chronic pain

If you suffer from arthritis and have come to rely on nonsteroidal anti-inflammatory drugs (NSAIDs) to relieve chronic pain, don't be surprised if your doctor won't renew your prescription—at least not right away. In spring 2007, the American Heart Association issued new guidelines asking doctors not to prescribe NSAIDs or COX-2 inhibitors (a new generation of NSAIDs) for musculoskeletal pain unless their patient had tried all other possibilities.

For years, NSAIDs have been the pain reliever of choice for people with arthritis. In fact, in 2003 Americans spent $5.5 billion on COX-2 inhibitors (such as Celebrex) and $3 billion on other NSAIDs such as aspirin, naproxen (Aleve), and ibuprofen (Advil, Motrin). Still, the drugs have never been ideal—it's long been known that NSAIDs can cause serious gastrointestinal and kidney problems. And this new recommendation is based on several studies showing that these drugs, with the exception of aspirin, increase the risk of heart attack and stroke (see "Some NSAIDs More Risky Than Others," on opposite page).

Although the advice specifically pertains to people with or at risk for heart disease, some doctors are following the recommendations for everyone they treat. The upshot is that millions with arthritis are wondering if they can take the drugs and what they can do for pain and inflammation if they cannot.

Give Non-Drug Treatment Options a Try

If you are taking an NSAID or celecoxib (Celebrex), the only COX-2 inhibitor still on the market, the first step is to speak to your doctor about alternatives, particularly if you have heart disease or are at risk for heart problems. Non-drug alternatives your doctor may suggest include:

Physical therapy and exercise. Your doctor may refer you to a physical therapist who will design a series of exercises that will help condition your muscles, build strength, and increase your range of motion, all of which can help relieve pain and stiffness and improve fitness. The exercises could include:

- Range-of-motion exercises. These stretching exercises increase flexibility and lessen stiffness.
- Strengthening exercises. These may include isometrics, which involve flexing and relaxing the muscles without moving the joints, or isotonics, which may involve the use of small dumbbells or stretch bands. Both types strengthen muscles, which can then better support your joints.
- Aerobic exercises. Exercises such as walking or biking help strengthen muscles, improve oxygen flow, and help control your weight, which reduces pressure on your joints.

Heat. Use of heat increases blood flow, relaxes chronically sore muscles, and relieves pain. Try using warm towels or hot packs for 15–20 minutes three times a day. Warm baths or showers may provide relief as well. You can also buy disposable wraps or patches that heat up when exposed to air. Physical therapists may use electromagnetic waves (shortwaves or microwaves) or ultrasound—both of which produce heat—to relieve pain in inflamed joints.

Cold. Applying a cold pack reduces acute swelling, inflammation, and pain by numbing the nerves. Wrap a bag of ice or frozen vegetables in a towel and apply for 10–15 minutes every four to six hours.

Water therapy (hydrotherapy). Exercising in a heated pool or whirlpool takes weight off your joints while allowing you to do range-of-motion exercises. Some community centers and YMCAs or YWCAs offer water classes for people with arthritis.

Massage. The gentle kneading of soft tissues relieves tension, loosens tight muscles, and reduces pain and swelling. Ask your massage therapist to show you some techniques you can do at home between sessions.

Transcutaneous electrical nerve stimulation. Commonly known as TENS, this procedure relieves pain by sending a low electrical current through electrodes placed on the skin. Your doctor may recommend this procedure and can refer you to a qualified physical therapist who can teach you how to use the device.

Relaxation therapy. Your physical therapist can teach you these exercises, which help release muscle tension. With progressive muscle relaxation, for example, you tighten and then slowly release a group of muscles, proceeding group by group over the whole body.

Acupuncture. This ancient Chinese pain-relief method involves placing, short thin needles at various sites to relieve pain, and a number of studies have shown that it provides some pain relief. It's possible that the needles stimulate nerves that trigger the release of natural painkillers called endorphins. Acupressure is similar, although the therapist uses pressure instead of needles.

Acupuncture should be performed by a licensed practitioner, using sterilized, disposable needles. Talk to your doctor before getting acupuncture, and ask for a referral. You can also contact the National Certification Commission for Acupuncture and Oriental Medicine or the American Academy of Medical Acupuncture for names of acupuncture practitioners.

Some NSAIDs More Risky Than Others

All NSAIDs are not created equal—especially in terms of heart attack and stroke risk. Here's why. All NSAIDs work by targeting an enzyme known as COX. This enzyme comes in two major forms: COX-1, which protects the stomach lining, and COX-2, which is responsible for the inflammation in arthritis and other painful conditions. Traditional NSAIDs, such as aspirin, block both of these enzymes. However, because COX-1 helps protect the lining of the stomach, traditional NSAIDs can cause stomach upset, ulcers, and, most seriously, bleeding.

COX-2 inhibitors were designed to avoid this side effect, targeting the inflammation-related COX-2 enzyme while leaving the stomach-protecting COX-1 alone. Unfortunately, scientists now believe that this selective targeting of COX-2 can increase the risk of heart attack and stroke, especially in people with or at risk for heart disease.

So if NSAIDs are the only painkillers that offer you relief, the American Heart Association (AHA) recommends starting with aspirin, which actually has heart-protecting effects. If aspirin doesn't offer relief, the AHA advises next trying the NSAIDs that are least selective for the COX-2 enzyme. Naproxen (Aleve) is the first choice here, although fewer studies have been done on it than other NSAIDs. Ibuprofen (Advil, Motrin) and diclofenac (Voltaren) have somewhat more anti-COX-2 activity than naproxen, and high doses may increase the risk of heart attack or stroke by 50%. Celecoxib (Celebrex)—the most COX-2 specific—should be the NSAID of last resort in patients with known cardiac disease.

When These Alternatives Fail

If none of the above alternatives help, your doctor may suggest acetaminophen (Tylenol), which has a lower risk of gastrointestinal problems than NSAIDs. Another non-NSAID option is the prescription pain reliever tramadol (Ultram). Your doctor might also prescribe a narcotic for short-term pain relief only. Usually, however, the narcotic is taken in conjunction with an NSAID, since narcotic pain relievers do not decrease inflammation, which is the underlying source of the pain that occurs with arthritis.

You can also try using topical creams or ointments that contain capsaicin, an anti-inflammatory chemical that is also the "heat" in hot peppers. More traditional unguents, such as BenGay and Aspercreme, might also help. Or ask your doctor about the possibility of injections of hyaluronic acid products (Hyalgan or Synvisc) that mimic natural joint lubricants. For osteoarthritis, these temporary pain relievers are injected directly into the joint. Corticosteroids, taken orally or injected, may also relieve pain by reducing inflammation.

For some people, antidepressants such as paroxetine (Paxil), sertraline (Zoloft), amitriptyline (Elavil), imipramine (Tofranil), or duloxetine (Cymbalta) help relieve pain.

If none of those work and you are not at risk for heart disease, your doctor may continue to prescribe NSAIDs for you at the lowest effective dose. ■

In one study, an eight-week muscle-strengthening program improved muscle tone and decreased pain significantly in people with osteoarthritis of the knee. Isometric exercise—pushing or pulling against a fixed object—is also helpful for people with osteoarthritis. Isometric exercises can strengthen your muscles without damaging your joints because the joints remain immobile during the exercise.

Aerobic exercises. This form of sustained exercise increases the need for oxygen, improving overall body fitness. High-impact aerobic activities such as jogging are risky for people with osteoarthritis because they may accelerate the breakdown of cartilage in weight-bearing joints. But low- or no-impact aerobic activities, such as swimming, walking, and bicycling, are excellent ways to improve your fitness. Swimming and other aquatic exercises are particularly good choices because these activities put little stress on your joints, increase joint flexibility, strengthen muscles, and boost self-confidence while providing a good aerobic workout.

Rest

The treatment of arthritis requires both rest and exercise. The trick is getting the right balance between the two.

When it comes to your joints, resting involves more than simply avoiding an activity that causes pain. Some people find that relaxation techniques, stress reduction, and biofeedback improve their resting time. Another important aspect of rest is the use of assistive devices that reduce strain on your joints.

Here are some examples of assistive devices:

- Canes, crutches, walkers, shoe inserts, or special shoes to improve walking
- Splints, braces, taping, or slings to support affected joints
- Raised toilet seats, shower grab bars, electric toothbrushes, higher chairs with arms, Velcro-fastened shoes, cushioned cooking implements, and other devices that help make activities of daily life easier to perform.

Although many of these items are available without a prescription, consulting a physical or occupational therapist may keep you from selecting the wrong item or using it improperly and thus aggravating your arthritis.

Heat and ice

Using heat and cold to reduce pain is another strategy that can help you exercise in comfort. Heat can be applied to an affected joint before exercise to aid stretching and reduce minor aches. Cold packs are often used after exercise to reduce swelling and help relieve pain.

Heat relaxes the muscles around stiff joints, which often reduces osteoarthritis pain. You can apply heat in several ways: hot baths and showers or hot towels provide moist heat; for dry heat, try heating pads and mitts, heat lamps (diathermy), and microwavable collars and pads that maintain heat for hours. Some people with osteoarthritis dip their hands and feet into warm paraffin wax, which forms a temporary coating of heat.

Whichever heat treatment you choose, don't apply it for more than 15 minutes at a time, and be sure to follow all safety directions so that you don't burn your skin.

You may find that you prefer cold for osteoarthritis pain relief. Some people get the best results by alternating between cold and heat. For cold applications, you can use a wet towel soaked in ice water, a plastic bag full of ice cubes, or even a bag of frozen vegetables (which will mold around a joint).

Drugstores also sell special fluid-filled pouches that can be frozen or heated for use on painful joints. Whatever method you use, don't apply cold for longer than 20 minutes at a time. Also be sure to put a dry towel or cloth on your skin first to prevent frostbite from direct contact with the cold source. If you have poor circulation, check with your doctor before using any cold treatment.

Education

Learn all you can about your condition. Most chapters of the Arthritis Foundation offer a six-week Self-Management Program that teaches people how to reduce and manage their joint pain. Studies show that participants typically experience a decrease in pain, an increase in physical activity, an improved quality of life, plus significant reductions in healthcare expenses. Contact your local Arthritis Foundation chapter for information about courses in your area (see page 77 for contact information).

Drugs for Pain Management

Effective medications are available to relieve osteoarthritis-related pain. Oral medications are used most often, but research linking some to an increased risk of heart disease has made doctors less inclined to prescribe them first. Some people find that injections into the affected joint or topical products applied to the skin surrounding a painful joint also help reduce pain.

However, although pain relievers make you feel better, they cannot cure your osteoarthritis. Researchers have not yet identified any medications that can reverse or prevent worsening of the condition.

Oral pain relievers

Taking an oral pain medication is sometimes the first step in the medical treatment of osteoarthritis. However, in 2007, the American Heart Association (AHA) issued new guidelines asking doctors not to prescribe nonsteroidal anti-inflammatory drugs (NSAIDs) or COX-2 inhibitors (a new generation of NSAIDs) to patients at risk for having a heart attack—including those with established coronary heart disease or risk factors, such as high blood pressure or high cholesterol—until they have tried all other methods of relieving a patient's pain. (See "Pain Relief Without NSAIDs" on pages 14–15.) The most commonly used pain relievers are acetaminophen (Tylenol) and NSAIDs. Which drug your doctor recommends depends on the intensity of your pain and the potential side effects of the medication. Usually, the drug with the fewest potential side effects is tried first. If this drug doesn't relieve pain adequately, other pain medications can be added or substituted.

Acetaminophen (Tylenol). This over-the-counter medication is the initial drug of choice for osteoarthritis because it is just as effective as most NSAIDs and is less likely to cause side effects such as stomach irritation. It is also inexpensive. In addition, because inflammation plays only a minor role in osteoarthritis, the anti-inflammatory effect of an NSAID usually is not required.

The maximum recommended daily dosage is 4,000 milligrams (mg), generally taken as 1,000 mg four times a day. Because it is often included in other medications, such as cold remedies, people sometimes take more than they think. As is true with any drug, acetaminophen can cause dangerous side effects if you take it regularly at dosages exceeding the recommended amount.

Acetaminophen may be harmful for people who have liver disease or who drink large amounts of alcohol. To prevent liver damage, you should not consume alcoholic beverages while taking acetaminophen. The drug may also be dangerous if you are taking the blood-thinning drug warfarin (Coumadin). Several years ago, a study showed that, in rare cases, heavy daily use of acetaminophen increases the risk of severe kidney damage. Although acetaminophen appears to cause a slightly lower risk of heart disease than NSAIDs, if you use it on a regular basis you should see your doctor periodically to be monitored for these and other side effects.

Traditional NSAIDs. If acetaminophen fails to control your osteoarthritis pain, NSAIDs are the next option. (See the drug chart on pages 20–23.) Aspirin, the original NSAID, is an effective and inexpensive treatment for osteoarthritis pain and may actually reduce the risk of heart disease. Other NSAID choices include ibuprofen (Advil, Motrin), naproxen (Aleve), and ketoprofen. However, if you need an NSAID other than aspirin, the AHA recommends starting with naproxen. If necessary, your doctor may prescribe a stronger NSAID such as diclofenac sodium (Voltaren) or nabumetone (Relafen).

Because inflammation is generally not a major problem in osteoarthritis, NSAIDs work primarily as pain relievers in this circumstance. How well osteoarthritis symptoms respond to a specific NSAID varies greatly from person to person. As a result, finding the right drug depends largely on trial and error. It can take at least two weeks of treatment to know whether the drug is effective.

Regular use of NSAIDs may cause stomach irritation, bleeding, and ulceration because the drugs interfere with the formation of the protective mucus that normally coats the stomach. In fact, some degree of gastrointestinal bleeding occurs in more than 50% of NSAID users. If you develop gastrointestinal discomfort or blood in your stools while taking an NSAID, you should call your doctor.

To reduce the risk of gastrointestinal problems, your doctor may recommend a traditional NSAID that is less likely to affect your stomach (for example, enteric-coated aspirin, which dissolves in the intestine rather than the stomach) or a traditional NSAID in combination with a drug that helps to protect your stomach. (Misoprostol is approved by the U.S. Food and Drug Administration [FDA] for this use, but your doctor may prescribe others.)

If you are over age 65, take corticosteroids, have a history of stomach ulcers or adverse reactions to NSAIDs, or have heart disease, diabetes, or liver or kidney problems, you should be carefully monitored while taking NSAIDs or should avoid them completely. Regular monitoring can detect liver and kidney problems in their early stages, before they become serious. Your doctor may also monitor your blood pressure, blood counts, and potassium levels during long-term NSAID treatment. If you take oral diabetes drugs or warfarin, be vigilant while using an NSAID, because it can increase the effects of these other drugs. NSAIDs, especially aspirin, can also worsen asthma.

COX-2 inhibitors. A new type of NSAID was developed in the 1990s that avoided some of these side effects. But two of these new COX-2 inhibitors—rofecoxib (Vioxx) and valdecoxib (Bextra)—

Commonly Used Nonsteroidal Anti-Inflammatory Drugs (NSAIDs) 2008

Drug type: Brand (generic)	Average daily dosage†	How to take
Acetylsalicylic acid*		
Anacin, Bayer, Bufferin, Easprin, ZORprin (aspirin)	3,600–5,400 mg	Do not chew or crush extended-release forms.
Nonacetylated salicylates		
Disalcid (salsalate)	1,000–3,000 mg	*Disalcid:* With food if stomach irritation is an issue.
Trilisate (choline magnesium trisalicylate)	3,000 mg	*Trilisate:* With a large glass of water and with food or a large glass of milk to reduce stomach irritation. Do not lie down for 30 minutes after taking this medicine. Divide into two doses per day.
COX-2 inhibitor		
Celebrex (celecoxib)	*OA*‡: 200 mg *RA*‡: 200–400 mg	With a full glass of water. May be taken with food. Do not lie down for 30 minutes after taking this medicine.
Enolic acid		
Mobic (meloxicam)	7.5–15 mg	With or without food. Antacid or milk may help avoid stomach problems.
Fenamate		
(meclofenamate sodium)	200–225 mg	With or without food. Antacid or milk may help avoid stomach problems.
Acetic acid		
Arthrotec (diclofenac/misoprostol)	*OA:* 100–150 mg/0.6 mg *RA:* 100–200 mg/ 0.6–0.8 mg	*Arthrotec:* With food. Do not use antacids containing magnesium. Do not crush or chew.
Cataflam, Voltaren (diclofenac)	*OA:* 100 mg *RA:* 100–200 mg	*All others:* With a glass of water. Taking pills with food, milk, or an antacid may reduce gastrointestinal effects but may also delay the drugs' effectiveness. Do not lie down for 20–30 minutes after taking. Do not crush or chew extended-release forms such as Lodine XL.
Clinoril (sulindac)	300–400 mg	
Indocin (indomethacin)	50–200 mg	
Lodine (etodolac)	800–1,200 mg	
Tolectin (tolmetin sodium)	1,200–1,800 mg	

See legend on page 22

Precautions	Most common side effects	Call your doctor if...
Enteric-coated formulation lessens gastrointestinal problems. Alters blood-clotting function, which may lead to bleeding. Do not take if you have asthma or ulcers.	Heartburn, nausea, vomiting, possible involvement in formation of stomach ulcers and bleeding, small amounts of blood in stool, stomach pain, stomach upset.	You have a continuous or high fever or a severe or persistent sore throat, especially with a high fever, vomiting, and nausea, or if you experience ringing in the ears, hearing loss, upset stomach, dizziness.
Do not take if you have flu symptoms or chickenpox. Use with extreme caution if you have kidney disease or ulcers. Avoid alcohol while using. Inform dentists and surgeons that you are using this drug.	*Disalcid:* Hearing impairment, nausea, rash, ringing in the ears, vertigo. *Trilisate:* Constipation, diarrhea, heartburn, indigestion, nausea, ringing in the ears, stomach pain and upset, vomiting.	You develop signs of an allergic reaction (swelling of hands, face, or throat), symptoms in box above.
May increase risk of heart attack, stroke, and potentially fatal stomach and bowel problems. Elderly people are at higher risk for serious stomach problems. Not recommended for people with a history of severe kidney disease.	Stomach pain, constipation, diarrhea, gas, heartburn, nausea, vomiting, dizziness.	You develop chest pain, breathing problems, vision changes, slurring of speech, numbness or weakness, flu-like symptoms, tenderness in your right upper chest, blood in vomit or stools, sudden and severe changes in skin (including yellowing), swelling of hands, face, or throat.
May increase risk of heart attack, stroke, and potentially fatal stomach and bowel problems. Elderly people are at higher risk for serious stomach problems. Not recommended for people with a history of severe kidney disease.	Stomach pain, constipation, diarrhea, gas, heartburn, nausea, vomiting, dizziness.	You develop chest pain, breathing problems, vision changes, slurring of speech, numbness or weakness, flu-like symptoms, tenderness in your right upper chest, blood in vomit or stools, sudden and severe changes in skin (including yellowing), swelling of hands, face, or throat.
May (rarely) cause bowel irritation that could progress to more serious colitis. May cause drowsiness; avoid alcohol while taking.	Stomach pain, constipation, diarrhea, gas, heartburn, nausea, vomiting, dizziness.	You develop chest pain, breathing problems, vision changes, slurring of speech, numbness or weakness, flu-like symptoms, tenderness in your right upper chest, blood in vomit or stools, sudden and severe changes in skin (including yellowing), swelling of hands, face, or throat.
Arthrotec: Pregnant women must not take, as it has been associated with miscarriage and birth defects. *Indocin:* May aggravate psychiatric or other central nervous system disorders and may cause drowsiness, which can interfere with driving.	Stomach pain, constipation, diarrhea, gas, heartburn, nausea, vomiting, dizziness.	You develop chest pain, breathing problems, vision changes, slurring of speech, numbness or weakness, flu-like symptoms, tenderness in your right upper chest, blood in vomit or stools, sudden and severe changes in skin (including yellowing). Also watch for signs of an allergic reaction (swelling of hands, face, or throat). *Indocin:* You develop headache.

continued on the next page

Commonly Used Nonsteroidal Anti-Inflammatory Drugs (NSAIDs) 2008 (continued)

Drug type: Brand (generic)	Average daily dosage†	How to take
Naphthylalkanone		
(nabumetone)	1,000–2,000 mg	With or without food. With 8 oz of water.
Propionic acid derivatives		
Advil, Motrin (ibuprofen)	1,200–3,200 mg	With or without food, in divided doses 2–4x/day.
Aleve, Anaprox, Naprelan, Naprosyn (naproxen)	400–1,650 mg	
Nalfon (fenoprofen calcium)	900–3,200 mg	
Orudis, Oruvail (ketoprofen)	200–300 mg	

* Available over the counter without a prescription.
† These dosages represent an average range for the treatment of arthritis. The precise effective dosage varies from person to person and depends on many factors. Do not make any change to your medication without consulting your doctor.
‡ OA = osteoarthritis; RA = rheumatoid arthritis.

General precautions for NSAIDs: With the exception of aspirin, NSAIDs may cause an increased risk of potentially fatal blood clots, heart attacks, or stroke and are contraindicated before or after heart bypass surgery. All NSAIDs may cause bleeding, ulcers, and perforation in the stomach or intestines, a risk that is higher in elderly people. NSAIDs may also increase fluid retention and blood pressure and cause kidney damage, asthma attacks in people who already have asthma, and various skin conditions. Adverse effects vary by dose, duration of use, age of user, and factors such as smoking and alcohol use. Do not take aspirin while using an NSAID.

were withdrawn from the market after being linked to an increased risk of cardiovascular problems.

The FDA continues to have concerns about the safety of a third COX-2 inhibitor, celecoxib (Celebrex), which is still available. The drug now contains a strong warning on its label stating that it is associated with an increased risk of heart attacks and strokes and should not be taken by people who have just had heart surgery. Physicians at Johns Hopkins reserve Celebrex for people who either do not benefit or have adverse effects from other pain relief alternatives and who are at low risk for heart attacks and strokes. Typically in such cases, the lowest effective dose is used for the shortest time possible.

Opioids. If you have severe osteoarthritis, and acetaminophen or NSAIDs do not provide sufficient pain relief, your doctor may prescribe stronger oral drugs called opioid pain relievers. Some examples are codeine and hydrocodone. Opioids are also sold in combination with acetaminophen, such as oxycodone with acetaminophen (Percocet) or propoxyphene with acetaminophen (Darvocet). All opioids are effective against pain but can cause drowsiness, nausea,

Precautions	Most common side effects	Call your doctor if...
May be associated with adverse reactions to sun exposure.	Stomach pain, constipation, diarrhea, gas, heartburn, nausea, vomiting, dizziness, ringing in ears, headache, skin rash.	You develop chest pain, severe stomach pain, blood in vomit or stools, swelling of hands, face, or throat.
May be associated with adverse reactions to sun exposure. Advil, Motrin, Anaprox, Nalfon, and Naprosyn may cause drowsiness that impairs ability to drive safely. Oruvail is less likely to cause drowsiness. Ibuprofen may decrease the benefit of aspirin taken for heart attack or stroke.	Stomach pain, constipation, diarrhea, gas, heartburn, nausea, vomiting, dizziness, ringing in ears, headache, skin rash.	You develop chest pain, shortness of breath, weakness in one part or side of the body, slurred speech, severe stomach pain, heartburn, blood in vomit or stools, swelling of hands, face, or throat.

vomiting, constipation, and dizziness. Opiates can also cause psychological and physical dependence (addiction) when used over the long term. Consequently, doctors generally limit their use to several weeks.

Tramadol (Ultram), a strong opioid with a different mode of action, may be less addictive. A pill combining tramadol with acetaminophen (Ultracet) is available. Like the other opioid drugs, tramadol may cause drowsiness, constipation, nausea, and dizziness.

Injected pain relievers

Another approach to treating osteoarthritis is the use of corticosteroids and other drugs that are injected directly into painful joints (called intra-articular injection). If acetaminophen or NSAIDs do not relieve your osteoarthritis symptoms sufficiently, you may be a candidate for intra-articular injections.

Corticosteroid injections. Corticosteroids are powerful anti-inflammatory hormones that many people take in oral form to treat rheumatoid arthritis and other inflammatory diseases. They can also relieve pain when injected into a joint. Intra-articular injections of corticosteroids have proven particularly effective for relieving painful osteoarthritis of the knee. Unfortunately, frequent corticosteroid injections increase the risk of cartilage damage. As a result, they can't be used more than two or three times a year.

Corticosteroid injections can't reverse the underlying degenerative process in the joint, but they do relieve osteoarthritis pain for a few weeks or months. If your knees hurt, this temporary relief may allow you to begin physical therapy or even to dance at a wedding.

Hyaluronic acid injections (viscosupplementation). The synovial fluid in your joints contains a lubricating substance called hyaluronic acid. Studies show that some individuals with osteoarthritis have a lower-than-normal concentration of this substance, especially in their knees. A series of intra-articular knee injections of hyaluronic acid—also called viscosupplementation—performed over several weeks can provide pain relief and improvements in knee function for up to one year. Viscosupplementation doesn't work for everyone, and if the results of initial therapy are unsatisfactory, it may be necessary to repeat the round of injections several months later.

The FDA has approved four preparations of hyaluronic acid for the intra-articular treatment of knee osteoarthritis: Hyalgan, Orthovisc, Synvisc, and Supartz. One major advantage of these preparations is that they appear to cause few, if any, serious side effects, although temporary pain, swelling, and itching may occur at the injection site.

The long-term effects of viscosupplementation are unknown. No evidence indicates that it can reverse or delay the progression of osteoarthritis.

Other injections. Research on other intra-articular injections is still in the early stages. One small study found that an injection of 1 mg of morphine into the knee joints of people with osteoarthritis provided pain relief for at least a week.

Topical analgesics

Many of the nonprescription creams, gels, and ointments that are advertised for arthritis pain can provide some temporary pain relief. The three types of topical analgesics are:

Counter-irritants. Counter-irritant products contain compounds such as menthol, camphor, eucalyptus oil, or turpentine oil that mask pain by producing a warm or cool sensation. A frequent side effect is reddening of the skin, which is harmless and temporary. Some of these products also contain salicylates or capsaicin (for example, ArthriCare, BenGay, Flexall 454 Ultra Plus Gel, and Icy Hot Chill Stick).

Salicylates. Topical salicylates (such as Aspercreme and Sportscreme) work in the same way as the NSAID aspirin—by inhibiting the release of prostaglandins, fatty acids that perform a variety of regulatory actions but also cause inflammation. Topical salicylates appear to relieve pain more effectively than a placebo, but no studies have compared these products with oral pain medications. Because some of the medication is absorbed into the body, people who are sensitive to aspirin or are taking drugs that might interact with aspirin may need to avoid these products.

Capsaicin. Other topical preparations (such as Capzasin and Zostrix) contain capsaicin, the compound that gives hot peppers their "bite." Capsaicin was once considered to be a questionable "alternative" remedy but now is an accepted part of conventional medicine. Capsaicin reduces the amount of a neurotransmitter (chemical messenger) called substance P, which triggers transmission of pain impulses to the brain and can also provoke inflammation. Topical capsaicin appears to have no serious side effects, but burning, stinging, and redness occur in 40–70% of people who use the products. These side effects usually subside after several days of use. Capsaicin products must be applied three to four times a day. It may take several weeks before you notice any benefits.

In general, topical treatments for joint pain have few side effects, but some precautions apply. They are for external use only and should not come in contact with the eyes, nose, mouth, or any open skin. Wash your hands immediately after applying any of these products. Don't use topical treatments more than three or four times a day, and discontinue them immediately if severe irritation develops. Many topical products come with warnings not to bandage or apply heat to a treated area. With some formulations, manufacturers recommend that you stop using the product and see a doctor if your symptoms do not improve after seven days. And don't expect miracles or spend big bucks for "secret formulas." If it sounds too good to be true, it probably is.

Surgery

You've used analgesic creams, ice, heat, exercise, physical therapy, and assistive devices. You have tried all the pain medications, even opioids. Maybe you've even lost 20 lbs. But your joints are still so stiff and painful that you can't drive your car or participate in hobbies you enjoy. Should you consider surgery? If so, what are your options?

ASK THE DOCTOR

Q. *I am 82 years old and I'm thinking about knee replacement surgery. Am I too old, and how can I tell when this surgery is really needed?*

A. It used to be that patients between age 60 and 75 were the ideal candidates for knee replacements. But recent studies suggest that knee replacements in patients over age 80 lead to a substantial reduction in pain and a greater ability to function. So if you're in fairly good health with stable chronic conditions, age alone needn't be a deterrent. Although the risk of complications such as blood clots, bleeding, or stroke is higher in older patients and in those with other conditions such as heart disease or obesity, the overall rate of complications is only 5%.

To determine whether surgery is a good option for you, think about the following questions: How far can you walk? Can you get up without pushing up? What activities can you no longer do because of knee pain? Are you gaining weight because you're not as active as you once were? Does the pain keep you awake? If your answers indicate that you're not able to do as much as you used to or you're not sleeping well because of your knees, it may be time to consider surgery, particularly if you've already tried nonsurgical options such as rest, heat and ice, anti-inflammatory medications, cortisone injections, physical therapy, and stretching exercises.

Weighing the pros and cons

Joint surgery is not a quick fix, and it is not without risks. Serious complications, such as blood clots and infections, can occur. For example, more than 40% of people undergoing total knee replacement develop blood clots. In addition, the road to recovery can be difficult and time consuming, particularly with joint replacement surgery. But many people who undergo joint surgery experience decreases in their pain as well as significant improvements in psychological well-being and quality of life. Despite the risks of surgery, the expense, and the substantial commitment of time required for recovery, the potential rewards for your physical and mental health are great.

Many people put off having joint surgery, even when their doctor has assured them that surgery is an appropriate option. Often they feel their pain isn't bad enough to warrant joint repair. But studies show that waiting until your pain and loss of function are substantial can make joint surgery more difficult and reduce your chance of regaining good function. One good reason for postponing surgery, however, is obesity. Although joint replacement surgery is effective in the majority of people who are obese, being obese does make the surgery more risky (see "Obesity and Arthritis" on pages 28–29).

If you are interested in having joint surgery, and your doctor thinks you might be a candidate, it's time to look for a surgeon. When you speak with surgeons, be sure to ask how many procedures they do each year, what their success rate has been, and where they perform their surgeries. Studies show that surgeons who do the most operations each year generally have the highest success rates. Moreover, hospitals that are affiliated with medical schools (teaching hospitals) also tend to have the best track records. Because infections may occur following joint surgery, asking about the hospital's infection rate is also important.

Types of surgery

At your first office visit with your surgeon, the two of you will determine whether surgery is right for you. If it is, the next decision is which type of surgery best meets your needs.

Arthroscopy. An arthroscopic procedure involves making a tiny incision in the skin through which the doctor inserts surgical tools and an arthroscope—a thin, lighted tube with a camera attached to one end. Arthroscopic surgery can be performed on the knee, hip, shoulder, elbow, or hand. Arthroscopy is less costly and less painful than the other types of joint surgery, and the recovery time is shorter.

An orthopedic surgeon performs the procedure in a hospital operating room or an outpatient surgical suite.

Arthroscopy may be used diagnostically (to determine the type of arthritis or the amount of damage) or therapeutically (to perform debridement or lavage).

Debridement involves smoothing roughened cartilage and bone, whereas lavage involves flushing out the joint to remove debris such as loose pieces of bone and cartilage. A recent study found that neither debridement nor lavage is an effective treatment for knee osteoarthritis, but arthroscopy may still be useful for some people who have large pieces of debris or torn cartilage in a joint.

Osteotomy ("bone cutting"). In osteotomy, the bones are cut and re-aligned. An osteotomy requires a long recovery period, but it also relieves pain and the results are more long-lasting than those seen with other procedures. Recovery is 80% complete in about six weeks and 100% complete within six months.

Hemicallotasis. In this procedure, a bone is realigned by lengthening it on one side. This is done by cutting the bone and attaching an external fixation device to it with pins. The fixation device must remain in place for about 12 weeks, during which time the patient turns screws on the device to increase slowly the distance between the cut ends of bone. The body then produces new bone in this area, allowing the bone to lengthen by about 1 mm a day. The most serious complication of hemicallotasis is infection at the site where the pins enter the body.

When arthroscopy, osteotomy, or hemicallotasis is not feasible, your doctor may recommend arthrodesis or joint replacement.

Arthrodesis. In this procedure, the surgeon fuses two bones in a finger, wrist, ankle, or foot joint. Although the operation results in a loss of flexibility, it relieves the pain caused by two bones rubbing against each other in a damaged joint. The fused bone is also more stable and better able to bear weight.

Arthrodesis is an alternative to joint replacement for people whose bones are not strong enough to support an artificial joint or who have frequent joint infections that rule out the use of an artificial joint. It may also be used in small joints, such as in the thumb, where replacements are performed less often. Arthrodesis is very effective for controlling pain; however, fusing the joint limits function.

Joint replacement (arthroplasty). The most common type of arthroplasty is total joint replacement. In this procedure, the entire diseased or damaged joint is removed and replaced with an artificial one (a prosthesis) to relieve pain and restore function. Arthroplasty

NEW RESEARCH

Moderate Activity After Total Joint Replacements Appears Safe

Hip or knee replacements probably won't halt your golf game or drive you from the bowling lanes. A recent study finds that moderate activities like biking, bowling, and golf are fine for older people who have had such replacements.

A week before surgery (170 hip replacements and 184 knee replacements), the researchers measured pain and function—ability to walk, climb stairs, and do the routine actions involved in day-to-day living—and level of activity in 354 people whose average age was mid to late 60s. The same assessments were taken again at six and 12 months after surgery.

The researchers found that the average hip score on a scale of 1–100, measuring both function and pain, was 40 before surgery and 95 one year after surgery. The average knee score, measuring pain, on a scale of 1–-200 was 39 before surgery and 96 one year later. For function, the average knee score was 44 before surgery and 95 a year later. Importantly, the people who were functioning well after their joint replacements also returned to moderate physical activity.

If you do face a joint replacement or have had one, ask your physician about the risks of physical activity, such as a loosening or dislocation of the replacement and the possible need for a repeat surgery. But chances are your doctor will tell you to go ahead and polish up the golf shoes.

CLINICAL JOURNAL OF SPORTS MEDICINE
Volume 17, page 104
March 2007

Obesity and Arthritis

Is joint replacement too high a risk?

The percentage of Americans who are obese has tripled in the last quarter century, an "epidemic" that is fueling a boom in joint-replacement surgery. In part this is because obese people are more likely to develop arthritis, particularly osteoarthritis. In turn, obesity significantly increases the risks of joint surgery and worsens the results.

How Those Extra Pounds Can Stress Your Joints

The link between osteoarthritis and obesity—defined as a body mass index (a measure of body fat in relation to height and weight) of more than 30—isn't surprising. The force of a single footstep on a knee or hip is about three to six times a person's body weight.

That means that if you weigh 200 lbs, the force on your joints with each step amounts to at least 600 lbs. More strenuous activities, such as rising out of a chair or going up or down stairs increase the load even more.

Obesity not only multiplies the stress on joints; it also likely speeds the breakdown of cartilage. In fact, an obese person is 25% more likely to have hip osteoarthritis and three to four times more likely to have knee osteoarthritis than someone of normal weight.

Other factors related to obesity may also boost the risk of osteoarthritis. Obesity may increase the stiffness of the subchondral bone plate, the bone beneath the joint cartilage. This makes the bone less able to absorb impact, throwing even more burden on the cartilage.

Studies also suggest that leptin, a hormone linked to obesity, may contribute to the development of osteoarthritis by promoting inflammation. Researchers have found leptin in the joint fluid of osteoarthritis patients, and the levels are higher both in heavier people and in those with more severe arthritis.

Why Extra Weight Adds to Surgical Risk

Just as obesity increases the risk of developing osteoarthritis, it also makes joint replacement surgery more risky.

When Duke University researchers studied a database of one million people who had had major joint replacement, they found that nearly 4% of obese patients had complications during their hospitalization, compared with less than 3% of nonobese patients. And obese patients were 45% more likely than those of normal weight to require additional care in a health facility or at home.

Figures from other studies are even higher, indicating that obese patients are more than twice as likely to have complications or to need placement in a rehab facility after surgery.

Increases in the risk of infection are worrisome as well. A study in one Boston hospital found that although the obese made up only

requires hospitalization and, usually, general anesthesia. In some instances, such as knee replacements, regional anesthesia (spinal, epidural, or nerve block) may be used to numb the lower body.

Most joint replacement surgeries (80–90%) are done on the hip and knee, although joints in the shoulder, elbow, hand, ankle, and foot can also be replaced. New technology and improved operating techniques and materials have made joint replacement the best treatment for many people. According to *Consumer Reports,* more than 600,000 people in the United States have hip or knee replacement surgery each year, 70% of them because of osteoarthritis. A 2006 survey showed that even though recovery can be long and sometimes painful, 82% of people who had this kind of surgery were very or completely satisfied with the results.

39% of orthopedic surgery patients, they experienced 44% of wound infections. In part that's because the extra folds of skin make the wounds tougher to keep clean. Obese patients also tend to have high rates of diabetes, high blood pressure, and heart disease, all of which add to the risk of infection.

In addition, obese patients tend to have longer operations, larger incisions, more blood loss, and a greater risk of blood clots and pneumonia.

What's more, the results of joint replacement are not as good. Patients who are obese tend to gain weight following joint replacements. This increases the wear and tear on the new joints, which in turn raises the possibility that the joint will need to be replaced again in the future.

In a 2004 study at the Johns Hopkins University School of Medicine, the success rate of knee replacements in the obese was 88%, compared with 99% in people who were not obese.

How You Can Boost the Odds of Success

Most surgeons don't like to operate on patients weighing more than 300 lbs. Some, in fact, will set a surgery date a year in advance to give patients time to reach a safer weight.

Fortunately, there are ways to work with your doctor to make your surgery and its aftermath safer and more successful.

1. Lose some of that excess weight. Obviously, you'll need to focus on good nutrition and cutting calories. Depending on your pain level, a moderate exercise program can help you to lose weight. It can also improve your conditioning and strength.

2. Get your blood pressure under control. Medication may be required, but exercise and weight loss also can help.

3. Focus on better blood sugar control. If you have diabetes or prediabetes, diet and/or medication can help normalize your blood sugar levels during and after surgery, reducing the risk of infection.

4. Tell your doctor if you've had an infection with an antibiotic-resistant bacterium. You may need a special antibiotic before and during surgery.

5. Ask your surgeon what will be done to prevent deep vein thrombosis. This type of blood clot can form when you are bedridden after surgery and may travel to your lungs or even your brain. There are many effective approaches, including the use of blood-thinning medications and compression stockings (which inflate and deflate after surgery to keep blood flowing).

6. Continue to lose weight— and keep it off after the surgery.

The Bottom Line

Working with your doctor to minimize the risks of joint replacement surgery is worth the effort. After all, joint replacement succeeds in almost nine out of 10 obese people. What's more, the surgery is likely to lessen your pain, making it easier to move and therefore easier to get the exercise you need to lose those extra pounds. ■

If you choose to have arthroplasty, be sure to get as much information as you can about the procedure, the recovery time, and the rehabilitation process. In one study, people who participated in a two-hour educational program prior to knee replacement showed markedly greater and faster improvement after surgery than did people who did not participate in the program. People in the educational program also spent an average of two days less in the hospital and required fewer sessions of physical therapy to recover fully.

To ensure optimal satisfaction from arthroplasty, before the operation you and your surgeon should discuss the activities (including sports) you intend to continue afterward. The information will help the surgeon select the most appropriate prosthesis, implantation technique, and rehabilitation program and will make you aware of the risks and limitations of your activities. Recommended activities after surgery include golfing, swimming, cycling, bowling, and sailing. On the "not recommended" list are sports such as running, racquetball, and basketball.

Complications of joint replacement. Significant complications occur in about 40% of people who undergo joint replacement surgery. The most frequent is blood clots in leg veins. Surgeons take precautions to prevent this by prescribing blood thinners, such as aspirin or heparin, and using leg compression equipment (typically an air pressure device that repeatedly inflates and deflates to massage the leg and keep blood flowing).

A potentially more serious but less common complication is infection in the surgical wound or in the joint. Most infections can be treated with antibiotics, but infections deep in the joint may require removal of the prosthesis. Eventually, your surgeon can reimplant a new prosthesis. Individuals who have an arthroplasty have to guard against infection for as long as one to two years after surgery by taking oral antibiotics for even small infections and before dental work or urinary examinations. However, with preventive measures, the infection rate is no more than 3%.

Physical therapy after joint replacement. Successful joint replacement, especially of the knee, requires a considerable investment of time and energy in rehabilitation. Rehabilitation begins in the hospital, usually the day after surgery. During this period, a strict timetable of exercise, rest, and medication is crucial to the success of the surgery. You may feel considerable pain immediately after the surgery (from muscles disturbed during the operation, rather than from the joint itself), and that can make rehabilitation difficult at first.

Recovery from knee, hip, and all other types of joint replacement requires a series of sessions with a physical therapist. Physical therapy exercises focus on building strength and regaining flexibility. The physical therapist may also use techniques such as massage and application of cold to minimize swelling, which interferes with flexibility. In addition, every patient receives a regimen of exercises to perform at home. Use of continuous passive motion therapy using a machine for rehabilitation has not been shown to increase motion or to accelerate recovery.

Thanks to all this rehabilitation, recovery from a knee replacement is usually 80% complete within four weeks. Full recovery usually takes a year, sometimes even longer. Recovery from a hip replacement is usually 80% complete within four weeks and 100% complete within six months.

Less invasive types of joint replacement. Surgeons continually seek ways to make joint replacements and repairs easier, safer, and less arduous for the patient. A number of new techniques are currently under development.

Some surgeons have started replacing hips and knees through very small incisions, a procedure called minimally invasive joint replacement. This technique results in less damage to muscle, tendons, and ligaments as well as less pain and a faster recovery. However, minimally invasive procedures are more difficult to perform than standard joint replacements, and researchers don't yet know whether the long-term results will be as good. In addition, not everyone is a candidate, including individuals who are obese.

Another less invasive option is resurfacing, also referred to as joint resurfacing. It involves removing damaged cartilage at bone ends in a joint and then capping the surface with metal. However, surgeons don't often use this procedure due to a lack of information on long-term outcomes.

Another alternative to a total knee replacement is a unicompartmental knee replacement, which involves replacing only the damaged section of the knee. This may be an option for individuals with limited knee damage. However, it is very effective for only a small percentage of people with arthritis.

Alternative and Complementary Treatments

Many people with arthritis rely on complementary medicine, products and techniques used in combination with conventional treatments. For example, they may listen to soothing music or go to an arthritis support group to make living with arthritis easier.

This is very different from alternative medicine, in which certain products and techniques are used instead of conventional medicine. Examples of alternative therapies are taking an herbal supplement or following a special diet to treat your osteoarthritis, rather than or in addition to taking the medications your doctor has prescribed.

Whether you are using complementary or alternative treatments, letting your doctor know about them is always important, because they may change your osteoarthritis symptoms, test results, and responses to prescribed treatments.

What alternative remedies work for osteoarthritis? Despite increasing research in the field, neither the Arthritis Foundation nor the American College of Rheumatology officially recommends any nutritional or herbal supplements for the treatment of osteoarthritis. One reason is that supplements are not approved by the FDA. In

ASK THE DOCTOR

Q. *I had hip replacement surgery, but I'm afraid the implant is loose. What are the signs?*

A. A hip replacement fits into the thigh bone, or femur, and the pelvis so that the implant can't move. However, over time—usually no sooner than 10 years or so—it can loosen, more often on the pelvic side than on the thigh bone side, causing pain, often in the groin, and restricting hip movement. But you may also feel no symptoms. That's why it's important to see your surgeons every one to two years so he or she can check for any problems.

The most common cause of loosening is osteolysis, a degeneration of the bone surrounding an implant that doesn't show up immediately on an x-ray. Osteolysis is caused by the wearing away of the implant surfaces and is more likely to happen in very active or overweight people. Tiny fragments of the implant irritate the surrounding tissue, ultimately weakening the bone. However, the new materials—ceramic on polyethylene, ceramic on ceramic, and metal on metal—appear to have much smaller particles that break off as they wear, causing less irritation than the traditional polyethylene implants. Also, improved diagnostic tests, such as spiral computed tomograms are revealing osteolysis earlier, which means a simpler revision surgery and a better outcome.

Infection also can cause loosening. However, improvements in sterile techniques and treatments have lowered infection risk.

addition, product manufacturing often is not well controlled. That means the level of active ingredients may vary from batch to batch, with some batches containing significantly less of the active substance than the label indicates. Some supplements even contain harmful contaminants such as lead or mercury.

Despite these potential problems, some research suggests that one alternative remedy—glucosamine, taken alone or with chondroitin—may be as effective as ibuprofen in relieving osteoarthritis symptoms. But not all studies have shown a benefit.

Glucosamine and chondroitin

Glucosamine and chondroitin are compounds found in human cartilage tissue. They are believed to play an important role in the formation and maintenance of cartilage within joints and may be involved in joint repair. But can glucosamine and chondroitin supplements help to reduce osteoarthritis symptoms? Many research reports say they do. In a recent meta-analysis (a combination of data from many published studies), glucosamine produced significant improvements in joint narrowing, pain control, and mobility. Chondroitin was less effective in measures of joint narrowing but was equivalent to glucosamine in reducing osteoarthritis symptoms.

Another recent study measured the effects of glucosamine in postmenopausal women who took the supplement or a placebo for three years. Women in the placebo group showed increased joint-space narrowing (that is, worsening arthritis), whereas those who took glucosamine did not. The glucosamine group also showed significant improvement in osteoarthritis symptoms.

Despite these encouraging results, researchers still have much to learn about the supplements. In fact, in 2006, a large government-sponsored study called the Glucosamine/Chondroitin Arthritis Intervention Trial (GAIT) found that, overall, glucosamine and chondroitin, either alone or in combination, were no more effective than a placebo in easing symptoms of knee osteoarthritis. However, a subgroup of people with moderate to severe pain did experience significant pain relief with the glucosamine-chondroitin combination. The GAIT study, which is continuing, will address other aspects of glucosamine and chondroitin treatment, including its potential to prevent progression of joint damage.

Products containing glucosamine and chondroitin are available without a prescription. Although these substances appear to cause few or no side effects, they may not be safe for people with diabetes. Glucosamine, even in very low doses, has the potential to raise

Stem Cells for Cartilage Implants

Human trial now underway may hold promise for arthritis

Imagine treating your aging knee cartilage much as you would a spring garden—by planting seeds for regrowth. As the need for knee replacements soars—approximately 400,000 Americans will get knee replacements this year—scientists are exploring ways to "seed" the regrowth of cartilage using stem cells.

From Stem Cell to Cartilage

Cartilage has only one type of cell, called a chondrocyte. That simplicity makes cartilage a good choice for stem cell research. Stem cells are the source of all other kinds of cells, and they renew themselves indefinitely. Embryonic stem cells (ESCs), taken from eggs just fertilized, are essentially blank slates and, as such, are ideal sources for replacement tissue.

But use of human ESCs is controversial, and few are available for research in the United States. One alternative is to use adult stem cells, which are taken from organs or bone marrow. The drawback is that these stem cells are already programmed to develop into certain kinds of cells. Consequently, they are not as amenable as ESCs to manipulation or cultivation in the laboratory. Nevertheless, they are readily available, so researchers are working to tap their potential.

First Human Clinical Trial

Scientists at Johns Hopkins have already shown that adult stem cells can develop into chondrocytes that trigger repair in the damaged knee cartilage of adult goats. Those findings helped lay the groundwork for a study at the University of Southern California (USC) that researchers are watching closely. It is the first human clinical trial using adult stem cells to spur cartilage growth in damaged knees.

The USC researchers are zeroing in on injuries to the meniscus, the shock-absorbing cartilage that pads the knees. Injuries to the meniscus are common. Every year, about 800,000 Americans have injured meniscuses removed surgically. Although the surgery relieves pain, arthritis eventually develops in most cases.

The two-year USC trial involves 55 patients, each of whom underwent surgery to remove at least 50% of the injured meniscus from one knee. Eighteen of the participants already showed signs of mild arthritis. For this study, the researchers began by taking bone-marrow cells called mesenchymal stem cells (MSCs) from donors and placing them in a tissue culture to multiply. (Researchers already know that MSCs can morph into chondrocytes. And MSCs can match any tissue type, relieving concerns about tissue rejection.) They injected a mixture containing millions of the cultured stem cells into the knees of half the patients one week after surgery. The other patients received a sham injection.

Encouraging Results

Although none of the study's participants showed significant cartilage growth after six months, one third of those who received a stem- cell injection experienced some reversal of their arthritis symptoms—evidence of cell activity that researchers don't yet understand. By comparison, no one in the control group showed such a reversal.

The scientists remain cautiously optimistic that some cell growth may occur over the next six months. Importantly, the injected stem-cell solution appears to be safe—a finding that opens the door for research involving people with more severe arthritis symptoms.

Additional Research

Scientists elsewhere are working to develop stem cells that can regenerate articular cartilage, the cartilage that covers the ends of bones and wears away in people with arthritis.

In the first animal studies to use stem cells from muscles, scientists at the University of Pittsburgh genetically altered the cells to release the BMP-4 protein. This protein encourages the formation of chondrocytes. Stem cells carried in a medium of fibrin (protein) glue and injected into damaged cartilage in rats were able to settle into tiny breaks within the surrounding cartilage and grow new tissue integrated within the old cartilage.

In England, investigators successfully cultivated adult stem cells, taken from the bone marrow of osteoarthritis patients, into an extremely resilient type of cartilage. Another group converted ESCs into cartilage cells that were transplanted into mice. Although neither of these new forms of cartilage derived from human stem cells has been implanted into humans, experts in the field predict that new stem-cell based treatments for arthritic joints may be available within five to 10 years. ■

blood glucose (sugar) levels. There is also some concern that chondroitin might interact with the anticoagulant drug warfarin, causing excessive bleeding. In addition, people who are allergic to shellfish should not use glucosamine because it is derived from the shells of oysters and crabs.

If you are interested in taking glucosamine and chondroitin, and you have your doctor's permission, you can try taking these supplements either singly or in combination. But if you see no improvement in your symptoms after three months, you should stop taking them.

Other vitamin and herbal supplements

Some studies suggest that the progression of osteoarthritis may be slower in people who take supplements containing vitamin D and antioxidants such as vitamin C, vitamin E, and beta-carotene. The Arthritis Foundation states that vitamin supplements have not undergone sufficient testing for the treatment of osteoarthritis and thus are not recommended for this purpose. In addition, megadoses of some vitamins can be dangerous to your health. In a recent Johns Hopkins study, people who took more than 400 IU of vitamin E daily as supplements had a 10% greater risk of dying from a variety of diseases than did people who took smaller doses or no vitamin E at all.

Additional complementary and alternative options

The National Center for Complementary and Alternative Medicine (NCCAM), part of the government's National Institutes of Health (NIH), now funds research on complementary and alternative medicine. This means that in the coming years we will have more accurate information to guide decisions about nontraditional remedies.

In the meantime, here's a brief rundown of what we know now:

Yoga. An ancient Indian exercise and breathing technique, yoga has been proven to improve breathing, strengthen muscles, and improve flexibility, mobility, and stability. Yoga is also an effective stress-reduction technique.

Tai chi. This Chinese exercise program provides benefits similar to those associated with yoga. Tai chi and yoga have become increasingly popular in the United States. Both are safe.

Acupuncture. Used for centuries by the Chinese, practitioners of this ancient healing method insert, then manipulate thin metallic needles in specific anatomical points in the body. Several studies suggest that acupuncture is effective in treating osteoarthritis pain. A recent study of 570 older people with knee osteoarthritis found that those who had 23 acupuncture treatments showed a 40–45%

improvement in joint pain and function compared with people who were given sham (placebo) acupuncture treatments. Another study found that people who had acupuncture treatments once a week for 12 weeks felt less pain and stiffness and needed less pain medication than did people who did not undergo acupuncture. Yet results from a recent German study are perplexing: After 10 treatments (real or sham) over 26 weeks, half of each group had significantly less pain and stiffness and more joint function.

Acupuncture is not recommended for people who have bleeding disorders or take blood thinners like warfarin. Sterilization of the acupuncture needles is crucial, as use of unsterilized needles can lead to serious infections, including HIV and hepatitis. That's why it is important to select an acupuncture practitioner who is certified by a national accrediting organization such as the American Academy of Medical Acupuncture or the National Certification Commission for Acupuncture and Oriental Medicine.

Mind-body interventions. Meditation, prayer, and creative therapies using art, music, and dance are examples of mind-body interventions. Some other interventions that involve the mind, such as support groups and cognitive-behavioral therapy, have become elements of mainstream medical approaches to osteoarthritis.

Massage and other manipulation methods. These measures help relax the muscles, promoting overall relaxation.

Electromagnetic field therapy. Pulsed electrical stimulation is applied over the joints to reduce osteoarthritis symptoms. Some studies show this technique to be more effective than placebo treatments.

If you are interested in trying a complementary therapy for arthritis, ask your doctor or check with a nearby hospital or medical school for a referral to an experienced, licensed practitioner.

Treatments Not Recommended

Even though the American College of Rheumatology does not recommend complementary or alternative treatments for osteoarthritis, many people try them anyway. Some of these treatments can be dangerous; others won't harm you, but they are not worth spending money on.

Here's a list of some of the nontraditional treatments that the Arthritis Foundation says are unsafe and should not be tried: arnica *(Arnica montana)*; aconite *(Aconitum napellus)*; adrenal, spleen, and thymus extracts; autumn crocus *(Colchicum autumnale)*; 5-HTP (5-hydroxytryptophan); GHB (gamma-hydroxybutyrate); GBL (gamma-butyrolactone); L-tryptophan; chaparral; and Kombucha tea.

NEW RESEARCH

Hydrotherapy and Tai Chi Can Help Osteoarthritis Discomfort

Maybe you've given up on exercise because it just doesn't seem to help the discomfort in your knees and hips. But take heart, a recent study finds that two kinds of exercise can help pain and function in people with hip or knee osteoarthritis.

The researchers assigned 152 people with chronic osteoarthritis to one of three groups: a control group, a group assigned to hydrotherapy classes, and another assigned to classes in tai chi, traditional Chinese exercises that involve slow, flowing movements. Both sets of exercisers, all over age 59, worked out for an hour twice a week for 12 weeks.

After 12 weeks, people in both exercise groups were better able to do things like walk and climb stairs than were those in the control group. Although both types of exercise reduced pain, the hydrotherapy group showed significant improvement, and they had a greater lift in spirits and reduction in stress than the tai chi group.

Although hydrotherapy was the winner in terms of pain and stress relief, people in both classes said that their physical function was greatly improved.

Check with your local chapter of the Arthritis Foundation for information on aquatics classes if you'd like to give hydrotherapy a try. Your local Y also might be a source for these and tai chi classes.

ARTHRITIS & RHEUMATISM
Volume 57, page 407
April 15, 2007

SAMe. Also on the "not recommended" list is S-adenosylmethionine (SAMe). Pronounced "sammy," this naturally occurring compound found in all living cells has been available as an over-the-counter supplement in the United States since 1999. As with other supplements, the FDA does not regulate the effectiveness or safety of SAMe. A recent government-sponsored review of scientific studies on SAMe found that only one of 10 published studies showed a decrease in osteoarthritis pain. Because the quality of the studies on SAMe for osteoarthritis is questionable, the supplement is not recommended as a treatment for the disease. It is expensive and often causes diarrhea and other gastrointestinal problems.

Bracelets. Containing metals such as copper or "static magnets," bracelets are frequently marketed as pain relievers for osteoarthritis. Despite a few studies claiming they work, arthritis experts do not recommend them.

"Miracle" remedies. If you hear an ad on the radio or TV touting a new, secret, miracle remedy for arthritis that even the best doctors don't know about, keep your wallet closed and change the channel. If the remedy were that miraculous, everyone would know about it already, and it wouldn't need to be advertised. If no one knows about it, it hasn't been well tested and no evidence shows that it works.

Treatments Under Development

Researchers are conducting studies on a new class of disease-modifying osteoarthritis drugs (DMOADs). Much of the damage from osteoarthritis is believed to result from a disturbance in the natural cycle of cartilage destruction and rebuilding, DMOADs may eventually offer relief by inhibiting the release of enzymes that break down cartilage.

Gene therapy is another option researchers are studying as a treatment for osteoarthritis. They are also testing growth factors and stem cells for their potential to improve bone healing after joint repair surgery. Use of stem cells to grow new cartilage is also under investigation (see "Stem Cells for Cartilage Implants" on page 33).

RHEUMATOID ARTHRITIS

Rheumatoid arthritis affects approximately 2.1 million Americans. Unlike osteoarthritis, which occurs equally in both sexes, rheumatoid arthritis affects three times as many women as men. Osteoarthritis usually begins late in life; rheumatoid arthritis often begins between ages 30 and 50, but it can develop at any age. The major distinguishing characteristics of rheumatoid arthritis are that it is chronic, systemic (affecting the whole body), inflammatory, and autoimmune.

Autoimmune. This term describes an immune-system attack that the body launches upon itself. For some unknown reason, the immune system becomes "confused" and begins to interpret molecular signals from normal body tissues as if they are coming from harmful infectious bacteria or viruses. In rheumatoid arthritis, the chief target of this attack is the synovial membrane, the lining of the joints that connect parts of the skeleton.

Inflammatory. When the white blood cells of the immune system attack the synovial membrane, they begin to release the same poisonous substances that kill bacteria and viruses during an infection. The result is a series of chemical changes that produce the same local symptoms that occur with an infection: the combination of heat, swelling, pain, and redness known as inflammation.

Chronic. Like osteoarthritis, rheumatoid arthritis is a chronic disease; the autoimmune attacks can continue indefinitely. But it is more crippling than osteoarthritis. As time goes on, continued inflammation causes the synovial membrane to thicken. An area of inflammatory cells (called a pannus) often starts to form at the point where the synovial membrane joins the cartilage. Continued release of enzymes and growth factors by the white blood cells, along with growth of the pannus, can erode cartilage, tendons, ligaments, and even bones within the joint capsule. As rheumatoid arthritis progresses, the ever-growing pannus can further limit joint motion. Inflammation of tissues surrounding the joint may eventually cause permanent joint damage and deformities (see the illustration on page 3).

Systemic. Unfortunately, the effects of rheumatoid arthritis are not limited to the joints; they can have consequences throughout the entire body. As a result, people who have the disease are frequently fatigued, often lose their appetite, and tend to run a low fever and feel generally unwell, as if they have the flu. Without proper treatment, this serious systemic illness can lead to significant disability and premature death.

Causes of Rheumatoid Arthritis

The exact cause of rheumatoid arthritis is still unknown. However, researchers have identified some factors that may increase a person's risk of developing the disease.

Sleep Disturbances and Arthritis

A good night's rest helps put inflammation to bed

Sleep is often elusive for people with arthritis: Of the 42.7 million Americans with the condition, 32% have trouble sleeping. Unfortunately, lack of sleep increases pain and fatigue, dampens spirits, and is associated with a host of ills, including heart disease and diabetes. And now, a recent study at the University of California reveals that loss of an even small amount of sleep boosts inflammatory activity in the body. The news makes a good night's sleep—at least seven to eight hours—more important than ever for people with arthritis.

The Sleep-Inflammation Link

Scientists have known for some time that inflammation increases the risk of various diseases such as arthritis, heart disease, and diabetes. But the California study is the first to show how sleep loss affects the immune system. The scientists took blood samples from 30 healthy adults after three nights of uninterrupted sleep and also after a fourth night when the participants slept for only part of the night. The investigators found that certain white blood cells called monocytes—part of the immune system—produced significantly more of two inflammatory proteins following the night of little sleep than they did after a sound sleep. Although inflammation following injury promotes healing, chronic inflammation—as can occur over time with too little sleep—ultimately damages healthy organs and tissues.

What's Behind Those Sleepless Nights?

Depression and anxiety are the greatest predictors of sleep problems in those with arthritis, according to a study using data from the National Health Interview Survey of more than 31,000 people. In addition, pain, stress, medications, restless legs syndrome, and a variety of daytime behaviors can be responsible for difficulty falling and staying asleep (insomnia).

Depression. Normally, sleep has two states: non-rapid eye movement (NREM) sleep and rapid-eye movement (REM) sleep. As we sleep, our body swings back and forth between the two states.

Characteristically, people who are clinically depressed have intense and long versions of REM sleep. Also known as dream sleep, this stage of slumber consolidates memory and, normally, lessens the emotional impact of new memories. However, in people with depression, the part of the brain that deals with emotion stays aroused, and negative thoughts aren't calmed, as they normally would be. Instead of regulating a negative mood, REM sleep worsens it.

Staying asleep is also a problem. People with depression often wake early in the morning during the longest phase of REM sleep and are unable to go back to sleep.

Anxiety. Most of us can keep anxiety at bay during a busy day, but at night as we try to sleep, worries can surface, arousing our nervous system, which in turn stirs up muscle tension, pulse rate, and breathing. And it's not unusual for people with a chronic illness such as arthritis to have more anxiety than people without it. A 2007 Norwegian study of more than 200 people with rheumatoid arthritis, for example, found that 20–30% had high levels of anxiety, which was also associated with greater pain.

Pain. Not surprisingly, being in pain makes it difficult to get a good night's sleep. A recent study involving nearly 9,000 people found that those with rheumatoid arthritis were more likely to have sleep disturbances than those with noninflammatory disorders.

Stress. Another worry—stress. In a recent year-long British study of 129 people with rheumatoid arthritis, those who described themselves as feeling greater stress than others in the study had more frequent sleep problems. And those whose sleep was disrupted also reported feeling greater pain, fatigue, and morning stiffness.

Genetics

Rheumatoid arthritis can run in a family, but having the condition does not greatly increase the risk to a person's children.

A specific genetic marker called HLA-DR4 occurs in more than two thirds of white men and women who have rheumatoid arthritis.

Medications. Prescription drugs can contribute to sleep problems as well. Long-term use of anti-inflammatory corticosteroids, such as cortisone and prednisone, can cause sleeplessness, among other side effects. Opiate pain relievers, such as morphine or codeine, can cause the user to sleep lightly, resulting in more frequent awakening and, frequently, difficulty returning to sleep. Opiates also suppress REM sleep. In addition, the effects of pain medications can vary from person to person: The same medication that makes some people drowsy can stimulate others.

Restless legs syndrome. This disorder, which is sometimes associated with arthritis, causes unpleasant crawling or tingling sensations in the legs and an urge to move them to get relief. These movements result in repeated awakenings at night, interrupting the normal phases of sleep that are crucial for rejuvenation.

Caffeine and alcohol. Drinking coffee and other caffeine-rich beverages, such as tea or cola, may interfere with your ability to get a good night's sleep because caffeine acts as a stimulant on the central nervous system.

Although alcohol can make you drowsy, if consumed close to bedtime it can disrupt sleep. Initially, alcohol increases deep sleep and reduces REM sleep. But during the second half of the night, the alcohol causes fitful, light sleep, many awakenings, and vivid dreams or nightmares during REM sleep. The result: loss of a good night's sleep.

Other factors. Sleeping for more than 45 minutes in the afternoon can make it harder to snooze soundly at night. Regularly working, reading, or watching TV in bed may cause you to associate the bed with wakefulness, not sleep. Although pain and fatigue may make it difficult to exercise if you have arthritis, lack of physical activity also can contribute to a poor night's sleep.

How Can You Break the Sleeplessness Cycle?

The first and simplest step is to check what experts call your "sleep hygiene." If you're napping in the afternoon, smoking, or drinking alcohol close to bedtime, cut out those habits. If you treat your bedroom like an office, awhirl with activity, start doing those things elsewhere. And cut back on caffeine (remember it's in chocolate, sodas, and tea as well as coffee). A glass of milk or a light snack at bedtime is not a bad idea so you don't wake up feeling hungry.

A warm bath before bed helps, too, temporarily raising your body temperature: As your temperature drops again, your body naturally becomes drowsy. That's why a cool room may help as well.

Also, try putting yourself on a regular schedule, going to sleep each night and rising at the same time every day. And, with your doctor's okay, incorporate some exercise like walking daily, no closer than three hours before bed.

You should also talk to your doctor about the medications you are taking, and ask if they may be keeping you up. He or she may be able to prescribe a different medication or change your dose to solve the problem.

If you are depressed or anxious or you feel pain is keeping you from sleeping, your doctor needs to know that as well. Some antidepressants can effectively treat both depression and pain, which, in turn, will likely improve sleep. And the doctor may also suggest pain medication.

Newer nonbenzodiazepine sleep medications such as zolpidem (Ambien) and zaleplon (Sonata), which help you fall asleep faster, also may be an option but only for a short time and only as a last resort because of their potential for addiction. Two other prescription sleep aids, eszopiclone (Lunesta) and ramelteon (Rozerem) are approved for longer-term use.

Some doctors may suggest a combination of sleep or pain medications and cognitive-behavioral therapy. A cognitive-behavioral therapist can offer tips on sleep hygiene as well as relaxation training, using techniques such as abdominal breathing or meditation that reduce anxiety and muscle tension. ■

However, approximately one in five people who do not have rheumatoid arthritis also have the HLA-DR4 marker. Consequently, the presence of HLA-DR4 may indicate a risk of rheumatoid arthritis, but people who have the marker are not necessarily destined to develop the disease.

Infection

Several types of arthritis occur as a result of infections. The most familiar infection-related form can occur during or after Lyme disease, which is the result of a bite from an infected deer tick. The bacterium the tick transmits first causes a rash, fever, and neck stiffness. Weeks later, severe joint inflammation (Lyme arthritis) may arise and may last for months or even a lifetime. Some researchers think that, in a similar way, exposure to certain bacteria or viruses can trigger the abnormal immune response that causes rheumatoid arthritis among people who are genetically susceptible.

Environmental Factors

Several studies have found that heavy smokers and people who have been heavily exposed to cigarette smoke are more likely to develop rheumatoid arthritis than nonsmokers. Another study that involved more than 25,000 people ages 45–75 suggested that eating a diet too rich in red meat and other high-protein foods may increase the risk of rheumatoid arthritis. A convincing explanation for the existence of rheumatoid arthritis, however, still continues to elude researchers.

Prevention of Rheumatoid Arthritis

Because its cause is unknown, predicting how rheumatoid arthritis might be prevented is difficult. Because this form of arthritis is more common among women than men, some researchers are examining the role of hormones in triggering the disease. The fact that women who breast-feed for at least a year are less likely to develop rheumatoid arthritis also suggests that hormones might be involved, but as yet no conclusive evidence has led researchers to suspect any hormones in particular.

For several years, scientists have been working to develop a vaccine that might prevent the autoimmune reactions that cause rheumatoid arthritis. In 2006, a firm based in the United States bought the rights to test a vaccine against rheumatoid arthritis that has shown promise in preliminary human trials in the People's Republic of China, but doctors would use it as a form of therapy to reduce symptoms, not as a preventive strategy. A potential preventive vaccine has not yet moved from laboratory mice to studies involving humans.

Symptoms of Rheumatoid Arthritis

Morning stiffness and symmetrical joint pain are the most recognizable symptoms of rheumatoid arthritis. But most often, the first symptoms are fatigue, weakness, low-grade fever, or loss of appetite and weight. These conditions can arise even before joint problems develop. Because these symptoms occur in many other illnesses, you and your doctor may not initially suspect arthritis.

Prolonged Stiffness

When morning stiffness occurs with rheumatoid arthritis, it usually lasts longer than one hour and gradually improves during the day. (In osteoarthritis, morning stiffness lasts less than an hour.) Stiffness tends to last longer when rheumatoid arthritis is more severe and to increase after long periods of sitting.

Inflammation

With osteoarthritis, joints ache and feel tender, but there is little or no swelling. In people with rheumatoid arthritis, however, affected joints become inflamed (red, warm, swollen, and painful). Rheumatoid arthritis typically starts on both sides of the body at once and occurs in small as well as large joints, especially in the hands and fingers, wrists, knees, ankles, and feet. The symmetrical pattern and the presence of inflammation distinguish rheumatoid arthritis from osteoarthritis. Also, unlike osteoarthritis, rheumatoid arthritis rarely affects the top joints of the fingers (those closest to the fingernails).

About 20% of people with rheumatoid arthritis develop rheumatoid nodules—hard lumps of tissue under the skin, especially near the elbows. Rheumatoid nodules often indicate more severe disease activity (ongoing inflammation); they sometimes disappear when disease activity lessens.

Flares

Rheumatoid arthritis is a disease that waxes and wanes. It's marked by periods of increased disease activity called flare-ups or flares, which are characterized by worsening pain, stiffness, and inflammation. When rheumatoid arthritis is in a flare-up, the continuing inflammatory process can lead to irreversible joint damage.

Systemic Effects

Rheumatoid arthritis inflammation may spread to membranes and connective tissues through the body. For example, some individuals

NEW RESEARCH

New Clues to the Cause of Extra-Articular Rheumatoid Arthritis

Previous research has linked both rheumatoid factor and antibodies called cyclic citrullinated peptides (anti–CCP) to rheumatoid arthritis (RA). But few studies have been done on their connection to extra-articular RA, which affects parts of the body beyond the joints, such as the eyes and nerves. Now researchers have shown a strong link between both antibodies and extra-articular RA.

The researchers examined the levels of rheumatoid factor and anti–CCP in 35 people recently diagnosed with severe extra-articular RA, comparing them with 70 people who had RA without systemic complications. Of those with extra-articular RA, 94% tested positive for rheumatoid factor compared with only 71% of those without extra-articular RA. In addition, 77% with extra-articular RA tested positive for anti–CCP compared with 56% of those who did not have systemic complications.

The findings suggest that both rheumatoid factor and anti–CCP play a role in systemic RA, and high levels of rheumatoid factor are a likely indicator of severe extra-articular RA.

ANNALS OF THE RHEUMATIC DISEASES
Volume 66, page 59
January 2007

develop inflammation of the outer layer of the eye(scleritis), or inflammation of the membrane lining the chest wall (pleurisy).

Another systemic effect, nerve damage (neuropathy), may occur when an inflamed joint compresses a nerve. About one third of people with rheumatoid arthritis also develop mild anemia (decreased number of red blood cells), and in approximately 10–15%, primarily women, glands around the eyes and mouth are affected, causing decreased production of tears and saliva (a disorder known as Sjögren's syndrome).

Less frequently, rheumatoid arthritis sometimes causes inflammation of blood vessels throughout the body (vasculitis) or in the membrane surrounding the heart (pericarditis). A rare complication is Felty syndrome, in which the spleen enlarges and white blood cell count drops, leading to recurrent infections.

Advanced Effects

In later stages of rheumatoid arthritis, damage to cartilage, tendons, ligaments, and bones in the joints causes deformity, weakness, and immobility. As occurs with osteoarthritis, people with advanced rheumatoid arthritis often have trouble performing everyday tasks such as buttoning a blouse or shirt, combing their hair, tying shoelaces, holding a fork, opening doors, or turning the steering wheel of a car. Severe rheumatoid arthritis also makes people more susceptible to infection and increases the risk of developing heart disease.

Diagnosis of Rheumatoid Arthritis

Early diagnosis and immediate, aggressive treatment of rheumatoid arthritis are crucial, because only a brief window of opportunity exists to prevent permanent disability and lifelong complications. But early diagnosis is often difficult. First, the early symptoms of rheumatoid arthritis often mimic those of osteoarthritis, the flu, and other viral illnesses. Second, in the early stages of the disease, joints may not be red or swollen and may appear normal on x-rays.

Find the Right Doctor

To increase your chances of getting an accurate and early diagnosis, choosing the right doctor is important. Because rheumatoid arthritis is not common, your general physician may have little experience with the disease. When in doubt, ask for a referral to a board-certified rheumatologist—a physician who specializes in arthritis and other rheumatic diseases. Rheumatologists have extensive training and experience in diagnosing and treating these diseases and will recognize subtle clues that are the key to an accurate, early diagnosis.

Seven Diagnostic Criteria

Rheumatologists follow standardized guidelines for evaluating anyone who might have rheumatoid arthritis. No single laboratory test or diagnostic procedure can confirm the diagnosis.

Instead, seven diagnostic criteria are used:

- Morning stiffness
- Arthritis in three or more joint areas
- Arthritis in the hand joints
- Symmetrical arthritis
- Rheumatoid nodules
- Elevated serum level of rheumatoid factor
- Radiographic (x-ray) changes.

The diagnosis will be rheumatoid arthritis if the first four criteria have been present for at least six weeks, long enough to rule out the possibility that a virus has caused the arthritis symptoms.

Even if you don't meet the four-out-of-seven criteria standard, you still may have rheumatoid arthritis. If you have two or three of the criteria, more testing is necessary, because if you do have rheumatoid arthritis, even a short delay in beginning treatment can be harmful.

Medical History and Physical Examination

The doctor will take a medical history and perform a physical examination similar to the one used to diagnose osteoarthritis (see pages 10–11). One goal of the medical history and physical examination is to rule out other possible causes for your symptoms.

You may also be asked to rate your general health and your pain level on a 1–10 scale. These are called global assessments. Your doctor will make another global assessment based on your comments and the results of your physical exam. Global assessments provide a baseline measure for future comparisons.

After the question session, the doctor will examine you, looking for actively inflamed joints and rheumatoid nodules. Part of the examination is a count of the tender and swollen joints. This count provides an objective measure of your baseline level of disease activity, which the doctor can use to evaluate changes in your condition over time. The doctor also will check for mechanical joint problems, such as loss of motion, noisy joints, instability, poor alignment, and deformities.

ASK THE DOCTOR

Q. ***I heard that it's not safe to get vaccines if you have RA. Does that mean I should not get a flu shot?***

A. No. Flu shots are especially important for people with rheumatoid arthritis (RA) because the immunosuppressive drugs used to treat the disease can increase the risk of getting the flu and also slow recovery from flu in those who get it.

A vaccine deliberately exposes a person to an infectious substance so the immune system will create antibodies to ward off infection. Some vaccines are made from live viruses, and in people whose immune systems are compromised, such vaccines carry a small risk of causing the disease that the vaccine is designed to protect against. Fortunately, the injectable form of the flu vaccine is made with a killed virus and so is not dangerous for people with compromised immune systems. People with RA should avoid the FluMist nasal vaccine, however, which contains a live virus.

For the flu shot to work effectively, you should be vaccinated when your RA is well controlled with low-dose medications only (or no drugs at all). This is because high doses of immunosuppressive drugs—for example, more than 20 mg a day of prednisone—inhibit the body's ability to produce protective antibodies in response to vaccination. However, a recent study found that adalimumab (Humira) does not reduce the protective effect of a flu shot.

The Puzzle in Rheumatoid Arthritis Testing

A new test may point to a need for early treatment

Early treatment is essential to halt or slow bone damage in rheumatoid arthritis, most of which usually occurs within the first two years of diagnosis. It would be a boon to have a test that identifies people with early symptoms who will go on to develop rheumatoid arthritis, so that treatment can begin quickly.

Recent research hints that a test for antibodies to proteins called cyclic citrullinated peptides (CCP) may serve that purpose—but only for certain people.

The "gold standard" for diagnosing rheumatoid arthritis, the test for rheumatoid factor (RF), is relatively good at detecting the presence of the disease, but people may not test positive until six to 12 months after the onset of the disease.

Antibodies to CCP, however, can show up in the blood two or three years *before* rheumatoid arthritis symptoms first arise. In fact, one study suggests that the anti-CCP test is most accurate in the first three months after the onset of symptoms. Perhaps the test is specific for an early stage of rheumatoid arthritis.

RF vs. Anti-CCP

Statistically, the RF test is better than the anti-CCP test at identifying individuals who are developing rheumatoid arthritis. Some 70–80% of people with rheumatoid arthritis test positive for RF at some point. In contrast, only 50–70% of people who develop rheumatoid arthritis ever test positive for antibodies to CCP.

On the other hand, the anti-CCP test, although newer, appears so far to be much more specific. Although many people who test positive for RF never develop rheumatoid arthritis, the few studies done to date suggest that almost everyone who tests positive for anti-CCP antibodies and who has symptoms consistent with rheumatoid arthritis will eventually develop the disease.

Confusing Results

As many as half of people with rheumatoid arthritis test negative for antibodies to CCP, so it is difficult to know what to make of a negative test. It has also been unclear how to interpret a positive test, because the results are inconsistent.

In a recent Canadian study, among 384 people who had inflammatory arthritis for less than one year, there were just 26 who had no hint other than a positive anti-CCP test that they might be developing rheumatoid arthritis. Of these, only five developed erosion in their joints within two years, and only one progressed to severe rheumatoid arthritis. Evidently, for the other 379 people, the test had little or no predictive value. And a Boston study of 525 individuals with rheumatoid arthritis found that levels of anti-CCP antibodies did not correlate with disease severity.

However, a study in the Netherlands recently found that, among 110 people with early signs of arthritis who were assigned at random to take either methotrexate (a common rheumatoid arthritis drug) or placebo, the drug dramatically

Laboratory Tests

You will need to undergo an array of tests. Results from these tests will help the doctor diagnose your disease as well as provide baseline values that he or she can use to evaluate disease progression and the success of your treatment.

Rheumatoid factor

The most important laboratory test in diagnosing rheumatoid arthritis is a blood test for rheumatoid factor, an immune substance that is elevated in about 70–80% of people who have the disease. Many people with rheumatoid arthritis initially show no evidence slowed the progress of rheumatoid arthritis—but only in those who tested positive for anti-CCP. So the test may be a poor predictor of severe rheumatoid arthritis, but a good signal to start early treatment.

Clues From Genetics

Like a positive RF test, the presence of antibodies to CCP is evidence that the body is setting up an immune reaction against itself. Anti-CCP antibodies target proteins containing a molecule called citrulline, which is often found in the inflamed lining of joints affected by rheumatoid arthritis. Researchers suspect that the presence of citrulline may have something to do with the inflammatory process—at least in a subset of people with rheumatoid arthritis.

Recent genetic studies in Europe strengthen this idea. A study from Germany found that anti-CCP antibodies occur both more frequently and at higher levels in people with rheumatoid arthritis who have certain variants of a genetic subtype called HLA-DRB1.

Among people with the variant DRB1-04, more severe rheumatoid arthritis develops in those who test positive for anti-CCP. And a Swedish study found that anti-CCP was 100% accurate in predicting progression to rheumatoid arthritis in people who had another genetic marker called PTPN22 1858T. This may explain why anti-CCP testing works better in some studies than in others: Genetic differences that are not measured may skew the results.

The research that links anti-CCP testing to genetic types is not yet complete, and tests for the markers are not widely available. But some researchers suggest that it is time for a separate classification of early rheumatoid arthritis: Those who test positive for anti-CCP appear to have a different trigger for the disease, a different disease course, and a different response to treatment than those who test negative.

Interpreting Your Result

For now, doctors do not recommend the anti-CCP test when symptoms of inflammatory arthritis (such as joint pain and inflammation) are absent. But the test could be especially useful for decision making in the case of people who test negative for RF but continue to have joint pain and inflammation.

If you test positive for antibodies to CCP, even without a positive test for RF, you will likely develop rheumatoid arthritis. This is also true if you test positive for both anti-CCP and RF. And you may develop a more severe form of rheumatoid arthritis than if you lacked the anti-CCP antibodies.

Positive Result: Good News

The good news is that a positive anti-CCP test result means you may be able to slow the progress of rheumatoid arthritis with early treatment. So it's important to have the test quickly after symptoms begin.

If you test negative for both RF and anti-CCP, it's much less likely that your joint pain is a signal of rheumatoid arthritis. However, neither test offers a guarantee: Rheumatoid arthritis can develop in people who have negative results on both tests. ■

of rheumatoid factor but test positive six to 12 months later, as the disease progresses. This test alone is not a definitive indicator of rheumatoid arthritis because elevated levels may also occur in people with other autoimmune diseases as well as with many other unrelated disorders.

ANA test

Antinuclear antibodies (ANA) are another immune factor found in 30–40% of people with rheumatoid arthritis. (As is the case with rheumatoid factor, however, ANA may also be present in people who do not have rheumatoid arthritis.)

Anti-CCP

Some doctors now use a newer, more definitive test. The new test detects antibodies to cyclic citrullinated peptides (CCPs), signs of an immune reaction to the degradation of a protein that occurs in the synovium (the membrane that lines the joints). These antibodies are very specific to rheumatoid arthritis and often appear in the blood long before the onset of rheumatoid arthritis symptoms. Recent research suggests that this test may be most accurate within three months of the onset of symptoms. (See "The Puzzle in Rheumatoid Arthritis Testing" on pages 44–45.)

Sed rate

The erythrocyte sedimentation rate (sed rate) helps to differentiate rheumatoid arthritis from osteoarthritis. The inflammation in rheumatoid arthritis causes red blood cells to clump together and quickly fall to the bottom of a test tube. The sed rate measures the speed at which this occurs. It is elevated in rheumatoid arthritis but is normal in osteoarthritis.Your doctor may also test you for C-reactive protein (CRP), a substance that appears in the blood during many types of inflammation.

Blood count

Your doctor will order a complete blood count to measure levels of red blood cells, white blood cells, and platelets. People with rheumatoid arthritis often have anemia (a decreased level of oxygen-carrying red blood cells) and a high level of white blood cells (the infection-fighting cells that cause inflammation). Inflammation is also associated with an increased level of platelets, the cells that help the blood to clot.

Other lab tests

Additional tests may be needed to determine baseline values and to check for abnormal function of the liver, kidneys, and other organs. These tests may measure electrolytes (minerals that regulate body functions), creatinine (an indicator of kidney function), liver enzymes, and blood in the stool. Many drugs for rheumatoid arthritis can be toxic to the liver and kidneys. If tests indicate liver and kidney function abnormalities, your doctor will prescribe other drugs.

Synovial fluid

You may have a small amount of fluid withdrawn from one of your inflamed joints. The number of white blood cells in the synovial fluid is another helpful measure of inflammation. But because white cells also fight infection, high levels may also indicate the presence of infection or another type of disease.

X-rays

Early in rheumatoid arthritis, joints in the hands and feet often show structural damage on an x-ray. Baseline x-rays provide a starting point against which to measure disease progression.

Bone mineral density test

You may also need a bone mineral density test, an x-ray procedure that uses very low doses of radiation to detect osteoporosis (bone thinning). Because of inflammation and immobilization of the joints, as well as certain medications (corticosteroids, for example), osteoporosis is a significant risk for women and men with rheumatoid arthritis, especially for postmenopausal women (see "Osteoporosis: A Common Complication of Rheumatoid Arthritis" on pages 50–51).

Treatment of Rheumatoid Arthritis

The goals of treatment for rheumatoid arthritis are to relieve pain, reduce inflammation, maintain function, and prevent joint damage and systemic illness. Unfortunately, there is no cure for rheumatoid arthritis, but disease-modifying antirheumatic drugs (DMARDs) can help produce long-term remission of the disease. Using the right medications and starting them as early as possible are the keys to achieving treatment goals.

Assessing Prognosis

Most people with rheumatoid arthritis are treated with a combination of drugs. Deciding which drugs to use involves an assessment of your prognosis (predicted disease progression). To determine your prognosis, your doctor will take into consideration your age when the disease began, level of rheumatoid factor, sed rate, number of swollen joints, and the presence of systemic conditions, such as rheumatoid nodules, Sjögren's syndrome, scleritis, vasculitis, pericarditis, or Felty's syndrome.

People who develop rheumatoid arthritis before age 40 and have high levels of rheumatoid factor, an elevated sed rate, more than 20 swollen joints, and one or more systemic conditions are considered

NEW RESEARCH

Remicade May Prevent Bone Loss in Rheumatoid Arthritis

Even if infliximab (Remicade) does not lessen disease activity in people with rheumatoid arthritis, it may keep them from losing bone. These findings are from a new study—the first to examine the effect of the drug on bone mineral density (BMD).

Remicade is an antibody that blocks the action of tumor necrosis factor (TNF)-a, a protein that promotes inflammation and joint damage in people with RA. Remicade has been shown to reduce joint destruction, but its effect on bone has been unclear.

Researchers looked at the baseline and one-year BMD readings in 90 patients with RA who took Remicade with methotrexate, another commonly used drug for the condition. The control group consisted of RA patients who took only methotrexate.

After one year, the control group had lower spine and femoral neck (upper thigh bone) BMD levels compared with their baseline readings. But in people who took Remicade, BMD levels did not change, even in those whose disease activity—number of swollen and tender joints, sense of health, and level of inflammation—seemed unchanged by the treatment.

If you're taking Remicade for RA, it could be a boon to your bones as well.

ARTHRITIS RESEARCH & THERAPY
Volume 9, page 1
June 2007

to have a poor prognosis. Studies demonstrate that these individuals have more than a 70% chance of developing joint damage or joint erosions within two years of disease onset.

Thanks to the advent of disease-modifying drugs, an unfavorable prognosis does not mean an inevitable downward spiral. But these people do need more aggressive treatment, and they need it quickly. They also require more frequent visits to their doctors, more frequent tests, and more help in adjusting to the physical, occupational, and emotional consequences of their condition.

The long-term prognosis for all people with rheumatoid arthritis also depends on controlling the other conditions that may develop. People with rheumatoid arthritis have a shorter lifespan than the general population, largely because of an increased risk of coronary heart disease, infection (especially lung infection), and osteoporosis. If you have rheumatoid arthritis, you need to take extra steps to prevent, detect, and treat these diseases.

Measuring Treatment Effects

After you have taken your medication for several weeks, your doctor will repeat the same tests and assessments used to establish your baseline. Repeating the tests will help the doctor to assess the treatment's effectiveness.

The American College of Rheumatology (ACR) has developed a scoring system that doctors use to rate any changes. The ACR standard for a 20% "clinical improvement" (referred to as ACR 20) requires 20% improvement in the count of tender and swollen joints and 20% improvement in at least three of the following five measures:

- Your assessment of pain
- Your global assessment of disease activity
- Your physician's global assessment of your disease activity
- Your assessment of physical function
- Your sed rate or other markers of inflammation.

The same criteria are used to identify improvements of 50–70% (known as ACR 50 and ACR 70, respectively).

The maximum level of improvement is called a complete remission. A remission occurs when there is an absence of the following: symptoms of active inflammatory joint pain, morning stiffness, fatigue, white blood cells in the synovial fluid, progression of joint damage (as judged by x-rays taken at each examination and compared with baseline x-rays), and elevated sed rate or C-reactive protein levels.

NEW RESEARCH

Change Treatment? No Way

That's the verdict from many people with rheumatoid arthritis (RA)—even if they still experience symptoms, according to a new study.

Using questionnaire responses from more than 6,000 people with RA, researchers found that 64% would not change therapy as long as their condition did not worsen, and 77% were happy with their medications. Yet more than 70% of people who were satisfied with their therapy also had at least moderate disease activity, indicated by several clinical measures of pain and inflammation.

The main reason most would hesitate to change: Concerns about the risk of side effects, cited by nearly 73%. About 71% didn't want to switch because their doctor didn't feel they needed to, and almost that many believed that no better medications were available, including 58% of those who were not taking relatively new medications like etanercept (Enbrel) and infliximab (Remicade). Worry that the disease would spiral out of control on a new regimen was a concern of 69%.

Insurance and monetary concerns were also an issue. More than half didn't want the hassle of getting insurance approval for new medications, and 43% said they could not afford them.

If you're not getting the relief you need from your current regimen, in most cases, other options are available. Talk with your doctor about your concerns.

ARTHRITIS & RHEUMATISM
Volume 56, page 2135
July 2007

At an ACR 20 rating, you may notice a modest improvement in your arthritis symptoms. If you reach an ACR 50 or ACR 70, you will definitely experience a meaningful, positive change. If you achieve complete remission, you may feel as if you never had rheumatoid arthritis. Unfortunately, however, these improvements may not be permanent.

Drug Treatments

Few people achieve permanent remission, making it likely that you will have to take rheumatoid arthritis medication for the rest of your life. Your treatment will probably require a combination of medications from three drug categories: nonsteroidal anti-inflammatory drugs (NSAIDs), corticosteroids, and DMARDs.

In the past, people with newly diagnosed rheumatoid arthritis were treated first with an over-the-counter pain reliever, such as acetaminophen (Tylenol) or one of the over-the-counter NSAIDs such as aspirin or ibuprofen (Advil, Motrin). Only when the disease worsened would doctors begin to prescribe stronger medications, and by the time a DMARD was started, some joint damage was already permanent.

In recent years, the prognosis for rheumatoid arthritis patients has improved dramatically, thanks to earlier use of powerful new DMARDs. Rheumatoid arthritis guidelines now specify DMARDs as the first drugs to use in newly diagnosed people. This more aggressive approach makes long-term remission an attainable goal for many more rheumatoid arthritis patients.

However, the newest disease-modifying drugs—called biologic response modifiers (BRMs)—are very expensive. They typically cost more than $1,000 per month. When you add this cost to the expense of your other arthritis medications, x-rays, blood and urine tests, visits to your doctor, physical therapy, treatment for depression (which is common in rheumatoid arthritis patients), and indirect costs related to disability and missed work, it is obvious that having rheumatoid arthritis can be a significant financial burden.

Unfortunately, insurance companies often press for the lowest-cost drugs and treatment. Your doctor can help you balance monetary concerns with the need to prevent disability.

Disease-modifying antirheumatic drugs (DMARDs)

DMARDs have anti-inflammatory properties and, more important, the ability to slow the disease process by suppressing the immune

NEW RESEARCH

Combined RA Therapies Have Edge Over Single Drug Treatment

Combination therapy for early rheumatoid arthritis (RA) isn't just for people who don't respond to a single-drug therapy. According to a new study, it may be a good option for treatment of all patients with this condition.

Flemish researchers followed 508 people with early RA for two years. One group was given a single therapy, beginning with methotrexate and followed by other one-at-a time drugs; a second group took methotrexate followed by a mix of combination therapies; a third started with combination therapy that included tapered, high doses of prednisone; and a fourth began with a combination therapy that included infliximab (Remicade).

All four approaches lowered disease activity. In fact, 79% of the participants had a low level of disease activity after two years and were better able to function. However, during the first year of treatment, participants in groups three and four had substantially lower levels of disease than those in groups one and two. And their joints showed less damage at the end of two years. Medications also had to be adjusted less often in groups three and four than in groups one and two.

Because better control over the RA in the first year is an important factor in controlling disease progression, combination therapy should be considered early on.

ANNALS OF INTERNAL MEDICINE
Volume 146, page 406
March 2007

Osteoporosis: A Common Complication of Rheumatoid Arthritis

Taking proactive measures can reduce your risk

When you think about who's at risk for osteoporosis, a stereotypical portrait probably comes to mind: a thin Caucasian or Asian woman who's over age 50. But if you have rheumatoid arthritis (RA), add yourself to that picture. Women—and men—with RA also have a significantly increased risk of osteoporosis and for fractures, not only of the hip, but also the arms, legs, pelvis, and spine.

In fact, according to a 2006 British study, people with RA are 50% more likely to develop osteoporosis and bone fractures than those who don't have RA. Women face the greatest odds: They are two to three times more likely to have RA than men and have four times the risk of osteoporosis.

The study of about 30,000 people with RA and 91,000 without it found that the risk existed even if no other risk factors for osteoporosis, such as the long-term use of corticosteroids, smoking, and being thin, were present. In fact, the risk posed by RA alone was as great as the risk caused by taking corticosteroids.

What Raises the Risk of Osteoporosis?

Although scientists are still trying to sort out why people with RA are more likely to develop osteoporosis than others, they do know some of the factors that heighten risk.

Disease activity. In addition to the joint damage that the disease's chronic inflammation may cause, RA itself appears to trigger bone loss in the affected joint as well as other bones throughout the body. Some studies suggest that proteins that control inflammation (cytokines) also regulate cells called osteoclasts that are responsible for breaking down bone.

Corticosteroids. These medications are frequently prescribed to slow the progress of RA. Examples of medications in this category include prednisone, prednisolone, dexamethasone, and cortisone. Unfortunately, corticosteroids (also called glucocorticoids) jumpstart bone loss by suppressing bone formation and increasing bone breakdown. They also interfere with the way the body uses calcium and lower the levels of sex hormones (estrogen and testosterone), both of which add to bone loss. Although short-term use doesn't appear harmful to bones, anyone taking corticosteroids for more than three months raises his or her risk of osteoporosis.

Lack of exercise. The pain and damage caused by RA can limit both your ability and your desire to exercise. But making the effort to do some exercise is important: The tug of muscles on bones whenever you move strengthens your bones.

How Strong Are Your Bones?

To find out, you will need to undergo a simple, painless test called dual energy x-ray absorptiometry (DXA). It uses low doses of radiation (lower than a regular x-ray) to measure your bone density in comparison to that of young, healthy people without osteoporosis or RA. If your score (called a T-score) is less than -2.5, you have osteoporosis. A score of -1 to -2.5 means you have osteopenia, the first stage of bone loss.

Doctors generally recommend a baseline DXA scan for anyone planning to take corticosteroid therapy for six months or more. At Johns Hopkins, people with or at risk for osteoporosis are usually advised to get a scan every 18–24 months to monitor changes and the effect of any treatment. The cost of a DXA scan ranges from about $125–350; Medicare and most private insurers will pay for testing every two years.

Proven Ways To Prevent Bone Loss

You can take steps to help prevent or halt bone loss and, hopefully, keep your T-score out of the danger zone. If you use corticosteroids, studies show that most bone loss occurs in the first months of treatment—followed by slower continuous loss. Therefore, beginning a prevention program when you start taking the medication is best. Even if you aren't a long-term corticosteroid user, if you have RA it's still a smart move to follow these recommendations for osteoporosis prevention.

Take calcium and vitamin D supplements. Calcium helps develop and maintain bone structure, and vitamin D helps the bones absorb calcium and hold onto minerals. The higher a bone's mineral content, the stronger it is. Your doctor can check your vitamin D level to make sure that you are not deficient. In general, women and men should take 1,500 mg of calcium and 800 international units (IU) of vitamin D daily. Again, check with your rheumatologist to see what dose he or she recommends for you.

You can also boost the amounts of vitamin D and calcium you get by eating low-fat dairy products, dark green leafy vegetables, and calcium-fortified foods and drinks. A walk in the sunshine will also boost your vitamin D: The skin produces vitamin D from ultraviolet light.

Get some weight-bearing exercise. Weight-bearing exercise like walking, climbing stairs, and lifting weights forces muscles to push against bone and to work against gravity, which strengthens bones. Movement also helps keep muscles flexible and improves balance so that you're less likely to fall and break a bone.

Take medications. Studies show that several medications can help prevent or halt bone loss.

• ***Bisphosphonates.*** Risedronate (Actonel), approved in 2000 for the prevention of osteoporosis in women using corticosteroids and for the treatment of postmenopausal osteoporosis, was also approved for use in men at risk for corticosteroid-induced osteoporosis in 2006. Actonel is from a class of drugs called bisphosphonates, the leading treatment for osteoporosis. Alendronate (Fosamax) and ibandronate (Boniva) are two other commonly prescribed bisphosphonates for osteoporosis prevention and treatment. These medications slow the breakdown of bone and improve bone density.

Bisphosphonate use has been associated with osteonecrosis of the jaw—a serious condition in which bone cells in the jaw die because of decreased blood flow, most often following a dental extraction or some other trauma to the jaw. While reports of this condition in people taking bisphosphonates are uncommon, it is advisable to get regular dental checkups and let your dentist know if you are taking a bisphosphonate.

• ***Hormone replacement therapy (HRT).*** Hormonal replacement with estrogen or estrogen plus progestin also slows bone loss in postmenopausal women. However, HRT is controversial because it increases the risk of estrogen-fed breast cancer and, in women over age 60, heart disease.

An alternative is raloxifene (Evista), one of a new class of drugs called selective estrogen receptor modulators (SERMs) and the only one approved for the prevention and treatment of postmenopausal osteoporosis. SERMs appear less risky than traditional estrogen replacements—and in some women may actually lower breast cancer risk—but they are not as effective for osteoporosis prevention as either bisphosphonates or HRT.

In men, abnormally low levels of the hormone testosterone can cause osteoporosis. For men with this problem, testosterone replacement therapy (TRT)—available in injection, patch, and gel formulations—helps preserve bone mass by increasing testosterone to normal levels. However, high levels of testosterone are associated with an increased risk of prostate cancer. If you have a documented testosterone deficiency and are considering TRT, discuss the risks versus the benefits with your doctor.

• ***Calcitonin.*** This natural hormone is involved in regulating calcium and bone metabolism and has also been approved for the treatment of osteoporosis, but not prevention. Although it is not considered as effective as bisphosphonates, it may be a reasonable option if you can't or don't want to take that type of medication. Calcitonin can be taken as a nasal spray or as an injection.

• ***Forteo (Terlparatide).*** Approved by the FDA in 2002, this synthetic form of the parathyroid hormone (PTH) is the first medication approved for osteoporosis that stimulates the formation of new bone.

It's given by self-injection in the thigh or stomach once or twice daily, but it is reserved for the treatment of people with severe osteoporosis and fractures.

Stop smoking. Last, but certainly not least, if you smoke, quit. Not only is it harmful for your heart and lungs, but it's also bad for your bones. Smoking can trigger early menopause, which in turn ups bone loss, and it interferes with calcium absorption. Coupled with RA, that's "a perfect storm" for osteoporosis. ■

system. Because DMARDs reduce your immune response, once you start taking one of these medications it's important to check with your doctor before getting any vaccinations and to notify your doctor if you develop any signs of an infection, such as chills, fever, sore throat, or cough.

Older vs. newer. Doctors divide DMARDs into two main groups: the older DMARDs that they have been prescribing for decades, such as methotrexate, and the newer biologic response modifiers, the first of which was approved less than 10 years ago. The newer group of DMARDs act directly on the immune system by inhibiting proteins called cytokines, which are involved in inflammation. The drug chart on pages 56–59 describes the actions and effects of each of the DMARDs.

Rheumatologists have not yet agreed on which type of DMARD is best to give first: an older, less expensive, oral DMARD or a newer, more powerful, injectable biologic response modifier. Most rheumatologists choose oral methotrexate as the initial therapy because of its long track record of effectiveness, its low risk of side effects, and its low cost. However, a recent study found that the antibiotic doxycycline, when given with methotrexate, relieved symptoms better than methotrexate alone. Doxycycline has been shown to inhibit the rapid reproduction of cells.

According to one recent study, an added benefit of the traditional DMARDs is that over five years, they lower heart attack risk by 20%. The researchers found no such protection from the newer DMARDs. However, many of the older DMARDs also have rare but dangerous side effects. They should not be taken during pregnancy, and it is crucial to notify your doctor immediately if you develop a skin rash, mouth sore, abdominal pain, unusual fatigue, yellowing of the skin, easy bruising, recurrent infections, or fever. When you use one of these drugs, you must be monitored closely by your doctor.

The new biologic response modifiers have dangers too. They can increase the risk of lymphoma (a type of cancer), demyelinating syndromes (such as multiple sclerosis), and serious bacterial infections such as pneumonia, especially in people over age 65. You should not take one of these drugs if you have an active infection or an immune system disorder or are taking other immunosuppressive drugs.

Biologic response modifiers. These new medications often work for people who have not been helped by older DMARDs. They are typically added to the treatment regimen when methotrexate does not relieve symptoms.

Three of the biologic DMARDs—adalimumab (Humira), anakinra (Kineret), and etanercept (Enbrel)—are self-injected subcutaneously (into the layer of fat directly under the skin). If you take one of these injectable drugs, a healthcare professional will teach you or your caregiver the correct injection technique and help with the first few injections. These drugs must be stored in the refrigerator.

Abatacept (Orencia), infliximab (Remicade), and rituximab (Rituxan) are administered via intravenous (I.V.) infusion (that is, the drug flows through an I.V. line placed in your arm) at your doctor's office or an outpatient clinic. This usually takes about two hours.

During these infusions, some people have severe allergy-like reactions, with fever, chills, nausea, and shortness of breath. That's why a doctor or nurse should always monitor you during the infusion. Some doctors advise taking an antihistamine, acetaminophen, and/or prednisone before the infusion to help prevent these reactions.

Nonsteroidal anti-inflammatory drugs (NSAIDs)

NSAIDs reduce pain and inflammation, but they don't prevent joint destruction or worsening of rheumatoid arthritis. That and recent findings that NSAIDs can elevate the risk of heart disease are why they are no longer recommended as the sole treatment for rheumatoid arthritis. Instead, NSAIDs are used with DMARDs to provide additional relief from pain and inflammation when other avenues of pain relief have been tried without success.

Aspirin, however, is an exception. It is less expensive than other NSAIDs and may lower the risk of heart disease. Unless there is some reason not to use it (such as an allergy), aspirin is the NSAID of choice to reduce rheumatoid arthritis inflammation. The dosage can range from 2,400–5,400 mg per day, taken in divided doses. However, gastrointestinal irritation often limits the amount of aspirin people can tolerate.

People with rheumatoid arthritis, especially older people, are twice as likely as those with osteoarthritis to develop gastrointestinal ulcers and other serious complications from NSAIDs. Some (but not all) studies suggest that newer NSAIDs called COX-2 inhibitors might have fewer gastrointestinal side effects. But in light of recent concerns that COX-2 inhibitors can increase the risk of heart attacks and strokes—and the resulting removal of two of these three drugs (Vioxx and Bextra) from the market—your doctor may not prescribe Celebrex, the one COX-2 inhibitor that remains available. (See "Some NSAIDs More Risky Than Others" on page 15.)

NEW RESEARCH

RA: If One Anti–TNF Drug Doesn't Work, Another Might

When one anti-tumor necrosis factor (anti–TNF) medication doesn't work or produces ill effects, switching to another may be a good idea, a British study suggests.

The study involved almost 7,000 people with rheumatoid arthritis who took either adalimumab, (Humira), etanercept (Enbrel), or infliximab (Remicade), the three available anti–TNF medications. Over approximately 15 months, 856 switched to a second anti–TNF; 503 because of ineffectiveness and the remainder as a result of adverse effects.

Of those who switched medications, 73% were still taking the second medication after an average of six months. People who discontinued the second medication usually did so for the same reason they stopped taking the first. However, those who stopped taking both the first and second medication because of side effects did not necessarily experience the same problems with both drugs. It's not clear whether people who have no response to two anti–TNF medications should try a third or try another class of drugs.

If you've tried one anti–TNF medication but stopped taking it because it didn't work or you could not tolerate the side effects, you may want to try another. If you've tried two without success, discuss with your doctor whether a trial with a third might be beneficial or if it's time to move on to another type of medication.

ARTHRITIS & RHEUMATISM
Volume 56, page 13
January 2007

As in the treatment of osteoarthritis, the goal is to use the NSAID that provides the greatest benefit while producing the fewest risks and side effects. It may require trial and error to find the best option, because some people respond better to one NSAID than to another. (For more on NSAIDs, see pages 20–23.)

Corticosteroids

Typically, corticosteroid drugs are given in pill form, but as with osteoarthritis, injecting corticosteroids into the most affected joints is safe and highly effective for rheumatoid arthritis.

Low oral doses of the corticosteroid drug prednisone usually produce a rapid and dramatic improvement in rheumatoid arthritis symptoms by reducing inflammation and suppressing the immune system. Recent studies suggest that corticosteroid treatment may also slow the rate of joint damage. However, inflammation and joint damage frequently recur or get worse once a corticosteroid is discontinued. For that reason, you and your doctor may be tempted to continue corticosteroid use for long periods of time. But doing so can result in serious side effects: stomach ulcers, weight gain with fat deposits in the trunk (especially the upper back), diabetes, high blood pressure, thinning of the skin with easy bruising and poor wound healing, acne, weakness, muscle wasting, cataracts, increased susceptibility to infections, psychiatric disturbances, and osteoporosis.

Corticosteroids are best reserved for short-term treatment in people who are waiting for a DMARD to take effect. Corticosteroids are also used for incapacitating flares, for severe manifestations of rheumatoid arthritis affecting other organs (such as vasculitis and scleritis), or when alternative drugs are unsuccessful or cause intolerable side effects.

Because osteoporosis develops in as many as 50% of people taking corticosteroids, the American College of Rheumatology recommends using the lowest effective dose, supplemented with 1,500 mg of calcium and 400–800 IU of vitamin D daily. It's also important to avoid smoking and alcohol, to maintain a healthy weight, and to get regular weight-bearing exercise such as walking. A baseline bone mineral density test should be done before beginning treatment, with follow-up scans every one or two years to monitor changes in bone density. An osteoporosis treatment, such as Fosamax or Actonel, is often recommended as well.

The adrenal glands stop producing steroids when you are taking a corticosteroid, so when the medication is discontinued after being used at high doses or for a long time, the dosage must be reduced

NEW RESEARCH

Low-dose Steroids May Slow Damage From RA

Doctors have long debated whether low doses of steroids actually slow disease progression or simply provide symptom relief. Now, after reviewing 15 studies involving more than 1,400 people, researchers report that steroids in low doses, when given with other disease-modifying antirheumatic drugs (DMARDs), do indeed appear to inhibit rheumatoid arthritis progression in its early stages.

Most of the studies involved people who had had RA for less than two years who were given an average of 2,300 mg of prednisone in their first year of treatment, along with other DMARDs. The studies compared the results from people taking low-dose steroids with those of people taking a placebo or another drug by examining x-rays of the hands, hands and feet, or feet only. All of the trials except one showed that the steroids reduced the rate of erosion seen in the x-rays. It is not clear whether steroid use is effective in people with long-standing RA.

Recent findings suggest that some of the side effects associated with corticosteroid use may be less serious than previously believed, and others, such as osteoporosis, can be readily treated. So if you've had active rheumatoid arthritis for less than two years and are taking a DMARD, adding a low-dose steroid to your regimen may be a reasonably safe way to help prevent severe joint damage.

COCHRANE DATABASE OF SYSTEMATIC REVIEWS
Volume 1, CD006356
January 24, 2007

very slowly to give the adrenal glands a chance to resume steroid production. This will also help to prevent a disease flare.

Rest and Exercise

It is crucial that people who have rheumatoid arthritis get enough exercise of the right kind and sufficient rest. Physical therapy and the joint protection offered by products such as braces, splints, and assistive devices are often helpful, especially during flares.

Rest

Fatigue can be the most incapacitating aspect of rheumatoid arthritis. Taking frequent rest breaks when your joints are inflamed can help. In the short term, complete bed rest may be necessary when severe inflammation occurs in multiple joints. You can take the following steps to relieve fatigue:

- Get ample rest—at least 10 hours of sleep a day, either all at night or about eight hours at night and two hours during daytime naps (unless naps disrupt your nighttime sleep).
- Relieve pain promptly, because continued pain causes fatigue. (Use pain medications, joint rest, and applications of heat or cold when necessary.)
- Prioritize daily activities and carry out only the most essential ones. Postpone nonessential activities until flares subside.
- Divide your work by thinking of your energy in terms of a budget that you must balance against your daily activities. Just as you would not spend all your money at the beginning of the month, don't carry out all vigorous work at one time of the day. Instead, spread it out with rest periods between tasks.
- Try not to waste energy. For example, instead of making numerous trips up and down stairs during the day, consolidate activities and complete all of the tasks on one floor before moving on to the next.

Even when your joints are inflamed, you can still do gentle stretching exercises while resting to keep your joints mobile and to prevent flexion contracture (loss of joint motion due to shortening of the surrounding tissues). This also helps to protect your joints while you are at rest. For example:

- Do not remain seated for a long time; stand up periodically.
- If your hip or knee joints are painful, lie in a face-down position on a firm bed for about 15 minutes several times a day.
- Apply removable splints to inflamed joints to alleviate muscle spasms and reduce the likelihood of deformities.

NEW RESEARCH

Guidelines Clarify When To Use Rituxan for RA

People with rheumatoid arthritis (RA) who have moderate or severe disease activity, particularly those who do not respond to TNF (tumor necrosis factor) blockers, may be candidates for rituximab (Rituxan), according to a group of European and Canadian experts. Rituxan, the first drug to target B-cells involved in joint inflammation for treatment of RA, is also used to treat a type of cancer known as lymphoma.

The panel also recommends the drug for people with RA who don't respond to methotrexate or other disease-modifying antirheumatic drugs (DMARDs) but not for those with infections or heart failure. The recommended dosage is two 200-mg intravenous infusions separated by two weeks and 100 mg of the corticosteroid methylprednisone (or its equivalent) given intravenously before the infusions to prevent infusion reactions. Methotrexate may also be taken weekly to increase the effectiveness of the treatment. Improvement is usually seen within four months.

Since the publication of these guidelines, the U. S. Food and Drug Administration has revised Rituxan's label to include a warning about the risk of progressive multifocal leukoencephalopathy (PML), a potentially fatal brain infection. People with lupus or who are undergoing chemotherapy or immunotherapy appear to be at greatest risk. At the time of the label change, no cases of PML had been reported in RA patients.

ANNALS OF THE RHEUMATIC DISEASES
Volume 66, page 143
February 2007

Commonly Used Disease-Modifying and Other Antirheumatic Drugs 2008

Drug type: Brand (generic)	Average daily dosage*	How to take
Traditional disease-modifying antirheumatic drugs (DMARDs)		
Arava (leflunomide)	100 mg/day for 3 days, then 10–20 mg/day	Dose may be reduced if side effects are bothersome.
Azasan, Imuran (azathioprine)	50–150 mg/day (gradually increasing)	Once or twice per day. Right after meals, to prevent stomach problems.
Azulfidine, Azulfidine EN-tabs (sulfasalazine)	500–1,000 mg 2–3x/day (1.5–4 g/day) (gradually increasing)	With full glass of water after meals to avoid gastrointestinal problems. Swallow tablets whole.
Cellcept (mycophenolate mofetil)	1 g 2x/day	On an empty stomach.
Cuprimine, Depen (penicillamine)	125–1,500 mg/day (gradually increasing)	On an empty stomach 1 hour before or 2 hours after meals and at least 1 hour apart from any other drug, milk, antacids, or supplements that contain zinc or iron.
Cytoxan, Neosar (cyclophosphamide)	1–3 mg/kg/day	On an empty stomach, or with small amounts of food or milk, to prevent stomach problems.
Gengraf, Neoral, Sandimmune (cyclosporine)	2.5–4 mg/kg/day	Twice a day, at the same time each day. Do not mix oral form with milk. Avoid grapefruits and grapefruit juice.
Plaquenil (hydroxychloroquine)	100–200 mg 2x/day	With meals or milk.
Rheumatrex, Trexall (methotrexate)	5–15 mg/week	1–2 hours before a meal. (Sometimes given in injectable form.)
Gold salts		
Myochrysine (gold sodium thiomalate)	25–50 mg every 2–4 weeks	Injection
Ridaura (auranofin)	3 mg 2x/day	Begins with low doses, increased slowly.

See legend on page 58

Precautions	Most common side effects	Comments
Do not take if you have liver disease or are a heavy alcohol user. Do not take live vaccines while using. Do not use while pregnant.	Diarrhea, skin rash, hair loss, weight loss, increase in blood pressure.	Takes effect in 4–8 weeks. More than 40% of users have a 20% reduction in symptoms. Blood tests required to monitor liver function.
Risk of serious infection, abnormal bleeding, and liver problems. May cause skin rash or mouth sores. Avoid alcohol. Frequent blood tests required. Do not use while pregnant or breast-feeding.	Nausea, vomiting, loss of appetite, diarrhea, fever.	May take 3 months to take effect. Used only for severe symptoms that do not respond to other drugs. Seek medical attention for fever or bleeding.
Side effects require close monitoring during first 3 months. Call your doctor if you develop sore throat, fever, or jaundice.	Abdominal cramps, diarrhea, loss of appetite, nausea, vomiting, dizziness, rash, headache, skin yellowing, sun sensitivity, decreased sperm count (reversible).	Usually takes effect in 1–3 months. Generally used in combination with methotrexate.
Increases susceptibility to infection. Do not get any vaccinations without your doctor's approval. May increase your risk of developing certain types of cancer, including skin cancer. See your dermatologist twice a year. Requires regular lab tests to monitor your response to treatment.	Abdominal pain and cramping, constipation, diarrhea, upset stomach, nausea, vomiting, headache, anemia, cough, chest pain, difficulty breathing, general weakness, high blood pressure, infection, swollen hands, feet, ankles or lower legs.	Call your doctor right away if any of these side effects is severe or does not go away; if you develop signs of infection, such as a persistent sore throat or fever, night sweats, painful urination; or if you experience any other unusual symptoms.
Blood and urine tests needed every few months. Do not use if you have a history of kidney disease. Do not use while pregnant.	Diarrhea, nausea, vomiting, loss of taste, mild stomach pain, loss of appetite, mouth ulcers, fever, rash.	May take 3 months to take effect. Not used for ankylosing spondylitis. Increases need for vitamin B_6: Take 25 mg daily. Users must be under close medical supervision.
Increases susceptibility to infection. May cause cancer after long-term use. Do not use while pregnant.	Nausea, vomiting, loss of appetite and weight, temporary hair loss, temporary reduction of sperm count, fatigue, dizziness, confusion.	May help those not helped by other drugs. Drink fluids to prevent bladder inflammation and bleeding. Call doctor immediately in case of fatigue, dizziness, or confusion.
May cause kidney damage and high blood pressure. Increases susceptibility to infection. Avoid alcohol. Available in two forms (original and modified); be sure your pharmacist gives you exactly what is prescribed.	Headache, tremors, unusual hair growth on body and face, diarrhea, gas, swollen or bleeding gums, sensitivity to sunlight.	May be combined with methotrexate. Call doctor if you develop flu-like symptoms, sore throat, difficulty or pain when urinating, skin abnormalities, long-term fatigue or weakness, night sweats, swollen glands, or stomach pain or fullness.
May cause visual disturbances.Users need to have eye exams twice a year.	Side effects are uncommon but may include diarrhea, loss of appetite, headache, stomach pain, itching, dizziness.	May take up to 6 months to be effective. Least potent but best tolerated among the traditional DMARDs. Often used in combination with methotrexate.
May increase susceptibility to infection or cause lung inflammation. Avoid alcohol. Do not take while pregnant. Blood tests required every 4–8 weeks.	Gastrointestinal bleeding, loss of appetite, nausea, vomiting, mouth ulcers, skin sensitivity to sunlight, acne, boils, skin rash.	Takes effect in 1–2 months. About 50% of users show significant improvement. Folic acid may reduce the risk of toxic effects.
To reduce diarrhea, eat a high-fiber diet. Periodic blood and urine tests required. Avoid alcohol.	Skin rash, mouth sores, diarrhea (more common with pills), kidney damage, loss of appetite, nausea, vomiting, indigestion, constipation, itching, transient joint pain shortly after injections.	Usually takes effect in 3–6 months. Effective in 60% of cases. Rarely prescribed because of side effects.

continued on the next page

Commonly Used Disease-Modifying and Other Antirheumatic Drugs 2008 (continued)

Drug type: Brand (generic)	Average daily dosage*	How to take
Biologic response modifiers (BRMs)		
Enbrel (etanercept)	25 mg 2x/week or 50 mg 1x/week	Self-injected under the skin, rotating site of injection each time. Store in refrigerator.
Humira (adalimumab)	40 mg every other week	Self-injected under the skin, rotating site of injection each time. Store in refrigerator.
Kineret (anakinra)	100 mg/day	Self-injected under the skin, at about the same time every day. Apply cold pack to minimize side effects. Store in refrigerator.
Orencia (abatacept)	500–1,000 mg per infusion, depending on body weight	30-minute infusion at 2 and 4 weeks after first infusion and every 4 weeks thereafter.
Remicade (infliximab)	3 mg/kg every 8 weeks once dose is stabilized (see Comments)	2-hour intravenous infusion (used in combination with methotrexate).
Rituxan (rituximab)	Two 1,000-mg infusions 2 weeks apart	Intravenous infusion. Glucocorticoids recommended 30 minutes before each infusion to minimize risk of potentially dangerous infusion reactions.
Corticosteroids		
Prednisone, Intensol, Sterapred (prednisone)	5–200 mg/day	First thing in the morning, with food to avoid upset stomach.

* Dosages represent an average range for the treatment of rheumatoid arthritis. The precise effective dosage varies from person to person and depends on many factors. Do not make any change to your medication without consulting your doctor.

† COPD=chronic obstructive pulmonary disease; RA=rheumatoid arthritis.

For information on nonsteroidal anti-inflammatory drugs (NSAIDs) used to alleviate symptoms of rheumatoid diseases, see the chart on pages 20–23.

Precautions	Most common side effects	Comments
Watch for signs of (rare) nerve damage: confusion, numbness, changes in vision, and difficulty walking. Also report fever, bruising, bleeding easily, paleness, shortness of breath, or rash. Stop using Enbrel immediately if you develop a serious infection. In those with RA, may increase risk of lymphoma.	Mild irritation (pain, swelling, or itching) at the injection site that usually decreases after a few weeks of use, headache, allergic reactions, sinus infections.	Takes effect in 2 weeks to 3 months. About 60% of users have a 20% reduction in symptoms. Contact doctor immediately if you develop high fever, chills, skin rash, sinus pain, difficulty or pain while urinating.
Rare side effects include serious infections, lymphoma, lupus-like symptoms, and allergic reactions. Do not take if you have multiple sclerosis or heart failure.	Mild irritation at injection site, rash, sinus infections, headache, nausea.	Used alone or combined with other DMARDs. About half of users have 50% reduction in symptoms. Contact doctor if you notice abnormal bleeding, bruising.
Periodic blood tests required. Stop using Kineret immediately if you develop a serious infection.	Mild irritation (swelling, bruising, itching, or stinging) at the injection site in 80% of users (usually decreases in 1–2 months).	For people who don't benefit from or can't tolerate other DMARDs. Takes about one month to be effective. About 40% of users have about a 20% reduction in symptoms.
May be associated with serious infection and allergic reactions. People taking Orencia should not take live vaccines. High risk of respiratory side effects in users who have COPD.† In rare cases, associated with certain kinds of cancer.	Infusion reactions (headache, dizziness, rise in blood pressure), cold-like symptoms, and nausea.	Prescribed after other BRMs have failed. About half of users have about a 50% reduction in symptoms.
May be associated with serious, even fatal infections. Very risky for people with heart failure. Tuberculosis test required before first infusion. Watch for signs of (rare) nerve damage: confusion, numbness, changes in vision, and difficulty walking.	Headache, indigestion, muscle aches, fever, rash, flu-like symptoms. Initial reactions to infusion (hives, blood pressure changes, chest pain, breathing problems) tend to diminish with time.	Given in combination with methotrexate, at 2 and 6 weeks after first dose and every 8 weeks thereafter. About half of users have at least a 20% reduction in symptoms.
Serious, sometimes fatal, infusion reactions include headache, nausea, chest pain, breathing and cardiovascular problems, hives, flu-like symptoms. Do not take live vaccines while using. Regular blood tests required.	Infections, stomach irritation, rash. About one third of users have a reaction to the first infusion (see Precautions); about 13% react adversely to the second infusion.	Originally used in cancer treatment. Given along with Rheumatrex to people who do not respond to other DMARDs. About half of users have a 20% reduction in symptoms.
Do not use if you have muscle or nerve disease, wide-angle glaucoma, ulcers, hypertension, heart failure, serious infection, diabetes, or high cholesterol. May cause osteoporosis. Long-term use may harm the adrenal glands.	Increased appetite, nervousness, sleep problems, stomach upset, weight gain, infection.	Often used in combination with other drugs. Can produce rapid, dramatic improvement but should be used only for severe joint flares or serious nonjoint complications of RA. Long-term use must be ended slowly to avoid a flare.

Exercise

When your joints are not inflamed, you should engage in moderate aerobic exercise to increase your endurance and keep your joints flexible. Even vigorous activity is fine if you feel up to it and if you do not already have significant damage in your large joints. After vigorous exercise, however, you may need to take additional medications, such as aspirin, to control pain and inflammation.

A gentler alternative for people with rheumatoid arthritis is water exercise in a heated pool. Exercising in water reduces stress on your weight-bearing joints, and the water's heat relaxes your muscles.

When your joints are inflamed, only gentle exercises such as bending and straightening the joint are appropriate. For example, gentle stretching exercises such as opening and closing your hand can help to maintain mobility in your hands. As joint inflammation subsides, you can gradually begin resistance exercises, which may involve light weights or working against your own body weight. (Avoid any exercise that causes increased pain an hour later.)

Braces, Splints, and Assistive Devices

Braces and splints help to relieve pain and stabilize and protect joints during periods of inflammation. At these times, your joints (especially those in the hands and wrists) are more prone to injury. Even when your arthritis isn't acting up, you will probably want to use assistive devices, such as faucet turners, jar openers, and easy-grip kitchen tools, to make everyday tasks easier. You may also need a cane or crutches to make walking easier.

Occupational therapists are experts in fitting braces and splints, recommending assistive devices, and instructing people on their proper use. Braces and splints are available over the counter or can be custom-made (the best choice for people with rheumatoid arthritis). Splints should be lightweight and easy to remove, allowing for range-of-motion exercises several times a day. They are most effective for the hands and wrists.

Prolonged or improper use of splints can increase stiffness and diminish muscle strength and joint mobility. For this reason, your doctor may instead recommend physical therapy or a corticosteroid injection into the painful joint.

Treating Depression

The pain and disability of rheumatoid arthritis can trigger depression. In fact, about 20% of people with the disease develop depression, compared with only 2–3% of men and 5–9% of women in the general population. That's why seeking help in coping with the emotional consequences of having rheumatoid arthritis is so important.

You may be reluctant to tell your doctor about an emotional problem, but it is just like any other arthritis symptom. In fact, depression may worsen your arthritis pain, and treating it can help relieve some rheumatoid arthritis symptoms. Treatment options include medication, psychotherapy, and exercise. Your rheumatologist will be able to recommend a psychotherapist or psychiatrist. Joining a support group can be helpful, too.

Research shows that becoming more educated about arthritis can help reduce or prevent depression. In a study of 202 older people with arthritis, those who attended a 10-week class about the symptoms, course, and treatment of arthritis had fewer symptoms of depression at the end of the class than those in the control group. The Arthritis Foundation offers a self-help education program for people with arthritis. Check with your local chapter for a schedule of courses in your area (see page 77 for contact information).

Surgery

If you take a combination of drugs for your rheumatoid arthritis but still have severe pain, poor range of motion, and joint damage that make activities of everyday life difficult, it may be time to consider surgery. Many of the procedures used to treat osteoarthritis also work for rheumatoid arthritis (see pages 25–31), such as total joint replacement and arthrodesis (joint fusion). Two additional options for people with rheumatoid arthritis are synovectomy and resection.

Studies show that people who have poorer functional ability before surgery usually take longer to regain functional independence after surgery. By not delaying surgery, you can increase your chances of a good recovery.

Synovectomy

This procedure involves removing the inflamed synovial membrane. It can be performed on the elbow, shoulder, hip, or knee. Depending on the size of the joint, synovectomy is performed through either a standard incision (open surgery) or several smaller incisions using special instruments (arthroscopy). Synovectomy reduces the joint stiffness and destruction of cartilage, ligaments, tendons, and bone caused by substances released from the diseased synovial cells.

Synovectomy is not as complicated as joint replacement, but it may not be permanent, because the synovial membrane can grow back. Medications such as DMARDs and NSAIDs are still required

ASK THE DOCTOR

Q. ***How long do hip and knee implants last?***

A. About 90–95% of hip implants last at least 10 years, and approximately 80–85% of knees last at least 20 years. Lab testing suggests that new implants could now last 20 to 25 years or longer. That's because older joint replacements made of plastic and polyethylene have now been replaced with those made of longer-lasting materials such as cross-linked polyethylene, a durable plastic; ceramic surfaces; or metal-to-metal ones that resemble ball bearings.

In the real world, how long a joint lasts depends on how much use it gets. Although implants allow a return to active sports such as golf, biking, and swimming, they're not designed for impact sports like jogging or tennis. The trade-off may be that joints wear out sooner.

If you do need a second implant, you will have what's called revision surgery. Sometimes people need new implants if the original plastic liner on the implant wears out, if the replacement loosens or breaks, or if they develop an infection. Not all revisions require a replacement of every implant part. A simple revision is the replacement of a worn liner with a new one. A complex revision might involve grafting more bone onto the joint or dealing with an infection. In the case of infection, the replacement joint would have to be removed, and you would need intravenous antibiotics for six to eight weeks before the replacement could be reinserted.

after the procedure to reduce the possibility of recurrent synovitis (inflammation of the synovium).

Resection

In this procedure, all or part of a bone is removed from a joint in the hand, wrist, elbow, toe, or ankle, largely to relieve pain. Recovery times vary but may be as long as several weeks.

Alternative and Complementary Treatments

People with rheumatoid arthritis often turn to therapies that are outside the medical mainstream, especially when conventional medications are not working or are causing troubling side effects. The problem is that few of these nontraditional treatments have been evaluated in well-designed studies. If you do try any alternative or complementary treatments, tell your doctor. Do not stop your regular therapies without your doctor's advice.

Which nontraditional therapies are safe to try? The positive and negative recommendations discussed in the section on osteoarthritis (see pages 31–36) also apply to rheumatoid arthritis, except that glucosamine, chondroitin, and acupuncture, which may be effective for osteoarthritis, are not effective for rheumatoid arthritis.

A few small studies suggest that gamma linolenic acid (GLA) and fish-oil supplements may be helpful for rheumatoid arthritis. GLA is found in borage oil, evening primrose oil, and black currant oil. The usual dosage is about 1,800 mg a day. The active ingredients in fish oil are omega-3 fatty acids; the usual daily dosage is 3 g a day.

Both GLA and fish oil may cause bleeding in people taking warfarin or NSAIDs. Evening primrose oil can lead to gastrointestinal symptoms such as indigestion, nausea, diarrhea, and abdominal pain. Fish oil can cause indigestion, bad breath, and nosebleeds; nausea and diarrhea may occur at high doses. Because these supplements are not regulated by the FDA, lack of standardization is a potential problem. The safest bet is to buy supplements that meet U.S. Pharmacopeia standards (look for the USP symbol) or to check on supplements at www.ConsumerLab.com. (An independent organization, ConsumerLab tests supplements for a fee paid by manufacturers and provides the results of its testing to subscribers.)

Treatments Not Recommended

Most of the alternative and complementary treatments that are discouraged for osteoarthritis (see pages 35–36) are not recommended for rheumatoid arthritis, either. In addition, the following therapies are sometimes touted for rheumatoid arthritis, but scientific research has not documented their effectiveness:

Prosorba column

This therapy involves removing inflammation-producing proteins from a person's blood by pumping the liquid plasma part of blood through a plastic cylinder containing protein A. Protein A binds to the inflammation-causing antibodies. The procedure is similar to kidney dialysis, but no studies have yet indicated whether it has long-term effectiveness.

Glucosamine and chondroitin

These supplements have shown some promise in people with osteoarthritis. However, no evidence indicates that they are effective for rheumatoid arthritis.

Acupuncture

Inserting fine needles into specific places in the body appears to hold some promise as a treatment for osteoarthritis. However, studies on acupuncture for rheumatoid arthritis have been disappointing.

Homeopathy

In homeopathy, an agent such as bee venom is greatly diluted and then administered as a remedy—a questionable strategy, because the remedies are so dilute that they contain almost none of the "active" ingredients. A controlled trial testing 42 homeopathic remedies found that they were no more effective than a placebo for treating rheumatoid arthritis.

Treatments Under Development

Rheumatoid arthritis is the focus of intensive research, and new drugs and treatments are on the horizon.

Monoclonal antibodies

In 2006, the FDA approved the newest biologic DMARD, rituximab (Rituxan), for rheumatoid arthritis that has not responded to other medications. Rituxan is a monoclonal antibody. Antibodies are the proteins that the immune system uses to recognize its targets; monoclonal antibodies are highly specific, purified copies of a single antibody, designed to target only one type of cell involved in a particular disease. Because monoclonal antibodies are so specific, other types of cells remain unharmed. Moreover, the antibodies can be

ASK THE DOCTOR

Q. ***How do fish oil and other natural medicines compare with DMARDs for the treatment of RA?***

A. Fish oil, as well as flaxseed, soybeans, and walnuts, contains omega-3 fatty acids, natural anti-inflammatories that, like aspirin, boost the production of resolvins (fats that appear to inhibit the action of inflammatory cells). People with RA often have lower levels of omega-3 fatty acids than do people without the disease. You can add omega-3s to your diet by eating a serving of fatty fish like salmon twice a week or by taking a fish-oil supplement.

Other natural remedies sometimes touted for RA are antioxidants, the nutrients in fruits and vegetables that appear to limit damage by free radicals, the off-balance molecules that damage healthy cells. Free radicals are thought to worsen cartilage erosion in arthritis. Bromelain, an anti-inflammatory ingredient in pineapples; pomegranates; ginger; and tumeric also are considered anti-inflammatories.

Although it's important to eat a healthy diet full of fruits and vegetables and to take a multivitamin when you have RA, omega-3s, antioxidants, and spices can't control the amount of inflammation associated with RA and cannot take the place of disease-modifying antirheumatic drugs (DMARDs). DMARDs, such as methotrexate, are proven to reduce the symptoms of RA and to slow or even stop its progression. If you do decide to take a supplement of any kind while taking DMARDS or other medications for RA, speak to your doctor first.

manufactured in large quantities. Scientists are testing other monoclonal antibodies for rheumatoid arthritis.

Stem cell transplants

The strategy behind using stem cell transplants in rheumatoid arthritis is to replace the immune cells that attack the synovium with cells that do not, using either donor bone marrow or embryo tissue as a source of stem cells. Although there are few reports of attempts to use stem cells from embryos, there is evidence of success using stem cells taken from adults—and even from patients themselves.

In 2004, doctors published a case report of one woman whose rheumatoid arthritis went into remission after a transplant of blood marrow stem cells from her healthy sister. Researchers have proposed another approach—albeit a risky one—for patients who find no relief in any other treatment. This involves removing all immune cells from the patient's body, filtering out those that do not attack the synovium, and reinjecting just these cells. A clinical trial of this strategy for people with rheumatoid arthritis began in 2006 at Northwestern University in Chicago.

The same year, a research team from the same medical center reported success using this strategy to treat patients with lupus (see pages 68–69), an autoimmune disease similar to rheumatoid arthritis. The participants were severely ill individuals for whom no other treatment had been effective. Two of the 50 patients died during the operation, the team reported in the *Journal of the American Medical Association*, but 25 of the study participants went into complete remission for five years.

Gene therapy

The effort to cure diseases by inserting new genes into human cells fell into public and medical disfavor after a patient died during a gene therapy experiment in 1999. But the concept is showing new promise against rheumatoid arthritis. Animal studies are under way to find out whether inserting new genes into people with rheumatoid arthritis can prevent the effects of their disease without causing them harm. The hope is that such treatments will provide permanent relief.

In 2005, researchers at the University of Pittsburgh injected cells containing a new gene into the joints of rheumatoid arthritis patients shortly before they were due to have these joints removed. The injected cells contained a gene modified to create a substance that blocked tissue-damaging cytokines from binding to synovial cells. Microscopic tests after the joints were removed indicated that the cells were having the intended effect, and the patients showed no evidence of harm from the experiment.

Although much remains to be learned before gene therapy can become an accepted treatment, scientists are working hard to develop such a therapy for rheumatoid arthritis.

GOUT

Gout is an extremely painful rheumatic disease caused by deposits of uric acid in a joint or in the surrounding connective tissue. Uric acid is a waste product produced as the body breaks down purines, common substances found in meats, fish, and many other foods. Normally, uric acid dissolves in the blood, passes through the kidneys, and is eliminated in the urine. But overproduction of uric acid or its inefficient removal by the kidneys allows uric acid levels to build up, causing a condition called hyperuricemia. The excess uric acid then accumulates as needle-like crystals inside a joint.

The symptoms of a gout attack are impossible to ignore—sudden stabbing pain and swelling in one joint, which often begins in the middle of the night. The affected joint is warm, red, and very tender to the touch. An initial gout attack typically involves a joint in the foot, especially at the base of the big toe. Other common sites of gout attacks are the ankle, instep, heel, knee, wrist, finger, or elbow. A gout attack may be triggered by alcohol, certain medications (aspirin, some diuretics, niacin, immunosuppressants, levodopa), an illness, or a stressful event.

Gout is believed to have a genetic component, as nearly one in five individuals who develop gout has a family history of the disease. Other risk factors are gender (men outnumber women by nine to one); age (it is more common in adults than in children); being overweight; excessive consumption of alcohol; the presence of kidney disease, high blood pressure, high cholesterol, or diabetes; and exposure to lead. A high consumption of purine-rich foods also increases the risk of having a gout attack. Purine-rich foods include certain meats and fish, poultry, liver, dried beans, asparagus, mushrooms, cauliflower, peas, and spinach.

An acute attack of gout typically is treated with high doses of NSAIDs or with corticosteroids (oral or injected). If these medications do not relieve the symptoms, an older drug named colchicine

NEW RESEARCH

Coffee May Lower the Risk of Gout

Worried about gout? Feel free to order another cup of joe. Canadian researchers sorting through data on more than 14,000 men and women from the six-year Third National Health and Nutrition Examination Survey found that people who drank four or more cups of coffee a day lowered their risk of gout by 40–60%.The participants, who filled out questionnaires about their diets over the previous month, ranged in age from 40 to 75 and had no history of gout.

Coffee—and, to a lesser extent, decaffeinated coffee—significantly lowered the amount of uric acid in the blood. The build up of uric acid causes gout. However tea and other caffeinated beverages had little effect, leading researchers to conclude that elements other than caffeine in coffee, like an antioxidant called chlorogenic acid, caused the uric acid levels to drop.

Researchers aren't suggesting that you drink four cups of coffee a day to ward off gout. But if you have the condition or are at risk for it, go ahead and enjoy your morning brew.

ARTHRITIS & RHEUMATISM
Volume 57, page 816
June 15, 2007

New Guidelines Question Existence of Chronic Lyme Disease

Extended antibiotic treatments don't help

Some physicians believe that people with Lyme disease (see pages 72–73) can develop a chronic illness that is relieved by long-term use of antibiotics. But new guidelines for the treatment of Lyme disease, issued by the Infectious Disease Society of America (IDSA) in November 2006, have raised a stir by questioning this assertion.

The IDSA guidelines, which are in their first revision since 2000, say that 95% of people with Lyme disease are cured by a 14- to 28-day course of oral antibiotics and that no credible scientific evidence suggests that the infection itself continues past the recommended initial treatment.

Although the guidelines state that physicians should use their own judgment in treating people who appear to have chronic Lyme disease, some specialists note that asserting their judgment in the face of the new guidelines is difficult because of possible repercussions from both state medical boards and insurance companies. In fact, doctors in New Jersey, Michigan, Nevada, and elsewhere have either had their medical licenses revoked or are being investigated by their state medical boards for treating post-Lyme disease symptoms with long-term doses of antibiotics.

A Challenging Diagnosis

There is no question that Lyme disease, the most common infection caused by tick-borne bacteria (it affected more than 25,000 Americans in 2005), can result in arthritis and other conditions if left untreated. And it is sometimes challenging to diagnose and deal with.

Caused by the bacterium *Borrelia burgdorferi,* the infection's symptoms can be confused with those of other diseases such as fibromyalgia, Parkinson's disease, Lou Gehrig's disease, or multiple sclerosis. The most common and only definitive symptom is a circular "bull's-eye" rash that appears seven to 14 days after a tick bite. Other symptoms range from flu-like joint and muscle pain, fatigue, fever, and swollen lymph nodes to arthritis, neurological problems (memory lapses, facial paralysis, inflammation of the lining of the brain, or meningitis), or heart problems such as abnormal rhythm or slowed heart rate.

Further complicating diagnosis is the fact that the same tick that transmits Lyme disease may also carry other bacteria, including the ones that cause human granulocytic anaplasmosis (HGA), an infectious disease that also causes flu-like symptoms, and babesiosis, a sometimes fatal illness. Both of these can be identified by blood tests. Among people who develop Lyme disease but who do not get prompt treatment with antibiotics, 60% develop arthritis (usually affecting the knees), 10% develop facial nerve palsy or facial paralysis, and 5% experience heart-related complications. Although blood tests can verify the presence of antibodies to *Borrelia burgdorferi* after weeks or months of infection, early results are unreliable.

Chronic Lyme Disease vs. Post-Lyme Disease

The issue in contention, however, is not the initial diagnosis; it is the ISDA's assertion (which many mainstream physicians endorse) that "chronic Lyme disease syndrome" is a misnomer. A more accurate label, it says, is "post-Lyme disease syndrome." The largest trial to study the syndrome described it as including any of a number of symptoms—

may be prescribed. Colchicine, which has a number of unpleasant side effects, is more effective if given within 12 hours of the onset of the attack. Someone who has repeated gout attacks will probably be placed on a preventive medication, such as allopurinol (Lopurin, Zyloprim), probenecid (Probalan), or febuxostat. Losing weight if overweight, exercising, drinking plenty of fluids, and avoiding high-purine foods also will help prevent future attacks.

muscular pain, pain radiating down an arm or leg, tingling, numbness, or cognitive difficulties—that appear within six months of initial infection and persist for at least six months.

In a step-by-step review of more than 400 studies, the new guidelines lay out what might explain the difficulties that persist past initial treatment in a minority of patients. Some symptoms may be due to inflammation unrelated to the Lyme disease infection, the guidelines say, or inflammation that does result from Lyme disease infection may simply be slow to improve. But the guidelines are quick to add that at least three randomized trials and one retrospective study indicate that extended antibiotic treatments don't help.

Ongoing difficulties may also be due to a simultaneous tick-borne infection such as babesiosis or HGA. And the aches and pains that trouble people after Lyme disease may be nothing unusual: Studies show that 20–30% of the general population experiences chronic fatigue, and 11% of people report chronic pain accompanied by depression, anxiety, and fatigue. About one in five adults is diagnosed with arthritis, and 2% have fibromyalgia, another condition that affects some patients infected with the Lyme bacterium. Unfortunately, no reliable study has been done to compare these figures with the numbers of people who appear to have post-Lyme disease syndrome.

Physicians opposed to the guidelines, however, note that the assertions run counter to the patterns of post-Lyme disease illness they see in their patients and have been relieving with long-term doses of antibiotics. Some also feel the trials cited in the guidelines did not last long enough to establish reliably whether or not the antibiotics were helpful.

If You Suspect Lyme Disease

The best course of action is preventive. Before going into tick-infested areas like the woods, put on protective clothing and tick repellant, and check your body for ticks afterward. If a tick has bitten you, remove it and let a doctor know about the bite within 72 hours.

For now, the best route to avert post-Lyme disease syndrome is early (but limited) antibiotic treatment. If you are in an area where Lyme disease is prevalent or if the tick is recognized as one that carries the Lyme disease bacterium, the doctor will likely offer a single dose of the antibiotic doxycycline and watch you closely for a month. If you develop either a bull's-eye rash or a flu-like illness within a month of being bitten, let your doctor know. If you do have Lyme disease, your doctor will prescribe a 14- to 28-day course of antibiotics, depending on the antibiotic.

If your symptoms are slow to improve, see a rheumatologist, who may then recommend a second four-week course of antibiotics. Some patients with post-Lyme disease syndrome do improve with continued use of antibiotics. But that may have to do with the anti-inflammatory effects of the drugs, not their antibacterial properties. The guidelines and most mainstream physicians agree that using antibiotics long term can be harmful. Overuse of antibiotics can make some bacteria more resistant to drugs and can lead to longer-lasting (or even fatal) illnesses and the need for more toxic drugs.

If you continue to have arthritis-like symptoms well beyond an episode of Lyme disease, seek the advice of an infectious disease specialist or rheumatologist in your area. ■

BURSITIS

Bursitis is an inflammation or irritation of a bursa, one of the small, fluid-filled sacs found between bones, muscles, tendons, and skin near joints. These sacs cushion and lubricate the tissues and allow them to glide across one another. The irritation that causes bursitis can arise during overuse or repetitive stress on a joint caused by, for example, painting a house, gardening, or playing tennis. Bursitis also may develop after an injury to an area, prolonged pressure on the tissue (as when kneeling for an extended time), improper body mechanics, or general lack of conditioning. In some instances, an infection in the bursa causes bursitis.

The pain from an inflamed or irritated bursa may seem to be coming from the joint itself, a misperception that sometimes leads people to believe they have arthritis in that joint. Bursitis-related pain can be dull and aching or sharp and intense. It increases with movement and may be especially bothersome at night. Sometimes the area around the joint is swollen, and the surrounding skin may be red and warm to the touch.

Bursitis usually responds well to rest, NSAIDs, and application of ice or cold gel packs during the first 48 hours and heat in the days after. A doctor should be consulted if symptoms persist beyond a week to 10 days or if the pain is accompanied by fever and chills. Use of a splint, brace, or sling to immobilize the area will allow the tissue to rest and heal. If pain and inflammation continue for several weeks, it may be necessary to inject a corticosteroid into the joint.

Prevention of bursitis involves stretching and strengthening the muscles in the area and improving overall conditioning. People who have bad posture and improper body mechanics (which place undue stress on joints) may need physical therapy to correct body alignment. Knee and elbow pads or other cushioning materials will help prevent bursitis related to pressure on certain tissues. It's also important to take frequent breaks when performing repetitive tasks, such as vacuuming or raking leaves, and to stop the activity if pain occurs.

LUPUS

Systemic lupus erythematosus (SLE), or lupus, is an autoimmune disease, in which the immune system mistakenly attacks the body's own organs and tissues. The sites most often affected are the joints, skin, kidneys, heart, lungs, blood vessels, and brain.

What causes the disease is not clear, but researchers suspect that it arises through the interplay of genetic, environmental, and, possibly, hormonal factors. Lupus is much more common in women than in men, and its onset typically occurs between the ages of 15 and 45.

Lupus can be difficult to diagnose because of its varied symptoms, the different body systems that can be affected, and its proclivity to flare and subside. The most common symptoms are painful or swollen joints, muscle pain, fever, and rashes (typically on the face, especially the so-called butterfly rash across the nose and cheeks). Other possible symptoms include hair loss, chest pain when taking a deep breath, sun sensitivity, fingers that turn pale or purple when exposed to cold or stress, and mouth ulcers. Lupus may affect only one body system, such as the joints and skin, or it can have system-wide effects such as anemia and extreme fatigue. Arriving at a firm diagnosis may take months or even years. It requires not only a physical exam and a detailed medical history, but also an array of laboratory tests to rule out other diseases that cause similar symptoms.

Lupus has no cure. Treatment is aimed at preventing flares and minimizing organ damage. Corticosteroid medications such as prednisone are a mainstay of lupus treatment. NSAIDs and antimalaria medications also are important in easing inflammation, joint pain, fever, skin rashes, and fatigue. Some patients will require immunosuppressant medications or DMARDs such as azathioprine (Imuran) or cyclophosphamide (Cytoxan, Neosar).

Because of the challenges involved in diagnosing and treating lupus, it is important to seek treatment from a physician who has experience in managing the disease. Lupus treatment is a partnership between the physician and the patient, who plays an important role in recognizing and heading off flares. If you are a fully informed patient dedicated to maintaining your overall health, you will likely achieve a good quality of life, despite having lupus.

ANKYLOSING SPONDYLITIS

Ankylosing spondylitis (AS) is a form of inflammatory arthritis. It primarily affects the joints and ligaments in the spine and in the sacroiliac area (where the spine connects to the pelvis). The disease typically begins in early adulthood, usually before age 35, and is more common in males than in females.

Genetic susceptibility plays an important role in AS. Most people who have the disease carry the genetic marker HLA-B27. However, HLA-B27 is a common marker in the population as a whole, and only about 2% of people who have HLA-B27 will develop AS. Researchers believe that HLA-B27 provides a genetic susceptibility to AS and that an infection or environmental factor triggers the disease. In some individuals, AS develops after a gastrointestinal or urinary tract infection.

The severity of AS varies greatly from one person to another. The most prominent initial symptoms are low back pain and stiffness in the spine and hips. Some AS patients experience only intermittent back pain. For others, the pain and stiffness progress to other joints, such as those in the knees, feet, and shoulders. The disease may advance to other organs, causing complications such as inflammatory bowel disease, eye inflammation, and inflammation in the heart and lungs.

The most worrisome spinal complication is spinal fusion. This results when chronic inflammation damages the vertebrae, joints, and ligaments in the back. As the body attempts to repair the damage, new bone grows and may fuse the vertebrae. Spinal fusion renders the spine immobile (sometimes "frozen" in a stooped position) and can also stiffen the rib cage, restricting lung capacity and interfering with breathing.

Because back pain is so common in the general population, an AS diagnosis is easy to miss early in the course of the disease. The diagnostic workup includes a physical exam, a review of family history, blood tests, and imaging studies, such as x-rays, a computed tomography (CT) scan, or magnetic resonance imaging (MRI). NSAIDs are usually the first-line therapy. DMARDs and corticosteroids are of limited use. Tumor necrosis factor (TNF) blockers, such as adalimumab (Humira), etanercept (Enbrel), and infliximab (Remicade), have proved quite effective when NSAIDs fail.

Exercise and physical therapy play an important role in AS treatment. Daily exercise is essential to improve posture, spinal mobility, and chest expansion. Swimming is an excellent exercise for people who have AS, because it is non–weight bearing, provides a good aerobic workout, and helps improve lung function. Walking, weight training, yoga, and Pilates are other good activities. People with AS also should work with a physical therapist to strengthen the back and abdominal muscles. Physical therapy will help achieve and maintain ideal posture and appropriate sleep positions. These measures will help keep the body upright, and that can limit disability if spinal fusion occurs.

FIBROMYALGIA

Fibromyalgia is a syndrome characterized by widespread muscle pain, fatigue, and the presence of what are called "tender points"—18 specific sites on the body that are exceptionally sensitive to pressure.

Fibromyalgia is not a type of arthritis because it does not cause inflammation or damage the joints. But it is included under the broad umbrella of rheumatic disorders, health conditions that affect the joints or soft tissues and cause chronic pain. Fibromyalgia affects three to six million Americans, mostly women, and appears to be more common among people with rheumatoid arthritis and other rheumatic conditions.

In addition to chronic muscle pain, tenderness, and fatigue, fibromyalgia symptoms may include sleep problems, morning stiffness, headaches, cognitive and memory problems ("fibro fog"), irritable bowel syndrome, painful menstrual periods, restless legs syndrome, numbness or tingling in the extremities, and temperature sensitivity.

It's not clear what causes fibromyalgia. Heredity may play a role, perhaps through genetic differences in pain perception. Other possible triggers include abnormal pain processing through the brain and spinal cord, an injury, or a viral infection. Sleep disturbances may be both a symptom and a contributing factor in fibromyalgia.

Diagnosis of fibromyalgia can be difficult, sometimes involving a process of elimination, as testing rules out other conditions that share the same symptoms. No laboratory tests or imaging procedures are available, and some people see several physicians before they receive a correct diagnosis. If your doctor suspects fibromyalgia, he or she will use a set of criteria developed by the American College of Rheumatology to make the diagnosis. These criteria are:

- Widespread pain for at least three months
- Pain on both sides of the body, above and below the waist
- Pain in at least 11 of the 18 tender points.

The physician evaluates the tender points by applying pressure to each spot with one or two fingers or with a device called a dolorimeter.

The treatment of fibromyalgia involves managing the symptoms. Drugs typically used include antidepressants, pain relievers, sleep medications, muscle relaxants, antianxiety agents, antiseizure medications, and medications used to control headaches. Last spring, the FDA approved pregabalin (Lyrica) for the treatment of fibromyalgia. In clinical trials, Lyrica reduced pain better than placebo. This medication is also approved to treat neuropathic pain (pain from damaged nerves) in people with diabetes and pain in people who have had shingles (postherpetic neuralgia). It is also used to treat certain types of seizures.

Self-care is crucial to managing fibromyalgia. Restful sleep and

NEW RESEARCH

Neurontin: A New Option for Fibromyalgia?

Treatment options for the pain and fatigue of fibromyalgia are limited. But results from a 12-week study suggest that the epilepsy drug gabapentin (Neurontin) could offer some relief.

The researchers randomly assigned 150 individuals with fibromyalgia to take gabapentin (1,200–2,400 mg) for 12 weeks or placebo (inactive) pills. They found that compared with placebo, gabapentin significantly reduced pain and fatigue and improved the quality of sleep, as measured by several standardized tests. In fact, more than 50% of the gabapentin group reduced their pain severity score by at least 30% compared with only 31% of those taking placebo.

Currently, the FDA has not approved gabapentin for the treatment of fibromyalgia. However, pregabalin (Lyrica), a drug with a similar mechanism of action, was recently approved. If nothing else has helped alleviate your symptoms, ask your doctor about trying one of these medications.

ARTHRITIS & RHEUMATISM
Volume 56, page 1336
April 2007

regular exercise are especially important. Daily walks build endurance, reduce stress, and promote better sleep. Gentle stretching and strength training also are recommended. Deep breathing or meditation relieves stress and anxiety and may improve the quality of sleep. Scheduling regular rest periods during the day can combat fatigue (although napping may disrupt nighttime sleep). Cognitive-behavioral therapy allows some people with fibromyalgia to reframe beliefs about their illness and their responses to pain. Acupuncture may also be helpful in relieving pain, fatigue, and anxiety.

LYME DISEASE

Lyme disease arises in someone infected by the bacterium *Borrelia burgdorferi* after being bitten by either a deer tick or a black-legged tick that itself was infected by the bacterium. Ticks that carry the disease are tiny—about the size of a sesame seed or the head of a pin. Most cases of Lyme disease in the United States occur in the northeastern states, in northern areas of the Midwest, and in the northern Pacific Coast region (although the disease has been reported in other areas of the country).

In humans, the disease causes a range of symptoms, including a form of arthritis now referred to as Lyme arthritis. The first symptom of Lyme disease usually is a rash that appears between three days and a month after the tick bite. The rash begins with a small red bump at the site of the bite and then spreads outward. Sometimes the center of the rash fades, creating the so-called bull's-eye rash. Because tick bites often occur in areas of the body that aren't easy to see, the rash may be overlooked. In addition, some people have multiple red bumps instead of a rash. Other early symptoms may be mistaken for the flu: fever, chills, headaches, muscle aches, neck stiffness, and fatigue.

Lyme disease needs quick treatment with antibiotics. If the disease is left untreated, joint pain will develop in more than half of affected individuals. Some doctors believe that Lyme disease may persist for years, although a number of experts have begun to question this assertion (see "New Guidelines Question Existence of Chronic Lyme Disease" on pages 66–67). The infection may also spread to the nerves or heart. Nerve involvement can lead to Bell's palsy (a temporary paralysis on one side of the face), meningitis (inflammation of brain membranes), muscle weakness, and cognitive problems (such as memory loss or inability to concentrate).

Prevention of Lyme disease involves taking precautions when hiking or working in high grass or woods in areas of the country where Lyme disease is common. Ticks found within 48 hours usually will not have transmitted the infection.

You can significantly reduce your risk of contracting Lyme disease if you:

- Cover exposed skin (and tuck your pant legs into your socks)
- Use an insect repellent containing DEET
- Check your entire body (including your scalp) for ticks at the end of the day and remove them immediately with tweezers. ■

GLOSSARY

aerobic exercise—Sustained lower-intensity exercise that increases oxygen consumption and improves the functioning of the cardiovascular and respiratory systems.

anemia—A decreased number of red blood cells. This condition sometimes occurs in people with rheumatoid arthritis.

ankylosing spondylitis—A rheumatic disease that can cause arthritis of the spine and sacroiliac joints as well as inflammation of the eyes, lungs, and heart valves.

antimalarials—Drugs normally used to treat malaria but sometimes effective in the treatment of rheumatoid arthritis. The most commonly used antimalarial is hydroxychloroquine sulfate (Plaquenil).

arthrodesis—A procedure in which a surgeon fuses two bones together in a finger, wrist, ankle, or foot joint.

arthroplasty—Implantation of a mechanical joint to replace a diseased or damaged joint. Also called total joint replacement surgery.

arthroscope—A thin, lighted tube with a camera attached to one end that is used in arthroscopy.

arthroscopy—A surgical technique that uses a thin tube with a light and tiny video camera at one end to view the inside of a joint.

articular cartilage—The cartilage that covers the ends of the bones.

autoimmune disorder—A disorder, such as rheumatoid arthritis, that results when the body's tissues are attacked by its immune system.

biofeedback—A technique used to by a person to control certain body functions, such as blood pressure and heart rate, by monitoring one's own brain waves, muscle tension, etc.

bisphosphonate—A class of drugs used to maintain or improve bone density.

bone mineral density test—An x-ray procedure that uses very low doses of radiation to detect osteoporosis (bone thinning).

Bouchard's nodes—Knobby overgrowths of the middle joint of the fingers in people with osteoarthritis.

bursa—A small, fluid-filled sac between a tendon and a bone that protects muscles and tendons from coming into direct contact with bones.

bursitis—Inflammation of a bursa, especially in the shoulder, elbow, hip, knee, or foot.

cartilage—The connective tissue that covers the ends of bones and acts as the body's shock absorber by cushioning the bones from weight-bearing stress. Cartilage is composed mainly of water and a fibrous protein called collagen.

chondroitin—A compound found in human cartilage tissue believed to play an important role in the formation and maintenance of cartilage within joints and that may be involved in joint repair.

collagen—The major protein of connective tissue, cartilage, and bone.

connective tissue—A type of supporting tissue found throughout the body. The tissue helps to form membranes that hold internal organs in place.

coronary heart disease—A narrowing of the coronary arteries that results in inadequate blood flow to the heart.

corticosteroids—Potent drugs that are used to reduce the pain and inflammation associated with rheumatoid arthritis and other autoimmune disorders. Corticosteroid injections are sometimes used to relieve joint pain in people with osteoarthritis. Also called steroids.

creatinine—A component of blood protein; an increase can indicate kidney problems.

cyclooxygenase-2 (COX-2) inhibitors—Anti-inflammatory drugs that work by blocking the COX-2 enzyme (which plays a role in inflammation) but have no effect on the COX-1 enzyme (which helps protect the digestive tract).

cytokines—Proteins secreted by cells in the immune system that are involved in inflammation.

cytoprotective drugs—Medications that decrease the acid content of the stomach, reducing the risk of developing an ulcer when taking NSAIDs.

debridement—A procedure that involves smoothing roughened cartilage and bone.

disease-modifying antirheumatic drugs (DMARDs)—Anti-inflammatory drugs that not only help relieve the pain and inflammation of rheumatoid arthritis but also slow the progression of the disease. Once considered a treatment of last resort, they are now the first drugs prescribed.

disease-modifying osteoarthritis drugs (DMOADs)—A class of medications aimed at preventing joint damage in people with osteoarthritis by inhibiting the release of enzymes that break down cartilage. To date, no agent has been shown to have this effect in humans.

dolorimeter—A device a physician uses to evaluate tender points by using it to apply pressure to each spot.

electrolytes—Minerals that regulate body functions.

Felty syndrome—A rare complication of rheumatoid arthritis in which the spleen enlarges and the white blood cell count drops, leading to recurrent infections.

fibromyalgia syndrome—A rheumatic disorder characterized by body aches, pain, stiffness, sleep disturbances, and fatigue, as well as tenderness in specific sites on the body. It occurs predominantly in women.

flare-ups (or flares)—Periods of increased disease

activity in rheumatoid arthritis, characterized by worsening pain, stiffness, and inflammation.

flexion contracture—Loss of joint motion due to shortening of the surrounding tissues.

glucosamine—A compound found in human cartilage tissue believed to play an important role in the formation and maintenance of cartilage within joints and that may be involved in joint repair.

gout—A disease characterized by increased blood levels of uric acid, which produces pain and inflammation in the joints, particularly in the foot, ankle, or knee.

Heberden's nodes—Knobby overgrowths of the joint nearest the fingertips in people with osteoarthritis.

hemicallotasis—A procedure in which a bone is realigned by lengthening it on one side.

hemochromatosis—Excess iron in the body that can lead to secondary osteoarthritis.

hyaluronic acid—A lubricating substance in the synovial fluid of the joints.

hyperuricemia—The condition of having excess uric acid in the blood.

immunosuppressant—A medication that suppresses the body's immune response.

isometric exercise—Pushing or pulling against a fixed object.

joint aspiration—A procedure used to obtain a sample of synovial fluid from an affected joint to help determine if osteoarthritis is responsible for symptoms of pain and stiffness.

joint capsule—A sac-like envelope that encloses a joint and consists of an inner synovial membrane and an outer fibrous membrane.

joint space—The narrow open area between two bones that meet at a joint.

lavage—A procedure that involves flushing out the joint to remove debris such as loose pieces of bone and cartilage.

ligament—A band of fibrous tissue that connects two bones.

lupus—An inflammatory disease of connective tissue that causes skin rash, arthritis, and inflammation of different organs. It occurs primarily in women.

meniscal cartilage—Fibrous cartilage that acts as an additional shock absorber between the bones of the knee.

muscle—strong fibrous tissues that work in pairs, flexing and contracting, to produce movement in the joints.

neuropathy—nerve damage that may occur when an inflamed joint compresses a nerve, a possible systemic effect of rheumatoid arthritis.

nonsteroidal anti-inflammatory drugs (NSAIDs)—Medications that relieve joint pain and stiffness by reducing inflammation. Examples are aspirin and ibuprofen.

osteoarthritis (OA)—A type of arthritis characterized by pain and stiffness in the joints, such as those in the hands, hips, knees, spine, or feet, due to the breakdown of cartilage.

osteophyte—A bony outgrowth, also called a spur, that can result from friction between bones.

osteotomy—A procedure in which a wedge of bone in the knee, hip, or spine is cut away, and the remaining bones are realigned.

pannus—A thickening of the synovial membrane resulting from an overgrowth of synovial cells and an accumulation of white blood cells that occurs as rheumatoid arthritis progresses.

pericarditis—Inflammation of the blood vessels in the membrane surrounding the heart, sometimes caused by rheumatoid arthritis.

placebo—An inactive substance such as sugar or starch that may be used in a research study to compare its effects to those of active medications.

platelet—A component of blood that helps it clot.

pleurisy—Inflammation of the membrane lining the chest wall, which sometimes occurs with rheumatoid arthritis.

podagra—Severe pain in the big toe caused by gout.

primary osteoarthritis—The gradual breakdown of cartilage that occurs with age and is due to stress on a joint.

prosthesis—A device or apparatus used as a substitute for a missing part of the body or as an aid for a diseased part of the body.

purine—A substance that can be converted to uric acid in the body.

range-of-motion exercise—Moving a joint as far as possible in every direction without causing pain.

resection—A pain-relieving procedure in which all or part of a bone is removed from a joint in the hand, wrist, elbow, toe, or ankle.

resurfacing (bone relining)—A less invasive option than traditional bone replacement, this procedure involves removing damaged cartilage at bone ends in a joint and then capping the surface with metal. The joint capsule is sometimes lined with plastic as well.

rheumatoid arthritis—A chronic autoimmune disease characterized by pain, stiffness, inflammation, swelling, and, sometimes, destruction of joints.

rheumatoid nodules—Hard lumps of tissue under the skin, especially near the elbows.

rheumatologist—A physician who specializes in arthritis and other rheumatic diseases.

scleritis—Inflammation of the outer layer of the eye that sometimes occurs with rheumatoid arthritis.

secondary osteoarthritis—Osteoarthritis that results from conditions that cause damage to joint cartilage, such as a joint injury, chronic joint inflammation, overuse of a joint, or obesity.

sed rate (erythrocyte sedimentation rate)—A blood test that helps differentiate rheumatoid arthritis from osteoarthritis by measuring the speed at which clumped red blood cells fall to the bottom of a test tube. The rate is elevated in rheumatoid arthritis but normal in osteoarthritis.

Sjögren's syndrome—A disorder affecting the glands around the eyes and mouth, causing decreased production of tears and saliva, which sometimes occurs in people with rheumatoid arthritis.

spur—A bony growth that may form on joints affected by osteoarthritis.

synovectomy—A treatment for rheumatoid arthritis that involves the removal of the synovial membrane from a joint.

synovial fluid—A lubricating fluid secreted by the synovial membrane.

synovial membrane—Connective tissue that lines the cavity of a joint and produces synovial fluid.

synovitis—Inflammation of the synovial membrane.

tender point—A specific spot on the body that will elicit pain if touched in people with fibromyalgia.

tendon—A fibrous cord that connects muscles to bones.

tophi—Deposits of uric acid crystals in the skin or around joints.

tumor necrosis factor—A protein that plays a major role in the development of rheumatoid arthritis.

unicompartmental knee replacement—An alternative to a total knee replacement that involves replacing only the damaged section of the knee.

vasculitis—Inflammation of blood vessels throughout the body sometimes caused by rheumatoid arthritis.

viscosupplementation—A treatment option for people with osteoarthritis of the knee. It involves the injection of hyaluronic acid, a natural component of synovial fluid, directly into the knee joint.

white blood cells—Infection-fighting blood cells that cause inflammation.

HEALTH INFORMATION ORGANIZATIONS AND SUPPORT GROUPS

American Academy of Orthopaedic Surgeons
6300 N. River Rd.
Rosemont, IL 60018-4262
☎ 800-346-AAOS/847-823-7186
www.aaos.org
Professional organization concerned with skeletal deformities. Publishes information on orthopedic disorders; see their website or call for information.

Arthritis Foundation
P.O. Box 7669
Atlanta, GA 30357-0669
☎ 800-283-7800
www.arthritis.org
Provides information about causes, symptoms, diagnosis, and treatment of arthritis; offers support groups and supports arthritis research.

The Arthritis Society
393 University Ave., Ste. 1700
Toronto, Ontario
M5G 1E6 Canada
☎ 416-979-7228
www.arthritis.ca
Not-for-profit organization dedicated to finding the cause of (and ultimately the cure for) arthritis. Publishes informational pamphlets and videos.

Lupus Foundation of America
2000 L St. NW, Ste. 710
Washington, DC 20036
☎ 800-558-0121/202-349-1155
www.lupus.org
Nationwide charitable foundation that provides support groups, seeks funding for ongoing research, and helps locate doctors by area.

National Institute of Arthritis & Musculoskeletal & Skin Diseases Information Clearinghouse
National Institutes of Health
1 AMS Circle
Bethesda, MD 20892-3675
☎ 877-22-NIAMS/301-495-4484
www.niams.nih.gov
A branch of the NIH. Provides information about diseases of the bone, joint, muscle, and skin.

LEADING HOSPITALS
as Ranked by *U.S. News & World Report*

ORTHOPEDIC MEDICINE

1. **Hospital for Special Surgery**
New York, NY
☎ 212-606-1000
www.hss.edu

2. **Mayo Clinic**
Rochester, MN
☎ 507-284-2511/507-538-3270
www.mayoclinic.org

3. **Massachusetts General Hospital**
Boston, MA
☎ 617-726-2000
www.massgeneral.org

4. **Cleveland Clinic**
Cleveland, OH
☎ 800-223-2273/216-444-2200
www.clevelandclinic.org

5. **Johns Hopkins Hospital**
Baltimore, MD
☎ 410-502-4003/410-955-5464
www.hopkinsmedicine.org

6. **Duke University Medical Center**
Durham, NC
☎ 888-ASK-DUKE/919-416-3853
www.mc.duke.edu

7. **New York-Presbyterian University Hospital of Columbia and Cornell**
New York, NY
☎ 877-NYP-WELL
www.nyp.org

8. **Rush University Medical Center**
Chicago, IL
☎ 312-942-5000/888-352-RUSH
www.rush.edu

9. **University of California, Los Angeles, Medical Center**
Los Angeles, CA
☎ 310-825-9111/800-825-2631
www.healthcare.ucla.edu

10. **New York University Hospital for Joint Diseases**
New York, NY
☎ 212-263-7300
www.nyumedicalcenter.org

RHEUMATOLOGY

1. **Johns Hopkins Hospital**
Baltimore, MD
☎ 410-502-4003/410-955-5464
www.hopkinsmedicine.org

2. **Mayo Clinic**
Rochester, MN
☎ 507-284-2511/507-538-3270
www.mayoclinic.org

3. **Hospital for Special Surgery**
New York, NY
☎ 212-606-1000
www.hss.edu

4. **Cleveland Clinic**
Cleveland, OH
☎ 800-223-2273/216-444-2200
www.clevelandclinic.org

5. **University of California, Los Angeles, Medical Center**
Los Angeles, CA
☎ 310-825-9111/800-825-2631
www.healthcare.ucla.edu

6. **Brigham and Women's Hospital**
Boston, MA
☎ 617-732-5500
www.brighamandwomens.org

7. **Massachusetts General Hospital**
Boston, MA
☎ 617-726-2000
www.massgeneral.org

8. **University of Alabama Hospital at Birmingham**
Birmingham, AL
☎ 205-934-9999
www.health.uab.edu

9. **University of California, San Francisco, Medical Center**
San Francisco, CA
☎ 888-689-UCSF
www.ucsfhealth.org

10. **University of Pittsburgh Medical Center**
Pittsburgh, PA
☎ 800-533-UPMC
www.upmc.edu

INDEX

S

T

U

V

W

Y

Z

NOTES

NOTES

NOTES

NOTES

NOTES

NOTES

NOTES

NOTES

The information contained in this White Paper is not intended as a substitute for the advice of a physician. Readers who suspect they may have specific medical problems should consult a physician about any suggestions made.

Please address inquiries on bulk subscriptions and permission to reproduce selections from this White Paper to Medletter Associates, LLC, 6 Trowbridge Drive, Bethel, CT 06801.

The editors are interested in receiving your comments at whitepapers@johnshopkinshealthalerts.com or the above address but regret that they cannot answer letters of any sort personally.

ISBN 978-1-933087-57-3
1-933087-57-9

Printed in the United States of America

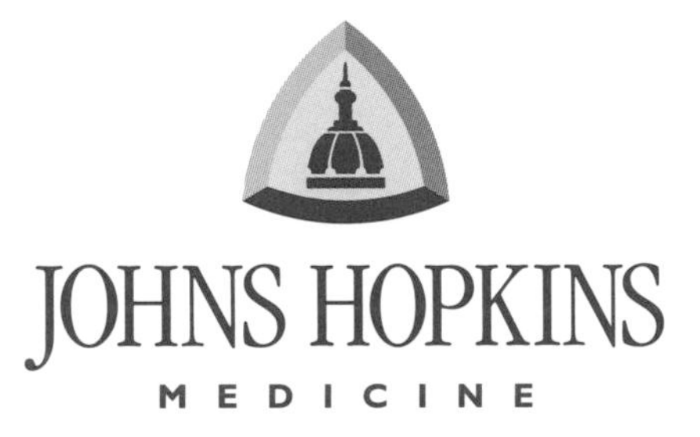

The Johns Hopkins White Papers are published yearly by Medletter Associates, LLC.

Visit our website for information on Johns Hopkins Health Publications, which include White Papers on specific disorders, home medical encyclopedias, consumer reference guides to drugs and medical tests, and our monthly newsletter *The Johns Hopkins Medical Letter: Health After 50*.
www.JohnsHopkinsHealthAlerts.com

BACK PAIN AND OSTEOPOROSIS

Lee H. Riley, III, M.D.,

and

Suzanne M. Jan de Beur, M.D.

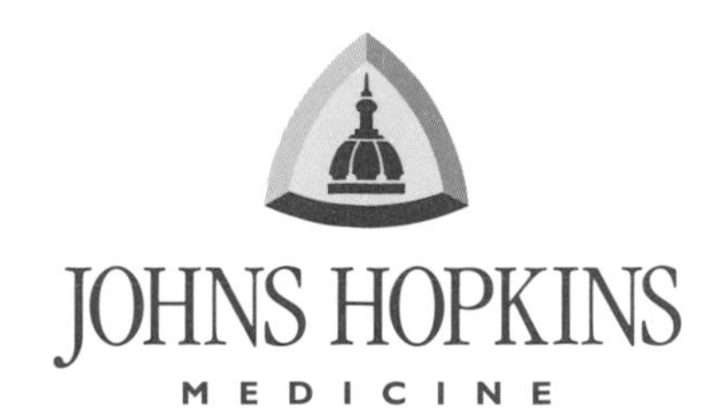

Dear Reader:

Welcome to the 2008 *Back Pain and Osteoporosis White Paper*—your Johns Hopkins guide to the prevention, diagnosis, and management of back pain and osteoporosis.

This year's highlights include:

- How to keep back and neck aches from **cramping your travel plans**. (page 10)
- How to ensure a **good night's sleep** when you have back pain. (page 18)
- Are fears of **addiction** overblown? Good advice if you take **opioids** for chronic back pain. (page 31)
- Who should have **surgery** to repair a **herniated disk**? (page 34)
- What's new in **artificial disks**, and are you a candidate? (page 40)
- The popular **diabetes drug** that may be **bad for bones**. (page 47)
- Why **depression** and **osteoporosis** may go hand in hand. (page 54)
- The dangers of **frailty**, and how to prevent them. (page 60)
- Is it ever okay to **stop taking your osteoporosis medicine**? (page 72)
- **Mending a cracked back**: New options to relieve pain and restore mobility after vertebral compression fracture. (page 76)

You'll also find a new "Ask the Doctor" column on pages 25, 37, 57, 59, and 63. This year's questions came from our patients, but next year we'd like to answer a few of yours. If you have any queries related to back pain or osteoporosis that you want answered in the White Papers or comments about the White Papers in general, please e-mail the editors at whitepapers@johnshopkinshealthalerts.com.

Wishing you the best of health in 2008,

Lee H. Riley, III, M.D.
Chief, Orthopedic Spine Division
Johns Hopkins Medicine

Suzanne M. Jan de Beur, M.D.
Director of Endocrinology
Johns Hopkins Bayview Medical Center

P. S. Please visit www.HopkinsBackPain.com for the latest news on back pain and osteoporosis and other information that will complement your Johns Hopkins White Paper.

THE AUTHORS

Lee H. Riley III, M.D., received his M.D. from the Johns Hopkins University School of Medicine. He completed his residency in orthopedic surgery at Johns Hopkins and was a fellow in spine surgery at the University of Miami. He is an Associate Professor of Orthopedic Surgery and Neurosurgery and Chief of the Orthopedic Spine Division at Johns Hopkins Medicine.

■ ■ ■

Suzanne M. Jan de Beur, M.D., received her M.D. from Weill Medical College of Cornell University in New York City. She completed her internal medicine residency at Johns Hopkins Hospital and was an endocrinology fellow at Hopkins. Currently, she is Director of Endocrinology at Johns Hopkins Bayview Medical Center and an Assistant Professor of Medicine at the Johns Hopkins University School of Medicine. She has special clinical expertise in metabolic bone disease and brings this clinical perspective to her laboratory research on molecular determinants of osteomalacia, disorders of phosphate homeostasis, and parathyroid hormone resistance syndromes. She has published extensively in leading journals, such as *The New England Journal of Medicine, The Lancet,* and the *Journal of Bone and Mineral Research.*

CONTENTS

BACK PAIN

Four out of five adults experience significant low back pain at some point in their lives. This figure is not surprising, given the amount of stress placed on the back throughout the day. It not only supports the weight of the body during standing, walking, and lifting, but also turns, twists, and bends. These movements are affected by the strength, flexibility, and alignment of many body parts. As a result, seemingly simple movements—how we habitually stand or sit, for instance—can adversely affect our backs, sometimes to the point of injury.

This White Paper describes the major causes of back pain in adults, including:

- Sprains, strains, and spasms
- Degenerative changes of the spinal bones and disks
- Herniated disks
- Vertebral compression fractures
- Spinal stenosis
- Spinal deformities.

Also discussed are sciatica and cauda equina syndrome, two conditions caused by spinal stenosis or disk herniation.

Anatomy of the Spine

The human spine is composed of 33 interlocking bones, called vertebrae, which stack upon each other at a slight angle to form the spine's S-shaped curve. This distinctive curvature helps the spine act as a shock absorber when we move while still supporting the body's weight. The vertebrae grow progressively larger and stronger from top to bottom. The seven delicate cervical (neck) vertebrae support the head; the larger 12 thoracic (chest) vertebrae bear the weight of the arms and trunk; and the five thickest and sturdiest lumbar (lower back) vertebrae carry the weight of the entire body. Because the lumbar region endures the greatest stress, it is the most vulnerable to strain or other problems. At the base of the spine are nine fused vertebrae that make up the sacrum (the back wall of the pelvis) and coccyx (tailbone).

Each vertebra consists of an oval body and seven bony projections, called processes, that jut out to the rear. Four of these processes meet with those from the adjacent vertebrae to form facet joints, which, with the aid of ligaments running down the length of the spine, connect the vertebrae to one another. The other three processes connect to some of the 140 overlapping back muscles that allow the back to move. Together, the vertebrae, ligaments, and muscles in the back and abdomen help to maintain erect posture.

Between each vertebra and the next is a flexible pad of cartilage-like tissue. This pad, which is called an intervertebral disk, cushions the vertebrae as the body moves and prevents them from grinding against each other. The high water content of the disks makes them very elastic—as we bend, twist, and move, they can expand, contract, and then return to their original shape. Thus, the disks, working in conjunction with the interlocking facet joints, give the spine its tremendous flexibility.

Yet another crucial function of the spine is to form a protective shell around the delicate spinal cord. At the rear of each vertebral body is a hole; when the vertebrae are stacked upon each other, these holes create a channel known as the spinal canal, through which the spinal cord runs. Spinal nerves, which branch off from the spinal cord through spaces (foramina) between adjacent vertebrae, extend to all parts of the body. The spinal cord ends at about waist level, dividing into a bundle of nerves that continues downward—the cauda equina (Latin for horse's tail, since its structure resembles the tail of a horse). Because of this intricate interweaving of bone and nerve tissue, problems with the vertebrae can cause symptoms from pressure on the spinal nerves or the spinal cord.

Causes of Back Pain

Most of the time, the exact cause of back pain is not easily determined. Fortunately, about 90% of cases improve on their own.

People under age 60 generally have acute backaches—that is, backaches that are sudden and short lived. These most often occur as pain limited to the back and result from a sprain or strain (it can be hard to distinguish between the two), a spasm, or, less frequently, a degenerated or herniated disk. In older people, chronic conditions such as degenerative changes of the spinal bones and disks, vertebral compression fractures, spinal stenosis (narrowing of the spinal column), and spinal deformities are the most common sources of back pain.

How Disks Herniate

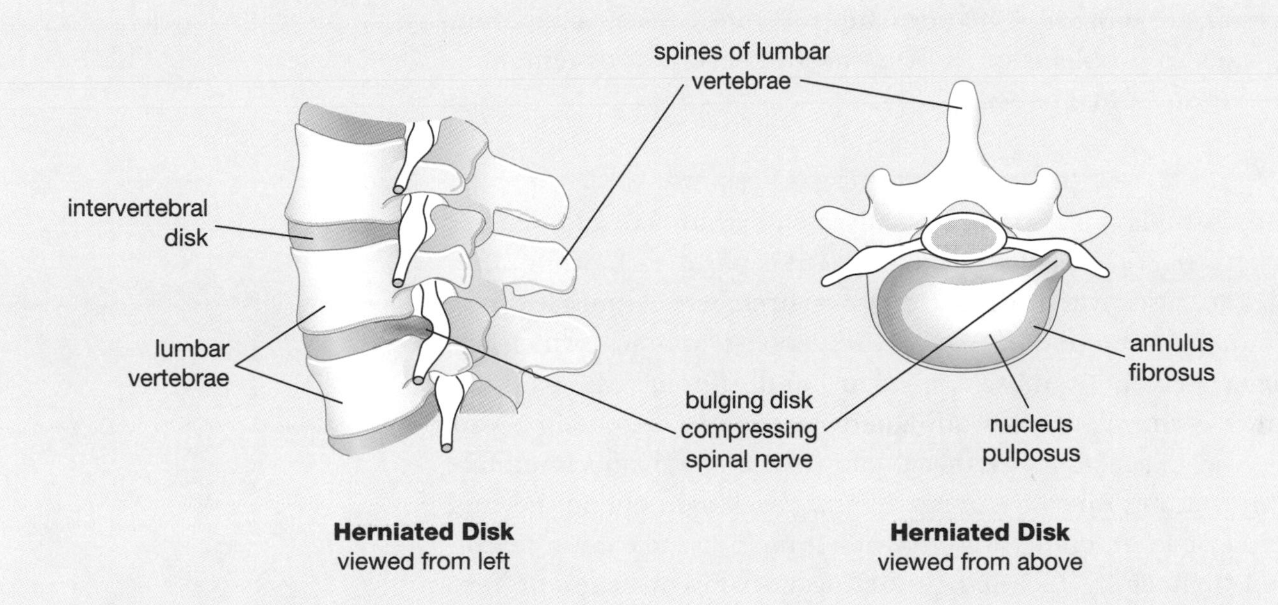

Herniated Disk
viewed from left

Herniated Disk
viewed from above

Each intervertebral disk is composed of two distinct regions: a tough, fibrous outer ring made up of many overlapping layers of collagen fibers (called the annulus fibrosus), and a soft, gel-like core (the nucleus pulposus). In a normal, healthy disk, these tissues contribute to the remarkable flexibility of the spine: As the body moves, the annular fibers expand and contract, while the gel-like nucleus changes shape.

Although each individual disk can only bend to a limited degree, their combined flexibility throughout the spine provides a great range of motion.

As we age, however, the disks gradually lose their resiliency. The annulus weakens, while the nucleus loses its water content, becoming progressively drier and more brittle. These changes make the disk more vulnerable to herniation—commonly known as a slipped disk.

Herniation may produce only local back pain, or pain may radiate down the path of a spinal nerve if the nerve is compressed by the protruding disk. There are varying degrees of herniation, ranging from mild to severe. ■

Other back-related disorders may cause symptoms that are not limited to back pain, however. For example, sciatica—pain that radiates into the buttocks, down the thighs to below the knees, and into the calves and often even the feet—is caused by irritation of a nerve leaving the spinal canal (the hollow channel through which the spinal cord runs) in the lumbar region of the back. Stiffness and loss of muscle strength may accompany back pain.

Although it may seem that back pain occurs suddenly (such as when bending down to pick up something), underlying problems—including normal aging, a weak back and weak abdominal muscles, obesity, and postural imbalances—set the stage for such "back attacks." The frequency of sprains and strains tends to decline after age 60, in part because older adults are less likely to participate in the kind of vigorous activities that lead to these problems. Also, the disks between the vertebrae become less pliable in older adults and, as a result, are more likely to herniate (protrude). Such rigidity, however, leads to problems of its own, mostly because of degeneration of the various spinal bones.

Sprains, Strains, and Spasms

Sprains, strains, and spasms usually result from activity or injury. The term *sprain* is used when a ligament is partly torn, while *strain* applies to cases when a muscle is overstretched. A muscle spasm refers to a contraction of muscles in response to injury, which may occur in a ligament, muscle, disk, or joint. Although the pain may be intense, muscle spasms ultimately protect you. The pain is your body's way of making sure that the injured area remains immobile, thus preventing further damage. Unlike back pain due to the compression of a nerve, the presence of a muscle spasm cannot be confirmed by imaging technology such as an x-ray or magnetic resonance imaging (MRI).

Degenerative Changes

Degenerative changes to the disks and facet joints in the lumbar spine, often referred to as degenerative osteoarthritis or spondylosis, are an inevitable consequence of aging. They usually begin around age 20, but imaging studies have detected changes within the disks of teenagers. Degenerative changes, along with vertebral compression fractures (see page 6) and kyphosis (see page 8), are responsible for the loss of height experienced by many people over age 50.

As we age, lumbar disks wear out because they are subjected to such large loads. Depending on what you do for a living and what types of activity you engage in during your leisure time, pressure on the lumbar spine can range from one to 11 times your body weight. Standing erect places a load on a lumbar disk equivalent to your body weight; bending, twisting, and lifting increase the load in proportion to the activity and the amount of weight lifted. Age-related loss of strength in the back muscles—which normally bear about one third of the load on the spine—also increases the stress on the disks and facet joints.

Over the years, the center of the disk slowly loses its water content and shrinks. This flattening of the disks leads to a narrowing of the space between the vertebrae. Further, as a result of supporting heavy loads, the vertebrae may develop bone spurs (osteophytes) that can press on a spinal nerve and cause pain. Another possible cause of pain is deterioration of the facet joints due to disk wear and vertebral changes.

In addition, arthritic changes (caused by a gradual erosion of the cartilage that lines the facet joints of the spine) can lead to pain and impair the smooth and coordinated movement of the spine. Pain also can occur if the nerves in the outer portion of the disks themselves are irritated.

Disk Herniation

About 10% of people experience symptoms from a herniated disk at some point in their lives. Autopsy studies reveal, however, that most people actually had a herniated disk during their lifetime but never experienced any symptoms.

Over the years, the demand of supporting the body's weight causes the outer layer of the disk to weaken, become thinner, and develop microscopic tears. At the same time, the center of the disk slowly loses its water content, so that it becomes progressively drier. These changes make the disk susceptible to herniation (protrusion), in which mild trauma such as lifting an object or even sneezing causes the center of the disk to bulge through the weakened outer layer (see "How Disks Herniate" on page 3).

Symptoms usually occur when the protruding disk presses on one or more of the spinal nerves emerging from the spinal column. In some individuals, the disk presses on the spinal cord itself or on the cauda equina. This causes pain not only in the back, but also in the part of the body served by the compressed and inflamed nerve. In some cases, disk fragments may break free, a condition referred to as sequestration. Although any disk can herniate, about 90–95% of cases occur in the two lowest disks because they bear the greatest weight.

When a disk herniates, the site and extent of the rupture determine the location and severity of the symptoms. For example, a herniated lumbar disk may cause pain, numbness, or weakness in one leg (sciatica), while a herniated cervical disk may produce similar symptoms in one arm or hand (less commonly, both sides can be affected). In general, a spasm of the back muscles plus difficulty walking or standing straight indicate a herniated disk; the spasm creates a recognizable leaning to one side in about half of those affected.

NEW RESEARCH

Steroid Injections on the Rise in Older People

Older people with back pain are receiving steroid injections for a growing number of conditions, despite limited evidence about how well the injections actually work and limited agreement on when they should be used.

A look at Medicare claims for steroid injections from 1994 through 2001 showed a 271% increase in injections into the lower back (epidural) and a 231% increase in injections into facet joints (small stabilizing joints located between and behind adjacent vertebrae). The majority of the injections were given to treat conditions for which there is little documented evidence of benefit. Women were 1.5 times more likely than men to receive an epidural steroid injection.

Expenditures associated with these injections have risen as well. The total inflation-adjusted reimbursed costs (professional fees only) for lumbosacral injections rose from $24 million to more than $175 million, and costs per injection doubled, rising from $115 to $227 per injection.

According to the researchers, at least part of the reason for the rise may be profit related. They note a 32% increase per year in steroid injections at ambulatory surgery centers, which are reimbursed at a higher rate than injections administered in a hospital or doctor's office.

SPINE
Volume 32, page 1754
July 2007

Pain due to a herniated disk usually strikes suddenly. The person may "feel something snap" before the pain begins—and the pain may start as a mild tingling or a "pins and needles" sensation before increasing in severity. If the herniated disk compresses the sciatic nerve, pain later radiates into a specific area of one leg. A decrease in back pain may be accompanied by increasingly severe pain, numbness, and weakness in one leg, along with changes in reflexes. In fact, a herniated lumbar disk is the most common cause of sciatica. If a ruptured disk compresses nerves in the neck, pain may radiate down the arms and be accompanied by weakness and numbness in the arms and hands.

Vertebral Compression Fractures

A healthy vertebra will not break unless it is subjected to a forceful injury, such as that occurring in a car accident. By contrast, even minor trauma—such as a sneeze—can cause a compression fracture of a vertebra that has been weakened by other conditions, such as:

- Osteoporosis (reduced bone mass), the most common cause of vertebral compression fractures. (Vertebral compression fractures related to osteoporosis are discussed in greater detail in the osteoporosis section; see page 51.)
- Paget's disease, which is most common in older individuals. It is characterized by excessive breakdown of bone and the formation of weaker, disordered bone, especially in the spine, pelvis, skull, and femur (thighbone). This unorganized bone is weak and prone to fracture, although the condition may produce no symptoms.
- Hyperparathyroidism, which can also cause bone problems. People with hyperparathyroidism have a benign tumor of the parathyroid gland that produces excessive amounts of parathyroid hormone, which weakens bones by stimulating osteoclasts, the cells that break down bones, and by promoting the loss of calcium from bone.
- Cancer. Vertebral compression fractures, although rarely a first sign of cancer, can occur in people with cancer that has spread to the spine. This spread occurs most often with breast cancer, prostate cancer, and multiple myeloma.

Spinal Stenosis

Spinal stenosis—a narrowing of the spinal canal—is usually caused by degenerative changes in the spine or may also develop as a complication of surgery, trauma to the spine, or involvement of the spine in Paget's disease. It typically affects people in their 50s and 60s and is about twice as common in men as in women.

As the body ages, gradual deterioration of the disks and facet joints in the spine causes the bones to rub together. This increased friction may eventually lead to the formation of overgrowths or bone spurs (called osteophytes) at the facet joints and around the rims of the vertebrae.

The two most common types of stenosis are:

Central spinal stenosis. This occurs when these overgrowths of bone gradually narrow the central canal of the spine; ligaments may thicken and cause narrowing of the spinal canal as well. Central narrowing leads to symptoms as the spinal cord or the cauda equina becomes compressed. Narrowing of the exit canals causes pain as the nerves branching off from the spinal cord become compressed or their blood supply is interrupted.

Lateral spinal stenosis. This condition, in which bone spurs narrow the bony canals that contain the nerves of the spinal cord, may develop alone or may accompany central stenosis. The characteristic symptom of nerve entrapment due to lateral stenosis is severe pain along the path of the affected nerve. Bed rest does not relieve the pain from lateral stenosis, and the person may pace the floor at night or keep changing positions while sitting.

Symptoms of spinal stenosis usually start slowly and are mild at first. Central stenosis can cause back pain, but usually the pain radiates into both legs. The pain does not follow the distribution of specific nerves but rather seems to involve the buttocks, thighs, calves, and, occasionally, the entire length of both legs.

The pain feels like cramping and may be associated with weakness, a "rubbery" feeling, numbness, and a sensation of loss of power in the legs. As a result of this weakness, people are prone to falls. Because the nerves controlling the bladder emerge from the lower spine, spinal stenosis may also cause urinary incontinence.

Intermittent Claudication

The pain of either type of spinal stenosis may be confused with that of another condition known as intermittent claudication. This condition produces a cramping pain in the buttocks, thighs, or calves caused by impaired blood flow to the legs due to atherosclerosis (hardening of the arteries). However, the two conditions can be distinguished from each other by the pattern of the pain. Pain due to intermittent claudication stops quickly when you rest, while pain due to spinal stenosis is related to body position and may continue for as long as you remain standing. Bending forward or sitting down usually relieves the pain, but even then the pain of spinal stenosis does not stop as quickly as pain resulting from insufficient blood flow. Another tip for telling the two conditions apart: Individuals with intermittent claudication find it easier to walk downhill, while walking uphill is easier for people with spinal stenosis.

Bed rest may increase spinal stenosis pain by exaggerating the natural curve of the lower back, which puts more pressure on the spinal cord. A person with spinal stenosis may feel more comfortable when sitting in a forward-leaning position, which flexes the lower spine and relieves some of the pressure on the nerves. Likewise, when people with spinal stenosis stand, they may be more comfortable leaning slightly forward. Many people with spinal stenosis find themselves leaning forward on a shopping cart while buying groceries. As spinal stenosis worsens, pain may occur while sitting, or it may wake the person at night.

Spinal Deformities

The three basic types of spinal deformities are kyphosis, lordosis, and scoliosis. These conditions usually develop during childhood or adolescence and worsen over time. However, these deformities may develop in older people solely as the result of degenerative changes that occur with age.

Kyphosis

This condition is characterized by extensive flexion (bending forward) of the spine. It usually affects the upper back (the thoracic spine) but may also occur in the neck or lower back. Thoracic kyphosis is sometimes referred to as dowager's hump, humpback, or hunchback. Kyphosis is particularly common in older women and can result from disk degeneration (in which the disks lose moisture and shrink), vertebral fractures due to osteoporosis, or both.

Severe thoracic kyphosis reduces the amount of space for the lungs and other organs, potentially leading to breathing problems or a protruding abdomen. It can also lead to difficulty finding clothes that fit properly.

Lordosis

In lordosis, or swayback, the abdomen is thrust too far forward and the buttocks too far to the rear. This condition is common in overweight people with weak abdominal muscles. Overly tight hip muscles can also contribute to lordosis.

Scoliosis

Defined as an abnormal sideways bend to the back, scoliosis is caused by a twisting of the spine. It can occur at any location in the spine. The amount of pain caused by scoliosis usually depends on the degree of the deformity; more pronounced bends tend to be more painful. Most scoliosis in our society is inherited and develops in childhood, but it may progress later in life because of disk degeneration. Scoliosis that arises during adulthood can be traced to asymmetrical changes in the disks. The scoliotic curve tends to be short and angular and is often associated with either kyphosis or spinal stenosis. Scoliosis occurring from degenerative changes alone tends to create fewer problems than childhood scoliosis.

Sciatica and Cauda Equina Syndrome

Sciatica, which affects 40% of adults during their lifetime, can occur when lateral spinal stenosis or a herniated disk irritates some part of either sciatic nerve. Each large sciatic nerve is formed by nerve roots that emerge from the lower spine, join together in the hip region, and run down the back of each thigh. Near the knee, the sciatic nerves branch into smaller nerves that extend into the calves, ankles, feet, and toes.

Sciatica results from irritation of one of the nerve roots in the lower back, most often those emanating from the fourth lumbar vertebra (L4), fifth lumbar vertebra (L5), or first sacral vertebra (S1). Pain or numbness develops along the path of the sciatic nerve; the precise location of symptoms depends on which spinal nerve root is affected. Compression of the sciatic nerves can also diminish leg strength.

After age 50, sciatica is more commonly caused by spinal stenosis than by disk herniation. About 90% of the time, sciatica caused by a herniated disk resolves within six weeks with little or no treatment. In up to half of all cases, sciatica from spinal stenosis resolves by itself within a month, but one in four people may have pain for as long as four months.

Compression of the cauda equina may result in the sudden onset of impaired bowel and bladder function (usually an inability to empty the bowel or bladder or, conversely, incontinence); loss of sensation in the groin, buttocks, and legs; and severe weakness or paralysis in the legs. These symptoms—known as cauda equina syndrome—indicate an emergency situation that requires immediate surgical attention. People who cannot reach their doctor quickly should go to the emergency room of a nearby hospital for treatment. Sciatica or cauda equina syndrome is usually due to one of the major disorders

NEW RESEARCH

Guidelines Recommend Limiting Steroid Injections for Sciatica

Epidural steroid injections do not provide long-term pain relief in people with sciatica and their use should be limited, according to new guidelines issued by the American Academy of Neurology.

After analyzing several high-quality scientific studies on the effectiveness of epidural steroid injections for sciatica, the guideline authors found that these injections did provide some—albeit limited—pain relief. However, that relief was apparent only from the second to the sixth week after the injection; there was neither immediate nor long-term relief. In addition, the injections failed to improve the ability to function and to reduce the need for surgery.

If your doctor recommends an epidural steroid injection for sciatica, it's important to understand that your respite from pain is likely to be short lived.

NEUROLOGY
Volume 68, page 723
March 6, 2007

Tips for Pain-Free Travel

Don't let back or neck pain cramp your travel plans

Traveling by car or plane can be a pain in the neck, literally, as well as a pain in the back. Sitting for prolonged periods adds strain to the structures of the lower back and neck, and poor posture while sitting puts even more stress on your spine. Regular travel with back or neck pain can be a challenge, but you can take measures to reduce or avoid pain and discomfort while on the road or in the air.

Traveling By Car

If you drive for extended periods you may be at risk for back and neck pain, sciatica, and herniated disks. However, you can make adjustments in the way you sit to limit spine and neck problems.

What's the optimal way to sit while driving? That question was answered in a study in the *Journal of Manipulative and Physiological Therapeutics*. After an exhaustive review of scientific journals and automotive engineering reports, here's what the authors recommend. The seat back should be almost straight up at a 100-degree angle from the floor. Your knees should be only slightly higher than your buttocks. Your head should tilt back very slightly (only 10%).

Current guidelines recommend that the elbows rest on the armrests as you grip the wheel with your hands in the 9 o'clock and the 3 o' clock positions (instead of at 10 o'clock and 2 o'clock positions) to avoid injuring the hands if the airbag deploys. The illustration below shows the recommended driving position for optimal back support.

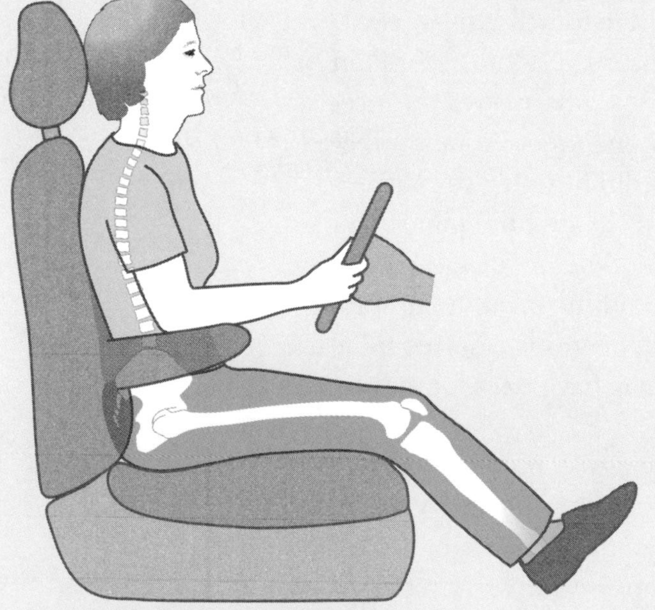

Proper Driving Position

Here are some additional tips:

- Make sure that your back is aligned against the back of your seat in an upright position and that your headrest is supporting the middle of your head.
- Use a lumbar support pillow to make your seat more comfortable and to support your lower back.
- Adjust the seat and steering wheel to a comfortable position to avoid reaching for the wheel.
- Consider using cruise control for long drives. Resting both feet on the floor provides more support for your lower back than if one foot is on the gas.
- Get out of the car and stretch every 20–30 minutes, if possible. See the inset box on the next page for suggestions.
- If back pain flares up while you're driving, apply a cold pack to the painful area. Wrap a small bag of ice in a towel and place it between your lower back and the seatback. Or if it feels better, alternate ice and heat from a disposable, portable heat pack every 15–20 minutes.

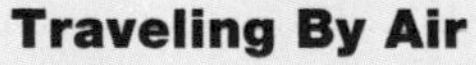

Traveling By Air

Air travel can be mentally taxing, but it can also take a toll on your body—especially your back. Lugging heavy bags, carrying young grandchildren, waiting for long periods in airports, and sitting in cramped conditions all may aggravate an existing back problem or create a new one. But by taking some precautions and performing simple stretching exercises, you can protect your back during air travel.

Here are some essential do's and don'ts.

• Don't carry heavy suitcases. Instead, pack lightly (it's better to use two smaller suitcases than one large one) and buy wheeled luggage or use rental baggage carts that are available in the terminal.

• Do check all heavy luggage. This way, you won't have to lift it into the overhead compartment on the plane.

• Don't twist or turn your head when you place a carry-on bag into the overhead compartment.

• Do place a pillow or rolled-up blanket behind your lower back and neck to maintain the natural S-shaped curve of the spine while sitting.

• Don't sit on a worn and hollowed seat. Put a folded blanket over the worn area for additional support.

• Do carry resealable plastic bags with you on the plane. If your back becomes sore during the trip, ask the flight attendant for ice. Put the ice in the plastic bag, wrap in a paper towel, and place it on your back.

• Don't sit in cramped quarters. When you book a flight, request an aisle or bulkhead seat so that you will have more room.

• Do take a muscle relaxant or an anti-inflammatory medication before and, if it's a long trip, during the flight.

• Don't sit still for an extended period. If you're on a long flight, get out of your seat. Walk up and down the aisle of the airplane and do some of the stretching exercises described in the inset box above. Moving about can help keep your joints loose and has the added benefit of reducing your risk of developing a blood clot. ■

Stretching Exercises

Experts who treat back pain recommend that you stretch regularly while you're in flight or when you take a driving break. Stretching can help relax tense muscles and overly tight ligaments in the back and neck.

Neck and shoulder stretches. A. To loosen your neck, rotate your head to the left and maintain this position for about five seconds. Turn your head forward again; then turn to the right and hold for five seconds. Repeat five times.

B. To loosen your shoulders and neck, shrug your shoulders up while holding your arms at your sides. Stay in this position for about five seconds, then return to a resting position. Repeat five times.

Back stretches. A. Begin in an upright seated position and gradually lower your torso toward your knees. Let your arms drop down and then wrap them around your thighs. Hold this position for about 20 seconds while breathing deeply, then return to your normal, seated position. Repeat five times.

B. While standing, put your hands on your lower back and slowly stretch backward from the waist. Hold for 10 seconds, then relax and straighten up. Repeat five times.

C. Place your hands on your hips and bend to the left. Maintain this position for five seconds. Return to an upright position, then bend to the right and hold for five seconds. Repeat five times.

Leg stretch. While sitting, keep the balls of your feet on the floor and raise your heels. Hold for 10 seconds. Lower your heels back down, and repeat 10 times. Although this is really a calf stretch exercise, you'll feel the stretch all the way up into your lower back.

of the spine, such as disk herniation, degenerative changes of the spinal disks, spinal stenosis, or vertebral compression fracture.

Additional Causes of Back Pain

Other medical conditions that affect the spine and can lead to back pain include ankylosing spondylitis, osteomalacia, spondylolysis, spondylolisthesis, and vertebral osteomyelitis.

Ankylosing spondylitis

This condition is a chronic inflammation of the facet joints and the joints between the back wall of the pelvis and the hip (the sacroiliac joints). Inflammation may also involve locations where ligaments and tendons attach to bone. In severe cases, the vertebrae may become fused together, resulting in rigidity. Because fusion can be painful, the person tends to lean forward and develop a stooped posture.

Osteomalacia

Bone is mostly made up of collagen but requires the minerals calcium and phosphorus for strength. Osteomalacia is a softening of bone that results from a lack of these minerals. The most common cause of osteomalacia is vitamin D deficiency, which is prevalent in older people. Vitamin D is essential for absorption of calcium and phosphorus. Fractures due to osteomalacia are more common in the pelvis and ribs but may also involve the spine.

Spondylolysis

Spondylolysis is a defect and weakness in a portion of the spine called the pars interarticularis, a small segment of bone joining the facet joints in the back of the spine. The condition is basically a stress fracture in the pars interarticularis and is either congenital (present at birth) or may be caused later in life by trauma.

Spondylolisthesis

Spondylolisthesis, in which one of the vertebrae slips forward onto an adjacent vertebra, causes a gradual deformity of the lower spine and narrowing of the vertebral canal. It may develop in people with spondylolysis (see above), can be congenital, or may develop later in life because of disk degeneration associated with abnormal facet joints.

Vertebral osteomyelitis

This disorder is a serious and increasingly common bacterial infection of the spine that causes pain in the neck or back and may or may not be accompanied by fever. It is often associated with autoimmune disorders such as type 1 diabetes (which is sometimes called juvenile or insulin-dependent diabetes).

Cancer

In rare instances, back pain is caused by cancer in the spine. Malignant tumors of the spine account for far less than 1% of all cases of back pain and occur more frequently in older people. Cancer can originate in the vertebrae, as in the case of multiple myeloma (cancer cells that move from the bone marrow to the bones at numerous sites). It can also spread to the spine from other sites in the body, most often from the breast, prostate, lung, kidney, or thyroid gland.

Other causes

Not all back pain is caused by problems with the spine or back muscles. In some cases, pain originates in the abdominal organs and radiates to the back. Conditions such as pancreatitis (inflammation of the pancreas), peptic ulcers (lesions in the stomach or small intestine), or an abdominal aortic aneurysm (a ballooning of the wall of the body's largest artery, which carries blood from the heart to the rest of the body) may also cause back pain.

In addition, back pain may originate from gallstones, kidney stones, kidney infections, and endometriosis (a growth of the tissue lining a woman's uterus in places other than the uterus). Last, but certainly not least, emotional stress may induce back pain.

Diagnosing Back Pain

After the common cold, back pain is the problem that most frequently brings people to a doctor's office. It is often difficult to pinpoint the exact cause of back pain because so many different body structures can be involved.

Fortunately, most episodes of back pain—about 90%—clear up with little or no treatment in about six weeks, reducing the need for medical intervention. As long as you're not experiencing severe back pain or other symptoms (such as severe nighttime pain or pain that worsens with lying down, weight loss, bowel or bladder dysfunction, or fever) that might indicate a health condition such as cancer, infection, cauda equina syndrome, or an abdominal aortic aneurysm, you can safely try self-treatment (see pages 24–25).

NEW RESEARCH

Surgery Is Superior for Common Back Problem

Surgery is the superior treatment for back pain due to degenerative lumbar spondylolisthesis with spinal stenosis—a condition that occurs when one vertebra in the spine slips forward onto another over time, producing pressure on the spinal cord and causing pain in the buttocks or legs while walking or standing.

Researchers followed 601 people who had experienced pain from this condition for at least three months and who underwent surgery to relieve pressure on the nerves or received nonsurgical treatments such as physical therapy, steroid injections, and pain medications. People in the surgery group reported quick relief of symptoms, some as early as six weeks after the procedure. After two years, people in the nonsurgical treatment group reported modest improvements. But those who had surgery reported they felt significantly less pain and could function much better.

Many people worry that they might get worse if they postpone surgery, but this was not the case. So if you have degenerative spondylolisthesis, it's not necessary to make an immediate decision on treatment. Based on these results, however, you'll feel substantially better faster if you schedule surgery sooner rather than later.

THE NEW ENGLAND JOURNAL OF MEDICINE
Volume 356, page 2257
May 31, 2007

Back pain due to muscle injury typically subsides completely in about six to eight weeks. Back pain that lasts longer than this is usually due to spinal column changes and merits a visit to a physician.

Signs and Symptoms

Only about 2% of back pain episodes require immediate medical treatment. However, to rule out the possibility of a dangerous condition, doctors still need to ask certain questions routinely—for example, whether you can relieve the pain by changing your position and whether you feel pain when you're not moving.

Back Pain History

Some of the best clues to the cause of your back pain will come from your description of the pain. Obtaining an accurate account is a doctor's primary method of tracking down the cause and determining whether and what type of treatment is necessary. Questions your doctor will ask include:

- Where is the pain located? Is it confined to the lower back or does it radiate to the buttocks or legs? (These questions check for sciatica.)
- How severe is the pain? For example, is the pain so excruciating that any movement is difficult or impossible? Can you go about your normal daily activities, even though the pain prevents vigorous exercise or activities associated with a lot of bending and twisting, such as gardening or golf? (A good description of pain intensity can help the doctor determine its cause.)
- When did the pain begin? Was it related to an activity or an injury? (If the pain follows an injury, it is less likely to be due to a slowly progressing condition, such as spinal stenosis.)
- What makes your back feel better or worse? For example, does lying down make it feel better? Does bending forward to tie a shoe increase the pain? (The pattern of pain may indicate whether a nerve is involved, possibly because of a disk herniation.)
- Have you had a prior episode of back pain? If so, how was it treated and how effective was the treatment? (The condition may have recurred.)
- Do you have any other health problems? (Weight loss and poor appetite, for example, raise the concern that cancer has spread to the vertebrae. In addition, some disorders, such as hyperthyroidism, can cause osteoporosis.)
- What medications do you take? (Certain drugs, such as corticosteroids or anticonvulsants, can affect spinal bone mass.)

• What do you do for a living, and what kinds of exercise or other activities do you do? In what ways is the pain disabling? (Muscle injury is frequently related to a particular activity.)

Physical Examination

During a physical exam, your doctor will typically focus on your back, legs, and feet. The doctor will look at your posture and curvature of the spine; a hands-on examination of areas that are sore may provide clues to the origin of the pain. To observe muscles and joints during movement, the doctor may ask you to sit, stand, walk (including on your toes or heels), twist, or bend forward or sideways.

A neurological exam, including tests of sensation, strength, and reflexes, will be conducted as well. These tests are important to detect disorders such as disk herniation and spinal stenosis, as the nerves emerging from each level of the spine are responsible for sensation and muscle strength in specific parts of the body.

For example, the nerve issuing from underneath the fifth lumbar vertebra (L5) is responsible for sensation in a narrow band that runs down the upper leg and wraps around to the front of the lower leg and the top of the foot. By detecting loss of sensation in a particular area or diminished strength in certain muscles, the doctor may be able to determine which level of the spine is causing the pain. Reduced reflexes at specific areas also can provide vital clues to the source of back pain.

Another important component of the physical examination is the straight-leg-raise test, which can help the doctor determine whether disk herniation may be responsible for the pain. During this exam, you lie on your back while the physician lifts each leg separately without bending the knee. The test is positive if raising the leg produces the typical symptoms—pain or tingling below the knee. The straight-leg-raise test is also helpful in monitoring the progress of treatment once a diagnosis has been made.

Last, a rectal examination may be done to assess the nerve function of the anus, because the nerves of the anus arise from the lower lumbar spine.

Laboratory Tests

Routine blood tests help determine the cause of back problems in a few situations. Results may reflect the presence of inflammation and/or an infection. For example:

• Blood levels of alkaline phosphatase (an enzyme released by bone-forming cells called osteoblasts) are often extremely high in people with active Paget's disease (which can cause vertebral compression fractures and spinal stenosis).

- Blood calcium levels are elevated in people with hyperparathyroidism (which, along with osteoporosis, can lead to vertebral compression fractures).
- PSA (prostate specific antigen), which is elevated in men with prostate cancer, can be measured by a blood test to determine whether back pain is due to the spread of prostate cancer.
- Abnormal proteins in blood and urine are often present in people with multiple myeloma (cancer of the plasma cells, a type of white blood cell).

Imaging Studies

Diagnostic imaging studies provide a view of the bones and the soft tissues, which comprise muscles, ligaments, cartilage, tendons, and blood vessels. These studies are usually done when surgery might be necessary.

X-rays

For chronic pain and for new-onset back pain lasting longer than four to six weeks, x-rays should be the first imaging study. They are especially useful for detecting fractures and invasion of bone by multiple myeloma. Although x-rays tend to be overused, they are useful for people over age 50, because this age group has a greater risk of malignancy and vertebral fractures. There is no need to be concerned about the health risks of modern x-rays; the radiation doses are low and there is no evidence of harm even from repeated exposure. Conventional x-rays are available almost anywhere and are relatively low in cost ($150–200, depending on where you live).

Computed tomography (CT) scans

During a CT scan, also called a computerized axial tomography (CAT) scan, a thin x-ray beam is rotated around a specific area of the body to create a cross-sectional picture. CT scans are 10–20 times more sensitive than x-rays; they provide better soft-tissue detail and good detail of the vertebrae. Although MRI scans or CT myelograms (see page 17) are even more useful for examining the soft tissues (for example, herniated disks), CT scans are still best for studying bone problems—for example, bone destruction due to infection. CT scans are considerably more expensive ($550 on average) and deliver more radiation than conventional x-rays.

CT myelogram

This procedure combines a CT scan and a myelogram (also known as myelography), a diagnostic tool that uses contrast dye that is injected into the fluid of the spinal canal. The contrast dye illuminates the spinal canal, cord, and nerve roots during imaging. A CT scan is taken after the dye is injected; the images produced clearly show both the bony structures of the spine and the nerve structures. The injection carries the risk of infection and side effects such as nausea, headaches, and pain or discomfort at the site of injection. People are required to sit or lie with their head elevated for six to eight hours afterward. These scans offer the best detail of bone and soft tissue. CT myelograms are usually performed only prior to surgery or after failed surgery. The average cost is $600.

Magnetic resonance imaging (MRI)

In MRI, the most sensitive imaging technique available, a person is surrounded with a powerful magnet. The magnet causes atomic nuclei in the body to vibrate and give out characteristic signals, which are then converted into two- and three-dimensional images. No x-rays are involved. This test provides the clearest images of soft tissues and is completely safe. Despite its precision, studies have shown that MRI should be reserved either for preoperative evaluation or for people with a suspected herniated disk whose back symptoms have not responded after four to six weeks of nonsurgical treatments. These scans cost on average about $1,000.

MRI may not generate a useful image of the bones in the spine. Therefore, it is not recommended for early diagnosis of back pain unless the doctor suspects a serious condition, such as cauda equina syndrome. Even when an MRI is warranted, some drawbacks must be considered.

First, the abnormalities revealed may not necessarily be the cause of the back pain. Second, because people must lie perfectly still for a long period (anywhere from 30 minutes to two hours) in a relatively small space, the procedure may be uncomfortable and difficult to tolerate, especially for people who are claustrophobic. (An open MRI produces less claustrophobia than a closed machine, but generally does not provide high-quality views and is not recommended.)

In addition, MRI cannot be used in people with devices such as implantable cardioverter-defibrillators, pacemakers, or aneurysm clips. If you have any of these devices or questions about the safety of an MRI scan in your case, it's best to speak with your doctor about it.

Getting a Good Night's Sleep With an Aching Back

Why you should, and how you can

If you've ever woken up with an aching back after a night of tossing and turning, you know the value of a good night's sleep. On the other hand, if you've gone to bed feeling pain in your neck or back, you know how hard it is to get that good night's sleep.

There seems to be a reciprocal relationship between sleep and pain. It's unclear whether chronic pain is caused by or is an effect of disturbed sleep. What is clear is that pain worsens when you are deprived of sleep. So it's essential to do whatever you can to make sure you sleep as well as you can. And a good night's sleep can improve your overall quality of life.

Chronic Pain/Poor Sleep

Numerous studies show that chronic pain in the neck or lower back significantly affects how well you sleep. According to a recent study of 70 people reported in the *Journal of Sleep Research*, more than half of those with chronic back pain had insomnia severe enough to interfere with their daily functioning and to cause them distress. By comparison, only 3% of a similar group that didn't have chronic back pain reported sleep problems. Not surprisingly, the people who said they felt the most pain and were anxious about their health had the most severe insomnia.

A growing body of evidence also shows that lack of sleep worsens pain. Recent findings from the Behavioral Sleep Medicine Program at Johns Hopkins show that frequently awakening for extended periods, such as when someone experiences insomnia in the middle of the night, impairs the natural pain control mechanisms that may play a key role in the development and exacerbation of chronic pain.

The main take-home message from this research is that your chronic lower back or neck pain should be treated in conjunction with any sleep problems you may have. When you and your doctor deal with the two together, there appears to be a synergistic effect on relieving overall pain and discomfort and improving your quality of life.

Finding the Right Mattress

Good sleeping posture, like good standing posture, allows the body to follow the natural S-shape curve of the spine; by contrast, poor sleeping positions can strain muscles and ligaments and increase the risk of developing a compressed nerve and, consequently, back pain. Your mattress affects your sleeping posture.

One recent study in the *American Journal of Physical Medicine and Rehabilitation* examined sleep disturbances among 268 people who had chronic low back pain for at least six months. As you might expect, there was a significant increase in restlessness and light sleep once back pain set in at night. Unexpected was the finding that those who slept on a very hard, orthopedic mattress slept worse than those who used a mattress of medium firmness. This goes against the common belief that a hard mattress is better for back pain.

According to the Better Sleep Council (a manufacturer's group), a mattress is "good" if it supports the natural curves of your body, particularly the spine and knees. A mattress that is too hard, for example, will create gaps between it and your body. The result is pressure points that restrict circulation and interfere with sleep by causing the person who is asleep to move around to restore circulation. Also beware of an extra soft mattress. While it may feel plush, a mattress that is too soft may not give your back the support it needs.

The American Chiropractic Association advocates using a mattress that has innerspring coils, which move independently to adjust to body curves, thereby keeping the spine in its natural position. Or you may want to try one of the newer memory foam mattresses, like Tempur-Pedic, or an inflatable mattress, such as Select Comfort, which lets you choose a different firmness for each half of the bed. The bottom line for a good mattress is comfort.

While mattresses wear out at different rates, the Better Sleep Council suggests you may need a new mattress if you wake up with stiffness, numbness, aches, and pains; you had a better night's sleep somewhere other than your own bed (such as a hotel); or your mattress shows visible signs of overuse (it sags, has lumps, the interior is exposed). In general, a mattress set that has been in use for five to seven years may no longer provide you with the best comfort and support, says the Council. Keep in mind that people's bodies change over tlme, and the need for good comfort and support only increases with age.

Here are some tips for finding a mattress that is just right for you.

- Be sure your mattress supports your lower back and, to some degree, conforms to your body.
- Always "rest test" a bed before buying it—lie down and stretch out to see how it feels. Get into the position you normally sleep in and make sure your body feels supported and comfortable. *Consumer Reports* recommends spending at least five minutes on each side and on your back or stomach (depending on which position you sleep in). Some companies will let you try out a mattress at home. Be prepared to pay for this option, but it could be money well spent.
- If your mattress is in good shape but is too hard, a layer of foam or a feather bed may help.
- If you share a bed, you and your partner should try the mattress together to make sure there is enough room for both of you. A queen- or king-size mattress is recommended for two people.
- The box spring, which absorbs the wear and tear of nightly use, also should be in good condition, since it helps provide durability and support. Mattresses and box springs are designed to work together, so it's best to buy a matching set. A memory foam mattress, works best on top of a platform bed.

Don't Forget Your Pillow

Lying in certain positions while you sleep can throw the spine out of alignment; for example, sleeping on your stomach puts stress on your neck and exaggerates the curve of the lower back. A better choice that helps maintain the natural curves of your spine is to sleep on your side with your knees bent and a pillow placed between them (see illustration A below).

Another option is to sleep on your back, but keep your knees slightly raised by placing a pillow underneath them (illustration B). This prevents your lower back from overarching by supporting the weight of your extended legs.

If you can't break the habit of sleeping on your stomach, place a pillow underneath your abdomen to keep your spine aligned (illustration C).

If you have neck pain, consider using a neck support pillow. A recent study in the *Journal of Rheumatology* found that individuals with chronic neck pain who slept with a neck support pillow and performed simple isometric neck exercises (see the inset box above) five to 10 minutes a day reported significant improvement in their symptoms. However, use of heat or cold packs with gentle massage, exercise alone, or the neck pillow alone was not as effective.

Another benefit from combination treatment: Those who used both the neck pillow and the exercises continued to feel better up to one year later. If you're interested in such a regimen, ask your doctor to refer you to a physical therapist who can teach you the exercises and the appropriate way to use a neck pillow during sleep. ■

Isometric Neck Exercise

Here's an example of an isometric exercise for the neck: Tilt your head to the right while applying resistance with your right hand. Hold for 20 seconds. Repeat on the left side, then do the same exercise, tilting your head first forward and then backward.

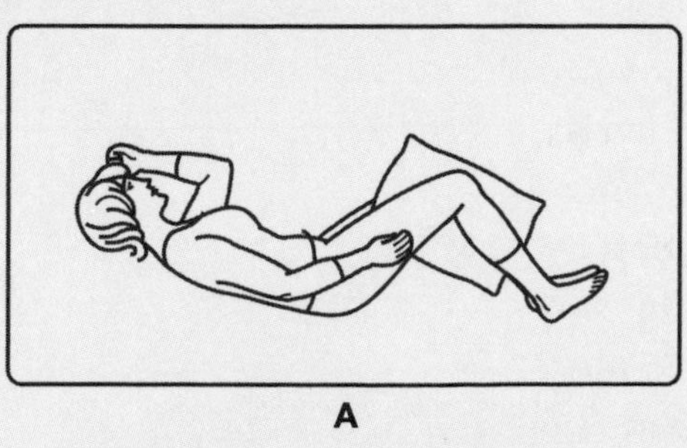

A

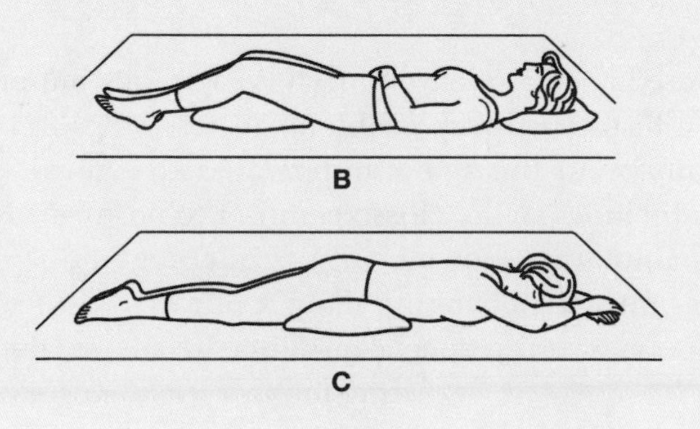

B

C

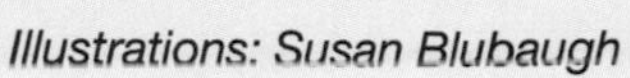

Illustrations: Susan Blubaugh

Bone scans

Bone scans measure the amount of radioactivity emitted from bone after an injection of a bone-seeking compound that contains technetium, a radioactive metal. The bone is scanned two to three hours after the injection, and information about the distribution of the radioactive compound in the bone is fed into a computer, which produces a two-dimensional image of the bone.

An area of bone that displays an increased uptake of technetium has a higher rate of bone turnover, which can be the result of a fracture not identified on an x-ray. It can also indicate the presence of metastatic cancer, Paget's disease, or osteomyelitis (a bacterial infection of the spine).

The amount of radiation delivered is similar to that of a CT scan. This technique can be used to identify fractures in both the central and peripheral areas of the body. The average cost is $500.

Electrical Tests

Three basic types of electrical tests may be used in difficult cases involving leg pain that has persisted for over a month. They may help the doctor pinpoint the source of pain or numbness or suggest the cause of pain (for example, whether it is due to disk herniation or nerve damage from an unrelated disorder, such as diabetes).

Electromyography. In this test, electrodes are used to measure muscle abnormalities.

Nerve conduction and sensory-evoked potentials. These two tests examine nerve function by measuring how fast the nerves conduct impulses.

All three of the electrical tests are used only when the diagnosis is in doubt. In addition, there is still some debate over their usefulness.

Preventing Back Pain

Because back pain may recur, it is especially important for anyone with a history of back problems to take steps to reduce their risk of damage to the spine and related structures. Preventive measures include paying close attention to posture and body mechanics (habitual ways of moving), stretching and strengthening particular muscles, changing daily routines to protect the back, and, if necessary, using special products to help reduce strain on the back.

Improving Posture

Contrary to popular belief, standing at attention like a military recruit—with the head and shoulders rigidly pulled back and the lower back excessively arched—is not correct posture and can be hard on the back. Good posture allows the body to follow the natural S-shaped curve of the spine. As simple as that sounds, however, poor habits, previous injuries, and even ill-fitting shoes can contribute to improper spinal alignment. Poor posture can strain muscles and ligaments and increase the risk of compressed nerves.

The easiest way to evaluate your posture is to stand sideways in front of a mirror when you're not wearing any bulky clothing. Ideally, it should be possible to visualize a vertical line running straight from the front of your earlobe through the front of your shoulder, down the center of your hip, just behind your kneecap, and just in front of your ankle bone. Your chin should be parallel to the floor, not thrust outward. Alternatively, stand with your heels against a wall. If the back of your head, shoulders, buttocks, and calves touch the wall—and you can slide your hand between the wall and your lower back—you have good alignment.

To check your posture while sitting, sit in an armless chair with your side to a mirror. You should be able to visualize a line running through the same points of your upper body down to the center of your hip.

Perpetual slouching with the shoulders rolled forward causes kyphosis. Mild kyphosis and lordosis (see page 8) can usually be corrected through a program of exercise, along with weight loss (for overweight people with lordosis.) More severe cases may require surgical correction.

Posture varies with age. As people get older and lose height because of disk changes, the curve in the lumbar region of the back tends to straighten, leading to a slight stoop, which is normal. In addition, the curve in the thoracic region tends to become accentuated with age.

The following tips will help to improve poor posture.

Standing

When standing, keep your head level and your chin slightly tucked in. Stand tall, stretching the top of your head towards the ceiling. Relax your shoulders and tighten your stomach muscles to tuck in your stomach.

Standing for long periods can be tiring and lead to bad posture. Distributing your weight so you are aligned vertically (a straight line from the point between your eyes to your chin, collarbone, breastbone, pelvis, and midpoint between your ankles) can relieve fatigue and maintain good posture.

Sitting and lying down

When sitting, use a straight-backed chair, and sit with your shoulders against the chair back, your chest lifted, your arms on the armrests, and your upper back straight. An ideal chair includes armrests to support the weight of your arms, thereby reducing the pressure on your back. Avoid low, soft chairs that are difficult to get into and out of. Your feet should comfortably touch the floor, with your knees positioned slightly higher than your hips. You may need to place a footstool or thick book underneath your feet. When sitting for any length of time, it is important to get up and move around every 30 minutes or so.

When driving, adjust your seat position so that your knees are slightly higher than your hips and in a position that you can comfortably reach the steering wheel, brakes, and accelerator. (See "Tips for Pain-Free Travel" on pages 10–11.) Shift your hand position on the steering wheel frequently to minimize stress on the muscles in the upper back and neck.

When in bed, lying on one side with knees bent and a pillow between them helps to maintain the natural curves of the spine. Place a pillow under your knees when sleeping on your back (see "Getting a Good Night's Sleep With an Aching Back" on pages 18–19).

Exercising To Protect and Strengthen the Back

Regular exercise helps people lose excess weight and improve their overall health. It can also help prevent back pain and injury. A review of numerous studies focusing on exercise to protect the back found that people who worked out regularly experienced less back pain and had fewer sick days due to back pain than those who didn't exercise.

Exercises for back pain focus on strengthening the muscles in the back and abdomen and stretching the muscles in the back. Flexibility exercises for your hips and even your shoulders may also be needed, because improving your flexibility in these areas will decrease the demands on your back.

Ask your doctor to refer you to a physical therapist, who can instruct you in exercises such as the pelvic tilt, cat stretch, and "crunches" (partial sit-ups). In addition, walking is an effective way to strengthen the back and improve posture.

Avoiding Back Strain

In addition to correct posture and exercise, many other aspects of your daily life influence the health of your back. Some people simply need to improve techniques used to perform everyday activities—lifting heavy objects, playing supports, or even getting in and out of a chair, for instance. Other people will need to avoid certain activities altogether.

Lift heavy objects properly

One study found that people who lifted objects improperly had twice the risk of a herniated disk as those who used the correct technique. To lift something safely, always bend at the knees and carry the object close to the body. The farther away from the body you hold an object, the more pressure placed on your spine. Holding objects at arm's length can increase the load on the lower spine by 15 times the original weight. For example, when a person carries a 10-lb box at arm's length from the body, it is putting 150 lbs of pressure on the spine.

Choose activities wisely

Depending on the severity of your back problem, you may need to avoid activities that require sudden twisting movements, including sports such as golf, bowling, football, basketball, baseball, weight lifting, and tennis and other racquet sports. If your physician approves, you may be able to continue some of these activities as long as you modify your technique.

In golf, for example, twisting movements during the swing must be minimized. In addition, golfers should keep their knees bent and spine straight when placing a ball on the tee or picking it up from the cup. Because improper serving and backhand techniques in tennis can strain the back, consider getting help with your technique from a tennis pro.

Maintain a healthy weight

Obesity places an extra burden on the lower back. It also increases the natural curve of the lumbar spine, forcing the vertebrae to bear weight at abnormal angles.

Quit smoking

Studies show that cigarette smoking decreases blood circulation in the intervertebral disks and speeds their degeneration. Smoking is also a major risk factor for osteoporosis.

Consider going to "back school"
Back schools are usually directed by a physical therapist, sometimes with the aid of a physician. They provide a safe, inexpensive, and effective way to learn more about how the back works and what can go wrong.

The school's director can analyze how your working conditions, daily activities, and even your sleeping habits may be harming your back. The school can customize an exercise program for you. Some schools also give instruction in relaxation techniques. A family doctor or physical therapist will have information about nearby schools.

Treating Back Pain

In most cases, back pain resolves quickly, regardless of the type of treatment. Fewer than 5% of people with back pain have a major medical problem that requires either intensive care or surgery. But if you experience severe back pain that doesn't improve after a couple of days of bed rest, or if your back pain is recurring or is accompanied by pain, numbness, or tingling that radiates into the buttocks or legs, it is important to see a doctor.

Self-Treatment

You can take the following steps on your own to help ease a backache.

Exercise
Back relaxation exercises—which involve gentle stretching to relax back muscles, lengthen the spine, and relieve compression of the vertebrae—are effective for alleviating stress and strain on the back. Ask your doctor for a referral to a physical therapist or for printed instructions on how to safely perform the exercises.

Rest
Lying down takes pressure off the spine and usually lessens pain. The best postures in bed are lying in the fetal position with a pillow between the knees, or on your back with knees flexed, using a pillow to support the legs. Most experts advise limiting bed rest to one or two days, however. The inactivity associated with longer periods of bed rest may do more harm than good by weakening muscles.

It is better to get out of bed and move around as soon as you can do so with reasonable comfort, even if some pain persists. Until the pain fully disappears, you should avoid lifting, bending, vigorous exercise, or other activities that place stress on the back.

While it may seem risky to move around when you are still experiencing back pain, medical research supports limiting the amount of bed rest. One study, for instance, found that people with acute back pain who continued ordinary activities recovered more rapidly than those for whom bed rest was prescribed. In fact, within a week, just 20% of the normal-activity group were still absent from work, compared with 41% of those on bed rest. After three months, people in the bed-rest group accumulated an average of 9.2 sick days, compared with 4.7 sick days in the normal-activity group.

Ice

After a sudden back injury that causes pain limited to the back area, immediately applying ice can be therapeutic. In addition to relieving pain, ice reduces internal bleeding and swelling by decreasing blood flow. An ice bag, commercial cold pack, or even a package of frozen vegetables should be used for 10–20 minutes every two hours for the first 48 hours after injury (while you're awake). The 20-minute limit is important to avoid the risk of frostbite. Another approach to relieving pain is to massage the painful area with an ice cube.

Heat

After an acute back injury, it is best to wait 48 hours before applying heat. But chronic back pain or a more widespread backache that begins some time after a back injury may be eased by relaxing muscles with a hot bath, a heating pad, a heat lamp, or hot, moist compresses.

Over-the-counter medications

Nonsteroidal anti-inflammatory drugs (NSAIDs)—such as aspirin, ibuprofen (Advil, Motrin), naproxen (Aleve), or ketoprofen (Orudis)—or the pain reliever acetaminophen (Tylenol) may help alleviate discomfort, reduce inflammation, or both. Check with your doctor if you are concerned about gastrointestinal or other side effects.

Traction, corsets, and braces

Little evidence supports the use of traction or corsets, although temporary use of a corset with built-in supports may be helpful during the recovery period following surgery or during activities that have to be performed even when you are still experiencing pain. Whether back braces help in treating back pain is unclear, and seemingly contradictory findings continue to be published.

ASK THE DOCTOR

Q. ***What are passive and active physical therapy modalities, and how do they work?***

A. Passive physical therapy is called passive because the modalities are done to you, whereas with active physical therapy you take an active role in the modalities.

Passive modalities typically are heat packs and/or ice massage and ultrasound. Heat and/or ice, the most commonly used type of modality, help reduce muscle spasm and inflammation. This usually works best over the first few days of back pain. You may find one or the other works better for you, or you can alternate them. Generally, you apply heat and/or ice for up to 20 minutes every two hours. Ultrasound uses sound waves applied to the skin to penetrate into and deeply heat soft tissues to enhance tissue healing. It is particularly useful to relieve acute pain.

Active physical therapy usually includes exercises to stretch and strengthen back muscles. Often, these exercises include a simple daily routine that may include knee pulls, hurdler stretches, modified toe-touches with and without rotation, abdominal curls, pelvic tilts, and back and hip extensions. Your physical therapist may also ask you to perform a spinal stabilization program consisting of progressive exercises that emphasize muscle strengthening to support the spine.

Commonly Used Drugs for Relieving Back Pain 2008

Drug type: Brand (generic)	Typical daily dosages*	How to take	How they work
Analgesic			
Tylenol, other brands (acetaminophen)	1,300–6,000 mg	In several doses per day, with water.	May inhibit receptors that transmit pain signals. Does not reduce inflammation.
Nonsteroidal anti-inflammatory drugs (NSAIDs)			
Advil, Motrin (ibuprofen) Aleve, Anaprox, Naprosyn (naproxen) Anacin, Bayer, other brands (aspirin) Dolobid (diflunisal) Actron, Orudis, Oruvail (ketoprofen) (meclofenamate)† Celebrex (celecoxib)	800–2,400 mg 220–440 mg 1,950–3,900 mg 500–1,000 mg 200–225 mg 200–400 mg 200–400 mg	*All except Celebrex:* Take with a full glass of water along with food, milk, or antacid. Limit alcohol while taking. Do not chew or crush pills. *Meclofenamate:* After taking, do not lie down for 30 minutes. *Celebrex:* Take with or without food.	Decrease inflammation and relieve pain by blocking prostaglandins, substances that induce pain, swelling, and fever.
Muscle relaxants			
Flexeril (cyclobenzaprine) Robaxin (methocarbamol) Soma, Vanadom (carisoprodol)	15–30 mg 4,000–6,000 mg 1,050–1,400 mg	2–4x/day. Exactly as directed. 3x/day and at bedtime.	Relax skeletal muscle and relieve spasm without interfering with muscle action.
Anticonvulsant			
Neurontin (gabapentin)	1,200 mg (individualized)	With or without food.	Seems to decrease sensitivity of spinal nerves that transmit pain signals.
Antidepressants			
(amitriptyline)† Norpramin (desipramine)	50–150 mg 100–200 mg	4x/day; largest dose at bedtime.	Enhance levels of neurotransmitters (such as serotonin) in the brain that are believed to reduce pain sensations.
Opiates			
Darvon (propoxyphene) Demerol (meperidine) Dolophine, Methadose (methadone) Avinza, Kadian, Oramorph, Roxanol (morphine) Endocet, Percocet, Roxicet, Roxilox, Tylox (oxycodone/acetaminophen) Percodan (oxycodone/aspirin) Ultracet (tramadol/acetaminophen) Ultram (tramadol) ***Long-acting:*** MS Contin (controlled-release morphine) OxyContin (controlled-release oxycodone)	210–390 mg 300–1,200 mg 15–40 mg 40–180 mg 4–6 tablets 4–6 tablets 4–8 tablets 50–200 mg 30–60 mg Highly individualized	*Percocet, Ultracet:* With food or milk. *Long-acting opiates:* Do not chew, break, or crush. This could cause a fatal overdose.	Depress the nervous system to inhibit perception of pain. *Percodan:* Also inhibits prostaglandins that cause inflammation. *Ultracet:* Also inhibits receptors that transmit pain signals.

Precautions	Most common side effects	Tell your doctor if...
Exceeding recommended dosage may cause liver or kidney damage, especially when combined with alcohol. Check with your doctor before taking any over-the-counter analgesic.	Fewer than most other drugs, except for rare allergic reactions (see symptoms at right).	You need to take it for more than 10 days. You have had ulcers or develop rash, hives, swelling, breathing difficulty.
May cause ulcers or internal bleeding. All drugs in this class (with the exception of aspirin) may increase the risk of heart attack and stroke. Avoid if you have asthma or liver, kidney, or heart problems. Check with your doctor before taking any over-the-counter NSAID.	Stomach irritation and many kinds of digestive problems (occur less with enteric-coated or buffered types); rash; itching, headache. Dolobid may cause insomnia or drowsiness.	You develop rash, hives, swelling, difficulty breathing, vision problems, stomach cramps, heartburn, indigestion, you have had ulcers or internal bleeding in the past, you need to take the drug for more than 10 days.
Do not use if you have arrhythmia or heart failure. Use alcohol with caution. Drowsiness may interfere with driving and use of machinery. *Soma:* Has addictive potential. *Flexeril:* Should be used for no more than 2 or 3 weeks. Do not use if you take MAO inhibitors.	Drowsiness, dry mouth, dizziness, clumsiness, headache, rash, upset stomach, nausea, vomiting, blurred vision.	*Robaxin:* You have kidney or liver disease, vision or digestion changes, urinary problems, dizziness, sudden mood changes. *Flexeril or Soma:* You develop severe drowsiness, confusion, hallucinations, heart palpitations, seizures.
People over age 50 may need to take lower doses to avoid drug build up. May impair ability to use machinery. When ending treatment, taper off usage over 5–7 days.	Dizziness, vision problems, clumsiness, sleepiness, shaking or tremor, swelling of hands or feet, weakness.	You have had kidney problems.
May take several weeks before effective. Avoid alcohol. May impair ability to use heavy machinery. *Amitriptyline:* Do not take while taking MAO inhibitors. Inform dentists and surgeons when taking. May cause sun sensitivity. *Norpramin:* May cause anxiety, agitation, or other mental changes including suicidal thoughts.	Rapid heartbeat, constipation, dry mouth, blurred vision, drowsiness, dizziness, confusion, susceptibility to falls, nausea, sedation, vomiting, rash.	You have a history of heart or thyroid disease, urinary retention, glaucoma, seizure disorder. You develop confusion, blurred vision, heart palpitations, stiffness or trembling, problems urinating.
Potentially addictive; used only for short-term relief of moderate to severe pain. Avoid alcohol. Avoid tranquilizers and sedatives except under doctor's direction. Use caution while driving or operating heavy machinery. Potentially fatal drug reactions. *Demerol:* Do not take if you have been taking MAO inhibitors.	Dizziness, lightheadedness, nausea, sedation, sweating, vomiting. Less common: constipation, mood changes, rash. *Ultracet:* anorexia, prostate disorder.	You have a history of drug abuse or alcoholism, breathing disorders such as asthma or chronic obstructive pulmonary disease; head injury; liver, kidney, intestine, or prostate disorders; history of seizures. You develop slower breathing, faintness, confusion, any other unusual problems.

MAO = monoamine oxidase inhibitor.

* Dosages represent an average range for treatment of back pain. Precise dosage varies from person to person and depends on many factors. Do not make any change to your prescription medication without consulting your doctor.

†Available only as a generic.

Alternative Therapies

A major study on the use of alternative therapies found that almost 60% of people who consulted a medical doctor for back pain had tried some sort of alternative therapy. When contemplating one of these options, it is important to remember that the treatments are considered alternative precisely because there is not enough scientific evidence to prove that they work consistently. Be particularly cautious about undertaking any treatments that are expensive and require more than half a dozen visits.

Be sure to tell your doctor if you are using any type of alternative therapy. Commonly used alternative methods for relieving back pain include acupuncture, acupressure, massage, relaxation therapy, spinal manipulation, yoga, and biofeedback.

Acupuncture

This treatment is based on the traditional Chinese medical theory that pain and disease occur when the body's natural energies (chi) are out of balance. The Chinese believe that chi is conducted through the body along pathways called meridians, which intersect at specific points in the body. Stimulating these points through acupuncture needles is meant to correct the improper flow of chi, thereby relieving the problem. Acupuncture is one of the few alternative therapies that are commonly covered by many insurance companies. Check with your insurer.

The needles used in acupuncture are as thin as a hair. In general, 10–15 of these needles are inserted into the back to treat pain. Sometimes they are stimulated with electricity or heat or are turned after insertion. Acupuncture may relieve pain by triggering nerves to send out natural, pain-blocking chemicals (endorphins) within the body.

A recent analysis of 33 published studies of acupuncture and back pain found that acupuncture effectively relieves chronic low back pain. However, the researchers noted that there is no evidence that acupuncture is more effective than other therapies. To find a reputable practitioner, contact one of the acupuncture organizations cited on page 82.

Acupressure

This therapy is similar to acupuncture in that it is based on the same theory of energy channels in the body. Continuous pressure is exerted on a trigger spot for three to five minutes to stimulate the flow of healing energy. This pressure may temporarily alleviate the pain, but it usually returns.

Massage therapy

In addition to relaxing muscles and easing tension in the back, massage is believed to temporarily overpower pain signals going to the brain. Massage therapy should only be performed by a trained, licensed massage therapist.

Relaxation therapy

High levels of stress not only adversely affect overall health, but can also contribute to back pain. Relaxation therapy teaches muscle relaxation and breathing techniques for coping with the stress of everyday life.

Another relaxation technique is meditation, designed to calm the mind as well as the body. Researchers have theorized that the metabolic response to meditation—the opposite of the response to stress—may counter the negative effects of stress.

Biofeedback

Using electronic sensors, biofeedback measures a person's automatic, stress-responsive body functions—such as breathing patterns, pulse rate, and muscle tension—while the person practices different relaxation methods. Data from the sensors can show which relaxation techniques are most effective for that individual. Biofeedback can also help train a person to regulate his or her body functions consciously, reducing the impact of stress on the body.

Yoga

Mounting evidence suggests that yoga can relieve chronic back pain. There are many schools or types of yoga. They feature precise alignment and props such as mats, blocks, and straps. The props help in achieving correct yoga poses. The poses, combined with breathing techniques, help relax muscles and calm the mind.

Spinal manipulation

For treatment of back pain lasting less than a month, spinal manipulation can be a good choice, provided there is no evidence of a spinal nerve root disorder (such as a herniated disk or spinal stenosis). If symptoms do not improve after four weeks, however, use of spinal manipulation should be re-evaluated.

A chiropractor, osteopath, or physical therapist may provide spinal manipulation, adjusting the vertebrae to reduce pain caused by poor alignment. The health care professional must be sure that back pain is not due to bone or joint disorders, since manipulating a spine that has been damaged by osteoporosis, for example, could result in further, more serious injury. X-rays of the area are usually taken before spinal manipulation to rule out vertebral fractures.

In properly screened people, spinal manipulation by a trained professional appears to be safe. Some people may experience discomfort, headache, or tiredness after treatment, but these effects are usually only temporary. Serious complications of lower-spine manipulation, such as paralysis and death, are rare. Complications, when they do occur, are more common with manipulations of the neck.

Medical Treatment

If you have severe back pain that lasts more than a few days, or if you have mild to moderate back pain that does not respond to self-treatment, it is important to visit your primary care physician. Regardless of the cause of the pain, a doctor will probably recommend the self-treatment techniques described on pages 24–25. In general, limiting the amount of bed rest and pain medication is the preferred approach to back pain management among primary care physicians—a strategy supported by current research.

In one study of more than 1,000 people, doctors were divided into three groups according to whether they had a low, medium, or high frequency of prescribing pain medications and bed rest. After a month, people seeing the physicians who least often prescribed drugs and bed rest improved more quickly than those in the other groups. Only 30% of these people had to make moderate to severe cutbacks in their daily activities, compared with 37% of people seeing doctors in the medium-frequency group and 46% in the high-frequency group. After a year, however, there were no differences among the three groups in pain levels or ability to function.

Many doctors feel that the successful treatment of back pain with minimal bed rest and minimal medication is a result of the self-care practices they recommend and teach their patients. The above study supports this belief: People whose physicians were least likely to prescribe bed rest and pain-relief medications reported being more satisfied with their personal knowledge of how to treat back pain and just as satisfied with their medical care as those whose doctors prescribed drugs and rest.

Prescription NSAIDs

When over-the-counter medications do not relieve back pain, the doctor might need to prescribe a stronger NSAID such as diflunisal (Dolobid) or meclofenamate (available in generic form only).

While a certain type of NSAID known as COX-2 inhibitors have been shown to treat pain and inflammation as effectively as traditional NSAIDs, they have come under scrutiny for their adverse effects, including an increased risk of heart attack and stroke in people with or at risk for cardiovascular disease. As a result of these concerns, the U.S. Food and Drug Administration (FDA) has strengthened the warnings on the labels of all prescription NSAIDs, including the COX-2 inhibitor celecoxib (Celebrex). Currently, Celebrex is the only COX-2 inhibitor still on the market in the United States.

Muscle relaxants

Studies have shown that muscle relaxants are an effective treatment for acute low back pain. Their usefulness for chronic low back pain requires further study, however.

Muscle relaxants appear to work by depressing the activity of nerves in the spinal cord and brain. Common muscle relaxants are baclofen (Lioresal), carisoprodol (Soma), cyclobenzaprine (Flexeril), and methocarbamol (Robaxin). The anticonvulsant gabapentin (Neurontin) also is used often. A few studies suggest that a combination of a muscle relaxant and an NSAID may be more beneficial than a muscle relaxant alone.

The use of muscle relaxants is controversial because they are potentially addictive. Therefore, you should not take them for more than one or two weeks, and people with a history of substance abuse or other mental health conditions should use them with great caution. Possible side effects include dizziness, drowsiness, dry mouth, headache, stomachache, and nausea or vomiting.

Opiates

Highly addictive painkillers such as opiates (morphine, codeine, meperidine) should also be used with a great deal of caution and only when all other treatments have failed. People who need opiates for more than a few days sometimes take controlled-release formulations of oxycodone (OxyContin) or morphine (MS Contin). These long-acting drugs provide more consistent control of back pain than standard, short-acting narcotics. (The chart on pages 26–27 gives an overview of oral medications prescribed for back pain.)

Disease-modifying antirheumatic drugs

The medication Etanercept (Enbrel), a disease-modifying antirheumatic drug (DMARD), is used to treat ankylosing spondylitis.

NEW RESEARCH

Long-Term Narcotics Use for Back Pain May Lead to Abuse

Narcotic drugs, or opioids, may be an effective short-term treatment for chronic low back pain, but there's a potential risk of substance abuse, a new study says.

The authors reached this conclusion after reviewing 38 studies of adults with back pain that lasted for at least three months. The investigators found that use of opioids for chronic back pain was effective for only about four months. What's more, evidence suggests that up to 25% of the patients who took opioids, such as Oxycontin, for chronic back pain may have been abusing them.

If you have chronic back pain, there is a wide range of nonopiate medications to choose from, including NSAIDs and tricyclic antidepressants. Nondrug options include exercise therapy, acupuncture, and electrical stimulation. Ask your doctor about trying these treatments initially, and use opioids only as a treatment of last resort. If all else fails, consider getting a referral to a pain treatment facility.

ANNALS OF INTERNAL MEDICINE
Volume 146, page 116
January 16, 2007

The drug works by interfering with an immune system protein known as tumor necrosis factor, which contributes to inflammation. Possible side effects of etanercept include reactions at the site of the injection and respiratory infections.

Exercise

If your back pain is mild, it is safe to get back to an aerobic exercise routine as soon as treatment eases your pain. After two weeks, exercises to strengthen the back and abdominal muscles can be started slowly. Building core strength in the back and abdomen is very beneficial in preventing recurrence.

Not recommended or unproven treatments

Prolonged bed rest (more than four days) is not recommended as part of treatment. Although still used occasionally, transcutaneous electrical nerve stimulation (TENS)—the application of low-energy electrical radiation to "numb" the nerves—is declining in popularity. Support belts and back machines have not been found to be of any benefit in the treatment of back pain.

Treating a Herniated Disk

About 80% of people with classic symptoms of a herniated lumbar disk—sciatica and back spasm—respond within six weeks to rest and pain medication. This conservative approach to treatment likely works because it gives the swelling around the nerve root a chance to subside. The limitation on physical activity helps the herniated disk material remain in place, reducing the risk of it fragmenting. A disk fragment that lodges in the spinal canal and presses on a nerve can cause significant loss of function.

Surgery

Surgery for a herniated disk may be unavoidable in cases of impaired bowel or bladder function, persistent or increasing sciatica despite bed rest, progressive leg weakness, and recurring episodes of incapacitating pain from sciatica.

Diskectomy. The traditional surgical treatment of a herniated disk, called diskectomy, is used only when at least six weeks of nonsurgical treatment offers no pain relief or when there is a problem in nerve function that causes a loss of movement, known as a neurological deficit. The procedure relieves pressure on the pinched nerve by making an incision into the distended annulus fibrosus (the tough outer layers of the disk) and removing the protruding

NEW RESEARCH

Sciatica Pain Diminishes With or Without Surgery

Surgery can provide fast pain relief for sciatica, but you might do just as well without an operation, a study finds.

Sciatica refers to leg pain caused by a herniated disk in the spine that presses on the sciatic nerve. Researchers randomly assigned 281 people with the condition for at least six weeks to have surgery to decompress the nerve or to receive conservative treatments such as pain medication and exercise.

On average, people who had surgery felt their leg pain was better after four weeks while it took about 12 weeks for those who did not have surgery to note improvement. But within one year, 95% of the study participants said they felt significantly better, no matter what treatment they had.

If you are experiencing searing pain or numbness in your leg and conservative treatment is not working, then surgery may be right for you. On the other hand, if you feel you can handle the leg pain and are willing to postpone surgery, you just might find that you don't need it.

THE NEW ENGLAND JOURNAL OF MEDICINE
Volume 356, page 2245
May 31, 2007

nucleus pulposus (the gel-like center). General anesthesia is required. Depending on the location of the herniation, the surgeon may need to remove a small part of the vertebra (open laminectomy) to gain access to the herniation site.

Although highly effective for pain relief, diskectomy leaves behind the weakened disk, which is less able to bear normal loads, so that the adjacent spinal vertebrae may continue to deteriorate.

In general, diskectomy produces improvement more rapidly than conservative treatment. After having a diskectomy, sciatica is relieved completely in about 80% of people and partially in another 15%, and back pain is eliminated in about 70% of people, often within days. The long-term results of surgical and nonsurgical treatment, however, are about the same (see "Who Needs Disk Surgery, Anyway?"on pages 34–35). How well you do during the first three months of conservative care may help you decide about surgery.

One day of hospitalization may be required after an open diskectomy (a procedure in which the surgeon makes a large incision in the patient's back to gain access to and operate on the spine). Over the subsequent several weeks, the treated disk gradually restabilizes as scar tissue fills the empty space. Almost all people can return to work six to eight weeks after the operation. Repeat surgery is not as effective at relieving pain as the first surgery.

Spinal fusion. In some cases, a spinal fusion is also performed. This procedure involves using bone grafts to fuse together two or more adjacent vertebrae. It should be considered in cases where chronic back pain was present before the herniated disk led to leg pain. Spinal fusion is not always reliable, and guidelines as to when it should be done are not as clear as those for diskectomy. Fusion may be recommended when back pain is greater than leg pain and is chronic. It is also recommended when a repeat operation is necessary, either because the first one was not effective in relieving pain or because herniation has recurred.

Unfortunately, spinal fusion alters the way the spine moves and may promote degenerative changes as well.

Artificial disks. Although artificial disks have been available in Europe for at least 20 years, the FDA did not approve their use in the United States until 2004. The first artificial disk available in this country, called the Charité, was authorized for use in single-level disk problems (where one disk is affected) after clinical trials revealed that the device preserved motion and was as effective as spinal fusion in relieving pain, with shorter healing and rehabilitation times. In 2006, the FDA approved a second artificial spinal disk, the ProDisc-L.

NEW RESEARCH

Device Improves Spinal Fusion Surgery Results

Spinal fusion surgery for herniated disks and other degenerative spine diseases is more likely to be successful when a system of plates is used to stabilize the vertebrae, particularly if more than one disk is involved.

This finding is from an analysis of 21 studies involving nearly 2,700 people who underwent spinal fusion surgery to grow two or more vertebrae together into a single bone. One of the goals of the surgery is to eliminate motion between the vertebrae, which is often the cause of significant pain for people with serious degenerative spinal disease.

The studies compared outcomes of five procedures—anterior cervical diskectomy (ACD), ACD with interbody fusion (ACDF), ACDF with a plate system (ACDFP), corpectomy, and corpectomy with the plate system. For a single disk-level fusion, success rates ranged from 85% for ACD to 97% for ACDFP. For fusions at two disk levels, rates ranged from 80% for ACDF to 96% for ACDFP. And for fusions at three disk levels, rates ranged from 65% for ACDF to 96% for corpectomy with plate placement.

If you have degenerative disease in your spine and are considering spinal fusion surgery, ask your doctor about the benefits and risks of using a plate system.

JOURNAL OF NEUROSURGERY: SPINE
Volume 6, page 298
April 2007

Who Needs Disk Surgery, Anyway?

New research suggests short-term gain but little advantage in the long run

Your back pain from a herniated disk is so bad that your doctor suggests surgery. Will an operation really ease your pain? The answer really depends on how and when you look at the results of treatment.

The most common surgery for back and leg pain is the removal of part or all of an intervertebral disk. For the most part, this procedure, known as diskectomy, is done electively—that is, when people choose to have it. But a protruding disk often improves over time on its own, without surgery. So what's the best course of action?

Actually, until now, what happened to people with back problems depended at least in part on where they lived, because rates of spinal fusion and diskectomy vary widely across the United States. For example, a look at Medicare recipients from 1992–2003, published recently in the journal *Spine*, found that rates of spinal fusion were 20 times higher and rates of diskectomy were eight times higher in some regions of the country than in others. The rates vary because there is no clear consensus on the what's the "best" treatment for disk problems.

Clear Outcome, Murky Conclusions

Researchers were hoping that the first large randomized trial comparing diskectomy with nonoperative treatment might help clear the air. Essentially, it was a draw—people with herniated disks improved substantially, and for the most part equally, within two years of treatment whether or not they had surgery, Dartmouth researchers reported in the *Journal of the American Medical Association*.

The 501 participants in this study—called the Spine Patient Outcomes Research Trial (SPORT)—had a herniated disk and persistent signs of nerve damage for at least six weeks. About half of the people were randomly assigned to have surgery and the others underwent nonoperative treatments, which included physical therapy; education and counseling, including home exercise instruction; use of nonsteroidal anti-inflammatory drugs (NSAIDs), opiates, and steroid injections; and restriction of activity. After two years, both groups had less pain and better physical function.

A companion study looked at 743 people who were eligible to participate in SPORT but declined to be randomized and instead made their own choice for either surgery or no surgery. After two years, the results were again similar for both treatments, although the people who had surgery felt better faster.

The researchers acknowledge that both studies were flawed, making it difficult to reach solid conclusions. For example, many people "crossed over" (switched to the other treatment) in the middle of the randomized study. In fact, only half those assigned to surgery actually had an operation within three months, while 30% of those not assigned to surgery had the procedure after all. Interestingly, those who were older, had higher incomes, higher education, and milder pain and disability were more likely not to have surgery. Patients who elected to have surgery tended to feel that their back problem was getting worse.

How To Decide About Diskectomy

When or if surgery for a herniated disk is appropriate remains controversial. As a general rule, if you have pain for three months and then have surgery, you're

Additional artificial disks are being tested in clinical trials in the United States. However, it will take five to 10 years to determine whether artificial disks can maintain long-term motion and prevent disk degeneration near the surgical site (see "Is an Artificial Disk for You?" on pages 40–41).

Candidates for disk surgery should have only minimal wear and tear in the facet joints.

likely to feel less pain and to function better two years later. If you use conservative, nonoperative treatments (see the inset box at right), it may take a little longer, but you will likely end up with the same good outcome after two years.

However, one clear finding in the SPORT study, was that there is no significant risk that either choice—surgery or nonoperative treatment—will actually make you worse.

How well you do during the first three months of conservative care may help you decide about surgery. At that point, you need to decide whether the pain is tolerable. If you can put up with it, then you may be able to get by without surgery. If the pain becomes intolerable, then surgery becomes more attractive since it can dramatically reduce the pain you are experiencing at that time. Ultimately, it's a quality-of-life decision.

Conservative Care

What effective conservative, nonoperative measures are available? Your doctor may suggest:

- Physical therapy with extension and flexion exercises
- Epidural injections of cortisone directly into the spine
- Acupuncture of the spine
- Spinal manipulation and massage
- Traction using a special device to decompress the spine (this seems to work better for bulging rather than herniated disks)
- Prescription-strength NSAIDs for two weeks
- Oral opiates
- Hot or cold packs—whatever makes your back feel better.

Learn As Much As You Can

If you have back pain, it's wise to learn as much as you can about the available options before deciding on any particular treatment. To make sure you're getting the best information and the right advice, find out the following:

- **What is your physical problem?** Have your doctor explain it in layperson's terms. If you don't understand, ask the doctor to explain it more simply. The more specific the anatomical location, the easier it is for imaging tests to pinpoint the location of the back pain, and the more likely that surgery will help you.
- **What would be a successful outcome of this intervention?** Be sure you have a clear understanding of the best result you can expect. Then consider whether that outcome is enough of an improvement to justify having surgery.
- **Understand the commitment surgery will require.** Have a good idea of what it will entail in terms of time, pain, recovery, and physical therapy. For example, diskectomy may be performed as an outpatient procedure or you may have to stay in the hospital for a day. Your pain may not be relieved immediately after the surgery, and you may also feel pain at the incision site. In addition, recovery from surgery can take days or years, depending on the type of operation you have.
- **Get a second opinion.** Before undergoing major, elective surgery of any type, seek out another surgeon's advice on the merits of the procedure in your situation. ■

Minimally invasive procedures. There are several less-invasive surgical alternatives that allow a smaller incision than traditional surgery.

- ***Microdiskectomy*** is performed by the surgeon using very small precision instruments placed inside an endoscope (a small lighted tube) and inserted through a miniscule opening in the back. The surgeon can view the disk and nerves through the endoscope as well as remove herniated disk material. Microdiskectomy appears to have a success rate similar to that of open diskectomy. Doctors may recommend this surgery to people who have leg pain for at least six weeks but do not experience relief with conservative treatments such as oral corticosteroids, NSAIDs, and physical therapy.

• ***Percutaneous arthroscopic diskectomy*** involves inserting a probe into the spine to scoop out the disk.

• ***Intradiskal electrothermal therapy*** (IDET) involves inserting a wire into the back that transmits heat into the collagen fibers of the disk, destroying pain receptors in the area. IDET initially appeared promising, but more recent reports have been disappointing.

• ***Laser diskectomy*** uses a laser to burn out the disk. This procedure has been the subject of considerable debate, as the results of the procedure have varied greatly. Some studies show no greater improvement in symptoms after laser diskectomy than in similar cases where no surgery was performed; in others, it is as successful as standard surgery.

Treating Vertebral Compression Fractures

Treatment of vertebral compression fractures includes minimal bed rest, pain medication, exercise, and osteoporosis treatment to reduce the risk of future fractures. In some cases, surgical procedures such as percutaneous vertebroplasty, kyphoplasty, or spinal fusion are performed.

Treating Spinal Stenosis

Nonsurgical treatment is appropriate if the symptoms of spinal stenosis are mild or if a person is not a good candidate for surgery—for example, an older adult with another serious illness. Treatment includes pain relievers such as acetaminophen (Tylenol) or NSAIDs, weight loss, and, especially, exercises to increase flexibility. Some success has been reported with the use of caudal epidural blocks—injections of pain relievers and a steroid directly into the base of the spine. Treatment with a bisphosphonate or injectable calcitonin (Miacalcin) may improve symptoms when spinal stenosis is due to Paget's disease.

If these measures fail to control symptoms, surgery is considered. Surgery is necessary when severe neurological deficits or impaired bowel or bladder function develop.

Surgical treatment

Decompression surgery for spinal stenosis enlarges the spinal canal to relieve pressure on the spinal cord. After the spinal column is opened at the narrowed points, the bone or fibrous tissue responsible for the constriction is removed. At times, a disk or fragments of a disk also may be removed. If an extensive amount of bone is removed, it may be necessary to fuse together two or more vertebrae to stabilize the spinal column (this may slightly decrease a person's flexibility).

The hospital stay for decompression surgery is typically three to five days. A person can get around using a walker the first or second day and then graduates to a cane, which he or she uses for six to 12 weeks. After that, walking without assistance is usually possible. Results tend to be excellent if the disease is limited to one or two vertebrae. Studies have shown that leg pain associated with stenosis significantly improves after surgery in 70–85% of people.

Risks of surgery

Older adults with spinal stenosis may have other health conditions, such as heart disease or arthritis, that increase the risk of surgical complications. These conditions do not necessarily rule out surgery as a treatment option, however.

In one study, researchers monitored 50 people, age 71–84, who had decompression surgery. Half of them had other disorders that severely limited their mobility. No complications involving anesthesia, the heart, or blood clots occurred during the procedure. After two years, 28 of the study participants (more than half) rated the procedure's effect on their leg pain as excellent (almost or totally pain free); nine reported fair relief (improved but residual pain); and nine said their pain was unchanged. Although the operation provided some relief, the rates of excellent outcomes were not as high as researchers had hoped. Therefore, although having other health conditions did not cause additional complications, it appeared to reduce the chances of obtaining the best results.

Treating Paget's Disease

Many people with Paget's disease require no treatment because they have no symptoms. The most clear-cut reasons for using drugs to treat Paget's disease are bone pain, bone fractures (such as vertebral fractures), and compression of nerves in the spine or elsewhere.

The FDA has approved injectable calcitonin, four oral bisphosphonate drugs (a class of drugs used to strengthen bone), and two intravenous bisphosphonate drugs for treatment of Paget's disease. Calcitonin (a synthetic version of a hormone that acts on bone) has pain-relieving properties and may be used in conjunction with a

ASK THE DOCTOR

Q. ***When can I resume sexual activity after back surgery?***

A. You may resume your normal sexual activity, within reason, as soon as you feel up to it. Lying on your side may be more comfortable at first. If you do lie on your back, use pillows to support your neck and knees. Also, try to avoid arching your back or rapidly shifting your spine.

Many people and their partners feel nervous about resuming sexual activity after back surgery. Keep in mind that a sexual relationship has both physical and emotional aspects. Talk openly with your partner and allow yourselves a gradual return to sexual activity.

Arrange to have sex when you are rested and physically comfortable. Create realistic performance expectations since it may take longer than you think to return to an active sex life. Anxiety on the part of either partner as well as some medications may interfere with sexual arousal or performance. Discuss any difficulties with your doctor, if necessary.

bisphosphonate, especially if additional pain relief is desired. No matter which drug is started first, it can be discontinued and replaced with another agent if it proves ineffective.

Calcitonin

Calcitonin (Miacalcin), which inhibits bone breakdown (resorption), is available for subcutaneous (under the skin) or intramuscular injection. Although it is also available as a nasal spray, the nasal formulation of calcitonin is not approved by the FDA for treating Paget's disease. Injections are initially given daily; after a month or so, symptoms may be controlled with less frequent injections (three times a week, for example).

After a variable period of time, calcitonin stops working in some people. Between 10% and 20% of those treated with calcitonin develop nausea, loss of appetite, and flushing of the face and ears. The drug is also expensive; depending on the dose, each injection costs between $4 and $8.

Bisphosphonates

The bisphosphonate class of drugs includes the oral medications alendronate (Fosamax), etidronate (Didronel), risedronate (Actonel), and tiludronate (Skelid). These medications are the first line of therapy for treating Paget's disease and are also used to prevent and treat osteoporosis.

For Paget's disease, alendronate (40 mg a day) and etidronate (200–400 mg a day) are both taken in a six-months-on, six-months-off cycle. Risedronate (30 mg a day) is taken in a two-months-on, two-months-off cycle and tiludronate (400 mg a day) is taken in a three-months-on, three-months-off cycle. If relapse occurs, a person may begin treatment again after a period of two or three months off the drug. (See page 66 for instructions on how to take alendronate and risedronate, as well as information on their side effects.)

If an oral bisphosphonate is no longer effective or cannot be tolerated because of gastrointestinal side effects or if Paget's disease is particularly severe, the intravenous bisphosphonate drugs pamidronate (Aredia) and zoledronic acid (Reclast) may be used. Reclast was approved by the U.S. Food and Drug Administration in April 2007 for the treatment of Paget's disease. Previously, it had been approved under the brand name Zometa for the treatment of cancer-related bone problems.

Pamidronate is administered using an injection schedule determined by the doctor. Possible side effects include abdominal cramps, chills, fever, nausea, pain, muscle spasms, sore throat, and muscle stiffness. Zoledronic acid is given in one 15-minute intravenous infusion. Potential side effects are similar to those of pamidronate.

Additional treatments

People with Paget's disease should also take 1,000–1,500 mg of calcium and 1,000 IU of vitamin D each day. People with signs and symptoms of spinal stenosis resulting from Paget's disease may require surgery if medication is ineffective in reducing the stenosis.

Treating Spinal Deformities

Most spinal deformities in adults, including adults over age 50, can be helped with flexibility exercises, posture maintenance, and general fitness. Mild anti-inflammatory medication and, occasionally, a rigid brace may help, although many older people cannot tolerate braces.

Surgery is recommended if the deformity is severe or will continue to worsen with age, if there are neurological problems associated with the deformity, or if pain does not respond to other measures.

Surgery usually involves the application of internal implants fixed to the bone (which allow for partial correction of the deformity) together with a spinal fusion. Old age should not prevent you from having this surgery if you need it, provided you are in good general health. Results are satisfactory 85% of the time.

Treating Cancer

Although myeloma and metastatic cancer cannot be cured, palliative treatment of back pain is often possible. Palliative care refers to treatment aimed at relieving pain and limiting any complications of a disease, rather than treatment aimed at curing a disease. Palliative treatment of back pain may include chemotherapy, radiation directed at the site of tumor invasion, and, at times, surgery.

For metastatic cancer of the spine, surgery may provide significant pain relief and preserve or restore nerve function. Bisphosphonate drugs are also used to reduce pain in metastatic cancer. People with metastatic prostate cancer may benefit from hormone therapies.

Managing Chronic Back Pain

Most cases of back pain resolve in a matter of weeks to months, but for some people the pain becomes a constant problem that interferes with their daily lives. If ignored, chronic back pain—generally

Is an Artificial Disk for You?

Spinal or cervical disks may ease pain but questions remain

Do you remember TV's Six Million Dollar Man—the wounded test pilot rebuilt with bionic body parts that made him stronger and faster than normal humans? What was science fiction in the 1970s is one step closer to reality today with the availability of artificial spinal and cervical disks. While these artificial disks don't impart super-human powers, they do mimic the function of real disks, in many cases allowing the recipient to move and bend in a near-normal manner. As such, they represent a promising alternative to spinal fusion surgery—the traditional treatment.

More than 5,000 Americans are now walking around with artificial spinal disks in place. Many say they feel better than ever, but no one in this country has had a disk for more than a few years. However, in spite of approval of two of these devices by the U.S. Food and Drug Administration (FDA), questions remain about their safety and durability over the long term.

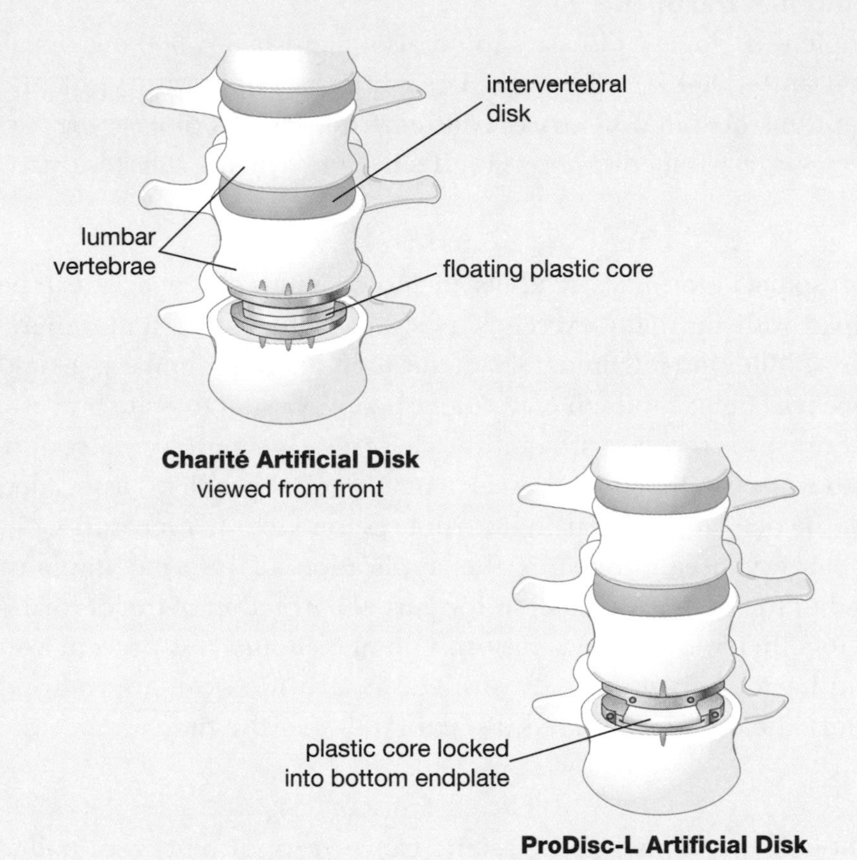

Charité Artificial Disk viewed from front

ProDisc-L Artificial Disk viewed from front

Artificial Spinal Disks

The two artificial spinal disk implants available for use in the United States are the Charité artificial disk and the ProDisc-L Total Replacement Disk (see the illustrations above).

Charité Artificial Disk. The FDA approved this device in 2004. The disk consists of a free-floating plastic core situated between two metal endplates that attach to the vertebrae. The core moves between the endplates and moves in and out as the spine bends forward and back. Studies show that two years after surgery in people with degenerative disk disease, the Charité disk relieved pain and improved the ability to function as well as (but no better than) spinal fusion.

ProDisc-L. This disk, which was approved by the FDA in 2006, consists of two endplates that are anchored to the top and bottom surfaces of the vertebrae and a plastic core that locks into the bottom endplate. The core moves with the upper endplate to permit motion. The portion of the core attached to the bottom endplate provides additional stability. A two-year randomized clinical trial that was the basis of the FDA's approval of this device showed that the ProDisc-L was better than spinal fusion in relieving pain and preserving motion in people with degenerative disk disease.

About the Procedure

To implant the artificial spinal disk, the surgeon makes an incision in the abdomen, removes the degenerated disk, and replaces it with the artificial one. The procedure, which is done in the hospital under general anesthesia, takes about two hours, and the typical hospital stay is two to four days. As with any surgery, the procedure can be hazardous, and the artificial disks may be hard to remove and replace if there is a problem with them.

The benefits. Compared with spinal fusion surgery, the potential benefits of an artificial spinal disk include quicker recovery time, more spine mobility after surgery, and less stress on adjacent disks.

Complications. As with any major operation, the procedure involves serious risks. In addition to the potential complications associated with surgery and general anesthesia (such as infection, uncontrolled bleeding, and pneumonia). Other complications, which occur rarely, include breakage of the metal plate and dislocation of the implant. There have been several reports of the disks slipping out of place—a complication that requires surgery for removal.

Experience counts. As you would expect, surgeons who have the most experience in inserting an artificial spinal disk seem to get the best results. This was documented in a study published in 2006 in the journal *Spine* that compared results from surgeons who had performed either more or fewer than 15 disk replacements before becoming involved in a major clinical trial of artificial disks. For patients with more experienced surgeons, surgery was 30 minutes shorter, there were fewer complications, and they left the hospital one-half day earlier.

"Lasting" Concerns

There is much debate in the medical community about the long-term durability of artificial spinal disks. Although they are designed to last for many years, like any artificial joint, these disks may eventually need to be replaced due to wear of the materials and loosening.

Because information about the safety and durability of the Charité artificial disk and ProDisc-L is limited, the FDA is requiring both manufacturers to perform five-year studies that evaluate the long-term safety and durability of their devices.

Are You a Candidate?

At present, spinal disk implants are not appropriate for everyone with low back pain. To be considered as a candidate, you must:

- Have degeneration in only one disk in the lumbar spine.
- Have undergone at least six months of treatment, such as physical therapy or use of pain medication or a back brace, with no improvement in symptoms.
- Not have significant leg pain.
- Be in overall good health with no signs of infection, osteoporosis, or arthritis.

Artificial Cervical Disks

The first artificial replacement for failing disks in the cervical spine was approved by the FDA in 2007. In clinical trials, the stainless steel device, called Prestige, relieved pain and improved ability to function at least as well as spinal fusion after two years.

If you have numbness in your arms in addition to severe pain and immobility associated with cervical disk degeneration, then the artificial cervical disk may be for you. Compared with surgery to insert an artificial lumbar disk, the cervical procedure appears to be less hazardous and involves techniques that are more familiar to surgeons. It is also easier to remove and replace the disk if necessary. As with spinal disks, these devices are meant to last for decades, but virtually all of the current information about them covers a much shorter time span.

A Final Caveat

If you're considering disk replacement surgery, discuss the risks and benefits with your doctor. If you get the okay, check with your insurance carrier before heading to surgery. Medicare will not pay for artificial disk surgery in people older than 60, and private insurers may have similar policies. ■

defined as unremitting pain that lasts at least six months and is not relieved by standard treatments—can lead to depression, disturbed sleep, poor balance, withdrawal from physical and social activities, inability to work, and a reduced quality of life.

The first step in relieving chronic back pain is careful medical evaluation by a doctor to assess the nature and degree of the pain and, if possible, to pinpoint the cause. Because pain is a subjective experience, the doctor will ask when and how often the pain occurs; what brings it on and how long it lasts; its location, intensity, and quality (for example, is it sharp, dull, or tingling?); and what treatments you have tried and how well they have worked. You may also be asked to rate the severity of your pain on a standard pain scale.

If your doctor is unable to identify a specific cause for the pain (such as nerve entrapment that can be relieved by surgery), a variety of medications may be tried, ranging from over-the-counter acetaminophen or NSAIDs to prescription antidepressants, muscle relaxants, or opiates (see the chart on pages 26–27).

Weight loss (if necessary) and exercise—stretching, flexibility, and muscle-strengthening exercises—are particularly helpful in treating chronic pain. Other strategies include self-application of heat and cold and cognitive and/or behavioral therapy. Spinal manipulation, acupuncture, acupressure, massage, relaxation therapy, or biofeedback may also help. If these measures fail to relieve the pain, your doctor may advise you to enroll in a pain treatment facility.

Pain Treatment Facilities

Currently, more than 1,500 pain treatment facilities in the United States offer programs for people with chronic pain, including back pain. These programs do not aim to cure the cause of pain. Rather, they use a variety of approaches to reduce or eliminate pain and its negative effects on daily life.

People generally turn to pain treatment facilities when they have run out of other options. These facilities can help individuals living with chronic pain to improve both their physical and mental coping skills. The programs focus on managing the following:

- Pain behavior—actions that worsen the quality of life, such as limping, moaning, moving slowly, or using a cane
- Self perception—perceiving oneself as impaired or having a disability
- Pain perception—a discrepancy between how much pain a person feels and how much his or her condition typically produces

• Mental health problems—depression, anxiety, drug or alcohol dependence (about 25% of chronic pain sufferers become dependent on pain-control medication), and impaired memory or concentration.

Pain facilities are generally not advised for people who have unstable medical conditions (such as uncontrolled high blood pressure or heart failure) or unrealistic expectations (such as finding a total cure) or those who are unwilling to participate in a formal program.

There are several types of pain facilities. Some focus on a single treatment method, such as acupuncture, while others target pain in a particular region of the body. There are also multidisciplinary pain centers or clinics, which doctors usually prefer because they offer a more comprehensive approach and have shown superior results in medical studies. Multidisciplinary centers view pain as a complex syndrome. Therefore, they provide an integrated treatment team that generally includes a primary care physician, surgeon, psychologist or psychiatrist, nurse, physical therapist, occupational therapist, vocational counselor, and social worker.

Since the quality of care varies from one program to another, finding the right one can take some time. Your doctor may be able to recommend a facility, or you can contact the Commission on Accreditation of Rehabilitation Facilities, which will provide a list of accredited programs near you (see page 82 for contact information). Although accreditation is not required, accredited programs tend to be comprehensive. In addition, some insurance plans only cover accredited facilities. The American Pain Society also can provide information about pain centers in your area (see page 82). In addition, the following tips may be helpful in your search:

• Programs located in hospitals and rehabilitation centers are most likely to offer comprehensive treatment. For the most specialized care, they should be located in a separate unit specifically set aside for the pain program.

• The program should include most of these features: biofeedback training, individual and family counseling, group therapy, occupational therapy, assertiveness training, regional anesthesia (nerve blocks), physical therapy, relaxation training and stress management, educational programs on medication and other aspects of pain management, and follow-up care after program completion.

• Make sure the program encourages family involvement. Educational sessions and joint counseling for your family members can help them to better understand your pain and the best ways to support you.

NEW RESEARCH

What's the Best Exercise for Chronic Back Pain?

Doctors commonly prescribe exercise for lower back pain. Now a new study sheds light on which type provides the greatest pain relief—at least for the short term.

The researchers randomly assigned 240 adults with low back pain for at least three months to one of three groups: general exercise, motor control exercise, or spinal manipulative therapy.

The general-exercise group performed strengthening and stretching exercises as well as exercises to improve cardiovascular fitness. The motor control–exercise group performed exercises aimed at improving the function of specific trunk muscles thought to be involved in movement of the spine. These included the diaphragm, the transversus abdominis, and the pelvic floor muscles. People in the spinal manipulative therapy-group were treated with joint mobilization or manipulation techniques applied to the spine or pelvis.

At eight weeks, people in the motor-control group and the spinal manipulative therapy group improved slightly more than those in the general-exercise group, with a better ability to function and a greater perception of benefit from treatment. However, at six and 12 months, there were no differences between any of the groups.

The bottom line: A variety of exercises can provide relief for chronic low back pain. Whichever you choose, you'll likely need to continue it for long-term relief.

PAIN
Volume 131, page 31
September 2007

• Find out what services your health insurance policy will reimburse.

• Try to meet with several staff members before you enter a program. The medical director should have board certification and training in pain management. Ask about the physical setup, whether the program is inpatient or outpatient, the duration of the program (and length of any inpatient stay), and whether job retraining is involved. You may also consider asking whether any current participants would be willing to speak to you about their experience.

• Make sure the program reviews your previous medical records and gives you a complete physical exam before entry. Bring copies of your recent medical records.

Neck Pain

The cervical spine, located in the neck, is subject to many of the same problems that plague the lower back—muscle strains and spasms, disk degeneration and denervation, and spinal stenosis. About 10–15% of people experience neck pain at any given time. Most neck pain is short lived and gets better on its own or with simple self-care measures. But sometimes neck pain is a red flag for a more serious problem.

Causes

The neck supports the weight of the head, which can be 10 lbs or more. Although the head should be centered over the spine when we sit or stand upright, countless activities—such as sitting at a computer, reading, watching television, or eating—cause people to slump, rounding their upper back and tilting their head forward. This can lead to muscle strain or spasm in the neck. Muscle strain or spasm can also arise from constantly looking over or under one's glasses, having poor sleeping posture, or taking long car trips.

General wear and tear from everyday activities and normal aging can cause changes in the disks of the neck that lead to pain and stiffness. For example, herniation of the intervertebral disks in the neck can decrease the space through which nerves exit the spinal canal, leading to pinched nerves and consequent pain. Bony outgrowths on the vertebrae (called osteophytes) also can pinch nerves. Spinal stenosis can put pressure on the spinal cord, causing pain or paralysis. Despite these possible causes of neck pain, most people with the problem do not have a herniated disk, osteophytes, or a disease that affects the spinal cord. Rather, neck pain is typically the result of muscle strain or spasm, as described on the previous page.

On occasion, neck pain can result from acceleration/deceleration injuries, commonly known as whiplash. It can also stem from serious problems like arthritis or cancer or from problems that originate in other areas of the body such as the shoulder. Chronic neck pain unassociated with any physical problem may result from associated stress or depression.

When To See a Doctor

Many cases of neck pain get better on their own. If neck pain is linked to a recent recreational or work-related activity, the pain will likely decrease within two weeks, and treatment from a doctor is usually unnecessary. However, you should see a doctor if your neck pain follows a serious injury, lasts longer than two weeks, or is accompanied by the following:

- Headaches, fever, or weight loss
- Pain that worsens at night
- An inability to touch your chin to your chest
- Difficulty walking, clumsiness, or weakness
- Pain, numbness, or tingling sensations in your fingers, arms, or legs
- Problems with bladder, bowel, or sexual function
- Discomfort or pressure in your chest.

Diagnosis

If you do seek help for neck pain from a physician, your evaluation will include a medical history, a physical examination, and, if needed, imaging tests. During the physical exam, the doctor will likely measure your reflexes, range of motion, sensation, strength, and muscle and nerve function in your neck, arms, and legs.

If pain is the only symptom, and it does not radiate beyond the neck, imaging studies are usually not necessary. In this instance, the neck pain is likely temporary and requires no invasive treatment. However, for people with a traumatic injury, rheumatoid arthritis, or a physical exam that does not pin down the cause of the pain, imaging studies may be needed. Imaging tests include x-rays, MRI scans, and CT scans. Further options may include electromyography and nerve conduction tests to assess the combined function of the muscles and nerves. People with intense pain that lasts for months may need further evaluation to rule out cancer.

Treatment

Treatment may be needed if neck pain does not get better on its own. If this is the case, noninvasive measures are generally tried first, beginning with over-the-counter medications such as acetaminophen (Tylenol) to treat pain or NSAIDs for pain and inflammation. Applying cold (especially in the initial stages of pain) and heat (in the later stages) can be helpful. Bed rest, reducing physical activity, and immobilizing the neck with a cervical collar may relieve pain in some people. (Cervical collars are available at surgical supply stores but should be used for no more than 10 days to avoid weakening the neck muscles.)

Range-of-motion exercises and massage also can be helpful. A physical therapist can teach you appropriate neck stretches and exercises for the shoulders and upper back to help ease neck pain and prevent future episodes. (Warning: Traditional neck-rolling exercises are not recommended.) Your doctor or physical therapist may also instruct you on how to correct detrimental aspects of your posture or the setup of your office.

If two weeks of conservative treatment do not alleviate your neck pain, muscle relaxants, ongoing physical therapy, or spinal manipulation (chiropractic) may be recommended. Another option is a cervical traction device, which uses weights and pulleys to help relieve pressure on the neck. The device is available at surgical supply stores.

For those whose neck pain appears to be caused by stress or depression, stress-management techniques or antidepressants are often useful. In addition, your doctor may prescribe corticosteroid medications (either oral or injected) to reduce inflammation.

Even people with disk herniation or mild spinal stenosis should be treated first with conservative measures if the pain does not radiate beyond the neck. If no treatment has successfully relieved the neck pain after eight weeks or if imaging studies indicate serious structural problems, you may need to consult with a spinal surgeon (a neurosurgeon or an orthopedic surgeon). Surgery involves relieving pressure on the spinal cord or the pinched nerve. Up to 90% of people who undergo surgery for neck pain experience significant pain relief.

OSTEOPOROSIS

The word osteoporosis means porous bone. A person with osteoporosis typically has low bone mass, poor bone quality, and fragile bones. This combination, together with the increased risk of falling among older people, leads to painful fractures and other health problems.

About 10 million Americans—eight million women and two million men—already have osteoporosis, and 34 million more are at increased risk because of low bone mass (osteopenia). Osteoporosis-related fractures are estimated to account for $13.8 billion in hospital and nursing home costs each year, and these costs are increasing. As our population continues to age (more than 35% of Americans will be age 50 or older by 2011), osteoporosis is expected to become an even greater health problem.

Structure of the Bones

Bones are not stable, solid structures that do not change with time, although that's what many people think. Bone is actually a living tissue that undergoes a constant process of renewal and rebuilding. In this process, called bone remodeling, old bone is resorbed (broken down) and new bone is formed (see "How Bones Form and Repair" on page 49).

The framework of each bone is a matrix, or scaffold, that is primarily composed of collagen. Collagen is soft but hardens as calcium and phosphorus are deposited. A regular supply of these minerals, which enter the bone from the bloodstream, is required to keep bones strong.

In the resorption stage of bone remodeling, special cells called osteoclasts invade the surface of the bone and remove both the matrix and minerals, leaving small cavities in the bone surface. This stage is followed by bone formation, which is carried out by another set of special cells, called osteoblasts, which fill in the cavities with new bone. The entire process takes three to six months, which is why broken bones take some time to heal—and why it takes time to assess whether an osteoporosis treatment is working.

When the rate of bone loss exceeds the rate of bone formation, the result is low bone mass. Because bone mass is difficult to measure noninvasively, the closely related value of bone mineral density (BMD) is used instead. BMD can be measured with a variety of x-ray techniques.

Bone quality also plays a role in bone strength. Bone quality refers to the overall architecture of bone, which can vary from person to person. Because no noninvasive procedure currently can determine bone quality, measuring BMD is the best way to identify osteoporosis and predict a person's risk of fractures.

NEW RESEARCH

Diabetes Drug Accelerates Bone Loss in Postmenopausal Women

The diabetes drug rosiglitazone (Avandia) appears to inhibit bone formation and accelerate bone loss in postmenopausal women, according to a recent study.

Researchers recruited 50 healthy postmenopausal women age 55 or over to take Avandia (8 mg daily) or placebo (inactive drug) for 14 weeks. Within one month in those who took Avandia, two markers of bone formation—P1NP and osteocalcin—fell by 13% and 10%, respectively. However, these markers remained stable in the placebo group. Both groups experienced a decline in bone mineral density (BMD) at the hip, but the reduction in the Avandia group was nearly 2% greater. And while women taking placebo saw little change in spine BMD, for those in the Avandia group, spine BMD dropped significantly from baseline.

Avandia and similar drugs, called thiazolidinediones, are used in conjunction with diet and exercise to improve blood sugar control in adults with type 2 (non-insulin-dependent) diabetes. The U. S. Food and Drug Administration recently added warning labels about the risks of heart failure for all thiazolidinediones and is also investigating information that Avandia may increase the risk of heart attacks.

If you're postmenopausal and take Avandia for diabetes, talk to your doctor about the implications for your bone health.

THE JOURNAL OF CLINICAL ENDOCRINOLOGY AND METABOLISM
Volume 92, page 1305
April 2007

Causes of Osteoporosis

Many women are at risk for developing osteoporosis, and that risk increases as they grow older. Women are more susceptible than men, because they have less total bone mass to begin with and because estrogen plays a vital role in bone health. As the production of natural estrogen drops off during menopause, the rate of bone loss begins to pull ahead of the rate of bone formation. Yet age and gender aren't the only risk factors to consider.

While some risk factors for osteoporosis can be controlled, others cannot. Risk factors that cannot be changed include:

- A history of fracture as an adult (especially after age 40)
- A history of fracture in a first-degree relative (male or female)
- Ethnicity (white and Asian women are at greater risk than women in other ethnic groups).

Risk factors that *can* be changed include:

- Smoking
- Low body weight (under 127 lbs)
- Low levels of estrogen in women and low levels of testosterone in men
- Prolonged low calcium and vitamin D intake
- Eating disorders
- Lack of exercise (or its opposite, excessive exercise that leads to missed menstrual periods during a woman's premenopausal years).

One of the main determinants of osteoporosis risk is family history. The genes that are important in determining susceptibility to osteoporosis have not been fully identified, but they may account for as much of 70% of osteoporosis risk. If you have a family history of osteoporosis, you should have your BMD measured to help determine your risk.

In addition to the factors listed above, osteoporosis can be caused by certain medications or other diseases. This is referred to as secondary osteoporosis. For instance, many people with severe asthma, rheumatoid arthritis, inflammatory bowel disease, or multiple sclerosis take corticosteroids, which are a common cause of osteoporosis. Other drugs that can cause osteoporosis include anticonvulsant drugs, which are used to treat epilepsy, and inappropriately high doses of thyroid hormone replacement. Studies have linked a high intake of vitamin A from retinol with increased risk of fractures among both men and postmenopausal women, although vitamin A from beta-carotene does not appear to affect fracture risk.

How Bones Form and Repair

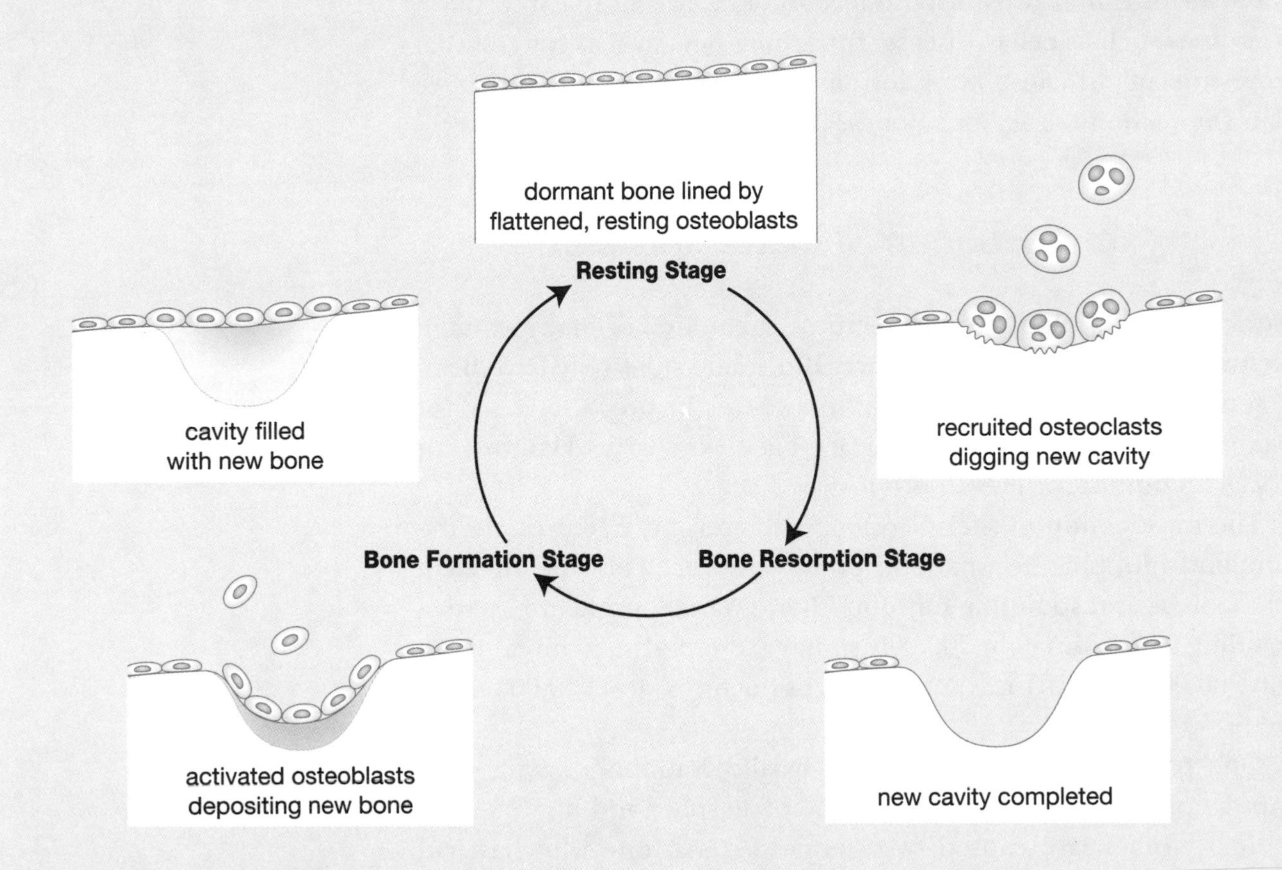

Many people think of their bones as stable structures that do not change with time. But bone is a living tissue that undergoes a constant process of renewal. In this process, called bone remodeling, old bone is resorbed (broken down) and new bone is formed.

The framework of each bone is a matrix, or scaffold, that is mostly made up of collagen. Although collagen is soft, it hardens with the deposition of calcium and phosphorus, which enter the bone from the bloodstream. A regular supply of these minerals is required to keep bones strong.

In the resorption stage of bone remodeling, special cells called osteoclasts invade the surface of the bone and remove both the matrix and minerals, leaving small cavities in the bone surface. Resorption is followed by the bone formation stage, which is carried out by another set of special cells, called osteoblasts, which fill in the cavities with new bone.

When bone loss outpaces bone formation, the result is low bone mass. When there is less bone, bones become more fragile and are more prone to fracture. Osteoporosis is a disease of severely low bone mass. ■

Certain other hormonal disorders, including an overactive thyroid gland (hyperthyroidism), Cushing's syndrome, and an overactive parathyroid gland (hyperparathyroidism), can cause bone loss in men and women. Inflammatory diseases such as inflammatory bowel disease (Crohn's disease and ulcerative colitis), lupus, and rheumatoid arthritis can also contribute to bone loss, as can malabsorption syndromes such as celiac disease. Intriguing new studies suggest that depression might cause bone loss, and ultimately, osteoporosis (see "Can Depression Break Your Bones?" on pages 54–55).

Complications of Osteoporosis

Osteoporosis is a silent, usually painless, saboteur. For many women, the first sign of trouble is a fracture. But subtle signs may have been present for some time—a gradual loss of height over the years, for instance, the rounding of the upper back (known as kyphosis, or dowager's hump), or even tooth loss.

The most common sites of osteoporosis-related fractures are the spine and hip, but the wrist and other bones may also be affected. Osteoporosis is responsible for more than 1.5 million fractures a year, including approximately 700,000 spinal (vertebral) fractures, more than 300,000 hip fractures, 250,000 wrist fractures, and 300,000 other fractures.

One panel of experts convened by the National Osteoporosis Foundation estimated that at least 90% of all spine and hip fractures in older women are caused by osteoporosis. Anyone who has had one osteoporosis-related fracture is at very high risk for a second.

Some people think that men can't get osteoporosis. That is simply not true. Before age 60, fractures are more common in men than in women, likely because of injuries related to sports and accidents. Although the prevalence of fractures increases in men after age 60, their rate is still less than half that of women of the same age. This is because men enter adulthood with greater bone mass than women—and women rapidly lose bone mass during the first three to five years after a natural or surgical menopause (or any other cause of estrogen deficiency).

The most commonly identified risk factors for osteoporosis in men are excessive alcohol intake, use of corticosteroid drugs (such as prednisone or dexamethasone), and hypogonadism (testosterone deficiency). If a man does develop osteoporosis, a thorough medical evaluation should be performed to determine the underlying cause.

Osteoporosis in a premenopausal woman or in any woman who is not responding to treatment also warrants evaluation for secondary causes of the disease.

Vertebral Compression Fractures

Compression fractures in people with weakened vertebrae are usually caused either by falling or by placing a load on outstretched arms (for example, by raising a window or lifting a small child or bag of groceries). Such spinal fractures typically cause the front of the vertebrae to collapse.

Bone loss in the spine takes place rapidly around the time of menopause, and estimates suggest that 25% of American women over the age of 50 experience one or more compression fractures of their vertebrae in their lifetime. Men account for approximately one seventh of the vertebral compression fractures associated with osteoporosis.

A vertebral compression fracture due to osteoporosis is accompanied by intense, localized back pain in about 80% of cases, though there may be no pain until a few days after the fracture. When pain does develop, it can be severe enough to incapacitate a person for several weeks. The pain worsens during activities that involve twisting or bending and initially does not ease up, even with bed rest.

Typically, the pain will resolve after several weeks with the use of mild analgesics and rest. The pain may continue and get worse, however, if the bone fails to heal because of a loss of blood supply or if the vertebral deformity that results from the fracture either accelerates degenerative changes in the facet joints or compresses a nerve root.

A frequent problem immediately following a fracture in the lower lumbar region is difficulty with urination and bowel movements. Fortunately, this is temporary.

Longer-term repercussions include stooped posture as well as loss of height. These structural changes reduce the amount of space available for vital organs such as the stomach and lungs. Compression of the stomach causes the abdomen to protrude and creates a sensation of indigestion or fullness that may lead to weight loss, while compression of the chest cavity leads to a reduction in lung capacity that can contribute to breathlessness or lung disease.

Structural changes caused by vertebral compression fractures also weaken the spinal extensor muscles, leading to fatigue. In addition, they can cause concerns about physical appearance and

NEW RESEARCH

Six Factors Predict Need for X-ray in Suspected Vertebral Fracture

A simple assessment can help doctors determine whether an older woman with osteoporosis and back pain needs an x-ray of the spine to detect a vertebral fracture.

For this study, investigators recruited 410 postmenopausal women, average age 74, who had osteoporosis and back pain. Using a 16-point index, which gave a numerical rating to each of six factors—age, loss of height, intensity of back pain, pain in the middle or upper back, sudden onset of pain, and a history of nonvertebral fractures—the researchers were able to estimate the probability of vertebral fracture.

They found that in women with a score of 7 or higher, the probability of fracture was at least 43%. The strongest predictors of fracture were sudden pain and a loss of height of about 4 inches.

Vertebral fractures due to osteoporosis are common, but they often go unrecognized. But if you have osteoporosis and have been experiencing back pain—especially of sudden onset—ask your doctor whether a spine x-ray is in order.

ANNALS OF RHEUMATIC DISEASE
Volume 66, page 81
January 2007

make it difficult to find clothes that fit properly. All of these problems may lead to depression as well as difficulty sitting or sleeping. Rarely, a severe vertebral collapse may cause paralysis by exerting pressure on the spinal cord.

Hip Fractures

Many women fear hip fractures—and with good reason. Of all types of fractures, hip fractures have the most significant impact on the quality of life. An alarming 20–25% of people over age 50 who break a hip will die within a year.

In addition, 40% are unable to walk independently a year after they've broken a hip, and 60% are unable to perform basic activities of daily living, such as dressing themselves. Because of these devastating consequences, preserving and boosting bone mass and preventing falls and fractures are crucial.

A hip fracture usually occurs when a person falls from a standing position, with the hip taking the impact of the fall, although less traumatic falls also can cause hip fractures. Ninety percent of the 350,000 hip fractures that occur each year in the United States are the result of a fall.

The rate of hip fracture begins to increase at age 50, doubling every five to six years. Nearly half of the women who reach the age of 90 have suffered a hip fracture. Men account for nearly 30% of hip fractures.

The risk factors for a hip fracture are:

- Being older than 65
- Being female
- Having a family history of fractures later in life
- Low body weight
- Poor nutrition
- Smoking or excessive alcohol use
- Mental impairment
- Poor eyesight
- Unsteady balance
- Frailty (see "Are You Frail?" on pages 60–61).

The symptoms of hip fracture are not subtle. They include pain in the groin or buttock, inability to put weight on the leg on the affected side, or pain when trying to bear weight. Hip fractures may also interrupt the nerves or blood vessels that supply the leg.

All hip fractures require surgical repair or replacement, and treatment is often required for injuries related to the fall, such as head injuries.

Other Osteoporotic Fractures

Because osteoporosis affects bone mass throughout the skeleton, it can lead to fractures anywhere in the body. The type and location of the trauma usually determine the kind of fracture involved.

For example, falling on an outstretched hand can lead to a specific type of wrist and forearm injury known as a Colles' fracture (a break at the end of one of the bones in the forearm). The wrist, toes, and ribs are among the most common sites of osteoporotic fractures.

For someone with severe osteoporosis, simply sneezing or coughing may be enough to cause painful fractures of the ribs and spine. Such fractures can sometimes lead to deformities as well as pain.

Diagnosing Osteoporosis

The National Osteoporosis Foundation recommends that all women age 65 and older get screened for osteoporosis. In addition, postmenopausal women who are under age 65 but have additional risk factors for osteoporosis (such as use of corticosteroids or a family history of osteoporosis) or who have recently had a fracture should be screened. Although widespread screening of premenopausal and perimenopausal women is not generally recommended, it might be appropriate depending on your individual health profile.

An individualized approach to screening based on advancing age and risk factor profile is optimal. For instance, if you are a perimenopausal woman in your early 50s with several significant risk factors, such as smoking, low body weight, and white ethnicity, your doctor may feel that testing is warranted.

There are no official guidelines on when to screen men for osteoporosis, but some experts have suggested routine osteoporosis screening in some older men (see the "New Research" column at right).

Medical History and Physical Examination

During an osteoporosis examination, the doctor will take an inventory of risk factors, including family history, history of fractures, menstrual history, dietary history, medications, habits such as cigarette smoking and alcohol consumption, and a review of past illnesses. The physical exam includes an assessment of spinal tenderness and curvature, height measurement, and a search for signs of other medical conditions that may contribute to osteoporosis.

NEW RESEARCH

Is Osteoporosis Screening and Testing Worthwhile for Men?

Routine testing and treatment for osteoporosis may indeed make sense for certain older men, according to a new study.

Researchers used a computer program to estimate the risk of hip fracture for white males over age 65—the group of men with the highest risk of osteoporosis. They also estimated the direct medical costs and indirect costs, such as lost productivity, associated with an osteoporotic fracture in these men.

They found that it may be cost-effective to perform routine bone mineral density testing in men older than 65 years if they had had an earlier fracture and to test men over 80 regardless of their fracture history. Treatment with bisphosphonates, if needed, also would be cost-effective if the price of therapy were less than $500 per year.

Routine screening for osteoporosis is currently not recommended for older men in the United States. But if you have risk factors for the condition (long-term steroid use; chronic disease that affects the kidneys, lungs, stomach or intestines and alters hormone levels; low testosterone level; smoking; drinking excessive amounts of alcohol, consuming too little calcium or getting insufficient physical exercise) talk to your doctor about whether you might be a candidate for bone mineral density testing and medication for osteoporosis prevention or treatment.

JOURNAL OF THE AMERICAN MEDICAL ASSOCIATION
Volume 298, page 629
August 8, 2007

Can Depression Break Your Bones?

More and more evidence suggests it can. Here's what you can do about it.

Depression and osteoporosis often go hand in hand. Being depressed increases the risk of spine and hip fractures, and aging men and postmenopausal women who have fractures are more likely to be depressed than healthy people of the same sex and age who don't.

Doctors don't know which comes first, the depression or the osteoporosis. But most experts agree that diagnosing and treating this emotional problem is important to the health of your bones.

Examining the Link

There are many reasons why depression and osteoporosis might be related. For instance, when you are depressed, you might not follow a healthy lifestyle (such as eating right and being physically active), which could lead to bone loss. If you have osteoporosis and are also depressed, you may be less likely to take your medications, including the osteoporosis treatment and calcium pills your doctor prescribed. Another school of thought suggests that in people with depression, a complex interplay among certain hormones, the brain, and bones may actually induce osteoporosis. What's more, the two conditions share many risk factors. Not only poor nutrition and physical inactivity but also corticosteroid use and decreased estrogen and testosterone levels.

The Research Accumulates

How strong is the link between osteoporosis and depression? The evidence began to build in the early 1980s, and now there's little doubt that depression in women and men is intertwined with bone health. Just consider the following recent studies:

• The large National Osteoporosis Risk Assessment study identified risk factors for fractures in more than 170,000 postmenopausal women. In addition to traditional risk factors, such as a history of fractures, low BMD, and poor overall health, the researchers found that they could also use depression to predict who was more likely to develop a fracture. Women with depression were 26% more likely to suffer a fracture over a five-year period than were women who weren't depressed.

• Depression was also associated with hip fracture in a sample of more than 6,000 adult men and women who were interviewed as part of the National Health and Nutrition Examination Survey (NHANES). Those with a higher level of depressive symptoms were about twice as likely to have a hip fracture as those with lowers levels, even after taking into account other risk factors for a hip fracture.

• The Multiple Outcomes of Raloxifene Evaluation study included about 3,800 postmenopausal women who had osteoporosis and who had also been assessed for depression. The researchers reported that women who had at least three vertebral fractures were more than three times as likely to have symptoms of depression as were those without fractures (13% vs. 4%).

• A study of 320 postmenopausal women examined the effects of depression on bone mineral density (BMD). The

Laboratory Tests

In select cases, blood and urine tests may be required to evaluate for medical conditions that can lead to osteoporosis. Blood tests include those that measure levels of calcium, thyroid-stimulating hormone, parathyroid hormone, the enzyme alkaline phosphatase, and vitamin D, as well as kidney and liver function tests. Calcium and cortisol may be measured in the urine.

When active bone resorption occurs in people with osteoporosis or Paget's disease, the urine shows increased amounts of collagen byproducts—pyridinium cross-links and N-telopeptides—created by women who were the most depressed were also more likely to lose BMD in the hip than women who weren't depressed, even after the researchers took into account the influence of exercise, calcium supplements, and weight loss. After one year, the effect on BMD from depression was generally small (about 2%), but if such a loss persisted year after year, it could become substantial.

Are You Depressed?

If you're like many people, you may be reluctant to talk about depression with your doctor. But receiving treatment for depression can have a positive impact on your emotional and overall health, including your bones.

You have major depression if you have either of the first two symptoms below, plus any four others for more than two weeks:

- Feel depressed with overwhelming feelings of sadness and grief
- Lose interest and pleasure in activities you used to enjoy
- Have difficulty sleeping
- Feel less energetic or fatigued
- Experience significant changes in appetite or weight
- Have trouble concentrating
- Feel restless or run down
- Feel guilty or hopeless
- Have recurrent thoughts of death or suicide.

Treating Depression

If you have a major or milder form of depression, your treatment may include medication, psychotherapy (counseling or talk therapy), or a combination of both.

Medication. The most popular medications used to treat depression are the selective serotonin reuptake inhibitors, also known as SSRIs (for example, Prozac, Zoloft, and Paxil). Although doctors have traditionally believed that SSRIs are safe for people with osteoporosis, results from two studies published last year in the *Archives of Internal Medicine* raise some concerns. In the first study, involving more than 2,700 mostly elderly women, SSRI use nearly doubled the rate of bone loss at the hip compared with those who did not use these drugs. In the second study, which involved nearly 6,000 mostly elderly men, those who used an SSRI had lower spine and hip BMD levels, 6% and 4%, respectively, than men who did not use an SSRI.

The investigators speculate that a receptor common to both brain and bones is inhibited by the SSRIs, thereby increasing the chance that drugs in this category may affect bone density as well as feelings of depression.

SSRIs are not intended for long-term use. If your doctor prescribes an SSRI for depression, she or he can monitor you for bone loss while you are taking the medication. Alternatively, your doctor can prescribe another type of antidepressant.

Psychotherapy. Seeing a therapist for talk therapy can be helpful. It can improve the effectiveness of your antidepressant medication and you'll learn new ways of thinking about your problems that can help prevent depression from returning.

Other options. What else might help? Spending time with friends and family may be uplifting. Try to exercise. It can decrease your risk of developing depression and lower its severity when it occurs. An added benefit: Exercise is good for your bones, too. ■

the breakdown of bone. Urine tests for these substances (such as Osteomark) have been approved by the FDA and are commercially available, but their usefulness is not universally accepted.

Although tests for pyridinium cross-links and N-telopeptides are not required for a diagnosis of osteoporosis, they are useful in assessing a person's response to therapy, because they can gauge response after just a few months of treatment. By comparison, it takes much longer to assess response to therapy using x-ray tests such as DXA scans, which generally are not repeated until you have completed a full year of treatment.

Bone Mineral Density Tests

Bone mineral density (BMD) tests are performed in people who are at risk for osteoporosis or have experienced a suspicious fracture. These tests help doctors diagnose osteoporosis or osteopenia (low bone mass, a warning sign for osteoporosis). They can also predict a person's risk of fracture, monitor progression of bone loss over time, and observe how well osteoporosis treatments are working.

To measure BMD, your doctor can use a variety of techniques. Generally, these fall into two categories: tests that measure BMD in the central areas of the body (that is, the spine, hip, and total body) and those that measure BMD in peripheral areas (for example, the wrist, finger, shinbone, kneecap, and heel).

All of the BMD tests are painless and safe. While the central techniques are considered the most precise, they are more expensive than the peripheral tests, and the equipment is not portable. The type of test your doctor performs may reflect a balance between your needs and the availability of BMD equipment in your area.

After starting treatment for osteoporosis, you may undergo BMD testing at one year to monitor your response to the chosen therapy. After this point, retesting every two to three years is recommended. Your doctor may want you to be retested more often, however, if you're switching from one treatment to another or you continue to experience rapid bone loss.

Central techniques

Central BMD tests include dual-energy x-ray absorptiometry and quantitative computed tomography. (Dual-photon absorptiometry, an older test, is used only rarely today.)

Dual-energy x-ray absorptiometry (DXA). This technique is the "gold standard" for the measurement of BMD. As the name implies, it involves the use of two x-ray beams aimed at the bone. A computer analyzes the amount of energy that passes through the bone and uses the measurement to calculate BMD. The test takes about 20 minutes and involves a low radiation exposure.

In addition to providing an accurate baseline BMD measurement, DXA is a valuable test for monitoring BMD changes over time as well as a person's response to osteoporosis treatment. Although DXA is the best tool for measuring BMD in most people, it does not provide accurate spinal measurements in people with a spinal deformity, arthritis in the lower spine, or a history of spinal surgery. In addition, hip measurements are not accurate in a hip that has been replaced or contains metal hardware.

BMD results from DXA are given as a T-score, which reflects how much the BMD is above or below normal. In general, a T-score of -1.0 or higher is considered to be normal, and a T-score of -2.5 or lower indicates osteoporosis. A person with a score between -1.0 and -2.5 may eventually develop osteoporosis or be at risk for a future fracture. A person with a score in this range is considered to have osteopenia.

Quantitative computed tomography (QCT). This procedure is not well studied or standardized, but it is sometimes performed instead of DXA to analyze bone density in the spine. QCT is similar to a regular computed tomography (CT) scan, in which x-rays generate a series of cross-sectional pictures that create a three-dimensional image. QCT simply uses different software than standard CT to analyze BMD. It takes about 10–15 minutes to perform, exposes the body to more radiation than other central or peripheral bone measurement methods (including DXA), and generally costs more than DXA.

Peripheral techniques

Peripheral techniques used to measure BMD include quantitative ultrasound, peripheral dual-energy x-ray absorptiometry, radiographic absorptiometry, peripheral quantitative computed tomography, and single-energy x-ray absorptiometry. Quantitative ultrasound and peripheral dual-energy x-ray absorptiometry are the most widely used peripheral BMD tests. (Single-photon absorptiometry, an older test, is rarely used.)

In general, peripheral techniques are valuable for osteoporosis screening, but their lack of precision makes them less useful for following changes in BMD over time or tracking response to therapy. Moreover, they cannot measure BMD at the hip or the spine—the sites where fractures have the most serious consequences.

Quantitative ultrasound (QUS)

This new technique involves passing high-frequency sound waves through bone to measure its density in peripheral sites, such as the shinbone, heel, and kneecap. There is no exposure to radiation, and the screening takes less than five minutes. Recent research indicates that QUS may be as accurate as DXA in predicting fracture risk and diagnosing osteoporosis.

Peripheral dual-energy x-ray absorptiometry (pDXA)

This test is similar to a central DXA test except that it uses a portable machine and measures BMD in the finger, wrist, or heel. It takes less than five minutes to perform, and exposure to radiation is low.

ASK THE DOCTOR

Q. ***Why is it important to get my bone scans done at the same place, on the same machine, and preferably by the same technician?***

A. Your doctor is following recommendations from the International Society for Clinical Densitometry (ISCD)—a professional society dedicated to enhancing the knowledge and quality of bone densitometry among healthcare professionals.

The ISCD recommends that scanning be performed in this fashion to reduce the risk of inconsistencies in the way the test is performed and the results are interpreted. For example, even slight differences in the calibration of bone scanning machines could lead to different results. Also, technologists may use different techniques to perform the test. Even when the technique is performed in exact accordance with the manufacturer's recommendations, the results may vary from one operator to the next. Or technicians at one facility may not use the same terminology for reporting results as those at another location.

By consistently using the same machine, operated by the same technician, at the same facility, the chances for error in obtaining and interpreting your results are reduced, enabling your doctor to more accurately monitor your response to therapy.

Radiographic absorptiometry (RA)

Radiographic absorptiometry uses regular x-ray technology to determine BMD in the hand. The x-ray is taken with a "reference wedge" placed near the hand; this wedge has a known density with which the density of the bone in the hand is then compared. In general, the results of RA testing provide an accurate measure of bone density. RA takes just one to three minutes to perform, and the test involves only a small exposure to radiation.

Peripheral quantitative computed tomography (pQCT)

This test is similar to the central QCT scan, except that it is used to measure BMD in the wrist. The scan takes about 10 minutes, and the results are generally accurate. Peripheral QCT is less expensive than central QCT, and exposure to radiation is lower.

Single-energy x-ray absorptiometry (SXA)

This test is commonly used to determine BMD in the heel or wrist. The procedure is similar in principle to DXA, except that it uses one x-ray beam instead of two. SXA takes about 10–15 minutes, and the exposure to radiation is minimal.

Preventing Osteoporosis

Taking steps to prevent osteoporosis can help you avoid bone fractures and back problems later in life. Osteoporosis prevention relies on a three-pronged approach of exercise, proper nutrition, and—when appropriate—medication.

While women are more likely than men to develop osteoporosis, men, too, should get regular exercise, eat well, and minimize other risk factors.

Exercise

Exercise is extremely important for preventing osteoporosis. The more active you are, the stronger your bones will be. Certain types of exercise are more beneficial than others for preventing osteoporosis. Your exercise routine should include weight-bearing and resistance exercises and ideally should begin well before menopause.

In weight-bearing exercises—such as brisk walking, stair climbing, jogging, and dancing—the bones and muscles work against gravity and the feet, legs, and spine bear the body's weight. This type of exercise helps strengthen the lower body and spine. (In contrast,

NEW RESEARCH

Exercise Protects Against Hip Fractures in Men, Too

Older men who remain active have fewer hip fractures than their less active counterparts, and those who play sports regularly have the lowest risk of breaking a hip, according to a new study of more than 2,000 men followed for 35 years.

The men were divided into three groups based on how active they were during their leisure time. One group did mostly sedentary activities, a second group walked or rode bicycles for pleasure, and a third group played sports or did heavy gardening for three hours a week. Over the next 35 years, only 8% of the very active men had hip fractures compared with 13% of the moderate exercisers and 20% of the sedentary men.

Being active is an important way for postmenopausal women to prevent osteoporosis. Apparently, it's important for men, too. It doesn't take much—a brisk walk or bike ride for 30 minutes a few times a week—for men to get the benefits of exercise, including improved muscle strength and balance and a reduced risk of falls. If you want even more protection from a hip fracture, get into a regular tennis game or do some heavy gardening.

PLOS MEDICINE
Volume 4, page 1094
June 2007

while activities such as swimming and bike riding can be good for your joints and your heart, they are not weight-bearing activities and therefore should not be your only form of exercise.) Some reports suggest that people who perform weight-bearing exercises have bone mass that is 10% greater than those who do not exercise regularly.

In resistance exercises, the muscles work against weights. Either free weights (such as dumbbells) or weight machines can be used for resistance training. This type of exercise is ideal for building bone mass in the upper body, an area that is weak in most women. Proper instruction and technique for performing the exercises are essential to avoid injury.

Nutrition

While calcium is in the nutritional spotlight for its role in preventing osteoporosis, vitamin D also is essential. A number of other nutrients provided by a well-rounded, healthy diet play a role in building healthy bone as well.

Calcium

For men and women age 19–50, the recommended daily intake (known as the Dietary Reference Intake, or DRI) for calcium is 1,000 mg per day. After age 50, the recommended amount increases to 1,200 mg per day.

The best sources of calcium are low-fat milk and other dairy products. One cup of milk contains 300 mg of calcium, and one cup of plain, low-fat yogurt contains 415 mg. Low-fat dairy products contain slightly more calcium than their full-fat counterparts—low-fat milk actually contains slightly more than 300 mg of calcium per cup, while full-fat milk contains slightly less. But the real reason to choose low-fat products is to avoid excessive intake of saturated fat. If you have lactose intolerance (an inability to digest the naturally occurring sugars in milk) and dairy foods give you digestive problems, you will need to include other sources of calcium in your diet such as canned salmon with bones (3 oz contains 200 mg of calcium), leafy green vegetables, almonds, calcium-fortified cereals, and calcium-fortified orange juice.

Despite these dietary sources of calcium, surveys show that most people get less than the DRI for calcium from their diet. In fact, a dietary intake of only 400 mg of calcium per day is quite common. Although meeting the DRI is possible with careful dietary planning, most people need to take daily supplements that provide an additional 500–1,000 mg of calcium.

ASK THE DOCTOR

Q. ***I have osteoporosis. How should I limit my activity so that I do not break a bone?***

A. Contrary to what you might believe, most people with osteoporosis should actually do more physical activity, not less. Physical activity places an increased "load" or force, on bones. Bones respond by increasing in density. It's important to maintain a load on your bones to build up your bone density. That usually requires you to exercise at a moderate intensity for at least six months. Any gains in bone density will be lost if you stop working out.

Your workout should consist of weight-bearing exercises, such as walking, plus strength training using lightweight dumbbells, resistance bands, or exercise machines.

Before you start any exercise program, however, particularly if you are frail or have had a fracture, ask your doctor or physical therapist about the correct way to perform the exercises, and don't overdo it.

Also, the National Osteoporosis Foundation sells an exercise video titled "Be BoneWise—Exercise," which demonstrates routines designed specifically for people with osteoporosis. The exercises avoid movements that could be unsafe, such as twisting the spine or bending forward from the waist. Go to www.nofstore.org for more information.

Are You Frail?

Frailty is often preventable—and sometimes reversible

If you have osteoporosis or have suffered a broken hip or other fracture, you are susceptible to frailty. And being frail is more dangerous than you might think. Fortunately, however, the condition is not inevitable. Knowing the warning signs can help you correct or prevent problems before you become seriously ill or disabled.

Take this quiz to find out if you or someone you know is at risk.

- Have you lost 10 lbs without trying in the past year?
- Do you often feel exhausted?
- Is your grip strength weak?
- Do you walk very slowly?
- Do you get very little physical activity?

If your answer to two of these questions is "yes" you may be at risk for frailty. If you answered yes three or more times, you are frail.

A Downward Spiral

The five-question definition of frailty above was developed by Linda Fried, M.D., Director of the Center on Aging and Health at Johns Hopkins University, after evaluating more than 5,000 men and women age 65 and older. Initially, about 7% in the study met the definition of being frail. Three years later, twice as many in that group had been hospitalized or had fallen and three times as many had died, compared with those who were not frail. Why did this occur?

Older people often face a combination of factors that can set in motion a downward spiral that impacts their health and well-being. Multiple and complex illnesses and the medications used to treat them along with environmental factors, such as having difficulty shopping and cooking for yourself, may lead to poor eating habits. Ultimately, those poor eating habits lead to malnutrition, which leads to muscle weakness, which, in turn, causes a decrease in activity and even less incentive to eat well.

Muscle weakness can also lead to balance problems, falls, and subsequent injuries, including fractures. At the same time, the immune system becomes weaker with age and a poor diet, making recovery from illness or injury an even greater challenge. The situation becomes even more dire when memory or mental health issues complicate the picture.

The end result—if you are frail, you are more likely to become disabled, to be unable to live independently, to be admitted to the hospital, and to face an earlier death than a person of the same age who is not frail. Fortunately, experts on aging say that it is possible to forestall and, in many cases, prevent frailty from ever developing. It can even be reversed if caught in its earliest stages.

An Apple a Day

Good nutrition is one of the best ways to keep frailty at bay. U.S. Dietary Guidelines recommend that women over age 50 consume at least 1,600 and no more than 2,200 calories each day, depending on activity level. For men of the same age, the recommendation is 2,000–2,800 calories.

What should you eat? Ideally, you should eat at least 5 oz of grains (bread, rice, pasta, cereal—whole grains are best), two cups of vegetables, 1 1/2 cups of fruit, three cups of milk or yogurt (or 1 1/2 oz of cheese), and 5 oz of lean meat, poultry, or fish. One study by researchers from Tufts University found that frail older women who ate a wide variety of fruits and vegetables had more energy, had a higher intake of nutrients, weighed more, and had bigger arm muscles. If it's simply not possible for you to eat all of the food recommended, at least try to eat something from each of the five major food groups each day. Of course if you're on a restricted diet for medical reasons, follow your doctor's instructions.

While it's easy to say, "eat a balanced diet," it's not as easy to do, particularly as you age. If you're having trouble chewing, your dentist may need to adjust your dentures. Certain medications and age-related changes in your sense of taste and smell may reduce your appetite, so talk to your doctor about getting help for these problems. If you are unable to get to the store or to cook, find out if there are any programs in your neighborhood that serve or deliver meals. Also drink plenty of fluids to avoid dehydration. Water, low-sodium soups, and milk are all good sources.

Even if you eat right, and especially if you don't, it's smart to take a vitamin and mineral supplement. Dr. Fried's research suggests that the frail may have more vitamin and mineral deficiencies, in particular a lack of beta-carotene, than the general population.

Exercise Your Body and Mind

One of the keys to maintaining your health and independence is to stay physically and mentally active.

Be physically active each day. Exercise can improve many of the physical changes associated with frailty. That's because muscle strength, stamina, flexibility, and balance all improve with exercise. Multiple studies show that these improvements can occur within just weeks of starting to exercise. And the people who benefit the most are those who are the most frail. In one study of 100 frail nursing home residents, average age 87, Tufts University researchers found that those who did strength training exercises and took nutrition supplements for 10 weeks significantly improved their muscle strength. What's more, they could walk faster and climb stairs better than they could before startlng the exercise program.

If you're not active, start by increasing your physical activity, and build exercise into your day. For example, walk to the mailbox instead of driving to the post office or park further from the door and walk. Walking can improve heart fitness, balance, and muscle mass.

For the most benefit, follow an exercise routine consisting of:

- Resistance exercises, such as arm raises, using weights or bands to build muscle and increase bone strength
- Balance exercises, such as leg raises, to reduce your risk of falling
- Stretching exercises to improve your flexibility
- Aerobic exercises—any activity that increases your heart rate and breathing for an extended period—to improve your heart's ability to function.

Try tai chi. This ancient Chinese exercise consists of a series of movements and breathing exercises. Study results are mixed, but a number show that tai chi helps relieve pain, improve balance, and reduce the risk of falling in seniors.

While you're never too old to exercise, check with your doctor before starting an exercise program, especially if you have chronic conditions, such as diabetes or heart disease. Also, find out what precautions you need to take if you've had hip or knee replacement surgery.

Keep your mind active. Researchers report that significant mental deterioration is not inevitable as you age. However, older people with illnesses such as diabetes, depression, and hypertension are more likely than their healthy counterparts to experience memory loss. In addition to keeping your blood pressure, glucose, and cholesterol at normal levels, maintaining a cognitively challenged lifestyle can also help reduce your risk. For example, do crossword or number puzzles like Sudoku, read the newspaper or books, and play games like bridge or chess.

Fight Depression

A recent study from the *Canadian Journal on Aging* finds that elderly people with depression who live at home are more likely to be frail than those who aren't depressed. Other studies show that depression can cause frailty to progress quickly.

You have major depression if you experience either of the first two symptoms below, plus any four others for more than two weeks:

- Depressed mood and overwhelming sadness and grief
- Loss of interest in once pleasurable activities
- Sleep problems, such as insomnia, nearly every day
- Decreased energy or fatigue
- Significant weight loss or gain
- Inability to concentrate
- Feeling restless or run down
- Feeling guilty or hopeless
- Recurrent thoughts of death or suicide

The good news is that depression is treatable. If you think you might be depressed, talk to your doctor about treatment. Options include psychotherapy and medication. Even exercise can help relieve mild forms of depression.

Ward Off Infections

If you're a frail older adult, even a simple viral or bacterial infection can be dangerous because your immune system doesn't work as well as it used to. One of the most important things you can do is to get the recommended vaccinations. The Centers for Disease Control and Prevention (CDC) advises people over age 65 to get a flu shot yearly. The CDC also advises people over age 65 get a pneumococcal vaccination if they haven't received one previously and to get revaccinated five years after the initial vaccination. These vaccinations can help boost your immune system so you don't get the flu or pneumonia. And they could save your life; for example, the influenza vaccine can reduce the risk of serious complications or death from the flu by 70–80% in the elderly. ■

A variety of calcium supplements are available. Calcium carbonate and calcium citrate contain the highest percentage of calcium in each tablet, but calcium citrate is more readily absorbed from the intestine. You should take calcium carbonate pills with meals because this type of calcium is absorbed better in the presence of stomach acid.

Vitamin D

Many people neglect to take a proper amount of vitamin D. A recent study found that women with low blood levels of vitamin D were at increased risk for hip fracture. Without vitamin D, the body cannot absorb calcium properly.

A number of studies have confirmed that vitamin D intake helps prevent osteoporosis and lower the risk of fractures in older adults. Vitamin D not only helps with the absorption of calcium, but also aids in the biochemical process by which calcium turns into bone.

Most vitamin D is synthesized by the skin in response to sunlight. In nature, very few foods contain vitamin D. While some foods are fortified—especially breakfast cereals and milk products—studies have shown that the amount listed on the label does not always reflect the contents accurately.

The National Osteoporosis Foundation recommends that women and men under age 50 consume 400–800 IU of vitamin D per day. For people age 50 and over, 800–1,000 IU per day is recommended.

Other nutrients

A healthy diet rich in fruits and vegetables will provide plenty of phosphorus, magnesium, and vitamins C and K, all of which play a role in bone health.

Vitamin A caution

If you take a daily multivitamin, choose one that contains no more than 900 micrograms (mcg) of vitamin A for men and 700 mcg for women. Also make sure that at least 20% of its vitamin A is in the form of beta-carotene. As mentioned earlier, research suggests that a high intake of vitamin A from retinol might increase the risk of hip fractures in postmenopausal women; too much vitamin A has also been associated with fractures in men.

Hormone Replacement Therapy (HRT)

Among its many other effects on the female body, the hormone estrogen stimulates the bone-building ability of osteoblasts and suppresses the bone-destroying activity of osteoclasts. At menopause,

NEW RESEARCH

More Vitamin D May Maintain Muscle Strength

If you don't get enough vitamin D from the food you eat or from exposure to the sun, it may affect your ability to perform daily activities, a new study finds.

This study of nearly 1,000 people age 65 and over found that physical performance (ability to stand from a chair, stand in increasingly challenging positions, and walk at a normal pace) and grip strength were about 5–10% lower in those who had low levels of vitamin D.

Vitamin D deficiency is common; about one in four people over age 60 has low vitamin D levels. Older adults are particularly prone to low vitamin D levels because they may get less exposure to sunlight than younger adults and because their skin is less efficient in producing vitamin D from sun exposure.

The National Osteoporosis Foundation recommends that everyone over age 50 consume 800–1,000 IU of vitamin D each day. How can you get an adequate amount? Turn to vitamin-D fortified foods such as milk, juice, and cereals, and ask your doctor if you need a vitamin D supplement. But keep in mind that lengthy exposure to ultraviolet radiation from the sun is not a good way to get extra vitamin D because of the risks of skin cancer.

JOURNAL OF GERONTOLOGY: MEDICAL SCIENCES
Volume 62A, page 440
April 2007

when estrogen levels fall, women suddenly experience a rapid loss of bone and an increased risk of fractures.

Hormone replacement therapy (HRT) involves taking estrogen to treat menopausal symptoms, such as hot flashes, night sweats, and vaginal dryness. The most common HRT formulation also contains a synthetic form of progesterone to counteract the increased risk of uterine cancer in women who take estrogen alone. Women who have had a hysterectomy are able to take estrogen without progesterone.

In addition to easing the symptoms of menopause, HRT reduces the rapid loss of bone that accompanies it. The sooner HRT begins after menopause, the greater the preservation of bone.

However, the decision to use HRT should not be taken lightly. One of the most common forms of HRT, conjugated equine estrogen plus medroxyprogesterone (Prempro), has been found to increase the risk of breast cancer and cardiovascular events (such as heart attacks, strokes, and blood clots) when taken for several years. For this reason, women should not take HRT for any longer than needed to treat menopausal symptoms.

If a woman is concerned about bone loss and thinking about HRT, she should discuss her personal risk and benefit profile with her doctor. Despite the fact that HRT continues to be recommended for preventing osteoporosis, other drugs are available that can accomplish the same goal.

One final note: As soon as HRT is discontinued, bone loss will begin again. Thus it is important to assess the need for osteoporosis treatment before discontinuing HRT.

ASK THE DOCTOR

Q. ***Is there such a thing as too much calcium and vitamin D?***

A. Yes, there is. If your body gets too much calcium, the excess calcium can build up in the kidneys and put you at risk for developing painful kidney stones. Some people overdo calcium and vitamin D supplements, which can boost calcium levels higher than your body can handle. You are not likely to get too much calcium just from food, however.

If you're like most people, you may only get 400 mg of calcium in your daily diet. The National Osteoporosis Foundation recommends that you get 1,000 mg of calcium daily if you are under age 50 and 1,200 mg daily if you are over age 50. For vitamin D, the recommended daily amounts are 400-800 IU for those under age 50 and 800-1,000 IU for those over age 50.

In general, the safe upper limit for calcium is 2,500 mg per day and for vitamin D is 2,000 IU per day.

Testosterone in men

Men with abnormally low levels of testosterone, which can cause osteoporosis, can take testosterone replacement therapy to help preserve their bones. (For more information, see the "Treatment in Men" section on page 74.)

Osteoporosis Medications

Alendronate (Fosamax), risedronate (Actonel), ibandronate (Boniva), and raloxifene (Evista) are FDA approved for both preventing and treating osteoporosis, but they should be used for prevention only in people who are at high risk for osteoporosis. Zoledronic acid (Reclast) and calcitonin (Fortical, Miacalcin) are medications that are approved for the treatment, but not prevention, of osteoporosis.

Of the osteoporosis medications approved for prevention by the

FDA, alendronate, risedronate, and ibandronate belong to the bisphosphonate class of drugs, while raloxifene is a selective estrogen receptor modulator. (For more information on these drugs, see pages 66–67.) Even when taking medication to prevent osteoporosis, it is important to get plenty of exercise, calcium, and vitamin D.

Corticosteroid Caution

Because the prolonged use of corticosteroids such as prednisone can result in significant reductions in bone mass, the American College of Rheumatology (ACR) has issued guidelines for preventing osteoporosis in people taking corticosteroids for longer than six months (typically those with such disorders as severe asthma, rheumatoid arthritis, inflammatory bowel disease, or multiple sclerosis). Because prednisone dosages as low as 7.5 mg per day can result in bone loss and an increased risk of fractures, the lowest effective dose should always be used. In addition, corticosteroid formulations that are either applied to the skin or inhaled cause fewer side effects than those taken orally.

The guidelines suggest getting a BMD measurement when beginning steroid therapy (or as soon as possible thereafter), following the lifestyle recommendations, and possibly using one of the preventive medications discussed above. (The FDA has approved both alendronate and risedronate to prevent steroid-induced osteoporosis.) The ACR guidelines also suggest taking extra calcium—a total of about 1,500 mg a day—and 800 IU of vitamin D.

Treating Osteoporosis

Treatment of osteoporosis starts with the same three-pronged plan used for prevention: exercise, nutrition, and medication.

Exercise

Weight-bearing and resistance exercise can reduce fracture risk and build bone, even after osteoporosis is diagnosed. But you may need to take certain precautions. For instance, you may need to discontinue activities that put you at increased risk for falling, such as skiing.

While balance exercises do not help build bone, they can help you avoid falls and fractures. Be sure to discuss your exercise habits with your doctor. You may need to consult a physical therapist for guidance on developing an exercise regimen specifically tailored to your individual condition and ability.

Nutrition

Even if you are prescribed medication to treat your osteoporosis, a healthy diet still counts. In particular, continue to monitor your calcium and vitamin D intake.

Numerous published studies have shown that bone loss after menopause can be slowed or even stopped by calcium supplements, even when started as many as five years after menopause. There is no reason to believe that men don't derive similar bone benefits from calcium.

Perhaps even more important is the finding that bone fractures decrease when people's diets are supplemented with vitamin D alone or with a combination of vitamin D and calcium. (Older people tend to have low blood levels of vitamin D and its active byproducts, which promote the absorption of calcium from the intestine.) As previously noted, men age 50 and older and postmenopausal women should consume 1,200 mg of calcium and 800–1,000 IU of vitamin D per day.

Medication

Drugs approved for treating osteoporosis fall into the following general categories: bisphosphonates, selective estrogen receptor modulators, and hormone and hormone-like preparations. (The chart on pages 66–69 gives an overview of drugs approved for osteoporosis treatment.)

Bisphosphonates

The bisphosphonates are the drugs most often prescribed to treat and prevent osteoporosis. Bisphosphonates help to preserve bone mass by slowing down bone resorption. Clinical studies of these drugs have focused on their effect on BMD and fracture risk.

Members of this drug class include alendronate, ibandronate, risedronate, and zoledronic acid. Alendronate and risedronate are indicated for the treatment of postmenopausal osteoporosis in women, for corticosteroid-induced osteoporosis in both women and men, and for other types of osteoporosis in men. Ibandronate and zoledronic acid are indicated for the treatment of osteoporosis in postmenopausal women. As mentioned previously, some of these drugs are also approved for the prevention of osteoporosis (see pages 63–64).

Although not approved for treating osteoporosis, three other bisphosphonates—etidronate (Didronel), pamidronate (Aredia), and tiludronate (Skelid)—are used for this purpose.

Combined estrogen replacement and bisphosphonate therapies

FDA APPROVAL

FDA Approves Once-Yearly Bisphosphonate for Osteoporosis

Taking your osteoporosis medication once a year might sound too good to be true, but the U. S. Food and Drug Administration has approved I.V. zoledronic acid (Reclast), the first and only once-yearly treatment for postmenopausal osteoporosis.

The approval was based on a three-year study showing that Reclast reduces the frequency of fractures in areas of the body typically affected by osteoporosis, including the hip, spine, wrist, arm, leg, and rib. In a trial of more than 7,700 postmenopausal women, Reclast reduced spine fractures by 70% and hip fractures by 41%. Investigators in this study also reported an increased risk of serious atrial fibrillation (abnormal heart rhythm), usually occurring more than 30 days after infusion, among Reclast users compared with the placebo group.

Reclast belongs to a class of drugs called bisphosphonates. Unlike other bisphosphonates taken in pill form, Reclast is given as a once-yearly 15-minute infusion into a vein.

More than half of all postmenopausal women taking daily or weekly bisphosphonates discontinue treatment at the end of one year, which may increase their risk of fractures. If you can't tolerate taking oral bisphosphonates or you find it difficult to remember to take your medication, ask your doctor about the benefits and risks of once-yearly treatment.

THE NEW ENGLAND JOURNAL OF MEDICINE
Volume 356, page 1809
May 3, 2007

Drugs To Treat Osteoporosis 2008

Drug type: Brand (generic)	Typical dosages*	How to take	How they work
Bisphosphonates			
Actonel (risedronate)	5 mg/day or 75 mg 2x/week on consecutive days	*Actonel and Fosamax*: Swallow pills whole with a full glass of plain water (not mineral water, juice, or coffee) at least 30 minutes before breakfast. Do not eat or drink anything but water and remain upright (sitting or standing) for 30–60 minutes after taking. Do not take with other medications. *Oral Boniva only:* Wait 60 minutes after taking before consuming food, more water, or other medications. *Intravenous Boniva:* 15- to 30-second injection into a vein.	*Actonel, Boniva, Fosamax, and Reclast*: Reduce fracture risk by inhibiting cells that break down bone tissue (osteoclasts) and helping preserve bone mass. Vitamin D in Fosamax plus D promotes calcium absorption.
Actonel plus calcium	35 mg 1x/week plus 500 mg elemental calcium 6x/week		
Boniva (ibandronate)	2.5 mg/day or 150 mg 1x/month		
Intravenous Boniva (ibandronate)	3 mg 1x/3 months		
Fosamax (alendronate)	10 mg/day or 70 mg 1x/week		
Fosamax plus D (alendronate/vitamin D)	70 mg plus 2,800 or 5,600 IU vitamin D/week		
Reclast (zoledronic acid)	5 mg 1x/year	*Reclast*: Administered intravenously over at least 15 minutes in a doctor's office, hospital, or clinic. On the day of treatment, eat and drink normally, which includes drinking at least 2 glasses of fluid, such as water, within a few hours of the infusion as directed by your doctor.	
Selective estrogen receptor modulator (SERM)			
Evista (raloxifene)	60 mg/day	Take any time with or without food.	Like HRT, replaces estrogen no longer produced by the ovaries. Acts selectively at the bone but not in the breast and uterus.
Recombinant human parathyroid hormone			
Forteo (teriparatide)	20-mcg injection 1x/day	Subcutaneous injection into thigh or abdomen.	Stimulates new bone formation, leading to increased bone mineral density and reduced risk of fractures.
Hormonal bone resorption inhibitors			
Fortical, Miacalcin (calcitonin–salmon)	200-IU spray 1x/day	Alternate nostrils daily.	Inhibits bone resorption and preserves bone mass.
Miacalcin IV (calcitonin–salmon)	100-IU injection 1x/day	Subcutaneous injection into thigh or abdomen.	

* These dosages represent an average range for the prevention or treatment of osteoporosis. The precise effective dosage varies from person to person and depends on many factors. Do not make any change in your medication without consulting your doctor.

Precautions	Most common side effects	Call your doctor if...
Actonel, Boniva, and Fosamax: Prevent esophagitis by taking pill as directed at left. Can (rarely) cause osteonecrosis of the jaw. Not recommended for those with kidney insufficiency or who cannot sit upright for at least 30 minutes (except intravenous Boniva). Consult your doctor to ensure that you are getting the appropriate amount of vitamin D and calcium in your supplements and diet.	*Actonel:* flu syndrome, chest pain, diarrhea, abdominal pain, nausea, constipation, difficult urination, swelling, joint pain, headache, dizziness, rash. Occasionally users have reported severe muscle or joint pain. *Boniva:* diarrhea, arm or leg pain, upset stomach. Intravenous form may cause mild reaction at injection site. *Fosamax:* abdominal pain, flu-like symptoms.	*Actonel, Boniva, and Fosamax*: You have kidney problems or a history of stomach problems, are taking NSAIDs or aspirin, develop chest or abdominal pain, heartburn, or difficulty swallowing, develop an exposed area on the jaw bone that fails to heal or is painful.
Reclast: You should not receive Reclast if you are already receiving Zometa. Reclast and Zometa are the same medicine. They both contain zoledronic acid. If you have severe kidney problems, you should not receive Reclast.	*Reclast*: Fever, flu-like symptoms, muscle and joint pain, nausea, fatigue, headache.	*Reclast*: You experience symptoms of low blood calcium (numbness or tingling, especially around the mouth, or muscle spasms) after receiving Reclast, or if you have persistent pain or a nonhealing sore of the mouth or of the jaw, or if any of the most common side effects persist.
Contraindicated in women with severe liver problems or a history of blood clots. May (rarely) cause blood clots in veins or lungs. Avoid extended immobility. Should not be used along with HRT.	Hot flashes, leg cramps.	You have a history of stroke or have stroke risk factors. You develop leg pain; swelling of hands, feet, or legs; redness; chest pain; shortness of breath; vision problems; hot flashes.
Use for more than 2 years is not advised. May predispose people to digitalis toxicity. Has caused cancer in rats. Not to be used in people with a history of skeletal radiation, cancer metastasis to bone, or Paget's disease.	Nausea, dizziness, leg cramps, gout, mild reactions at injection site.	You are taking digitalis, you have had bone cancer, bone radiation, Paget's disease, or high blood calcium, you develop nausea, vomiting, constipation, lethargy, muscle weakness.
Fortical: After 30 doses, spray bottle may not deliver accurately.	*Miacalcin:* nausea, flushing, redness at injection site. *Fortical:* nasal irritation or dryness, back pain.	You develop skin rash, hives, swelling of face or throat.

Chart continued on next page

Drugs To Treat Osteoporosis 2008 (continued)

Drug type: Brand (generic)	Typical daily dosages*	How to take	How they work
Hormone replacement therapy (HRT) for women			
Activella (estradiol/ norethindrone acetate)	1 tablet (1 mg/0.5 mg)/day	Continuously; do not skip a week.	Replaces the estrogen no longer produced by the ovaries in postmenopausal women, thereby preserving bone mass.
Cenestin, Premarin (estrogen, conjugated)	0.3–1.25 mg/day	Continuously or 25 days on, 5 days off, as prescribed.	
Estratest, Estratest HS, Menest (estrogen, esterified/ methyltestosterone)	1 tablet (1.25 mg/2.5 mg)/day; HS form: 1 tablet (0.625/1.25 mg)/day	Daily for 3 weeks, then no tablets for 1 week.	
Estrace, Gynodiol (estradiol)	0.5–2 mg/day	23 days on, 5 days off.	
Premphase (estrogen, conjugated/ estrogen, conjugated + medroxyprogesterone)	0.625 mg/day estrogen; 0.625 mg estrogen/5 mg medroxyprogesterone 1x/day	Estrogen pill for 14 days, then combined pill for 14 days.	
Prempro (estrogen, conjugated/ medroxyprogesterone)	0.3 mg/1.5 mg 0.625mg/2.5 mg	One pill daily.	
Alora Climara Estraderm Menostar Vivelle (transdermal estradiol)	0.75–3.0 mg 2x/week 2.0–7.6 mg/week 0.05–0.1 mg 2x/week 1 mg/week 2.19–8.66 mg 2x/week	Apply patch to abdomen, buttock, or hip. Use continuously if you have had a hysterectomy; 3 weeks on, 1 week off if you have a uterus.	
Hormone replacement therapy (HRT) for men			
Androgel 1% (testosterone gel)	5–10 g gel/day	Apply in the morning to upper arms. Let dry before you dress. Do not bathe, shower, or swim for 2 hours or more after applying Testim or for 5–6 hours after applying Androgel.	May help preserve bone mass by boosting testosterone levels, which decline in aging men.
Testim 1% (testosterone gel)	5–10 g gel/day		
Striant (transdermal testosterone)	30-mg pellet 2x/day	Apply pellet morning and evening to the gum, just above an incisor tooth. Alternate sides of the mouth.	

* These dosages represent an average range for the prevention or treatment of osteoporosis. The precise effective dosage varies from person to person and depends on many factors. Do not make any change in your medication without consulting your doctor.

have a modest additive effect in boosting bone mass. Several trials have shown that women with existing osteoporosis have a greater increase in BMD when treated with combination therapy than with either drug therapy alone.

Oral bisphosphonates are not easily absorbed, and they may lead to gastrointestinal side effects such as indigestion, diarrhea, stomach

Precautions	Most common side effects	Call your doctor if...
Estrogen products should not be used in women with a history of blood clots or stroke; cancer of the breast, uterus, or ovaries; or in women who are pregnant. May increase risk of dementia, although this association is controversial. Women who have not had a hysterectomy should consider using products with progesterone; women who have had a hysterectomy can take estrogen without progesterone. Prempro and Premphase may cause gallbladder disease. Estratest may cause hepatitis. Have mammograms yearly. Stop taking these medications before surgery to avoid blood clots. For the sole purpose of osteoporosis prevention, estrogen-containing drugs should be considered only if other medications are not an option.	Nausea, vomiting, headache, hair loss, change in sexual drive, redness or swelling of the skin, acne, vaginal bleeding, breast pain. *Prempro or Premphase:* high blood pressure, high blood sugar, depression.	You develop breast lumps, changes in your speech, chest pain, shortness of breath, pain in your legs, unusual vaginal bleeding, vomiting, dizziness or faintness, changes in vision. *Estratest:* You develop pain, tenderness, or swelling in your abdomen or ankles, yellowing of the skin, hoarseness, acne, facial hair.
For use by men only. Contraindicated in men who have had cancer of the breast or prostate. May increase risk of prostate cancer in healthy older men and may cause fluid retention in men with liver, kidney, or heart problems. Wash hands afterwards to avoid exposing others. Do not apply to the abdomen.	*Androgel or Testim:* redness at application site. *Striant:* gum or mouth irritation, unpleasant taste. Also, more rarely: sleep apnea, depression, difficulty urinating.	You have had prostate, liver, kidney, heart problems, or you develop nausea, vomiting, sleep or breathing problems, ankle swelling, erections that last too long or are too frequent. *Striant:* You have diabetes.

pain, heartburn, nausea, and peptic ulcers (nonhealing defects in the stomach or small intestine) as well as muscle cramps. Some people may experience side effects with one bisphosphonate, but they are able to tolerate another. Generally, less frequent dosing may lead to fewer gastrointestinal side effects.

To improve the absorption of oral bisphosphonates and to reduce the risk of gastrointestinal and esophageal side effects, it is important to follow proper dosing procedures. First, the drug should be taken immediately after getting up in the morning, at least half an hour before eating or drinking anything besides water (even tea, coffee, fruit juice, or mineral water can interfere with absorption), and before taking any other medication. Be sure to drink at least 8 oz of water when taking the tablet, and sit or stand upright for at least 30 minutes afterward.

If you dislike taking alendronate or risedronate every day, discuss less frequent treatment regimens with your doctor. Once-weekly regimens (70 mg of alendronate or 35 mg of risedronate) appear to be just as effective as conventional daily dosing, and the once-weekly routine may minimize the risk of esophageal irritation. Risedronate is also now available in a 75-mg tablet that can be taken on two consecutive days each month. Ibandronate can be taken orally just once a month but evidence of protection against hip fracture is lacking.

If you cannot tolerate oral forms of bisphosphonates because of gastrointestinal side effects, intravenous (I.V.) forms are available. In 2006, the FDA approved an I.V. version of ibandronate, which is given every three months, and in 2007, it approved an I.V. version of zoledronic acid, which is given once a year (see the "New Research" column on page 65). Another I.V. bisphosphonate is pamidronate (Aredia). Although this drug has not been approved by the FDA for the treatment of osteoporosis and limited data on fracture reduction have been published, it has been shown to improve bone mass.

Recent reports have linked bisphosphonates to osteonecrosis of the jaw (ONJ), a condition that is manifest by exposed areas of jawbone in the mouth. Invasive procedures, such as dental extraction, can increase the risk of ONJ. This condition is rare (about 1 in 100,000 for oral bisphosphonate users), and most reported cases have been in people taking I.V. bisphosphonates in high doses for the prevention and treatment of bone metastases. Some dentists recommend discontinuing use of these drugs for one to two months before and after a tooth extraction or implant surgery, but evidence to support this advice is limited. For now, it's wise to get regular dental checkups and to inform the dentist if you're taking a bisphosphonate.

Selective estrogen receptor modulators

Raloxifene (Evista) is a member of a class of drugs called selective estrogen receptor modulators (SERMs), which articles in the popular press sometimes call "designer estrogens." SERMs mimic some, but not all, of the actions of estrogen while apparently providing the beneficial effects of estrogen without some of its negative effects.

Although raloxifene appears to increase bone density in the spine and the hip, studies have found significant fracture reduction only in the spine. Thus, if you have osteoporosis in the hip, raloxifene may not be the ideal medication for you.

The FDA recently approved raloxifene for the prevention of breast cancer in postmenopausal women with osteoporosis who are at high risk for the disease. Approval was based on findings from three clinical trials comparing raloxifene with placebo and a fourth comparing it with tamoxifen, which was the first drug approved by the FDA for the chemoprevention of breast cancer. In the first three trials, raloxifene reduced the risk of invasive breast cancer by 44–71% compared with placebo. In the Study of Tamoxifen and Raloxifene (STAR) trial, raloxifene was as effective as tamoxifen for preventing breast cancer in postmenopausal women who were at high risk for it. Both drugs reduced the risk of invasive breast cancer by about 50%.

Because of its lack of estrogen-like action on breast and uterine tissue, raloxifene does not cause the breast tenderness and vaginal bleeding frequently seen with estrogen therapy. In addition, raloxifene does not increase the risk of uterine cancer when given without progesterone. An additional benefit of raloxifene is its estrogen-like effect of lowering "bad" low density lipoprotein (LDL) cholesterol. Furthermore, there appears to be no increased risk of heart attack. Although studies have shown no increased risk of stroke, the number of serious strokes associated with raloxifene use was greater than the number reported with placebo.

Taking raloxifene does have some risks. As with estrogen therapy, there is an increased risk of serious venous thromboembolic events (the blocking of a blood vessel by a particle that has broken away from a blood clot), particularly in the first four months of therapy. Unlike estrogen, raloxifene does not relieve menopausal symptoms. In fact, in some studies, it increased the incidence of hot flashes.

Hormonal preparations

Estrogen, used alone or with progesterone, continues to play a role in osteoporosis treatment, despite concern about its side effects (see pages 66–69). If you take estrogen for osteoporosis, you should use the lowest possible dose that can prevent bone loss effectively.

Teriparatide. The only "anabolic" (related to the hormone testosterone) therapy for osteoporosis is teriparatide (Forteo), a synthetic

NEW RESEARCH

Soy Compound May Boost Bone Density

Adding a soy-based product to calcium and vitamin D supplements may improve the bone density of postmenopausal women at risk for osteoporosis.

In a recent study, 389 postmenopausal women with low bone density but not osteoporosis were randomly assigned to take either genistein (54 mg per day), an estrogen-like compound found in soy, or a placebo (inactive) pill along with calcium and vitamin D supplements. After two years, the women taking genistein had higher bone density than those taking the placebo. What's more, blood and urine tests showed that those taking genistein were losing less bone. The researchers did not assess whether genistein lowered their risk of fracture.

The women taking genistein did not have any thickening of the uterus lining, a potentially precancerous effect of estrogen. However, because genistein has estrogen-like properties, the researchers caution against its use in women at high risk for endometrial or breast cancer.

In this study, women taking genistein were significantly more likely to experience digestive symptoms, including upset stomach and constipation, than those taking placebo.

ANNALS OF INTERNAL MEDICINE
Volume 146, page 839
June 19, 2007

Is it Ever Okay To Stop Taking Your Osteoporosis Medication?

Continuous use can reduce your risk of fracture

Have you ever run out of your osteoporosis medication and waited days, weeks, or even months before you refilled the prescription? Such behavior is all too common. Half of all individuals with osteoporosis stop taking their medication for months at a time, then begin using it regularly again. But just as yo-yo dieting isn't a good way to lose and maintain weight, stopping and restarting prescription medicine for osteoporosis is not the best way to build and maintain your bones.

The cornerstones of drug therapy for osteoporosis are oral bisphosphonates: alendronate (Fosamax), ibandronate (Boniva), and risedronate (Actonel). Some oral bisphosphonates are meant to be taken daily, while others should be taken once a week or once a month. By faithfully following the prescribed regimen, you can reduce your risk of fracture by up to 60%. For the best results, the latest research suggests you'll have to keep up with that regimen for at least five years before you can consider stopping.

I Need a Vacation

Why do some people stop taking their osteoporosis medication? There are many possible reasons. For instance, you may not see any visible benefit from drug therapy; therefore, you may not feel motivated to continue. Or you might experience gastrointestinal side effects, such as upset stomach or heartburn, which lead you to discontinue your medications. Also, the dosing instructions can be difficult to follow.

If regular use is a problem, ask your doctor if you can switch to a less frequent regimen. Many studies show that the fewer doses of bisphosphonates you need to take, for example, weekly rather than daily, the more likely it is that you'll use them regularly. If oral bisphosphonates upset your stomach, intravenous preparations such as I.V. ibandronate (given every three months) or I.V. zoledronic acid (given yearly) are available.

Three-Quarter Time

If you're using a daily or weekly medication and you take it at least three out of every four weeks each month, you can substantially reduce your risk of fracture.

A multicenter study of more than 35,000 postmenopausal women evaluated the relationship between adherence and nonadherence to bisphosphonate prescriptions and risk of fractures. The investigators found that just under half of the women refilled their prescriptions in two years, and only 20% of them kept taking bisphosphonates for that entire time. The women who continuously used their medications for two years had fewer fractures at all locations, including the spine and hip, and reduced their risk of these fractures by 20–45%, compared with women who took their medicine less frequently. Women who took the bisphosphonates two out of every four weeks each month also showed some reduction in fracture risk, but not as much as more frequent users.

version of human parathyroid hormone. A daily injection of teriparatide has been shown to increase BMD dramatically and to reduce fracture in the spine and hip. Teriparatide works differently from antiresorptive medications in that it stimulates bone formation rather than preventing bone resorption.

One troubling potential side effect of teriparatide is that it has increased the risk of bone cancer in rats that were injected with high doses of the medication. Although this type of cancer has not been observed in people treated with the medication, people at increased risk for bone cancer should not use teriparatide. This includes people with Paget's disease or an unexplained rise in alkaline phosphatase levels, which would show up on a standard blood

What that means is if you currently take bisphosphonates only half of the time, you will benefit only slightly from bisphosphonate therapy but if you want to significantly reduce your fracture risk, you'll need to take your medication at least three quarters of the time. Of course, all of the time is still best.

Just What the Doctor Ordered: A Drug Holiday

If you take a bisphosphonate for five years, you may be able to take a break from therapy—what doctors call a drug holiday. That's one of the results of the Fracture Intervention Trial Long-term Extension study of more than 1,000 postmenopausal women.

All of the women in the study had taken Fosamax for five years. Then they were randomly assigned to continue taking the medication for another five years (two thirds of the group) or to take placebo pills (the other one third). The women who stopped taking Fosamax over those five years had a moderate decline in bone mineral density (BMD), but no higher risk of nonvertebral fractures than those who continued taking the drug during that time. However, women who continued Fosamax beyond five years had a 55% lower risk of vertebral fractures. Consequently, say the authors, women who have a high risk of vertebral fractures, for example, those who had a previous vertebral fracture, should consider continuing bisphosphonate therapy.

How did the drug continue to work even though the women stopped using it? After taking a bisphosphonate for a long time, a residual amount continues to circulate in the blood and inhibit bone resorption. Retention of bisphosphonate in the bone may account for the slowed bone loss after the women discontinued taking the drug.

If you have had a good response to five years' worth of bisphosphonate therapy and are not at an increased risk for a vertebral fracture, ask your doctor whether you might be a candidate for a drug holiday.

You will still need to see the doctor regularly because it's important to monitor BMD level closely during this time. The recommendation at Johns Hopkins is a dual-energy x-ray absorptiometry (DXA) scan at one year after stopping therapy and if results show no change or an improvement, every two years thereafter. Bone turnover markers in the serum or urine may also be measured to detect early resumption of bone loss before it's seen on a DXA scan. If your BMD level drops, you may need to go back on osteoporosis therapy.

The Bottom Line

Long-term use of bisphosphonates appears to be safe and continues to reduce fracture risk. But research suggests that some patients who are not at increased risk for vertebral fracture can consider discontinuing bisphosphonate therapy after five years with the guidance of their doctor. Whether therapy is cyclical or continuous, adherence to the recommended treatment regimen is crucial for a good outcome. ■

test. It also includes people who have had radiation therapy targeting bone or cancer that has spread to bone. Teriparatide may also raise blood calcium levels, so anyone with high levels of calcium in the blood should not use it. Teriparatide should not be used for more than two years, and another osteoporosis medication must be used after teriparatide treatment to maintain the gain in bone density.

Calcitonin. Given by injection or nasal spray, calcitonin (Fortical, Miacalcin) is a synthetic version of a hormone produced by the human thyroid gland. It improves bone density and may slow bone loss in the spine. There appears to be a modest reduction in fracture risk in the spine, but calcitonin does not appear to protect against hip fracture. Overall, it is not as effective as the bisphosphonates, though it does have the particular benefit of relieving the pain of recent vertebral fractures. The usual dosage is an injection every day or every other day, or one puff of nasal spray daily. Although most people tolerate the nasal spray fairly well, some may develop rhinitis (nasal inflammation).

Treatment in Men

An underlying cause of osteoporosis can be identified in about half of the men who have the disorder. The most common causes include the use of corticosteroid medications, low testosterone levels, smoking, and excessive alcohol consumption. Treatment should be tailored to the underlying cause. For example, if testosterone levels are low, testosterone replacement therapy would be the appropriate course of treatment. In the past, testosterone could only be given by injection, usually every two weeks; today, newer preparations include skin patches (Striant) and testosterone gel (AndroGel, Testim), making hormone therapy far easier.

Bone medications that are approved for the treatment of osteoporosis in men include alendronate, risedronate, and teriparatide.

Preventing Fractures

Along with bone-strengthening medications, preventing falls is a crucial component of fracture prevention. There are a number of simple steps you can take to reduce the likelihood of falling. First, make sure that your floors are clear of any obstacles such as area rugs or extension cords. Hallways, stairwells, and bathrooms should be well lit (especially at night). Grab bars in showers and bathtubs are highly recommended.

Be sure that your eyeglasses or contact lens prescriptions are up to date. Review your medications with your doctor; some medications can increase the risk of falls by impairing balance and alertness. In some cases, lightly padded hip protectors may be recommended; these can reduce the risk of a hip fracture in the case of a fall.

Another way to reduce the risk of falls is to improve your muscle strength through resistance training and your balance through yoga or tai chi exercises. Check with a physical therapist or certified trainer to get recommendations that are appropriate and safe for you.

Treatment of Vertebral Compression Fractures

When symptoms from a vertebral fracture are severe, rest and pain medication are recommended. Over-the-counter pain relievers may be all that is needed, though applying ice to the painful area also may be helpful. If these measures do not provide enough relief, a short-term course of prescription pain relievers may be necessary. Some research suggests that alendronate also can reduce the pain associated with vertebral fractures. In addition, short-term use of a back brace may prevent painful movements of the spine and reduce the length of required bed rest.

Fortunately, in the vast majority of cases, the pain associated with vertebral fractures resolves over time with conservative measures. In cases that do not get better with these therapies, however, surgery may be required. Surgical techniques for treating vertebral compression fractures include percutaneous vertebroplasty, kyphoplasty, and spinal fusion.

Percutaneous vertebroplasty

This minimally invasive technique has had a high degree of success in repairing vertebral compression fractures caused by osteoporosis. The procedure, performed at Johns Hopkins and at many other institutions, involves injecting a special kind of cement called polymethylmethacrylate into both sides of the fractured vertebra. The cement strengthens the bone, preventing further collapse. Back pain subsides almost immediately after the procedure—usually in a matter of hours.

Percutaneous vertebroplasty is appropriate only for people who have suffered a recent fracture that is solely responsible for their back pain. Potential complications include soft-tissue damage and nerve-root pain and compression.

Kyphoplasty

To date, this technique appears to be as successful as vertebroplasty. Ideally, however, it should be performed within two to three months of the fracture. Using a special balloon, the recently collapsed vertebral body is expanded and then filled with cement (see "Mending a Cracked Back" on pages 76–77). As with vertebroplasty, possible complications include soft-tissue damage and nerve-root pain and compression.

Spinal fusion

In this procedure, bone grafts are used to join together two or more adjacent vertebrae. Spinal fusion may be necessary when back pain does not respond to more conservative treatments or when nerve pressure or severe deformity develops.

NEW RESEARCH

Prescription Vitamin D Lowers the Risk of Falls

Kidney function declines with age, and calcitriol is made in the kidneys. Calcitriol, given by prescription, may help prevent falls in older women with declining kidney function, a new study suggests.

For this study, 415 generally healthy women age 65 and older (106 of whom had impaired kidney function) took either calcitriol pills twice daily, estrogen and progestin with or without calcitriol, or placebo (inactive) pills for three years.

Overall, calcitriol reduced the number of falls by 46%. And in women with low kidney function, calcitriol alone and calcitriol plus estrogen and progestin reduced the rate of falls by 50–60%—an effect that was apparent by 12 months. Calcitriol may work by increasing muscle strength and improving balance. They caution that since the study participants were white women, their findings may not apply to women of other races or to men.

If your kidney function is declining, it may be worth asking your doctor about your need for vitamin D. Be aware that calcitriol interacts with some prescription drugs and nonprescription remedies, including calcium supplements and steroids. Thus, make sure your doctor knows all of the drugs and supplements you are taking. Also, when taking calcitriol, you must be monitored regularly and have your blood calcium checked every three months.

THE JOURNAL OF CLINICAL ENDOCRINOLOGY AND METABOLISM
Volume 92, page 51
January 2007

Mending a Cracked Back

Kyphoplasty offers new option for treating vertebral compression fractures

Like a skilled cat burglar, osteoporosis silently and stealthily robs its victims of bone. In this weakened state, bones are susceptible to fracture. When the fracture occurs in the bones in your spine, it can trigger a cascade of events, leading to the collapse or compression of your vertebrae (vertebral compression fracture). Ultimately with repeated fractures, you will start to get shorter and you will eventually appear to be permanently hunched over (kyphosis or dowager's hump).

Severe, focal, or prolonged pain in the back is often, but not always, the first sign of trouble. Most people improve with bed rest, reduced activity, pain medications, and strength training. But if you're one of the 20% who needs more aggressive treatment, vertebroplasty or kyphoplasty usually brings relief.

Both of these procedures entail injecting bone cement into fractured vertebrae to prevent further collapse. And both can significantly reduce your back pain, improve your quality of life, and enhance your mobility. However, it remains to be seen if one procedure is better than the other.

The Kyphoplasty Difference

During vertebroplasty, the physician makes a small incision in your back and, using x-ray guidance, passes a hollow needle through the muscles near the spine and into the fractured vertebra. Once the needle is correctly positioned, he or she injects bone cement through the needle into the vertebra. The cement hardens in about two hours.

The kyphoplasty procedure is similar, but it adds a step before the cement is injected into the fractured vertebra. For kyphoplasty, two small incisions are made in your back. Then a tiny probe is placed into the vertebral space where the fracture is located. Again using x-ray guidance, the surgeon inserts two miniature balloons, one on each side of the vertebra. Next, the balloons are carefully inflated to lift the collapsed bone and return it to its normal position. The balloons are then deflated and removed, and the spaces created by the balloons are filled with bone cement. The entire procedure takes from 30–45 minutes and is performed in the hospital.

How Kyphoplasty Stacks Up

Kyphoplasty appears to be significantly better than nonsurgical treatment at providing pain relief and improving the ability to function in people with this type of fracture and to be slightly better than vertebroplasty in relieving pain and restoring height. A recent review of 43 studies found that people with long-term pain from osteoporosis that didn't respond to medication and other nonsurgical treatments had less pain and functioned better after undergoing kyphoplasty. Also, they retained their restored vertebral height up to three years later. A review of 69 studies comparing vertebroplasty with kyphoplasty found that kyphoplasty was slightly better than vertebroplasty in relieving pain and restoring vertebral height, but neither was a clear winner.

The best way to determine whether kyphoplasty is better than vertebroplasty is through a head-to-head comparison in a study where patients are randomly assigned to one treatment or the other. Two such studies (one in the United States, the other worldwide) have begun in women with painful vertebral fractures caused by osteoporosis. Long-term results are expected by 2011.

Safety concerns. Studies in cadavers suggest that injecting bone cement into the vertebrae—a step performed in both vertebroplasty and kyphoplasty—may weaken adjacent bone and increase the risk of fractures. While recent studies report similar results in living patients, these findings are not absolute proof of cause and effect. The adjacent fractures might have occurred even if kyphoplasty or vertebroplasty had not been performed. At this point, you and your doctor should weigh the risks and benefits of either procedure for your particular situation.

Should You Consider Kyphoplasty?

You might be a candidate for kyphoplasty if, after a trial of conservative therapy, you have:

- Severe back pain that is poorly controlled with pain medication
- Severe functional limitations, for example, you cannot stand or walk.
- A fractured vertebra that has lost a great deal of height and shape
- Fractures located at the area of the spine between the lower back and the rib cage
- Multiple fractures, including a new fracture if you had a previous vertebral fracture that has healed.

Timing is crucial. Vertebral compression fractures are easy to overlook since back pain is often attributed to muscle strain, arthritis, or simply the normal aches and pains of aging. But prompt diagnosis is particularly important, since kyphoplasty is most successful when performed on relatively recent vertebral fractures, that is, those caught within two to three months.

So if you have osteoporosis and back pain that isn't relieved by medication and other conservative measures within a few weeks, talk to your doctor about tests to determine if you have a vertebral compression fracture.

An Ounce of Prevention

Remember, prevention is still the best medicine. If you are at risk for vertebral fracture, it's important to take advantage of all strategies to optimize your overall bone health, including drug therapy. But if preventive measures and conservative treatment options fail, kyphoplasty or vertebroplasty may help you walk pain free and a bit taller. ■

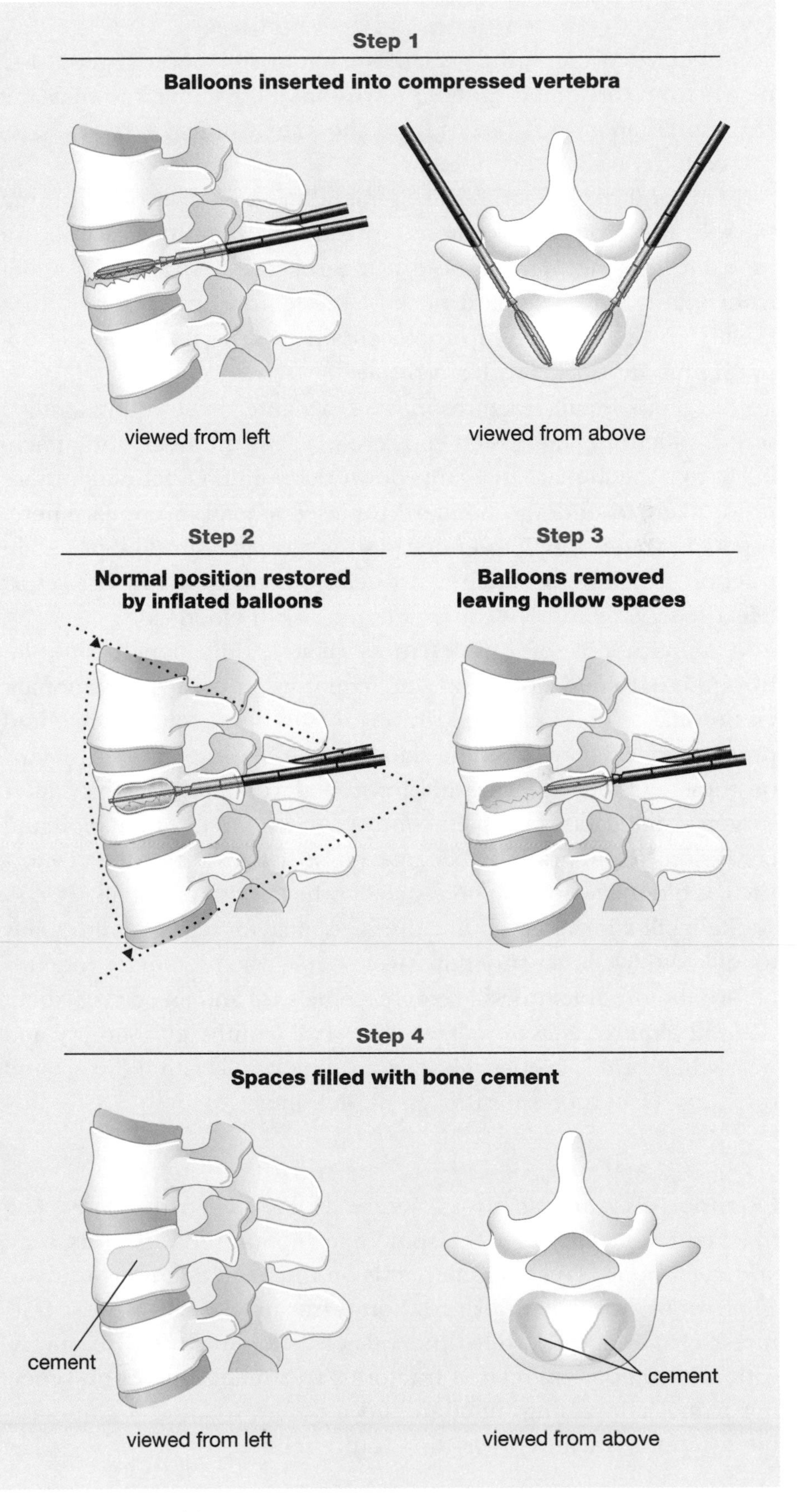

Treatment of Hip Fractures

Hip fractures occur in the neck of the femur (thighbone), about 1–2 inches from the joint or in the protrusion of the femur known as the trochanter, about 3–4 inches from the joint. Surgery is typically required to reposition the hipbone.

Femoral neck fractures are generally repaired in one of three ways. In the procedure known as internal fixation, metal screws are inserted into the bone to hold it together while it heals. In hemiarthroplasty, the head and neck of the femur are replaced with a metal prosthesis. Total hip replacement involves replacing the upper femur and socket with a prosthesis.

Surgeons repair fractures in the trochanter by inserting a metal screw, called a compression hip screw, across the bone and attaching it to a metal plate that runs down the femur. Older patients are more likely to undergo hemiarthroplasty or total hip replacement. A person who is too ill to undergo surgery may instead be placed in traction to allow the fracture to heal, but traction is a last resort because staying immobile increases the risk of blood clots.

Complications of hip fractures include infection, deep vein thrombosis (blood clotting in the deep veins of the leg), pulmonary embolism (a blood clot that travels to the lung), pneumonia, and pressure ulcers (breaks in the skin that can become infected). Many of these complications result from bed rest and inactivity after surgery. Medications for pain control can lead to disorientation and confusion. Complications become more serious with other factors such as older age and the presence of other health problems.

Rehabilitation after hip fracture is essential for regaining the ability to walk and live independently. Most people who lived independently before the hip fracture will require home care and assistance. About half will require canes or walkers for several months after surgery, and nearly half of this group will need a cane or walker to move around the house or outdoors for the rest of their lives.

Treatment of Other Osteoporotic Fractures

Osteoporosis can lead to a fracture at any site in the body. The most common sites after the spine and hip are the wrist, ribs, toes, and collarbone. Treatment depends on the bone that is broken and whether or not it is displaced. Some fractures (such as wrist fractures) require a cast, while others (such as toe fractures) do not. As with all osteoporosis-related fractures, treatment focuses on relieving pain, maintaining function and mobility, treating the underlying osteoporosis, and preventing future falls. ■

acupressure—Type of massage in which continuous pressure is exerted on a trigger spot for three–five minutes.

acupuncture—Traditional Chinese treatment in which thin needles are placed at specific spots along the body.

acute—Illness or symptoms that appear suddenly and have a short course.

alkaline phosphatase—Enzyme released by bone-forming cells called osteoblasts. Blood levels of the enzyme are elevated in people with Paget's disease.

analgesic—An agent that alleviates pain without causing loss of consciousness.

ankylosing spondylitis—Chronic inflammation of the facet joints and sacroiliac joints (between the sacrum and the pelvis).

annulus fibrosus—Tough, fibrous layers of tissue that cover an intervertebral disk.

balance exercise—A type of exercise that, when practiced regularly, can increase balance and help prevent falls; examples are tai chi and yoga.

biofeedback—Back pain treatment in which the person practices different relaxation methods while using electronic sensors to measure bodily functions, such as muscle tension, breathing patterns, and heart rate.

bisphosphonates—A class of drugs that help preserve bone mass by slowing bone resorption.

body mechanics—Habitual ways of moving that can affect back health.

bone mass—The amount of bone tissue in the body.

bone mineral density testing—Radiological testing to measure bone density. Testing gives accurate measurements of the amount of bone but not the actual structure or quality of bone.

bone quality—The architecture/geometry and the material properties of bone and bone tissue.

bone remodeling—Process by which old bone is resorbed and new bone is formed.

bone resorption—Breakdown of old bone.

bone scan—Imaging test that involves injecting radioactive technetium and then measuring how much radioactivity is taken up by specific areas of bone. This test can detect metastatic cancer, bony overgrowths in Paget's disease, bacterial infections of the spine, and small fractures that are not visible on x-rays.

bone spur—See osteophytes.

calcitonin—A naturally occurring hormone involved in calcium regulation and bone metabolism.

calcium carbonate/citrate—Forms of calcium used for calcium supplementation.

cauda equina—Bundle of nerve roots at the bottom of the spinal cord.

caudal epidural block—Injection of medication directly into the base of the spine.

cervical spine—Refers to the neck.

chiropractor—Healthcare professional who uses techniques such as physical manipulation and adjustment of the spine, massage, application of heat or cold, and electrical stimulation to treat back problems.

coccyx—A term for the tailbone.

collagen—A soft protein that hardens with the deposition of calcium and phosphorus; it is a main component of bone.

Colles' fracture—A common type of fracture in which the break occurs across the end of the main bone of the forearm.

compression fracture—Fracture of a vertebral body that results in loss of height or complete collapse of the vertebral body. This type of fracture usually occurs in bones weakened by osteoporosis.

computed tomography (CAT or CT) scan—Imaging technique in which the person lies on a special table while x-rays are passed through the body and sensed by a detector that rotates 360 degrees around the person. A computer combines the information into a cross-sectional picture that shows body structures and fluids, blood clots, tumors, and bones.

CT myelogram—CT scan carried out after contrast material is injected into the spinal canal; it offers good detail of bone and soft tissue.

decompression surgery—A procedure that involves enlarging the spinal canal to relieve pressure on the spinal cord.

deep vein thrombosis (DVT)—Blood clotting that occurs in the deep veins of the leg.

dietary reference intake (DRI)—Recommended daily intake of vitamins and minerals as determined by the Institute of Medicine.

disease-modifying antirheumatic drugs—Drugs that interfere with tumor necrosis factor, which contributes to inflammation.

diskectomy—Surgical treatment for a herniated disk that takes pressure off a pinched nerve by making an incision in the annulus fibrosus and removing the extruded nucleus pulposus.

disk replacement—Surgical procedure that replaces a herniated disk with an artificial one.

displacement—Movement of bone fragments from their original positions.

dowager's hump—Kyphosis in the upper back. Common in older women, it can result from disk degeneration, the collapse of vertebrae due to osteoporosis, or both.

dual energy x-ray absorptiometry (DEXA)—A test to

measure bone mineral density wherein two x-ray beams are directed at the spine or hip joint, and a computer calculates the amount of energy that passes through the bone.

electromyography—A test that uses electrodes to measure muscle abnormalities.

endorphins—Pain-blocking chemicals produced by the body.

facet joints—Joints formed by the interlocking of bony projections at the rear of adjacent vertebrae.

femur—Refers to the thighbone.

flexion—A forward bending of the spine.

foramina—Spaces between adjacent vertebrae.

fracture—A break in a bone caused by injury or osteoporosis.

hemiarthroplasty—An operation to repair hip fracture that involves replacing the head and neck of the femur with a prosthesis.

herniated disk—Bulging of the central part of an intervertebral disk (nucleus pulposus) through the fibrous layers of tissue (annulus fibrosus) that cover it.

hip replacement—Surgery to implant an artificial hip joint to replace a damaged hip joint. (See also total hip replacement, hemiarthroplasty, and internal fixation.)

hormone replacement therapy (HRT)—The administration of low-dose estrogen with or without progesterone to reduce the symptoms and rapid loss of bone that accompany menopause in women. Women who have had a hysterectomy do not need to take progesterone.

hyperparathyroidism—Excessive production of parathyroid hormone by the parathyroid gland; it weakens bones by promoting loss of calcium from bone.

hyperthyroidism—Excessive production of thyroid hormone that can result in osteoporosis.

intermittent claudication—Pain in the buttocks, thighs, or calves while walking. The pain, caused by impaired blood flow to the legs, stops promptly when the person rests. The pain of spinal stenosis may be confused with intermittent claudication.

internal fixation—An operation to repair a hip fracture that involves inserting metal screws into the bone to hold it together while it heals.

intervertebral disk—Flexible pad of tissue located between vertebrae that acts as a cushion during movement, preventing vertebrae from grinding against each other.

intradiskal electrothermal therapy—A minimally invasive procedure in which the nerves in the outer wall of the disk are destroyed with a heated wire.

ipriflavone—Synthetic isoflavone (structurally similar to isoflavones found in soy) that may prevent or treat osteoporosis.

isoflavone—A plant compound found in soy foods that has weak estrogen-like activity.

kyphoplasty—A new technique for treating vertebral compression fractures in which the collapsed vertebra is expanded using a special balloon and then filled with cement.

kyphosis—An abnormal accentuation of the usual curvature of the upper back and commonly referred to as a humpback or hunchback.

lactose intolerance—An inability to digest the naturally occurring sugars in dairy foods.

laser diskectomy—Surgical treatment for a herniated disk that uses a laser to burn out the inside of the disk; it is a less invasive alternative to diskectomy.

lordosis—Spinal deformity in which the abdomen is thrust too far forward and the buttocks too far to the rear; also called swayback.

lumbar spine—The lower back.

magnetic resonance imaging (MRI)—A sensitive imaging technique that surrounds a person with a powerful magnet while radio waves are passed through the body.

massage therapy—A therapy used to ease tension and relax back muscles.

microdiskectomy—A surgical treatment for a herniated disk that is done through a very small opening, it is a less invasive alternative to diskectomy.

muscle relaxants—Drugs that work by depressing the activity of nerves in the spinal cord and brain; they are used with caution as they cause drowsiness and are potentially addictive.

nerve conduction test—A test that examines nerve function.

n-teleopeptides—A by-product of the breakdown of bone that can be measured in urine tests.

nucleus pulposus—The central part of an intervertebral disk that, as a person ages, slowly loses its water content and shrinks.

open laminectomy—A surgical procedure for a herniated disk in which a small part of the vertebra is removed.

opiates—Drugs that depress the nervous system to block the perception of pain. As they are potentially addictive and have many side effects, they are used for back pain only when all other options have failed.

osteoblasts—Cells that fill small cavities in the bone surface with new bone during bone formation.

osteoclasts—Cells that invade the surface of bone and remove the matrix and minerals, leaving small cavities in the bone surface during bone resorption.

osteomalacia—A softening of bone that results from a lack of the essential minerals calcium and phosphorus.

osteopenia—Low bone mass.

osteophyte—A bony overgrowth, or spur.

osteoporosis—A disease marked by progressively decreasing bone mass; it results in weakened, brittle bones that can fracture easily.

Paget's disease—A condition characterized by excessive overgrowth of bone, especially in the spine, pelvis, skull, and femur.

palliative treatment—Therapy aimed at relieving pain and limiting disease complications rather than curing the disease.

parathyroid hormone—Hormone of the parathyroid gland that regulates calcium and phosphorus metabolism throughout the body.

pelvis—Basin-shaped structure in the lower part of the trunk composed of the two hipbones, tailbone (coccyx), and lower backbone (sacrum).

percutaneous arthroscopic diskectomy—Surgical treatment for a herniated disk that is less invasive than diskectomy; the procedure involves inserting a probe into the disk to scoop it out.

percutaneous vertebroplasty—A minimally invasive technique to treat vertebral compression fractures that involves the injection of cement into the fractured vertebra.

perimenopause—The time immediately before menopause begins.

peripheral dual-energy x-ray absorptiometry—A bone density test that is similar to DEXA and uses a portable machine to measure bone density in the finger, wrist, or heel.

peripheral quantitative computed tomography—A bone density test that is similar to QCT (see below) and measures bone density in the wrist.

peripheral sites—Bone sites other than those central to the body (spine and hip), such as the wrist, heel, and finger.

processes—Bony projections jutting out from the rear of a vertebra.

pulmonary embolism—A blood clot that blocks one of the blood vessels in the lungs.

pyridinium cross-links—A product created by the breakdown of bone that can be measured in urine tests.

quantitative computed tomography (QCT)—A test used to determine vertebral density by measuring the absorption of radiation by bone.

quantitative ultrasound—A technique that uses sound waves to measure bone density in peripheral sites.

radiographic absorptiometry—A technique that uses x-rays to measure bone density in the hand.

relaxation therapy—Treatment that teaches techniques of muscle relaxation and breathing so that a person can deal better with stress, a possible cause of back pain.

resistance exercise—A type of exercise that entails working muscles against weights.

sacroiliac joints—Joints on either side of the sacrum that join the sacrum to the other bones of the pelvis.

sacrum—The flat, triangular bone formed by the fusion of the lowest five vertebrae.

sciatic nerve—The nerve arising from the lower spine that extends into the leg and foot.

sciatica—Pain that radiates into the buttocks, down the thighs, into the calves, and often into the feet; the pain is caused by irritation of the sciatic nerve.

scoliosis—An abnormal sideways bend to the back caused by twisting of the spine.

secondary osteoporosis—Osteoporosis caused by certain medications or other diseases.

selective estrogen receptor modulators (SERMS)—A class of drugs that mimic the actions of estrogen in some tissues and block the effects of estrogen in others.

sensory-evoked potential—A test to examine nerve function.

sequestration—A condition in which fragments of a herniated disk break free.

single-energy x-ray absorptiometry—A test used to measure bone density in the wrist or heel, similar to DEXA, except that it uses one x-ray beam.

spasm—A sudden, involuntary muscle contraction that produces pain; spasms can occur when a muscle or ligament in the back is torn or when a disk or facet joint is injured.

trochanter—Part of the femur that protrudes below the bone's neck.

ultrasound—The use of high-frequency sound waves to detect osteoporosis and predict the risk of fractures.

vertebra, vertebrae (pl.)—Any of the 33 interlocking bones that form the spinal column.

vertebral compression fracture—Collapse of the front of a vertebra, often producing immediate and intense pain in the area of the fracture; it can be caused by even minor trauma in a vertebra weakened by cancer, osteoporosis, Paget's disease, or hyperparathyroidism.

vertebral osteomyelitis—A serious bacterial infection of the spine that can cause pain in the neck or back and is usually accompanied by fever.

weight-bearing exercise—Exercise such as walking, jogging, or stair climbing, in which the bones of the feet, legs, and spine bear the body's weight.

HEALTH INFORMATION ORGANIZATIONS AND SUPPORT GROUPS

American Academy of Medical Acupuncture
4929 Wilshire Blvd., Ste. 428
Los Angeles, CA 90010
☎ 323-937-5514
www.medicalacupuncture.org/findadoc/index.html
Provides referrals for physicians throughout the country who practice acupuncture. Promotes integration of acupuncture concepts with Western medical training.

American Academy of Orthopaedic Surgeons
6300 N. River Rd.
Rosemont, IL 60018-4262
☎ 800-346-AAOS/847-823-7186
www.aaos.org
Provides referrals to orthopedists in your area. Publishes information on orthopedic disorders.

American Osteopathic Association
142 E. Ontario St.
Chicago, IL 60611
☎ 800-621-1773/312-202-8000
www.osteopathic.org
National association of roughly 49,000 osteopathic physicians. Advances the practice and knowledge of osteopathic medicine, provides certification to osteopaths, and accredits osteopathic medical colleges and healthcare facilities.

American Pain Society
4700 W. Lake Ave.
Glenview, IL 60025
☎ 847-375-4715
www.ampainsoc.org
Provides information on pain centers throughout the country. Advances pain-related research, education, treatment, and professional practice.

Arthritis Foundation
P.O. Box 7669
Atlanta, GA 30357-0669
☎ 800-283-7800
www.arthritis.org
Provides information about causes, symptoms, diagnosis, and treatment of arthritis. Makes referrals to local chapters and offers services to improve quality of life for people with arthritis through support groups and social activities.

Commission on Accreditation of Rehabilitation Facilities
4891 E. Grant Rd.
Tucson, AZ 85712
☎ 888-281-6531/520-325-1044
www.carf.org
Nonprofit organization that provides accreditation in the human services field, focusing on the areas of rehabilitation, among others. Can provide a list of accredited rehabilitation facilities in your area.

National Certification Commission for Acupuncture and Oriental Medicine
76 South Laura St., Ste. 1290
Jacksonville, FL 32202
☎ 904-598-1005
www.nccaom.org
Provides an online directory designed for individuals seeking practitioners who meet national requirements for board certification in acupuncture and other types of Asian therapy.

National Institutes of Health Osteoporosis and Related Bone Diseases National Resource Center
2 AMS Circle
Bethesda, MD 20892-3676
☎ 800-624-BONE/202-223-0344
www.niams.nih.gov/bone
Provides information on bone diseases, including osteoporosis, Paget's disease, osteogenesis imperfecta, and hyperparathyroidism.

National Osteoporosis Foundation
1232 22nd St. NW
Washington, DC 20037-1202
☎ 202-223-2226/800-231-4222
www.nof.org
National volunteer health agency dedicated to reducing the prevalence of osteoporosis and promoting bone health. Information on osteoporosis prevention and treatment is available online or by request.

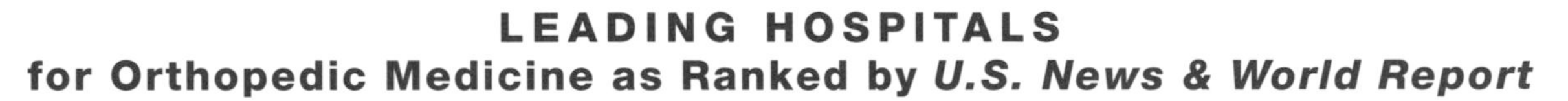

LEADING HOSPITALS
for Orthopedic Medicine as Ranked by *U.S. News & World Report*

1. **Hospital for Special Surgery**
   New York, NY
   ☎ 212-606-1000
   www.hss.edu

2. **Mayo Clinic**
   Rochester, MN
   ☎ 507-284-2511/507-538-3270
   www.mayoclinic.org

3. **Massachusetts General Hospital**
   Boston, MA
   ☎ 617-726-2000
   www.massgeneral.org

4. **Cleveland Clinic**
   Cleveland, OH
   ☎ 800-223-2273
   www.clevelandclinic.org

5. **Johns Hopkins Hospital**
   Baltimore, MD
   ☎ 410-502-4003/410-955-5464
   www.hopkinsmedicine.org

6. **Duke University Medical Center**
   Durham, NC
   ☎ 888-ASK-DUKE/919-416-3853
   www.mc.duke.edu

7. **New York-Presbyterian University Hospital of Columbia and Cornell**
   New York, NY
   ☎ 877-NYP-WELL
   www.nyp.org

8. **Rush University Medical Center**
   Chicago, IL
   ☎ 312-942-5000/888-352-RUSH
   www.rush.edu

9. **University of California, Los Angeles, Medical Center**
   Los Angeles, CA
   ☎ 310-825-9111/800-825-2631
   www.healthcare.ucla.edu

10. **New York University Hospital for Joint Diseases**
    New York, NY
    ☎ 212-263-7300
    www.nyumedicalcenter.org

INDEX

U

V

W

X

Y

Z

NOTES

NOTES

The information contained in this White Paper is not intended as a substitute for the advice of a physician. Readers who suspect they may have specific medical problems should consult a physician about any suggestions made.

Please address inquiries on bulk subscriptions and permission to reproduce selections from this White Paper to Medletter Associates, LLC, 6 Trowbridge Drive, Bethel, CT 06801.
The editors are interested in receiving your comments at whitepapers@johnshopkinshealthalerts.com or the above address but regret that they cannot answer letters of any sort personally.

ISBN 978-1-933087-58-0
1-933087-58-7

Printed in the United States of America

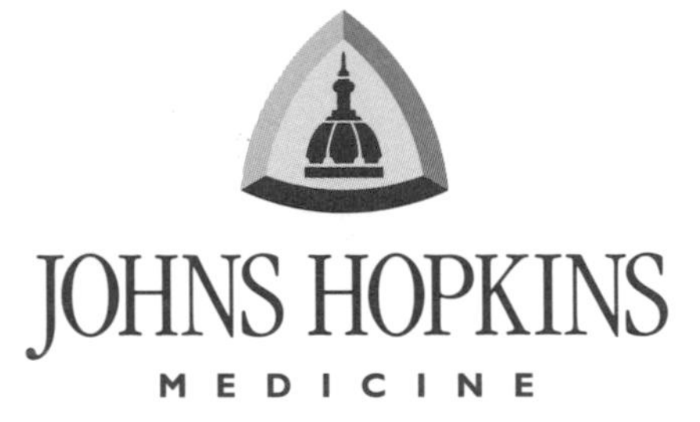

The Johns Hopkins White Papers are published yearly by Medletter Associates, LLC.

Visit our website for information on Johns Hopkins Health Publications, which include White Papers on specific disorders, home medical encyclopedias, consumer reference guides to drugs and medical tests, and our monthly newsletter *The Johns Hopkins Medical Letter: Health After 50.*
www.JohnsHopkinsHealthAlerts.com

COLON CANCER

Ross C. Donehower, M.D., F.A.C.P.

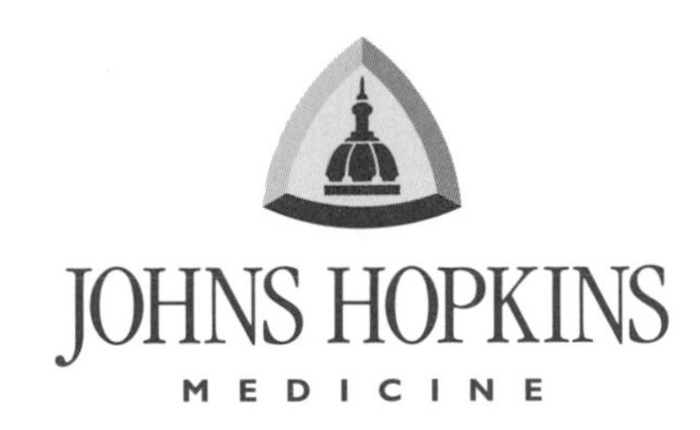

Dear Reader:

Welcome to the 2008 *Colon Cancer White Paper*—your Johns Hopkins guide to the prevention, diagnosis, and management of colon and rectal cancers.

This year's highlights include:

- Action plan for handling the **emotional aftershocks** of a colorectal cancer diagnosis. (page 6)
- Beyond colonoscopy: Promising new **state-of-the-art screening tests** for colorectal cancer. (page 10)
- Should you be concerned about **coffee and colon cancer**? (page 13)
- How soon should you get a **colonoscopy after polyp removal**? (page 17)
- **New research reveals** what factors make one colonoscopy more effective than another. (page 20)
- Does everyone need **regular colonoscopies** after age 50, or is there a point when you can safely stop? (page 24)
- Can you be "too old" for colorectal cancer surgery? How to **improve the outcome** in your 70s, 80s, and beyond. (page 34)
- Can massage and acupuncture **relieve pain after colon cancer surgery**? (page 37)
- Coping strategies for **"chemo brain,"** the mental fuzziness after chemotherapy. (page 52)
- **Focus on your diet** to help keep polyps and colon cancer from returning. (page 58)
- Seven key strategies for **preventing a recurrence** of colorectal cancer. (page 64)

You'll also find a new "Ask the Doctor" column on pages 29, 33, 49, 61, and 63. This year's questions came from my patients, but next year I'd like to answer a few of yours. If you have any colorectal cancer-related queries you want answered in the White Papers or comments about the White Papers in general, please e-mail the editors at whitepapers@johnshopkinshealthalerts.com.

Wishing you the best of health in 2008,

Ross C. Donehower, M.D., F.A.C.P.
Virginia and D.K. Ludwig Professor in Clinical Investigation of Cancer
Director, Division of Medical Oncology
Johns Hopkins University School of Medicine

P. S. Don't forget to visit www.HopkinsColonCancer.com for the latest news on colon cancer and other information that will complement your Johns Hopkins White Paper.

THE AUTHOR

Ross C. Donehower, M.D., F.A.C.P., is Director of the Division of Medical Oncology and the Medical Oncology Fellowship Training Program at the Johns Hopkins University School of Medicine and the Sidney Kimmel Comprehensive Cancer Center. He is a Professor of Medicine and Oncology and the Virginia and D.K. Ludwig Professor in Clinical Investigation of Cancer at that institution.

His professional activities have included membership on the American Board of Internal Medicine Medical Oncology Examination Committee and several positions with the American Society of Clinical Oncology, including the board of directors and chairmanship of the grant awards committee and the scientific program committee for the national meeting.

Dr. Donehower is a graduate of the University of Minnesota Medical School. He completed his internal medicine training at Johns Hopkins and his medical oncology training at the National Cancer Institute. He has been on the faculty at Johns Hopkins since 1980. His research and clinical activities relate to gastrointestinal malignancies and the development of new anticancer therapies.

CONTENTS

COLON CANCER

Although colon cancer is a more familiar term, doctors commonly refer to cancer that arises in the large intestine as colorectal cancer, a term that includes cancers of both the colon and the rectum. The American Cancer Society ranks colorectal cancer as the third most common cause of cancer (excluding skin cancer) and the second leading cause of cancer-related deaths among both men and women in the United States.

Yet when diagnosed and treated in the early stages, it is among the most curable of all cancers. The five-year survival rate for people whose colon or rectal cancer is discovered and treated in the early stages is more than 90%. In some cases, regular screening reveals precancerous growths that can be removed, thereby preventing cancer from developing in the first place.

This White Paper discusses the way colorectal cancer develops, how it can be detected early, and how you can reduce your risk. It will also describe new developments in screening, diagnosis, treatment options, and research, and ways in which people who have already been treated for colon cancer can lower their risk of having a recurrence.

What Is Colorectal Cancer?

Colorectal cancer occurs all over the world, with the highest rates in industrialized countries such as the United States, Canada, Australia, New Zealand, and the nations of western Europe. About 5% of the U.S. population will develop colorectal cancer. The lowest rates are found in developing countries in Africa and Asia.

In the United States, the death rate from colorectal cancer has been declining steadily over the past 20 years. Today, there are more than one million colorectal cancer survivors in the United States alone.

A major factor has been greater use of improved screening tests to detect cancer early, when it is treated best—and an increase in the number of people willing to have these tests, especially colonoscopy. Perhaps 80–90% of colorectal cancers could be prevented if everyone were screened and polyps identified and removed.

Many Reasons for Optimism

Colon cancer screening did not appear often in the news before the year 2000, when television personality Katie Couric had a colonoscopy that was broadcast on national television. Couric's husband, Jay Monahan, died of advanced colon cancer two years earlier, at the age of 42. After Couric publicized the importance of screening for early detection, colonoscopy rates rose by 20%.

Many improved treatments have also contributed to better survival and cure rates. Precancerous polyps and even small cancerous polyps can be removed during a colonoscopy. Cancers may be removed with laparoscopic surgery, which requires only a few small incisions rather than one very large abdominal incision.

Cancers that have moved beyond the very early stage may be treated with a combination of surgery and chemotherapy to reduce the chance of recurrence. Presurgical radiation may shrink some rectal cancers, allowing the surgeon to perform a less radical operation. Colorectal cancer that has metastasized (spread to other organs) or that comes back (recurs) locally is more serious.

Yet even in these cases, there are newer treatments, such as bevacizumab (Avastin), which can starve tumors of their blood supply. And techniques such as radiofrequency ablation (RFA) can pinpoint and destroy previously inoperable cancer that has invaded the liver.

In the past, some people feared screening because they believed that if colon or rectal cancer were discovered the consequence would be either bowel incontinence or a colostomy. (In a permanent colostomy, the rectum and anus are removed or bypassed and feces are eliminated through an opening created surgically through the abdomen. Bowel incontinence can result when a cancer that occurs low in the rectum or anus invades the sphincter muscles.)

Today, those concerns are less of an issue. Advances in surgical techniques and preoperative radiation have greatly decreased the need for colostomy. Newer imaging techniques such as rectal ultrasound can localize cancers in the rectum or anus precisely, so that surgeons can operate more carefully and preserve muscle function.

There is no question that colorectal cancer is a serious condition. But it is important to remember that there are treatment options at all stages.

How Does Colorectal Cancer Develop?

Because colorectal cancer may arise anywhere in the large intestine, cancers of the colon and the rectum are discussed together in the next few sections; but the treatment sections discuss them separately.

The Colon and Rectum: From Healthy to Cancer

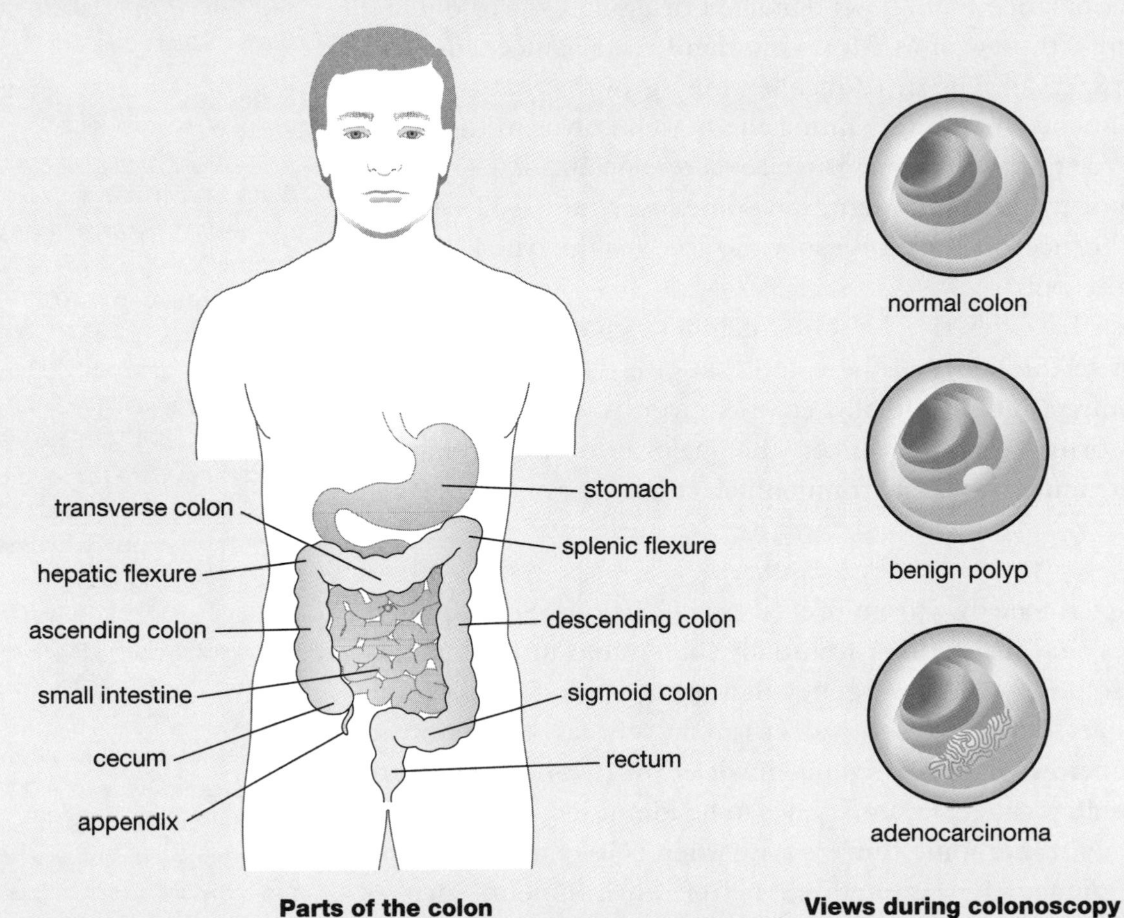

Parts of the colon

Views during colonoscopy

Your colon, or large intestine, is the last stop in the digestion process. The primary function of the colon is to absorb water. The rectum is a 5- to 10-inch canal at the end of the colon, where a ring of muscles holds undigested material in place before it is expelled.

The anatomy of your colon. Shaped like an upside-down letter "U", the large intestine is made up of six sections:

- The cecum, a small pouch about 2–3 inches long, located where the small intestine joins the colon
- The ascending colon, or right colon, which rises from the cecum up along the right side of the abdomen and makes a left turn at the hepatic flexure
- The transverse colon, which crosses the abdomen toward your left, and turns downward at the splenic flexure
- The descending colon, or left colon, which goes down the left side of your abdomen
- The short sigmoid colon, which looks like the letter "S"
- The rectum, where feces are stored before being expelled, and the anus, the opening at the end of the rectum.

How polyps become cancerous. The insets show: (1) the appearance of a normal colon during a colonoscopy; (2) a section of colon containing a polyp; and (3) a malignant cancer.

Polyps, which are benign (not cancerous), establish themselves in the upper (mucosal) layer of the colon and might not invade the underlying muscle or deeper layers of the wall of the colon. Malignant cancers penetrate the wall of the intestine. In advanced cancers, some tumor cells enter the bloodstream and have established secondary cancers elsewhere in the body. ■

Cancer occurs when cells grow out of control, somehow losing the normal balance that allows damaged or aging cells to die and be replaced with new ones. Most colon and rectal cancers develop from polyps, small benign (noncancerous) growths that protrude from the mucous membrane lining the bowel. Polyps in the colon or rectum are quite common, especially after age 50.

Many polyps remain benign, but some, over time, will become malignant (cancerous). This is especially true for the type known as adenomatous polyps.

Scientists have described a series of genetic changes in the DNA of the cells in the lining of the colon that give rise to the development of polyps and, eventually, colon cancer. Although there are inherited forms of colon cancer, the majority of these changes relate to age and various environmental factors.

Risk Factors

It's not known exactly why colorectal cancer begins. Some people carry genes that make them unusually susceptible to certain cancers, and some people have genes that are specific for colorectal cancer. In fact, because colon cancer is relatively easy to identify in the precancerous stage, the genes involved in colon cancer were some of the first cancer-related genes to be identified and studied.

It is thought that some cancers arise when cells containing these genes are damaged by something in the environment, such as exposure to toxins, or by lifestyle factors such as diet and smoking. As with many other cancers, aging also is a risk factor; the longer you live the more exposure you have to the influences that could trigger colorectal cancer.

Colorectal cancer was once considered to be a man's disease. But in terms of gender, it is actually an equal opportunity disease. Studies show that men develop these cancers only slightly more often than women, with men more at risk for colon cancer and women more at risk for rectal cancer.

The major risk factors for colon cancer are age, a personal or family history of cancer, lifestyle practices, and diet.

Age

The risks of developing many kinds of cancer increase as we age, and colon cancer is among them. More than 90% of people diagnosed with colorectal cancer are older than age 50.

Colorectal cancer only rarely affects young people, unless genetic factors or chronic inflammatory bowel disease are involved. This

NEW RESEARCH

Being Overweight Linked to Higher Colon Cancer Risk

Obesity has been connected with an increased risk of colon cancer, especially in men. Now a large study shows that simply being overweight also increases colon cancer risk for men of all ages and for women up to age 67.

Researchers examined data from more than 500,000 people in the National Institutes of Health (NIH) and AARP Diet and Health Study who were followed from 1995–2000. During that time 3,300 of the study participants developed colorectal cancer.

The researchers found that colon cancer risk in men rose in a linear fashion that corresponded with increasing body mass index (BMI). Risk was moderately increased for men who were overweight (BMI 25 to less than 30) and was doubled for those who were morbidly obese (BMI 40 or higher). Compared with men whose BMI was less than 23, men who were overweight had a 20–40% higher risk of developing colon cancer. For women, the findings were more variable, but there was still an upward trend with increasing weight, particularly for women younger than age 67.

If your BMI is higher than it should be—even if you're not obese—losing weight is a good idea for your overall health and for your colon in particular.

AMERICAN JOURNAL OF EPIDEMIOLOGY
Volume 166, page 36
April 21, 2007

could be in part because longevity gives cancers more time to develop. It is believed that colon and rectal cancers develop from adenomatous polyps over a span of seven to 10 years.

This is an incentive to have a colonoscopy regularly after age 50, because any polyps that the doctor finds can be removed while the examination is taking place. Screening for colorectal cancer is important. Whether it is best for you to begin at an earlier age in your own circumstance depends almost entirely on your family history.

Family history

It's estimated that about 15% of colorectal cancers run in families. For that reason, it's important to know the health history of your immediate family and to tell your children. A family history of colorectal cancer puts you at higher risk for developing the disease, which means you should have screenings more often than the average person.

Your risk of colorectal cancer increases if one or more first-degree relatives had it, and even more so if they developed it before age 60. A first-degree relative is a parent, sibling, or child. Your risk also increases if there is a family history of adenomatous polyps and of some other cancers, including endometrial, stomach, and bladder cancer.

In many cases, cancer that runs in families is caused by environmental or lifestyle factors, but some people inherit an increased genetic susceptibility to it. Currently, about 3–5% of all colorectal cancers can be traced directly to specific genes. The most common genetic causes of colon or rectal cancer are hereditary nonpolyposis colorectal cancer (HNPCC), and familial adenomatous polyposis (FAP).

HNPCC. Also called Lynch syndrome, HNPCC accounts for about 2–4% of all colorectal cancers. Most, but not all, people who inherit this genetic disorder will develop colorectal cancer. People with HNPCC tend to develop colorectal cancer before age 50.

FAP. People with FAP develop hundreds of polyps in the colon and rectum. Without treatment, FAP usually leads to colorectal cancer by age 40. Less than 1% of all colorectal cancers are due to this rare form of inherited cancer, which is caused by a change in the APC gene. A genetic variant of FAP, known as APCI1307K mutation, is found in about 6% of Ashkenazi Jews whose ancestors are from eastern Europe. About 10% of colorectal cancers in Ashkenazi Jews are associated with this mutation.

Genetic testing and counseling. If many people in your family develop cancer, a combination of inherited genetic factors could make you and your children especially susceptible to it. It's also

NEW RESEARCH

FAP Families Don't Follow-up With Surveillance

Despite knowing they are at heightened risk for colorectal cancer, some people with or at risk for familial adenomatous polyposis (FAP) fail to follow recommendations for endoscopic screening.

These are the findings from a survey of 71 people with FAP (an inherited condition that usually leads to cancer unless treated) or attenuated FAP (a related genetic condition that heightens the risk of developing colorectal cancer) and 79 close relatives.

The investigators found that only 54% of those with a personal history of FAP (all of whom had intact colons and/or rectums) and 42% of the at-risk relatives had recently followed current guidelines for colorectal cancer surveillance.

The major reason respondents gave for not following up with endoscopic screening was that their healthcare provider had not recommended it. Other reasons included a lack of health insurance or reimbursement and a belief that they were not at increased risk.

The benefits of early detection in preventing death from colorectal cancer are well known, but the advice bears repeating. If you or a family member has FAP or attenuated FAP, routine screening can improve your chances of preventing the development of colon cancer or identifying and treating it early, which will improve your chances for survival.

THE AMERICAN JOURNAL OF GASTROENTEROLOGY
Volume 102, page 153
January 2007

Surviving the Emotional Aftershock of Colorectal Cancer

Strategies to help you cope

Cancer changes everything. It turns a life upside down and shakes it, in just about every way. At first, the focus is on the physical disease and the many decisions around treatment. In that harried time, the psychological and emotional effects of having colon or rectal cancer may not even be on the agenda.

But cancer is a "mental" as well as a physical illness, says Eden Stotsky, a rectal cancer survivor and Education Program Coordinator at the Johns Hopkins Colon Cancer Center. The full emotional impact may not hit until after the initial crisis of treatment has passed, she says. And the emotions experienced, which may run the gamut from fear to anger to denial to depression, can literally knock you over. It may be a time of loss and grieving. Even those who have family and friends nearby may feel deeply lonely. Others may experience feelings of shame at having a cancer connected with bodily eliminations or guilt about surviving when others did not.

Some emotional fallout is to be expected and is normal, says Stotsky. It's important not to ignore or brush aside these feelings and to know that resources are available to help you and your family.

Professional Support

When reeling from a life blow such as cancer, professional support can be invaluable. Family and friends may offer emotional support, but they may be emotionally overwhelmed, too. In addition, you may discover that you are not able to be completely honest with loved ones about how you feel or you may worry that you will upset them if you express your true feelings.

That's why a professional counselor or therapist is often better suited than family or friends to help you sort through the emotions and issues associated with colorectal cancer survivorship. Counseling may even extend your life, according to results from a 10-year study recently reported in the *Journal of Clinical Oncology*.

For this study, investigators assigned nearly 300 people with various types of gastrointestinal cancer, including colon cancer, to receive hospital care only or hospital care plus formal counseling sessions with a psychotherapist. Ten years after treatment, the investigators found that people who had counseling lived significantly longer than those who didn't, even after accounting for tumor stage and location.

Results from this study are not definitive and need to be confirmed in larger studies by other researchers. In the meantime, cancer experts do agree that taking care of your mental health, whether through professional counseling or other means, can improve your quality of life, strengthen your recovery, and help you meet the challenges of living with cancer.

Choosing the Right Program for You

Professional counseling and group support are not for everyone. Some people get enough support from family and friends alone. Others feel uncomfortable sharing their emotions with strangers. If, however, you feel that you could benefit from professional counseling or group support, here are some tips for finding a program that will meet your needs.

Professional counseling. Many types of mental health professionals offer one-on-one or family counseling. Keep in mind that not every counselor has experience working with cancer survivors. Your doctor or treatment center may be able to recommend a mental health professional with the appropriate experience. These services are usually covered by insurance.

Support groups. As with professional counseling, support groups also can be a valuable tool for survivors and their families. Spending time with others who are going through the same process can be nurturing and empowering. You also may get ideas for coping from other group members or guest speakers.

Support groups come in many forms. Some are very organized, with a class-like agenda and sessions that meet for a set number of times, and they do not allow drop-ins; while others have a less formal structure. Some support groups are limited to people with a specific kind or stage of cancer, while others welcome people with various types of cancer.

Check with your doctor or healthcare team about finding a support group. Also, the National Cancer Institute offers a free fact sheet, *National Organizations That Offer Services to People With Cancer and Their Families,* which lists many organizations that can provide information about support groups. It is available online at www.cancer.gov/cancertopics/factsheet/support/organizations, or you can order it from the Cancer Information Service at 800–4–CANCER (800–422–6237).

Cancer buddy. Another option is to team up with a "cancer buddy" for mutual support. This can be someone nearby that you meet with in person or someone you connect with online or by phone. At Johns Hopkins, the coordinator of the "buddy network" matches newly diagnosed patients with those who have had the same type and stage of cancer and who share similar lifestyles.

Try it out. No matter what type of support you choose, it's a good idea to attend a few "trial" sessions to see if this is the type of help that best meets your needs. If you don't feel comfortable, the support is not going to be helpful, so don't be hesitant about leaving one therapist or group to try another.

Other Options

Many other options for support are available for cancer survivors.

Go online. The Internet is a valuable place to look for support, and you can participate anonymously, if you prefer. You can connect with a "virtual" cancer buddy or join online chat rooms. Again, it's good to have a referral from your healthcare team or to select a program offered by a respected organization such as your cancer center or the American Cancer Society (ACS), whose Cancer Survivors Network can be accessed at www.acscsn.org.

Try spiritual support. If you are so inclined, you may find that religion and spiritual practices bring you solace and comfort. Studies show that such practices may ease depression, stress, and anxiety and contribute to relaxation. The companionship of others who share your religious or spiritual beliefs can also be supportive.

However, do not expect to be cured by spiritual or religious practices, and avoid anyone who says your illness is caused by your thinking or a lack of faith. True spiritual and religious groups do not offer false promises or lay blame.

Visit a cancer retreat center. Special cancer retreat centers or camps located across the country provide a nurturing environment and offer support in dealing with the emotional aspects of a cancer diagnosis and treatment. Some are for cancer patients only while others are for family and caregivers as well. The stay varies from a day or two to a week or more. Insurance usually does not cover the fees charged by cancer retreat centers, but stays at some centers cost nothing for the person with cancer. Other centers may charge a fee but offer financial aid or scholarships to help defray costs.

Your cancer care team can help you locate a cancer retreat center. Or you can consult Cancer Matters, an online resource that lists contact information for a number of cancer retreat centers. For more information, go to www.cancermatters.com and click on "Find a Cancer Resource."

It's Your Life

You may find that others have plenty of advice about how and what you should do. All of this is usually well-meaning, but it can sometimes add to the stress of coping with cancer. It helps to remember that there is no right or wrong choice: What you do and how you do it is up to you, and resources are available to help. ■

possible that you have missed inheriting that particular combination of factors, so that even if other family members develop cancer, you may remain unaffected. If cancer seems to run in your family, consider consulting with a genetics expert, who can help determine your personal risk.

Your health history

The most important factor in determining your likelihood of developing colon cancer and how frequently you should be screened is your medical history. In helping to assess your needs, your doctor will want to know if you have:

A personal history of cancer. If you have had colorectal cancer, you have an increased risk of a recurrence or of developing a second primary cancer. Some other cancers increase the risk of developing colon cancer, including endometrial, bladder, and stomach cancer, especially if these appear to run in your family.

A personal history of polyps or other bowel diseases. Since most colorectal cancers develop from polyps, the more polyps you have had, the greater the risk that you will develop cancer of the colon. If you have had even one polyp that was of the adenomatous form (which has a high chance of becoming malignant) and that was 1 cm or larger, your doctor will recommend more frequent screening. Those who have a chronic inflammatory bowel condition such as Crohn's disease or ulcerative colitis also are at higher risk for developing colorectal cancer.

A personal history of type 2 diabetes. A diagnosis of type 2 diabetes increases the risk of developing colorectal cancer or polyps by 50%. The lifestyle risk factors for developing type 2 diabetes are the same as those for colorectal cancer, including inactivity, a diet high in calories, and being overweight or obese.

Your lifestyle and diet

Studies show that certain behaviors are associated with colorectal cancer. For example, the risk of developing colon cancer increases if you are physically inactive, obese, drink excessive amounts of alcohol, or eat a diet high in meat, refined grains, and fats, especially those from animal sources. In addition, smokers are 30–40% more likely to die of colorectal cancer than nonsmokers.

Ethnicity

The role of racial or ethnic factors in colorectal cancer is not well understood. People of all races and ethnic groups can get colorectal

NEW RESEARCH

Smoking Increases Colorectal Cancer Risk

Smoking has long been associated with the development of colorectal adenomas, but the link between smoking and colorectal cancer has been tenuous. Now, results from a large Hawaiian study show that smoking tobacco does increase the risk of colorectal cancer.

Researchers recruited nearly 4,000 people of Japanese, Hawaiian, Filipino, Chinese, and Caucasian ancestry and questioned them about their dietary and smoking habits. Half of the participants had colon or rectal cancer and the other half did not.

Women who had smoked were 27% more likely to develop colorectal cancer than women who had never smoked. The findings were similar for men; those who had smoked were 23% more likely to develop colorectal cancer than men who had never smoked.

The number of years a person smoked was also a risk factor: Men who smoked more than 40 pack-years (the number of tobacco products per day/20 x years of smoking) increased their risk by 48%, while women who smoked more than 30 pack-years increased their risk by 38% compared with never smokers. The risks were similar across racial and ethnic groups.

This study provides strong evidence that smoking tobacco increases the risk of colon and rectal cancer—adding one more reason you should try to kick the habit if you haven't already done so.

CANCER EPIDEMIOLOGY BIOMARKERS PREVENTION
Volume 16, page 1341
July 2007

cancer, and it's known that some Ashkenazi Jews carry a genetic mutation that makes them more susceptible.

Research shows that African American men and women have a higher risk of developing colorectal cancer before age 65 than the general population and a higher risk of dying of it. But it's not known whether this is related to heredity or to socioeconomic factors such as lifestyle and access to medical care. Currently, the American College of Gastroenterology advises that African Americans be screened for colorectal cancer beginning at age 45, rather than at age 50, the recommended age for those at average risk (see Screening and Prevention, on pages 14–26).

The Gastrointestinal Tract

To understand colorectal cancer diagnosis and treatments, it's useful to know how the gastrointestinal (GI) system works.

Your GI system is an efficient food-processing factory, working in assembly-line rhythm to digest food, absorb nutrients, and excrete the leftovers. When all is functioning well, it takes food little more than a day to move through the long tube of your digestive system, from intake to waste disposal.

The journey begins at the mouth, where food is chewed and softened with saliva before a trip down the esophagus into the kettle of the stomach. There, a mixture of gastric acids and enzymes begins to break down the food before it moves into the small intestine.

The small intestine is actually quite large—about 22 feet long—but is called small because it is only about 1 inch (2.5 cm) in diameter. This is where most of the food processing takes place and where most of the nutrients are absorbed. Digestive juices from the pancreas, gallbladder, and liver mingle here to reduce the food matter to the chemicals needed to nourish the body, including amino acids, fatty acids, and sugars. Wave-like contractions and relaxation of muscles called peristalsis keep the mixture moving along.

By the time this brew reaches the beginning of the lower intestinal tract, it is mostly liquid leftovers, from which all the nutrient value has been extracted.

The lower gastrointestinal tract is called by several names: the large intestine, the colorectum, the colon, or the large bowel. It's called the large intestine because it is wider in diameter than the small intestine, about 1–2 inches in diameter, although at 5–6 feet, it is only about one fourth as long.

NEW RESEARCH

Crohn's Disease Increases Chances of Developing Colon Cancer

Although some bowel diseases, such as ulcerative colitis, have been shown to increase the risk of colon cancer, the risk for people with Crohn's disease has been unclear. Now, a meta-analysis from the United Kingdom finds that people with Crohn's disease are at a significantly increased risk.

The investigators reviewed 34 studies involving more than 60,000 people with Crohn's disease and compared the findings with those in people who did not have the condition. They found that people with Crohn's disease had more than double the risk of developing colon cancer compared with the general population, and the risk was highest in people diagnosed before age 25. However, there was no increased risk of developing rectal cancer. The study also found that people with Crohn's disease were at increased risk for developing small bowel cancer, extraintestinal cancer, and lymphoma.

If you have Crohn's disease, particularly if you were diagnosed as a young adult, you may be at risk for colon cancer. Ask your doctor about the need for and frequency of surveillance colonoscopy examinations.

DISEASES OF THE COLON AND RECTUM
Volume 50, page 839
February 2007

2008 Update: State-of-the-Art Screening Tests for Colorectal Cancer

Coming soon to a doctor's office near you?

If swallowing a camera-containing pill sounds more like a scene in a James Bond movie than something your doctor might tell you to do, you're in for a surprise. A tiny camera-in-a-pill, known as the PillCam, is just one of a number of high-tech tests for screening and diagnosing colorectal cancer currently in use or under development.

Advances such as this could make screening and diagnostic tests safer, easier for doctors to perform, and in some cases, less distasteful for patients. Accuracy, however, is still a concern. For now, fecal occult blood testing coupled with flexible sigmoidoscopy is the most commonly used and most cost-effective method of screening, and colonoscopy remains the "gold standard" for screening and diagnosis. But the new tests described below may one day be contenders for those titles.

Candid Camera-Pill

Approved by the U. S. Food and Drug Administration (FDA) to detect abnormalities in the small intestine and the esophagus, the PillCam is now under investigation for use in the colon.

This disposable camera capsule is the size of a large vitamin pill and is swallowed with water. The minicamera is capable of taking four images per second for up to 10 hours, and it provides a 360-degree view of the folds and turns of the colon as it passes through the digestive system and is eventually excreted. Data from the camera are transmitted to a recording device worn on a belt around the waist, and images can then be downloaded to a computer for analysis by the doctor.

Study results are encouraging. Results from a small preliminary study show that the PillCam is as accurate as conventional endoscopic colonoscopy in finding polyps that are 6 mm (about the size of a pea) or larger. In addition, no adverse events, such as cramping, discomfort, or lodging of the camera in the colon, occurred.

Findings presented last year at a meeting of digestive disease specialists showed that the PillCam produced high-quality images in two thirds of the people, but the images were fair to poor in the remaining third. Nevertheless, the investigators say that the pill camera is sufficiently accurate to be used as a colon cancer screening tool. Larger trials are under way in the United States and in Europe to further evaluate its performance.

Even if results from those studies are favorable, however, two drawbacks limit the use of this technology for colon cancer screening. First, for the most accurate results, colon cleansing is required as it is with traditional endoscopy. Second, unlike conventional endoscopy, the camera-in-a-pill cannot be used to biopsy suspicious tissue or remove polyps, which means a follow-up colonoscopy would be required. Still, for people who are unable or unwilling to undergo conventional colonoscopy for screening, this procedure may offer a reasonable alternative.

Optical Biopsy

Can colon cancer be identified at its earliest stages—perhaps even before it develops—without performing a biopsy? Yes, it can, say researchers investigating a test known as Four Dimensional Elastic Light-scattering Fingerprinting (4D-ELF).

Using a special fiberoptic probe inserted into the rectum, researchers can see changes in cells that are 10–20 times smaller than the changes that can be seen by examining biopsied tissue under a microscope. Although only the rectum is probed, the examiner can predict whether colon cancer or a polyp is present anywhere in the colon. Another benefit: The test doesn't require bowel cleansing.

Early studies in more than 300 people show that 4D-ELF testing is accurate more than 90% of the time, and some investigators predict it could be commercially available within the next five years.

Safer, Standard Colonoscopy

Although colonoscopy examinations are very safe, there is a small risk of infection if the scope is not adequately disinfected, and a chance that the colon could be perforated during the procedure. In addition, some people experience discomfort during the procedure. A number of new products tackle these issues.

The ColonoSight, a disposable, air pressure–assisted colonoscope, has been cleared for marketing by the FDA. This system uses air pressure to pull the endoscope into the colon, which lessens the need for the operator to push it from behind for advancement and, in turn, reduces the risk of perforation. The device's disposable sheaths eliminate the need for disinfection between procedures, which reduces the risk of infection.

Another endoscopy system approved for marketing by the FDA is the NeoGuide. Unlike a conventional colonoscopy, in which the physician pushes a long flexible tube through the twists and turns of the colon, the NeoGuide uses computer sensors to construct a three-dimensional map of the colon that is used to guide a multisegmented endoscope through the lower gastrointestinal tract. Because the doctor is not applying pressure to the colon wall to steer the scope, colonoscopy with this procedure is less painful than one using a conventional scope.

The Aer-O-Scope is a self-propelling, self-navigating endoscope that is under investigation and is not yet available in the United States. This device contains a miniature camera embedded in a tiny balloon that is propelled by air pressure though the bowel. Sensors are used to change the size and shape of the balloon so that it adjusts to the contours of the colon as it passes through.

A preliminary study in 12 people showed that the device effectively made its way through the colon in 83% of the participants. Ten of the 12 comfortably underwent the procedure without needing pain medication or to be sedated.

The Virtues of Virtual Colonoscopy

Virtual colonoscopy uses computed tomography (CT) to construct three-dimensional images of the colon and rectum. It is noninvasive, no sedatives are required, and the scan takes only a few minutes to complete.

Some reports indicate that virtual colonoscopy performs as well as endoscopic exams in spotting polyps 6 mm or larger. Neither exam is perfect, however. In some studies, each test missed 10–14% of noncancerous growths of that size. Still, many doctors and insurers aren't yet ready to endorse it. Cost, convenience, and the patient's peace of mind are among the roadblocks.

A recent analysis argued that CT imaging screenings are more cost-effective and caused fewer complications than conventional colonoscopy, and they are just as likely to catch polyps that have reached a suspicious size. It's true that virtual colonoscopy costs half as much as a conventional endoscopic procedure—although that cost is not covered by Medicare or most private insurers—but by some reports, imaging can end up being more expensive than an endoscopic procedure because it may reveal suspicious but benign areas that lead to unnecessary testing. In addition, when polyps are found, an endoscopic procedure will have to be done anyway, which increases the costs and inconvenience.

For peace of mind, the tried-and-true endoscopic procedure wins again. A study in the *American Journal of Medicine* found that people at genetic risk for colon cancer or who tested positive in a fecal test preferred the endoscopic procedure over both barium tests and CT imaging because they felt it was most accurate.

In spite of its drawbacks, virtual colonoscopy offers an alternative for rare situations in which traditional colonoscopy cannot be performed because of technical issues. ■

The major job of the large intestine is to absorb salt and water from digested food and to maintain potassium balance. Friendly bacteria help break down any undigested food, carbohydrates, and amino acids. Peristalsis continues to move the leftovers along, as they gradually become formed into feces.

The next-to-last stop is the rectum, a 5- to 6-inch long canal that is wider than the colon. The processed feces are stored here, held in place by a ring of internal and external sphincter muscles, until they are expelled through the anus during a bowel movement.

Common Digestive Problems

When something goes wrong with the digestive system, it usually makes itself known pretty quickly, through pain or discomfort.

Common problems are upset stomach, constipation, and diarrhea, which are usually not serious and don't last long, although some can become chronic, as in irritable bowel syndrome (IBS). Other problems such as gastric reflux and ulcers appear only in the upper GI tract. None of these is known to contribute to colorectal cancer risk, though a change in bowel habits may be a sign of colon cancer.

Some kinds of inflammatory bowel disease (IBD) are connected with a higher risk of colon cancer. These include Crohn's disease and ulcerative colitis. These chronic conditions usually cause symptoms such as bleeding or pain that signal that the GI system has a functional problem.

However, colon or rectal cancer may generate few or no symptoms in the early stages. Cancer grows slowly, does not usually interfere with function in early stages, and can remain undetected for some time. This is bad news; by the time symptoms are noticeable, the disease can be advanced.

How Colorectal Cancer Begins

Almost all colorectal cancer starts in the mucosa, the innermost lining of the large intestine.

The wall of the large intestine is made up of four layers of tissue: the mucosa; the second layer—the submucosa, which carries blood vessels and nerves; the muscularis propria, which contains two sets of muscles; and the serosa, the outer membrane. The mucosa lining is lubricated with an alkaline mucus secreted from nearby glands to protect it from digestive juices, neutralize bacteria, and help move material along.

Colorectal cancers usually begin as benign polyps that grow from the mucosa. Some people are more prone than others to develop polyps, especially those with a personal or family history of colorectal cancer, those who carry specific genes for colorectal cancer, and those with type 2 diabetes.

Most of these polyps remain benign. But some known as adenomatous polyps (or adenomas) have a high potential for developing abnormal cells, becoming precancerous, and, eventually, evolving into cancer.

Adenomas usually grow on a stalk, resembling small mushrooms. They tend to grow very slowly over a decade or more. The risk of developing cancer increases with their increasing size and with the amount of time they have been growing in the colon.

Adenomas that are malignant are called adenocarcinomas. In the very early stages, abnormal cells are contained inside the polyp. If removed at this point, they may not develop into invasive cancer. However, as cancer cells multiply inside the polyp, they can invade deep into the wall of the colon or rectum and beyond. In advanced cases, the tumors grow through all tissue layers of the colorectal wall. They may also metastasize, shedding cells into the circulatory system and spreading the cancer to other organs, such as the liver and the lungs.

Polyps and Cancer

Fewer than 10% of all adenomas become cancerous. However, more than 95% of colorectal cancers develop from adenomas, and doctors now think some other types of benign polyps may become cancerous as well.

For this reason, doctors usually recommend removing all polyps. Small polyps can be removed easily and painlessly while you are having a colonoscopy or sigmoidoscopy. They are snared and severed with a retractable wire loop that is passed through the scoping instrument. Very small polyps may be destroyed with a small burst of electrical current.

Another precancerous condition seen in the colon is an abnormal cell growth or inflammation called dysplasia. The polyps and areas that look abnormal are biopsied and sent to be tested for malignant cells. If they are benign—as many are—no further treatment is needed, but you may be asked to have scoping exams within a few years to follow up.

If polyps are not benign but show signs of abnormal cells or cancer, your doctor will follow up with diagnostic tests and treatments.

NEW RESEARCH

Coffee—Not Tea—Reduces Risk of Colon Cancer

Green tea has gotten a lot of press for its healthy properties. But it turns out that coffee may be better for your colon.

When researchers reviewed data on the beverage-drinking habits of more than 96,000 Japanese men and women over a 10-year period, they found that coffee significantly lowered the risk of colon cancer in females. Women who regularly drank three or more cups of coffee a day had a 32% lower risk of colon cancer than those who almost never consumed coffee—even after taking into account factors that could have affected risk.

Colon cancer risk was not reduced for men, and neither women nor men had a reduced risk of rectal cancer.

Researchers are not sure why coffee appears protective, since caffeine is in green tea as well. The beneficial effect, they say, may have come from another substance in coffee.

The investigators caution that their results need to be confirmed by other researchers, but these findings do provide some degree of reassurance for women who savor a morning brew and have been concerned about possible adverse effects on the colon.

INTERNATIONAL JOURNAL OF CANCER
Volume 121, page 1312
September 2007

Very large polyps also may require surgery, whether they are benign or cancerous.

Other types of cancers occur in the colon, but these are much less common. They include lymphomas, which are cancers of immune system cells, and carcinoid tumors and gastrointestinal stromal tumors, which develop from specialized cells in the intestine.

Signs and Symptoms of Colorectal Cancer

There are usually no symptoms in the early stages of colorectal cancer. Many symptoms that do show up could be related to other digestive issues. If they are related to colorectal cancer, the disease could be advanced beyond early stages. Therefore, signs or symptoms of digestive problems that last more than a few weeks should be discussed with your doctor.

Some possible symptoms of colorectal cancer include:

- A change from usual bowel habits and appearance, such as constipation, diarrhea, or extremely narrow stools, that lasts for 10 days or more
- Bright red blood in the stools or black, tarry stools, which can be a sign of rectal or intestinal bleeding
- Pain or tenderness in the lower abdomen that doesn't go away
- Bloating, cramps, or gas pains
- A feeling that the rectum isn't completely empty after bowel movements
- Loss of appetite and weight
- Anemia, which can be a sign of blood loss from intestinal bleeding
- Vomiting
- Persistent fatigue, paleness, and heart palpitations, which can be signs of anemia
- Inability to pass stools at all for more than a week. This can signal an intestinal blockage, which is an emergency situation.

Screening and Prevention

Studies show that colorectal cancer can be controlled, cured, or even prevented if it is discovered early. Yet fewer than half of Americans over the age of 50 have had any kind of colon-cancer screening test, ever.

The "ick factor" plays a role. Many people regard the bowels and feces as unclean and are uncomfortable or embarrassed about fecal

Screening and Diagnostic Tests by Risk Level

Risk category	Age to begin	Recommended	Comments
Increased-risk groups			
People with a single adenoma or polyp smaller than 1 cm	3–6 years after first polyp removal	Colonoscopy	If the exam is normal, follow average-risk guidelines.
People with an adenoma larger than 1 cm, multiple adenomas, or adenomas with high-grade abnormalities	Within 3 years of first polyp removal	Colonoscopy	If normal, next exam in 5 years. If normal at that exam, follow guidelines for average risk.
Personal history of colorectal cancer surgery	Within 1 year of cancer surgery	Colonoscopy	If normal, next exam in 3 years. If normal at that exam, then exams every 5 years. For rectal cancer with no colostomy, proctoscopy every 6–12 months for 5 years.
Family history of colorectal cancer or adenomas in a first-degree relative before age 50 or in two or more first-degree relatives at any age	Age 40, or 10 years younger than the age when cancer or polyps showed up in a relative, whichever is earlier	Colonoscopy	Every 5–10 years.
High-risk groups			
Family history of familial adenomatous polyposis (FAP)	Puberty	Early colonoscopy and counseling to consider genetic testing	If the genetic test shows FAP, removal of the colon and referral to a center with experience in managing FAP.
Family history of hereditary nonpolyposis colon cancer (HNPCC)	Age 21	Colonoscopy and counseling to consider genetic testing	If the genetic test shows HNPCC or if there hasn't been genetic testing, every 1–2 years until age 40, then annually with referral to a center with experience in managing HNPCC.
Chronic bowel conditions, such as inflammatory bowel disease (chronic ulcerative colitis or Crohn's disease)	About 8 years after the onset of major colon inflammation, or 12–15 years after the onset of left-sided colitis	Colonoscopy with biopsies for abnormal tissue or polyps	Every 1–2 years, with referral to a center with experience in the surveillance and management of inflammatory bowel disease.

Adapted from American Cancer Society guidelines.

tests or rectal examinations. Some people are apprehensive about possible discomfort from an internal examination with sigmoidoscopy or colonoscopy or about the possibility of internal injury or infection, although these risks are very low.

Katie Couric's televised colonoscopy and other colon-cancer awareness campaigns have made more people willing to be tested. That's good news, because regular screenings starting at age 50 for people at average risk have a very good chance of catching polyps on their way to becoming cancer. Colorectal cancer is typically slow growing, taking five to 10 years to develop. When benign or precancerous polyps are removed during colonoscopy screenings, colon cancer may be prevented from developing at all. This is not just a matter of detecting cancer early; it prevents cancer from arising.

Types of Screening Tests

The type or frequency of screening tests depends on your individual risk situation, taking into account your age, health, history of cancer, and family history of cancer.

For people at age 50 with no symptoms and an average risk of colon cancer, doctors may recommend one or more of the following screening approaches that have been shown to be beneficial:

- Flexible sigmoidoscopy every five years
- Colonoscopy every 10 years
- Annual physical exam that includes take-home testing of the stool for fecal occult blood (FOBT) to complement endoscopic tests described above.

The ideal screening test for the entire population has not been determined, although an increasing number of doctors favor colonoscopy. If you are in one of the higher-risk groups or if you have had colon cancer or a related cancer, your doctor will recommend a more aggressive screening schedule.

Your doctor may recommend any of the following tests to monitor the health of your intestinal tract:

Annual physical exam and risk assessment

Routine physical examinations by your primary care doctor can help determine your risks of colorectal and other cancers, discover any conditions that may increase those risks, and identify signs or symptoms of disease.

The doctor assesses your overall personal health, including symptoms that could be related to colorectal cancer, such as anemia or gastrointestinal problems. You may be at higher risk for colorectal cancer if you have GI disorders such as inflammatory bowel disease (IBD; such as Crohn's disease) or a history of some cancers such as endometrial cancer (see the chart on page 15).

Your primary care doctor should also have a detailed history of any colorectal cancer, other cancer, or bowel disease in your immediate family, especially if a first-degree relative such as a parent or sibling had colorectal cancer.

The physical exam should include a digital rectal exam, in which your doctor examines the lower few inches of your rectum with a gloved finger, feeling for anything out of the ordinary. A stool sample taken at that time may show signs of colorectal cancer.

However, this exam alone is not enough to screen for colon cancer. The doctor cannot feel very far up the rectum, and a one-time stool sample is not adequate to reveal bleeding. Thus, a take-home fecal blood test should be part of the yearly exam.

Annual take-home fecal blood tests

These simple tests are painless, noninvasive, and done in the privacy of your home. The tests are inexpensive and can detect 30–85% of colorectal cancers.

Fecal blood tests look for evidence of blood. Blood vessels are more fragile in polyps and tumors, and the passage of feces can cause small amounts of blood to be released. This bleeding could be so slight that it would not be visible in your stool, especially in the early stages of tumor or polyp growth. A newer test, which is not yet widely available or covered by most insurers, can detect DNA from cancer cells in the stool.

The tests come in a kit with a specially treated test card and instructions on how to take tiny samples of stool from your bowel movements. The test kits are then sent to a lab for processing.

A negative test doesn't completely rule out colorectal cancer, because some polyps don't bleed. On the other hand, a positive test does not necessarily mean you have cancer. There are many other reasons for intestinal bleeding such as peptic ulcers, inflammatory bowel disease, or irritation from medications such as aspirin and nonsteroidal anti-inflammatory drugs (NSAIDs). If the test does show signs of bleeding, your doctor will probably want to prescribe a sigmoidoscopy or colonoscopy to check for its cause.

The standard: FOBT

The most widely used take-home test is called the fecal occult blood test (FOBT), which can reveal up to 50% of colon cancers.

NEW RESEARCH

Colonoscopy: Is It Safe To Extend the Interval After Polyp Removal?

Waiting five years between colonoscopies after polyp removal may be safe for people who had high-risk adenomas, according to a recent study from Germany. The same study suggests a 10-year interval for those with low- or average-risk adenomas.

The researchers examined the health records of 454 people (age 60–79 years) who had polyps removed endoscopically (by colonoscopy, sigmoidoscopy, or rectoscopy) and 391 who had not had an endoscopic procedure.

They found that having a polyp removed significantly reduced the risks of colorectal cancer for up to five years—even among people with high-risk adenomas. In fact, the lower risk was seen six to 10 years after the procedure. Overall, people with a polyp removal up to 10 years previously had a 60% lower risk of colorectal cancer than those who had not had an endoscopic procedure in the large bowel.

Traditionally, doctors have recommended waiting from one to three years between surveillance colonoscopies after polyp removal. But recent guidelines from a U. S. multispecialty scientific task force on colon cancer and the American Cancer Society recommend waiting five years between colonoscopies for people with low-risk adenomas, but they advise more frequent exams for people with moderate- or high-risk adenomas.

AMERICAN JOURNAL OF GASTROENTEROLOGY
Volume 102, page 1739
August 2007

It's based on a chemical reaction that reveals any hidden (or occult) blood in your stool. Since polyps in the colon tend to bleed slightly and intermittently, you will be asked to take a tiny sample from three bowel movements in a row.

To avoid false positives, this test requires some medication restrictions for up to 10 days and dietary restrictions for up to six days. You will be asked to avoid consuming:

- The pain medications called NSAIDs (such as ibuprofen and naproxen) and aspirin for seven days before the tests and during all the days when you are taking the test
- Red meat, including beef, pork, and lamb, and some fish for three days before and during the test, as these contain the animal blood protein hemoglobin
- Citrus fruits and juice and many raw vegetables, as they contain peroxidase that can create false positives
- More than 250 mg a day of vitamin C as well as iron supplements, as these can interfere with the chemical reaction in the test.

In addition, to collect the sample, most FOBT tests require that you prevent your fecal waste from having any contact with urine or water in the toilet bowl. Therefore, you have to pass your stool onto a sheet of plastic stretched over the toilet bowl or into a special container.

Doctors say it's important to complete the test and turn it in, even if you think you have consumed something on the "forbidden" list. However, if you want an accurate reading, it is best to follow the instructions exactly.

If you are taking a daily aspirin for heart health or NSAIDs for pain, be sure to check with your doctor before you stop taking them.

Risks and disadvantages. The FOBT test has no known risks. The disadvantage is that it catches only half of cancers: It doesn't detect polyps or tumors that are not bleeding. However, having FOBT done yearly improves the chance of detecting blood. It also has a high false-positive rate, meaning that it identifies some normal situations as cancer. If you test positive for hidden blood, you may need a colonoscopy to investigate further.

FIT: A new alternative

A newer version of the occult blood test, the fecal immunochemical test (FIT), does not require any dietary or vitamin restrictions, is easier to perform, and is specific for detecting the human form of the blood protein hemoglobin, so there are fewer false positives.

The FIT test detects an antibody (a sort of molecular "ID tag" used by the immune system) that is specific for the "globin" part of human hemoglobin deriving from the lower intestines only. It will not react to nonhuman hemoglobin in meat, to the peroxidase in raw vegetables or other foods, or to drugs or vitamins.

Like the FOBT test, the FIT test comes with a kit that includes a test card and a sampling tool. However, sampling doesn't require handling fecal material. Small disposable brushes are swiped across a portion of stool in the toilet bowl, then dabbed onto a test card. Only two samples from successive bowel movements are required. The test is then mailed to the lab for evaluation.

This test is more convenient than FOBT, and some studies show people prefer it. It has been available in Europe and Asia for about a decade, but it was only recently promoted in the United States. It is covered by Medicare, but it costs more than an FOBT, may not be available everywhere, and your health insurance plan may not cover it. Ask your doctor for more information.

Risks and disadvantages. FIT tests have no known risks. However, as with the FOBT, a negative result does not mean you do not have polyps, as not all polyps bleed. And a positive test for blood means you may be asked to have a colonoscopy to look for the cause.

Flexible sigmoidoscopy: The five-year test

A sigmoidoscopy uses an endoscopic instrument called a sigmoidoscope to examine the inside of the lower colon, which includes the descending colon, sigmoid colon, and rectum.

This procedure can catch nearly 100% of polyps and cancers in the lower colon, where some 60% of colorectal cancers as well as 60% of polyps with cancerous potential are found. However, it only covers one third of the colon.

This test is done as an outpatient procedure by a medical doctor or health professional such as a registered nurse who has been specially trained and certified to perform it. Sigmoidoscopy may be done in a doctor's office or at a clinic or hospital.

Your doctor's office will give you detailed instructions for a routine to clean out the lower part of your colon. You may be asked to take a laxative the night before and one or two enemas a few hours before the test. It's important that the lower bowel be clear of any feces so that the health professional can see any abnormalities.

The sigmoidoscope, a flexible tube about as wide as your finger, holds a light, a tiny video camera, an instrument to deliver small puffs of air to clear the visual field, and a hollow channel that can

NEW RESEARCH

Which Screening Test Is Preferred? Colonoscopy, It Turns Out

Colonoscopy is the source of many jokes and the cause of much squeamishness on the part of those scheduled for the test. But when 263 people at average risk for colon cancer were asked which colorectal cancer screening test they preferred—colonoscopy, fecal occult blood testing (FOBT), flexible sigmoidoscopy, flexible sigmoidoscopy plus FOBT, double-contrast barium enema, or stool DNA testing—51% chose colonoscopy.

The runner up was stool DNA testing, preferred by 28%. In third place was FOBT, chosen by 18%.

The respondents, who made their choices after completing a brief educational session on the different tests, cited accuracy as the main reason for choosing colonoscopy. Those who chose the noninvasive fecal tests cited concerns about discomfort and frequency of testing. Interestingly, most people stuck with their preference even if they would have to pay for it themselves.

AMERICAN JOURNAL OF MANAGED CARE
Volume 13, page 393
July 2007

What Makes a Good Colonoscopy?

An eye for detail and an aversion to haste help to catch early cancer

You invest a lot in a colonoscopy: time, inconvenience, discomfort, and money. It's a two-day commitment. Although colonoscopy itself is rarely uncomfortable, the preparatory diet and purging are often the worst part of the procedure. You may need to have someone drive you home after the procedure. And although most insurance plans cover this $2,000 screening test, it is seldom covered in full: Medicare recipients pay about $200.

So it is disheartening to learn from a recent study that not all colonoscopy exams are equally well done. The study, published in *The New England Journal of Medicine*, reveals that not all doctors use the same degree of care when they look for adenomatous polyps (those that have a risk of developing into colon cancer). In fact, some doctors were four times better than others at finding these adenomas.

Time Is of the Essence

Researchers concluded that success at detection of polyps depends on the amount of time doctors spend on the most crucial part of a colonoscopy—the slow removal of the endoscope, when most abnormalities are spotted and where there is the most variation in the examiners' speed of removal.

Experts recommend spending at least six to 10 minutes for this part of the procedure. Slower withdrawal times yield greater detection rates. But in this study, some of the doctors were not slow at all. The time spent ranged from three to 17 minutes for procedures in which no polyps were removed. Those gastroenterologists who spent more time—a minimum of six minutes—had more than double the detection rate of those who took less time: 28% vs. 12% for detecting any polyps and 6% vs. 3% for finding advanced adenomatous polyps.

Because the study looked at only 12 gastroenterologists in private practice, the authors were careful to say the results are preliminary. However, the researchers did review 2,053 colonoscopies performed on average-risk patients. What's more, this is not the first study to question the skill of colonoscopy examiners: Earlier studies have found that some doctors miss as many as 15–27% of polyps that have reached the adenoma stage. Still another study compared regular colonoscopies with so-called virtual colonoscopies, which image the interior of the colon using computed tomography (CT). Both procedures were done on the same day on the same patient. Both techniques

be used for instruments to biopsy tissue or to remove polyps.

The tube is advanced slowly through the anus up the rectum and colon about 25 inches (60 cm) to the first right-angle turn, which is called the splenic flexure. Enlarged images from the video camera are shown on a video monitor.

The health professional will look for polyps as well as anything out of the ordinary, such as areas of inflammation, ulcers, and signs of a bowel condition. These areas may be biopsied. All polyps will be removed as a precaution, and large polyps or those that appear cancerous or precancerous will be removed and sent to a laboratory for testing. If the polyps are found to be adenomatous or cancerous, you will be asked to have a colonoscopy.

The scoping part of the exam takes about 20 minutes. It may be uncomfortable but is not usually considered painful. You might experience some cramping: Deep breathing and relaxing can help missed some polyps. Also, recent research shows the detection rate of the examiner is more important than the patient's age or gender in determining how many adenomas are found. A task force of medical experts has estimated that, on average, a careful examiner will find precancerous polyps in at least 25% of men and 15% of women age 50 and older.

A Life-Saving Procedure

This information should not discourage you from having a colonoscopy. It is still the best way to check for colon cancer: The American Cancer Society says colorectal cancer deaths dropped 25% between 1990 and 2003, partly because more people are being screened and thus treated earlier.

And doctors want to do their best. When the 12-doctor study was published, the gastroenterologists involved began using timers to ensure longer examinations. Their detection rate has doubled.

Experience Counts

Evidence suggests that the best place to get your colonoscopy is a hospital and the best healthcare professional to perform it is a gastroenterologist. A Canadian study of more than 12,000 patients found that men and women who had their colonoscopies performed in an office by a family physician or an internist were more likely to have a new or missed colorectal cancer than people who had the procedure performed in the hospital by a gastroenterologist.

What Can You Do To Help?

Here is advice from gastroenterologists on getting an effective colonoscopy.

Ask questions before the procedure. You will have a mild sedative for the exam, so be prepared to discuss your concerns before you receive the medication—or even better, before the day of the procedure. Some practices and HMOs offer group educational sessions to explain the details of and the preparation for colonoscopy and to introduce people to the doctors who will perform the test. If this is not an option, contact the physician (or the nurse) in charge of your procedure in order to ask any questions you might have.

Do your part in the prep. If you haven't cleaned your colon thoroughly, the doctor will not have a clear view, and having the most skilled and careful examiner will not make much difference. In this situation, a responsible team will ask you to repeat the colonoscopy on another day, after you have done a better job of cleansing, or return sooner than recommended surveillance guidelines.

Does the doctor say the test was not complete? If you are told that it was not possible to reach or examine some part of your colon, ask for specifics. Then reschedule for a complete exam. ■

ease these sensations, which are usually temporary. Sedation is not usually used, and many people watch the progress of the sigmoidoscopy on the monitor along with the health professional. If you are very anxious, ask your doctor about prescribing a mild tranquilizer for the procedure.

Afterward, you should be able to drive and resume your usual activities, but you probably will want to take it easy for the rest of that day. If polyps or tissue were removed, you may have some minor bleeding. If you have heavy bleeding, fever, chills, or any concerns at all, contact your doctor or the clinic.

Risks and disadvantages. There is a very small risk of damage to the lower colon, such as infection or a perforation. The perforation rate is extremely low—approximately one to two per 10,000 colonoscopies. A disadvantage of a sigmoidoscopy is that it shows all of the rectum but less than half of the colon. So if anything out of the ordinary is seen in this area, you may need to have a colonoscopy to check out the entire colon.

Colonoscopy: The gold standard

This screening examination is considered the gold standard for finding and removing—and possibly preventing—colorectal cancer. It can detect up to 95% of colon cancers and can be used to remove precancerous polyps before they develop into cancer.

A colonoscopy uses the same technology as the sigmoidoscopy but examines the entire 5- or 6-foot length of the colon, from rectum to cecum (not just the lower part of the colon, as in sigmoidoscopy). The exam employs the same kind of long, flexible, narrow tube used for sigmoidoscopy, containing a light, a video camera, an instrument to deliver air puffs that clear the visual field, and a hollow channel for instruments to biopsy tissue or to remove polyps.

The flexible colonoscope is gently advanced up through the rectum, along the entire colon, and then slowly withdrawn. Images from the video camera are enlarged and projected on a monitor. Tissue or polyps can be biopsied or removed during the examination. The procedure takes between 30 and 60 minutes for the patient, sometimes longer if biopsies or polyp removal are necessary. The actual viewing time during the process is about 12–15 minutes (see "What Makes a Good Colonoscopy?" on pages 20–21).

All polyps are generally removed as a precaution, even if they do not appear to be precancerous. Larger polyps or abnormalities that cannot be removed are biopsied. The tissue is sent to a lab to be tested for cancer.

A doctor performs this test as an outpatient procedure. People are generally given a mild sedative, which creates a relaxed and drowsy state called conscious sedation. This is not a general anesthetic—you will be able to breathe on your own and may be able to respond when spoken to—but it does produce a short-term amnesia. You will probably not remember much about the procedure and should feel no pain or discomfort.

Indeed, most people think the worst part of this examination is the preparation, which involves purging your entire large intestine of fecal matter. Your doctor will give you detailed instructions about preparing for the test. These preparations are crucial: If your colon is not clear of feces, the doctor won't be able to see your colon lining clearly and may have to repeat the examination.

The whole process can take two days or more, during which you will want to be near a toilet for much of the time. The diet begins the entire day before the colonoscopy. It is limited to clear liquids only, such as chicken broth and clear fruit juices. It does allow black coffee or tea with sugar but no milk, and Jell-O in any color but red. You may also be asked to avoid blood thinners.

The laxative dosing begins during the evening before the colonoscopy. Laxatives are usually given in a liquid form, but a newer pill form that some individuals prefer is now available. Ask your doctor about it.

After your colonoscopy, you'll need to stay under observation until the sedation wears off. You won't be able to drive, so you should plan to have someone pick you up, or take a taxi home. Take it easy for the rest of the day, and drink plenty of fluids to replace those lost through laxatives.

If you had a biopsy or had some polyps removed, you may have some very mild bleeding from the rectum. This is normal. But if you begin to bleed heavily or have severe cramps, a fever, or chills, call your doctor.

Colonoscopies are recommended every 10 years after age 50 for people with an average risk of colon cancer. Since cancerous polyps tend to grow at a fairly slow rate, people who are not at increased risk who have shown no polyps at a base screening probably don't need colonoscopies more than every decade, as recommended. People at higher risk will have them more often.

Risks and disadvantages. Colonoscopy is an invasive procedure. Consequently, there is a very small risk (one to three per 1,000) of an adverse effect, such as an infection or a perforation from the flexible tube.

Colonoscopies are not foolproof: Because of the folds and turns of the large intestine, they can miss tumors, especially those that are flat and may be growing in the wall of the bowel. The annual fecal blood tests may help detect these tumors.

Dehydration can be an issue: If you have used an enema or oral laxative that contains sodium phosphate, you could be at risk for complications from dehydration. Be sure to drink plenty of fluids, and also consider drinking an electrolyte rehydration solution. There are several on the market. Ask your doctor for a recommendation.

Before you undertake a colonoscopy, be sure you discuss with your doctor your overall health, chronic conditions, and all medications you may be taking, including over-the-counter drugs and supplements.

NEW RESEARCH

For Colonoscopy, Location Matters

Not all colonoscopies are equal, a new study finds. Colorectal cancer is more likely to be missed if the colonoscopy is performed in a doctor's office rather than in a hospital or clinic.

These findings are from Canadian investigators who analyzed data from more than 12,000 people with colorectal cancer who had reportedly normal colonoscopies no more than three years before their diagnosis. They found that 3% of the people had a new or missed cancer, some within six months of their last colonoscopy.

And those who had a missed cancer were more likely to have had the procedure performed by an internist or family physician in an office setting. When looking specifically at colonoscopies performed by a family physician or internist in a doctor's office, they found that men were three times more likely and women were nearly twice as likely to have a new or missed cancer compared with those who underwent the procedure in a hospital.

The researchers also found that older men and women, people with diverticular disease, and women who had previously had abdominal surgery were at increased risk for a missed colorectal cancer.

For peace of mind, particularly if you're in one of the groups at increased risk for a missed cancer, have your next colonoscopy performed at a hospital or clinic by a doctor with experience performing the procedure.

GASTROENTEROLOGY
Volume 132, page 96
January 2007

Should You Have a Colonoscopy?

If you're over age 50, with few exceptions the answer is "yes"

Experts urge regular colonoscopy screening for everyone after age 50, and it seems to have paid off. Colon cancer rates are at a 14-year low, at least in part, due to increased screening that is identifying and removing precancerous polyps.

But a few studies are suggesting that some people, specifically the very elderly with multiple chronic diseases, may not need to be screened as often—or even at all. At this point, however, these findings are preliminary and need to be examined further before definitive recommendations can be made.

At Low Risk, 10 Years Is Often Enough

Most of us grudgingly accept the need for regular colonoscopy screenings but may wonder: Is it really safe to wait a decade before your next colonoscopy? Some researchers have wondered that as well.

The 10-year interval, the gold-standard period between screening colonoscopies for people at low risk, is based in part on the amount of time it usually takes a benign polyp to become cancerous. Until recently, there was little evidence to support this practice in people whose previous colonoscopies showed no evidence of cancer or polyps.

But new research suggests that the 10-year standard is more than adequate. In fact, it may be safe—although not recommended—to wait up to 20 years between colonoscopies. For example, a Canadian study that reviewed colonoscopy records of 35,975 people confirms that those with a negative (cancer-free) test result had a 72% lower risk of developing cancer over 10 years than the general population.

A German study that spanned more than a decade confirmed this finding and went even further: For people with a prior negative colonoscopy, the low-risk period can extend to 20 years.

We're not suggesting that you allow 20 years to pass between your colonoscopy screenings. But if you have a normal colonoscopy result, you can most likely wait at least a decade before undergoing the procedure again.

However, if a screening colonoscopy catches even one polyp, your risk of colon cancer goes up and so does the recommended frequency of screenings. The same is true if you have a family history of colorectal cancer or other risk factors for colorectal cancer.

For the Very Elderly, Perhaps Fewer Benefits

Is there an age beyond which it doesn't make sense to have colonoscopies anymore?

Research suggests the risk of colonoscopy may outweigh the benefits in octogenarians.

So far, there is no recommended cut-off age for a colonoscopy or for Medicare reimbursement. But as the number of Medicare recipients grows, along with the number of elderly people having regular colonoscopies, researchers are taking a look at the costs as well as the risks and benefits of this test in older people.

Two new studies reviewed the

Double-contrast barium enema: The old standby

Only a few decades ago, this x-ray examination was the only way to "see" the entire colon. It is still used instead of a colonoscopy in some cases, such as when a person refuses to have a colonoscopy or when a colonoscopy can't be performed because of an individual's unusual anatomy.

The exam involves coating the inside of the colon with a contrast solution of barium sulfate. The barium solution and a small amount of air (the double contrast) are slowly pumped into the colon results of more than 3,000 colonoscopies to address the question of when people might stop having these procedures. While the risks of developing colon cancer increase with age, the researchers observed, life expectancy decreases after age 80. Because colon cancers are slow to develop, and cancer rarely develops within 10 years of a negative colonoscopy, people over age 80 are likely to die of other causes even if colon cancer begins to develop.

In fact, the same German study that investigated the risks of a 20-year interval between colonoscopies also found that people who had a negative colonoscopy after age 55 probably have a very low risk for the rest of their lives. And in one study that reviewed colon exams in people age 50 and up, screening people who were at least the age of 80 only resulted in a 15% gain in life expectancy when compared with the benefit seen in the younger participants who were screened.

While a colonoscopy is safe for the elderly, it is never pleasant—even for the young—and research indicates that elderly people are less likely to cleanse their bowels adequately and are more likely to experience incomplete exams and complications. Putting all of these findings together, researchers suggest that doctors carefully consider the indications for colonoscopy in people who are over age 80. The test may not be needed or appropriate for everyone.

Chronic Illness May Alter Benefits

For people who have three or more long-term diseases, regular colonoscopy screenings may not offer much benefit, especially after about age 65.

A team of doctors at Yale University examined the health records of nearly 36,000 people age 67 or older who were diagnosed with colon cancer. They found that the presence of a chronic condition such as diabetes, heart disease, hip fracture, or dementia made a big difference in average life expectancy after a diagnosis of stage I cancer.

For example, for a 67-year-old man with stage I colon cancer and no chronic illnesses, average life expectancy was about 19 years; with one or two illnesses, it was 12 years; and with three or more, it dropped to eight years. Expected lifespans for a woman of the same age were similar, at 23, 16, and seven years, respectively. By age 75, men and women with three or more conditions and stage I colon cancer had an average life expectancy of about five years

What do all of these numbers mean? If you're in your late 60s or beyond and have a multitude of chronic health problems, having a colonoscopy may not improve your lifespan. As we've already mentioned, sporadic colon cancer grows slowly. As a result, you are more likely to die of one of your other health problems than of colon cancer, and this becomes more likely each year after age 67.

That said, the study results are based on group findings and are only estimates. Individual responses to aging, disease, and treatment can vary greatly. Thus, no matter what your age or health status, before deciding to stop colonoscopy screening, you should explore the issues in detail with your doctor. ■

through a small tube inserted into the rectum. The air distends the insides of the colon slightly, and the barium coats the lining. Because x-rays pass through the air but not through the barium, this provides an outline of the colon lining and shows polyps, growths, or other abnormalities.

Risks and disadvantages. This is not an invasive procedure, so there are very few complications.

Among the disadvantages are that it requires cleaning out the entire colon with a liquid diet and laxatives—just as is required with a colonoscopy—but it does not detect abnormalities with the same accuracy. The barium enema has a 70% rate of uncovering polyps one quarter of an inch (7 mm) or larger. And when these polyps are discovered, they cannot be removed or biopsied during this procedure. Consequently, if a barium enema shows that you have polyps, you will need a colonoscopy afterwards. Last, but not least, the test involves some discomfort, and fewer radiologists have experience performing it.

Newer Imaging Tests for Diagnosis and Treatment

Sophisticated imaging tests such as computed tomography (CT), positron-emission tomography (PET), magnetic resonance imaging (MRI), and ultrasound are rapidly evolving into better and more sensitive tools for examining the inside of the body and detecting abnormalities and disease.

So far, these imaging technologies are not commonly used for screening people who have no symptoms. Typically, they are used for detailed diagnosis after cancer is detected, including staging of the cancer, and for making treatment decisions.

Be wary of the full-body scan promoted by some imaging laboratories as an elective test to screen for hidden disease. The scan exposes you to radiation and is not adequate to screen for colorectal cancer. Also, insurance plans will not pay for full-body scans for that purpose.

Diagnosis and Pretreatment Evaluation

Diagnostic tests are performed when there are reasons to suspect cancer, such as signs and symptoms of colorectal cancer or laboratory studies that suggest a cancer may be present.

Sometimes, a doctor can make a preliminary diagnosis based on the endoscopic exam and on results of a biopsy of a tumor or polyp that was taken during the colonoscopy or sigmoidoscopy. This is especially true if there is a single precancerous or benign polyp and no family or personal history of cancer. However, doctors usually recommend a series of tests to consider all of the factors before making a diagnosis.

Diagnostic Tests

Together, the following tests can help doctors make a number of judgments. They can help to confirm or rule out cancer. If cancer is found, the tests can help to determine the grade (how aggressive it may be), to assess the extent of the cancer (the stage), and to tell whether it has spread (metastasized) beyond the colorectum.

Colonoscopy

In addition to being used for screening, colonoscopies are used for diagnosis when there are symptoms of colon or rectal problems.

If cancer is suspected, your doctor will want you to have a colonoscopy so that the lining of your entire colorectum can be examined carefully.

Biopsy

Polyps or areas that look suspicious can be biopsied or removed at the time of a colonoscopy or sigmoidoscopy, using a special instrument. If it appears cancer has spread, the doctor may also ask for a biopsy of the organ involved using CT or ultrasound guidance (see page 28). The tissue is then sent to a laboratory to be examined and tested.

Blood tests

If colon cancer is diagnosed, the medical team will draw some of your blood for a number of reasons, some of which are directly related to assessing the nature of the cancer.

CBC. A complete blood count (CBC) is a standard diagnostic test that determines the amount of red and white blood cells, whether infection is present, and whether you have anemia. Anemia can be a sign of cancer, as cancerous polyps tend to bleed easily, contributing to blood loss.

CEA. Some colorectal cancers may produce a high level of a protein molecule called carcinoembryonic antigen (CEA). This test is not reliable for detecting early colorectal cancers but is useful as a tumor marker and indicator of treatment progress. Levels are measured before and after treatments, because the levels should decrease when treatment is successful.

Imaging tests

These tests are rapidly evolving into ever more sophisticated diagnostic tools. There are several types of imaging tests that can help your doctors to make a detailed diagnosis, to determine whether cancer has spread and how far, and to plan and evaluate your treatment.

X-rays. Once, x-rays were the only way to see inside solid bodies. When colon cancer is being diagnosed, a chest x-ray may be taken to see if cancer has spread to the lungs.

NEW RESEARCH

Aspirin Inhibits Some—But Not All—Colorectal Cancers

Regular aspirin use reduces the risk of colon cancer, but only in people whose tumors are cyclooxygenase-2 (COX-2)–positive, according to a new study. COX-2 is an enzyme that may play an important role in the development of colon cancer.

Researchers reviewed the health records of more than 130,000 people who provided information on their aspirin use every two years throughout a 22-year study. From that group, 636 colorectal cancers developed that could be tested for COX-2 expression. About two thirds of those tumors were moderately or strongly COX-2 positive.

The investigators found that regular use of aspirin—defined as taking two or more standard aspirin tablets each week or using aspirin at least twice a week—reduced the risk of cancers that were COX-2 positive by 36%. However, it had no effect on tumors that were COX-2 negative.

The researchers predict that COX-2 may become a useful marker for identifying people with a history of colon cancer who could benefit from regular aspirin use. In the meantime, stick with aspirin to relieve your aches and pains or as directed by your doctor to prevent heart attacks, but don't use it to prevent colorectal cancer.

THE NEW ENGLAND JOURNAL OF MEDICINE
Volume 356, page 2131
May 24, 2007

Ultrasound. With ultrasound, sound waves are used to create an image. It is not used to show small polyps or growths in early-stage colon cancer. However, it is useful to evaluate the extent of some tumors, especially in cases of rectal and liver cancers.

Endorectal ultrasound can show the extent of rectal cancer, helping the doctor decide on a course of treatment. An ultrasound probe is inserted into the rectum to produce sound waves that create an image showing how deeply the tumor has penetrated the wall of the rectum and whether the cancer has spread to lymph nodes or other nearby tissues.

Intraoperative ultrasound is used during surgery to see whether cancer has spread to the liver. A special probe can be placed directly on the liver, giving doctors a much more accurate picture than one that is taken through the skin and muscles of the abdomen.

Computed tomography: CT, CAT, and spiral CT scans. A CT, or CAT, scan is a test taken by a kind of super x-ray machine linked to a computer that takes many images that give a detailed picture of internal organs. A CT scan may be used to see if colorectal cancer has metastasized to other organs.

A newer application is to use CT instead of a colonoscope to examine the colon in a so-called virtual colonoscopy. One drawback—exposure to radiation. Spiral CT scans provide three-dimensional images at a lower dose of radiation than regular CT scans.

Image-guided biopsy. CT scans and ultrasound can be used to guide a biopsy needle into the precise area where there is tissue that needs to be sampled.

Magnetic resonance imaging (MRI). This imaging procedure uses strong magnets to create images of the interior of the body. It may be used to look for cancer that has spread to other places in the body, beyond the region where it originated.

Positron emission tomography (PET). These scans are used, often along with CT scans, to search the body for metastasized cancer. They involve injections of a type of radioactive sugar. Cancer cells become visible because they absorb the sugar in higher amounts than do normal cells.

Issues Immediately After Diagnosis

People react in many ways to a diagnosis of cancer. Many people want to learn as much as they can about the disease and treatment, but others prefer to leave the treatment details to their medical team. The stress of a cancer diagnosis can make it difficult to decide how actively you want to be involved in the treatment process, and the sheer amount of information and decisions to be made may be overwhelming.

It's important at this time to have a support system to help you with the many decisions and questions. This can be a family member, close friend, or a counselor who specializes in helping people cope with cancer issues.

You will have a team of several medical specialists planning and directing your treatment. These may include a gastroenterologist, who specializes in diseases of the digestive system; a pathologist, who studies and evaluates biopsied tissue; a surgeon; a medical oncologist, to supervise cancer treatments; and a radiation oncologist, if radiation therapy is used.

It is useful to prepare a list of questions before you meet with your medical specialists and to take someone with you to help write down and remember the answers. Some people tape record the sessions to play over again later, for better understanding.

You may also want to consider seeking a second opinion for another evaluation of your options and choice of doctors. Some insurance companies require second opinions; most will pay for them on request. A second opinion is an opportunity to get another expert evaluation, to add to the diagnostic information, and to weigh treatment options and the choice of doctors.

What To Ask Your Doctor About the Diagnosis

If the doctor gives a diagnosis of cancer, here are some questions you may want to ask:

- What type of cancer do I have?
- Where is it located? Is it in more than one place?
- Are the lymph glands involved?
- Has the cancer spread outside the colon? Are other organs involved?
- What stage is the cancer, and exactly what does that mean?
- Is this type of cancer life threatening?
- Are there other tests I should have?
- How soon do I need to begin treatment?
- Who can I see for a second opinion?
- What are the side effects of treatment?
- Could this affect my relatives?

You may want to meet with a counselor trained to work with cancer patients, who can help you deal with the impact of your diagnosis.

ASK THE DOCTOR

Q. ***My doctor just told me that I have colon cancer and will need to undergo surgery. How can I get a second opinion?***

A. It is common for people to request a second opinion, especially before surgery or other involved treatment. Indeed, many insurance companies require a second opinion, and this is a good place to start. Ask your insurance company what your policy covers and if it requires you to see a doctor within that plan.

Also tell your doctor you would like to have a second opinion. Most doctors are accustomed to this and will be supportive. Ask for a referral and for copies of your medical records, including all test results, x-rays, and other imaging tests to take with you to the next doctor. You may have to sign a release and pay a copying fee, but there should be no problem in getting your records.

If a second opinion (or the doctor you wish to consult) is not covered by insurance, it may be worthwhile to pay for this examination out of pocket.

Staging Systems for Colorectal Cancer

Several different methods are in use that describe stages of colorectal cancer development according to the location and progression of the tumor or tumors. The TNM (tumor, node, metastasis) system, developed by the American Joint Committee on Cancer, is considered the most precise and descriptive, but your doctor may prefer the Dukes or Astler-Coller system. As you can see from the table, they all correlate in the same way with the more familiar Roman-numeral staging designations.

Stages	T	N	M	Dukes	Astler-Coller
Stage 0	Tis	N0	M0	—	—
Stage I	T1 or T2	N0	M0	A	A,B1
Stage IIA	T3	N0	M0	B	B2
Stage IIB	T4	N0	M0	B	B3
Stage IIIA	T1-T2	N1	M0	C	C1
Stage IIIB	T3-T4	N1	M0	C	C2,C3
Stage IIIC	Any T	N2	M0	C	C1,C2,C3
Stage IV	Any T	Any N	M1	—	D
Recurrent	—	—	—	—	—

What it means	Usual treatment (colon cancer)	Usual treatment (rectal cancer)
Earliest stage. Cancer is confined to inner lining of colon or rectum. Also known as carcinoma in situ or intramucosal carcinoma.	Surgery only, using polypectomy, local incision, or resection.	Surgery only, using polypectomy, local incision, or resection. No additional therapy.
Cancer has invaded middle layers but has not spread beyond the colon or rectum.	Surgery only, to remove cancer. No additional therapy.	Surgery only, using polypectomy, local incision, or resection. No additional therapy.
Has penetrated to outermost layers of colon or rectum. No spread to lymph nodes. No metastasis. Has grown through colon or rectal wall. No spread to lymph nodes. No metastasis.	Surgical resection. For some T4 cancers, radiation may be used. Selected patients may need chemotherapy. This is an area under active study.	Surgical resection, along with radiation and chemotherapy given before surgery and sometimes after surgery as well.
Has invaded submucosa and/or muscularis propria. Has spread to 1–3 lymph nodes. No metastasis. Has grown through colon or rectal wall or into nearby tissues or organs. Has spread to 1–3 lymph nodes. No metastasis. Has grown through colon or rectal wall or into nearby tissues or organs. Has spread to 4 or more lymph nodes. No metastasis.	Surgical resection with chemotherapy. Radiation if there is spread to adjacent tissues.	Surgery to remove rectal tumor. Radiation and/or chemotherapy before surgery. Chemotherapy after surgery.
Can be any level of tissue invasion or lymph node spread. Has metastasized to other organs, such as peritoneum or ovary.	Surgery, not expected to cure but to relieve blockage, symptoms. (If metastases in liver are small, surgery may lead to longer life or cure.) No surgery if patient's health is otherwise poor. Chemotherapy and/or radiation to relieve symptoms.	Surgery, not expected to cure but to relieve blockage, symptoms. Chemotherapy and/or radiation to relieve symptoms, contain metastases, and prolong life.
Cancer has been treated and has returned.	Chemotherapy is the mainstay of treatment unless recurrence is localized and can be surgically removed. Clinical trials should be considered.	Surgery, radiation, and/or chemotherapy to relieve symptoms, contain metastases, and prolong life. Options: Join clinical trial. Stop treatment.

Determining a Treatment Plan: Staging and Grading

As part of your treatment plan, the medical team may perform many tests to classify the stage and grade of the colorectal cancer.

Staging and grading are standardized ways to classify the extent and seriousness of a cancer. These systems use a universal shorthand to describe, evaluate, and compare cancer and its treatments in a way that helps health professionals communicate.

Grading refers to how aggressive a cancer may be, on a scale from 1 to 4, with Grade 4 being the most serious. It is based on how closely the tumor cells resemble normal cells. If the cancer cells look very similar to normal cells and are grouped together in an organized fashion, they are called well differentiated and classified as Grade 1. The less normal the cells look and the more undifferentiated (or abnormal appearing) they are, the higher the grade.

Staging refers to how far a cancer has spread, on a scale from 0 to IV, with 0 meaning a cancer that has not begun to invade the colon wall and IV describing cancer that has spread beyond the original site to other parts of the body.

In diagnosing and evaluating colorectal cancer, the size of the tumor is not as serious as how far it has grown into the wall of the colon and whether it has spread to lymph nodes and other parts of the body.

The stages describe whether the cancer is:

- in the inner lining of the colon only
- embedded in the colon wall
- penetrating through the colon wall
- involving lymph nodes
- metastatic (invading other organs).

Several different systems are used to describe the stages of colorectal cancer. The system most widely used today is called the TNM system. Developed by the American Joint Committee on Cancer (AJCC), the TNM system is considered the most precise and descriptive. T stands for the tumor and how deep it has penetrated into the colon wall, N stands for lymph node involvement, and M refers to metastases, or spread to other body parts.

Your doctor may use a different but compatible system, such as the Dukes or Astler-Coller systems. The chart on pages 30–31 shows how these systems relate to each other.

Doctors may not be able to determine the stage or grade of cancer until after surgery, when the abnormal tissue has been analyzed by a pathologist.

Although staging is a crucial step, in itself it does not completely define treatments. All treatment decisions are determined on an individual basis, because no two cancers and no two people are identical. Many other factors enter into your individual assessment, including your age, your general health, any other medical conditions you may have, your family history of cancer, and whether this is a new cancer or one that has recurred. Since your situation is unique, ask your doctor for a detailed explanation of the implications of the stage of the cancer.

Treatment Options

Cancer treatments and outcomes have greatly improved over the past few decades as a result of advances in surgery and medicine and also because of increased knowledge about how cancer progresses and responds to therapies. A diagnosis of colorectal cancer is serious, but there are options for treatment at any stage.

In most cases, a colon cancer diagnosis is not an emergency situation requiring immediate surgery or treatment. There is time to meet with a team of medical specialists to hear about treatment options and time to discuss and consider their recommendations. You also have time to interview doctors, to get a second opinion, and to choose a treatment center that is experienced in treating your type and stage of cancer.

Your treatment options depend on several factors, including the stage and location of the cancer, your general health overall, whether you have any coexisting health conditions, your age (see "How Old is Too Old for Colorectal Cancer Surgery?" on pages 34–35), and your preferences.

While cancer specialists are experts who can offer their best assessment of treatment options, your preferences and choices are an important part of the treatment plan. You have the right to decide how much treatment you want. In some cases, people opt to continue aggressive treatment as long as possible. Others decide to have limited treatment, no treatment, or only palliative treatment to control their symptoms.

While you are making these decisions, it can be helpful to consult with a counselor experienced in working with people who have cancer. You can find these counselors through major cancer treatment centers. Your doctor or treatment center staff may be able to refer you to a good one.

ASK THE DOCTOR

Q. ***Who should I tell about my cancer diagnosis, and how should I tell them?***

A. Your immediate family should know as much as possible; you may not be able to do all that you usually do, and they need to know that routines will change. Don't shrink from sharing bad news. Concealing the truth takes energy that you need to support each other and make decisions. Discuss ways to cope, which will help you work together effectively.

Tell close friends quickly. They may be hurt if they learn about your cancer from someone else and then find it difficult to be supportive. Most friends want to help; tell them what they can do, from cooking to dog walking to just coming over for tea.

However, you do not need to tell others every detail. Before you tell friends and acquaintances about your illness, think through your expectations and anticipate a variety of reactions. Friends may avoid you for fear of saying the wrong thing, become intrusive, or say something hurtful out of ignorance.

When telling young children, be honest and simple to avoid misunderstandings that may be equally upsetting. Be sure to let them ask questions and try to give them clear answers that they can understand. In some cases, it may help to have a social worker or psychologist talk to the child.

How Old Is Too Old for Colorectal Cancer Surgery?

Age is only one factor to consider

When a reasonably healthy octogenarian gets a diagnosis of colon cancer, the issue of age is bound to come up. How old is too old for colon cancer surgery? What are the risks? What kind of recovery and quality of life can the very elderly expect afterward? Is it worth it?

Few studies have looked at how the elderly fare after colorectal cancer treatment and pursued these hard-to-ask questions. But in the ones that have, the short answer is that octogenarians and even nonagenarians can fare as well as younger seniors, if they are in otherwise good health.

The Impact of Illness

It is true that the risks of surgery are higher for *some* older people. An analysis of 28 studies found lower survival rates among the elderly who have coexisting health conditions, are diagnosed at an advanced cancer stage, and have to undergo emergency procedures. Another study found that octogenarians with early-stage cancer survived 10 or more years after colorectal cancer surgery if they had no chronic illnesses.

Quality of Life

It appears that quality of life after treatment can be as good for octogenarians as it is for younger seniors—even in the face of coexisting illness, according to a recent Canadian study that compared the outcomes of people over age 80 with those in their 60s. The average age of the older group was 83 years at the time of surgery, while the "youngsters" ranged in age from 65–69. People in both groups underwent comparable surgical procedures and had similar coexisting health problems (such as hypertension and diabetes), although the older group had somewhat less advanced (lower-stage) cancers.

The responses to a survey on quality of life and functioning before and after surgery were remarkably similar in both groups. Before surgery, both worried about pain, becoming a burden, and death. After surgery, there were no major changes or differences between the groups in terms of their ability to perform daily functions or their overall health, sexual function, or quality of life.

While older people did have more concerns about stoma management (an opening in the abdomen that allows bodily wastes to pass through) and urination, and some had more difficulty walking up and down stairs, they also felt more energetic and vital than their younger counterparts. Not surprisingly, these researchers found that elderly people who reported a good quality of life after surgery were also mobile, active, and able to take care of themselves before their operation.

Though few in number, studies

Prognosis: A Prediction About Outcomes

In the course of treatment, your doctor will give you a prognosis, a prediction of the likely outcome of the cancer and treatments. The prognosis may change as more information about the disease becomes known and as your response to treatment is evaluated.

In colorectal cancer, prognosis is related to many factors:

- The stage of cancer: how deeply the tumor has invaded the bowel wall and any lymph node involvement (The size of the tumor is not as important as the stage.)
- Recurrent cancer: whether the cancer has returned after treatment
- Metastasized cancer: whether the cancer has spread to other organs

looking at the quality of life after other types of surgery in people over age 80 find—like the Canadian study—that in general elderly people report that their quality of life after surgery is good. This holds true even when their ability to function worsens.

Too Early To Draw Firm Conclusions?

The Canadian researchers emphasize that their study findings are preliminary, and some results may be biased. For example, the conclusions were based on responses from a very small number of respondents—only 29 in each group. Therefore, the results could be simply a matter of chance. In addition, the people who were willing and able to complete the survey in both groups were functioning at a high level—and were doing so before the surgery. Study results may have been different if people who responded to the survey weren't functioning at high levels before or after surgery, but it's impossible to know for sure.

While the results are preliminary, the study provides further ammunition for the argument that determining which patients are candidates for colon cancer surgery shouldn't be made solely on the basis of chronological age. High-functioning elderly people who undergo colon surgery appear able to retain their ability to function and maintain a good quality of life.

Improving the Odds

Experts note that regardless of age—but especially for the very old—the outcome is likely to be better under these conditions:

• The cancer is at an early stage. Most people in the study had stage 0, I, or II cancer; none had stage III or IV (see "Staging Systems for Colorectal Cancer" on pages 30–31).

• The person about to have treatment is functioning at a high level before surgery and in good general health, without multiple serious chronic diseases. People who have three or more chronic diseases—such as diabetes, rheumatoid arthritis, or heart disease—tend to have poorer outcomes.

• The surgery is seen as a positive action, and the person with cancer is aware of the procedures to be performed and the potential outcomes.

Other issues that could affect outcomes at any age include a family history of longevity and a good support system of family and friends.

Get a Geriatric Evaluation

The bottom line: Chronological age should not be the only factor considered when determining who will benefit from colorectal cancer surgery. But if you have concerns about how well you or a loved one might respond to surgery, ask the doctor to conduct a geriatric evaluation before surgery. This type of evaluation takes into account not only factors such as heart and lung function, but also other important considerations for older people such as nutritional and mental status. ■

- The age and overall health of the person with cancer
- Response or tolerance to therapy
- The postoperative blood levels of carcinoembryonic antigen (CEA), a substance that signals the existence of cancer cells.

You may see statistics about five-year survival rates and cure rates. Medical professionals use these statistics during clinical research as a way to compare the prognoses of different groups of people with cancer and also to project a likely prognosis for individuals with cancer. These statistics can be confusing and sometimes frightening.

It's important to know what the health team says about your prognosis, since prognosis relates to how much treatment is needed and how long people in your situation tend to survive after various treatment choices. It gives a framework for making decisions about treatments and about personal plans for your future.

However, it is more important to remember that these opinions and numbers are based on data collected about groups of people whose cancer is similar to yours. A prognosis is an educated estimate—not an absolute—about any individual's outcome.

Every cancer is unique, just as every person with cancer is unique. Sometimes a person who has a very poor prognosis does very well. Also, the prognosis can change over time and in response to treatments. Ask your doctor to explain in detail what your prognosis means.

Overview of Treatments

Treatment for both colon and rectal cancer almost always involves surgery and may include radiation, chemotherapy, or some combination of all three. In many ways, treatments for colon and rectal cancer are similar. The differences—and information about cancer that has metastasized—are discussed later in separate sections about treatments specific to colon and rectal cancer.

Surgery

The first line of treatment for colorectal cancer is to remove the primary tumor or tumors. If your cancer is confined to polyps or a small area, surgery is probably the only treatment that you need. For stage I or II cancers that have not spread to the lymph nodes, the expected five-year survival rate after surgery without chemotherapy is 80–90%.

Surgery usually involves removing the segment of the colon or rectum that has the primary cancer and a margin of healthy colon on either side of the cancer. The surgeon will also remove the tissue that holds the colon in place (mesentery) and the adjacent lymph nodes. The number of lymph nodes removed can be important in providing an accurate stage and prognosis.

What happens in surgery. Preparation for colon or rectal surgery involves taking laxatives and enemas and fasting for at least eight hours before the operation to empty the entire bowel as completely as possible. A general anesthetic puts you into a deep sleep, and a tube is inserted into your throat to regulate your breathing for the length of the procedure.

For abdominal surgery, an 8- to 12-inch incision is made into the abdomen to remove the cancer and some surrounding tissue and to reconnect the bowel ends, a process called anastomosis.

After major surgery, you will have some pain for two or three days, which is relieved with morphine or other pain medication. You will not be able to eat and will be given intravenous fluids. After a few days, you should be able to eat, and bowel function will resume, although it may take a few days to return to normal function. A typical hospital stay for colorectal surgery is between four and eight days, and full recovery takes about two months.

After rectal surgery, in which the procedure may be quite complex, it may take longer for bowel function to return and there may also be some drains (tubes inserted near the surgical site to allow draining of fluids) in place for a few days.

In some cases, it may be possible to have a minimally invasive procedure (laparoscopy) instead of abdominal surgery to remove the cancer. For a laparoscopic procedure, the surgeon uses a number of very small incisions to gain access to the colon or rectum. Laparoscopic surgery has a shorter recovery time than abdominal surgery. The preparation for a laparoscopic procedure is the same as for abdominal surgery.

In rare cases after either type of surgery, it may not be possible to reconnect the intestines to regain normal bowel function. In such cases, a surgical opening (ostomy) is created to allow waste to pass into a removable pouch located outside the body. (When the opening connects to the colon, this procedure is called a colostomy; when it connects to the small intestine, the procedure is called an ileostomy.) This pouch may be temporary, giving the surgical site time to heal. After six to eight weeks, it can usually be reversed. Occasionally, it is not possible to reconnect the colon or preserve the anal muscles, and the opening will need to remain in place permanently (see Living With a Colostomy on page 49).

Possible side effects of surgery. Surgical techniques have improved greatly in recent years. However, side effects can include bleeding, blood clots in the legs, infection, and damage to nearby organs, muscles, or nerves during the operation. This could result in problems such as irregular bowel movements, diarrhea, fecal incontinence, and urinary and bladder complications. Men may have erection and ejaculation problems following rectal surgery, but women do not usually see any effects on sexual function unless extensive pelvic surgery is needed. Other aftereffects of surgery can include blockages or other problems arising due to adhesions or scar tissue in the colon or rectum. These aftereffects can be temporary or permanent. Complications are more common after rectal surgery than after operations involving thc colon.

NEW RESEARCH

Massage and Acupuncture Relieve Pain After Cancer Surgery

Adding massage and acupuncture to the usual care provided after cancer surgery relieved pain and depression more than traditional postoperative care alone, according to a recent study.

Both massage and acupuncture were given for 10–30 minutes at the bedsides of 138 people who underwent surgery for intestinal and other cancers. Swedish massage was used along with an acupressure foot massage. Acupuncture was given at points related to the patients' symptoms, which included pain and nausea.

On a scale of 1–10, pain scores in the massage/acupuncture group declined by 1.4 points compared with 0.6 points in the usual-care group. Among people who reported pain of at least level 3 on the scale, pain scores declined by nearly 2 points compared with 0.3 points for those who received usual care. Therapy with massage and acupuncture was similarly effective in alleviating depressed moods.

These findings require confirmation in a larger study. Nevertheless, there is a growing acceptance among healthcare providers of complementary therapies such as these to help relieve the side effects of cancer treatment. If you're scheduled for colorectal cancer surgery, find out if your hospital or cancer center offers such therapies and whether some of these treatments are covered by your insurance.

JOURNAL OF PAIN AND SYMPTOM MANAGEMENT
Volume 33, page 258
March 2007

Colon Cancer Surgery

Removing a threat while preserving a vital function

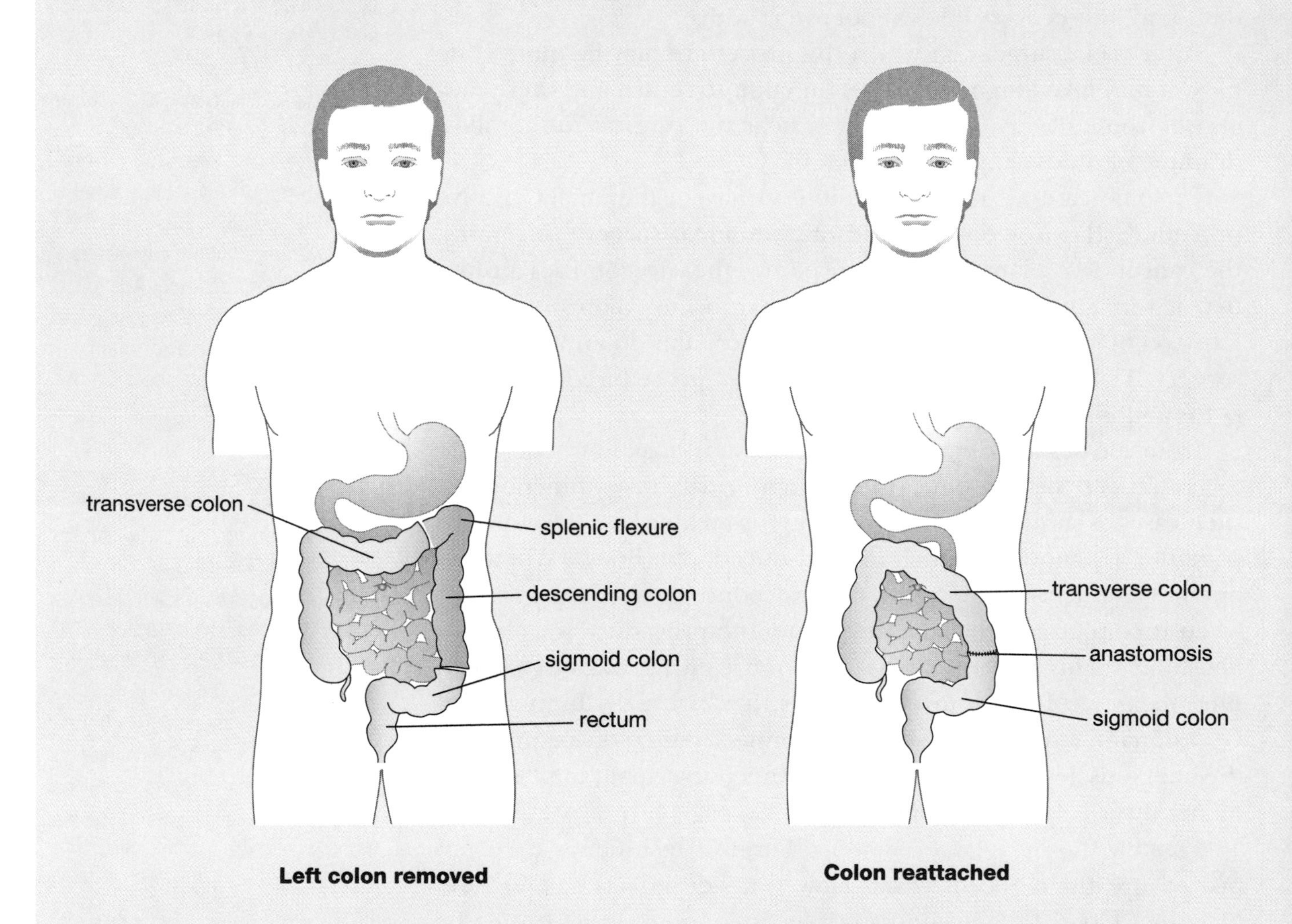

Left colon removed

Colon reattached

Surgery is usually the first line of treatment for colon cancer and may be all that is needed. There are many different types and degrees of surgery, depending on the location and extent of the cancer.

In most cases, one fourth to one half of the colon will be removed, regardless of the size of the tumor. This is because, when surgery severs the complex blood supply to a section of colon, that entire section would die anyway without oxygen and nutrients.

The remaining sections of the colon are sutured together to restore the digestive canal. When this is impossible, a colostomy is created to allow feces to

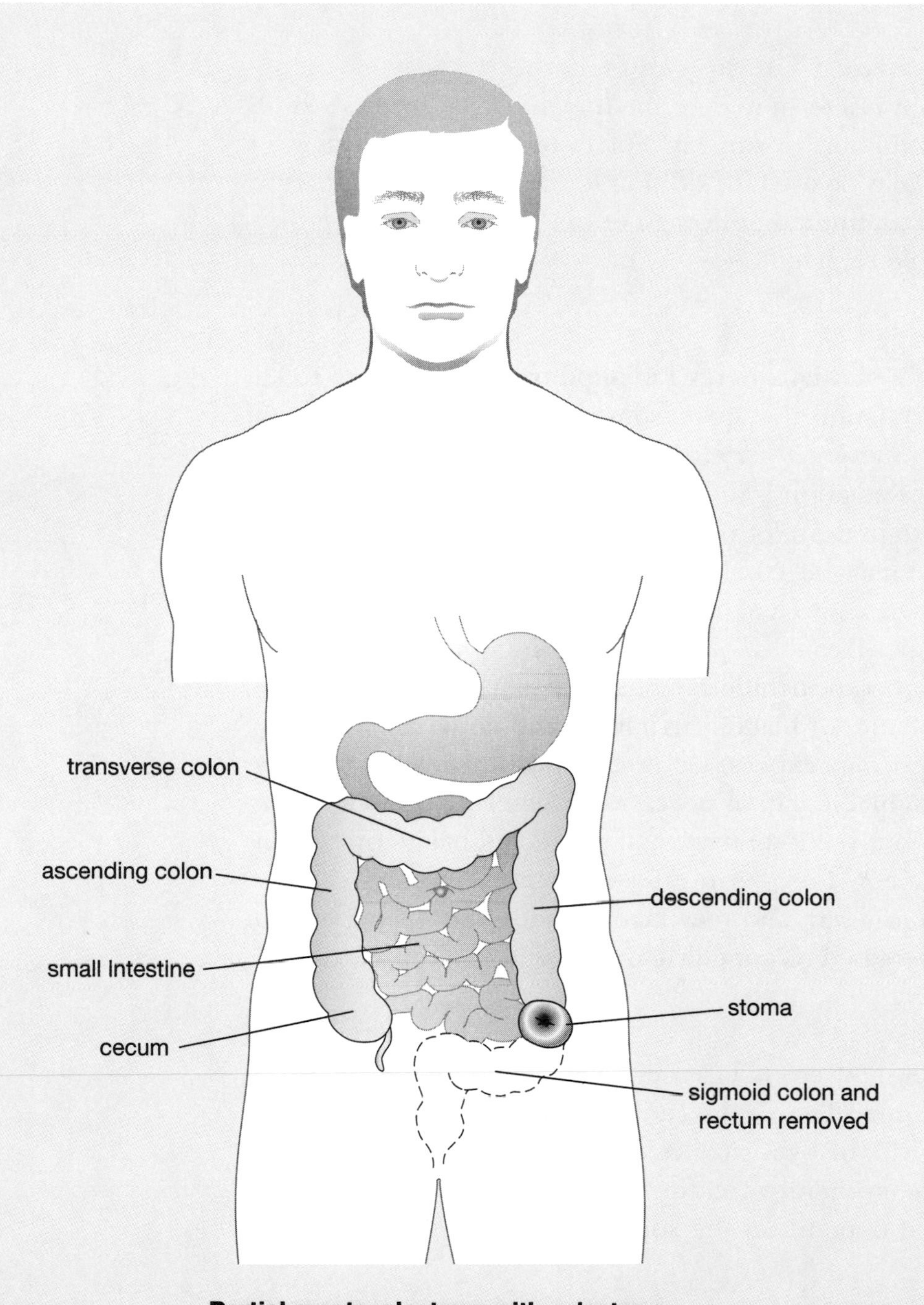

Partial proctocolectomy with colostomy

pass outside the abdomen into a pouch.

The illustration shows a left hemicolectomy, a typical procedure to remove cancer that arises in the left colon somewhere between the splenic flexure and the rectum. When a tumor occurs in a different part of the colon, the surgical procedure is similar but the colon is severed and reattached in a different location.

On the rare occasions where the location of the tumor makes it technically impossible to reattach the colon while preserving the function of the muscles in the rectum or anus, a colostomy may be the only option. ■

Adjuvant Therapies:
Radiation Therapy and Chemotherapy

Adjuvant therapy is a term to describe the use of one or more kinds of therapy in addition to surgery. For example, radiation and/or chemotherapy may be used in addition to surgery. Adjuvant therapy may be advised when there is no sign of cancer but there are indications that it could return.

Radiation therapy

With this treatment, high-energy radiation particles are used to kill cancer cells. Radiation therapy is sometimes used to shrink rectal tumors before or after surgery for rectal cancer that has penetrated the bowel wall. Radiation is rarely used for colon cancers. The goal of radiation is to prevent local recurrences near the primary tumor site. Radiation may be combined with or used alternately with chemotherapy. (See also Radiation on pages 55–57).

Possible side effects of radiation therapy. The side effects of radiation therapy can include fatigue, mild skin irritation, nausea, diarrhea, rectal and/or bladder irritation, and bowel incontinence. Afterwards, men may experience erectile dysfunction and women may develop vaginal irritation or scarring. Side effects lessen or disappear after therapy, but some sexual, rectal, and bladder problems may be permanent. Long-term effects can include other cancers, but these are fairly rare and may take decades to develop. Women may have an increased risk of pelvic fractures in the future.

Chemotherapy

Chemotherapeutic drugs kill cancer cells or stop them from dividing and spreading. The drugs can be given by mouth, by intravenous (I.V.) drip, or by injection into a vein (bolus). There is no one perfect chemotherapy treatment: The times, ways, and particular drugs used depend on the specific colorectal cancer and on the patient.

Used after surgery, chemotherapy is a kind of insurance to be certain all cancer cells have been killed. Combined with radiation, it may act as a booster to make treatments more effective. When used following surgery in patients who had cancer in the lymph nodes (stage III), it may reduce the risk of dying by one third and lower the risk of recurrence by 40%.

Chemotherapy is not usually used following surgery for colon cancers in stage I–II, unless there is a recurrence of cancer following previous treatment. It is used more often in stage III cancers that have invaded the lymph nodes. In advanced stage IV cancers or other cancers for which surgery is not an option, chemotherapy can be used as palliative therapy to prolong life, shrink tumors, and relieve symptoms.

Developing and improving chemotherapeutic agents for colorectal cancer are the focus of intensive investigation by scientists and medical professionals. In fact, many treatments in use today are based on results from large clinical trials aimed at optimizing the effectiveness of drug therapy. People with advanced cancers may have the opportunity to test a new drug by joining a clinical trial, which could lead to safer more effective treatment in the future (see page 62).

Currently, there are two basic kinds of cancer drugs: cytotoxics and biologics. Cytotoxics interfere with basic cell division. These are considered traditional cancer drugs and include 5-fluorouracil (5-FU)—often given with leucovorin to enhance its activity—irinotecan (Camptosar), and oxaliplatin (Eloxatin). The drug 5-FU was developed nearly 40 years ago; irinotecan and oxaliplatin are recently approved drugs.

Biologic drugs are a relatively new development. They are genetically engineered large proteins (antibodies) that "target" specific molecules, attempting to reverse the defects that have caused cells to become cancerous by destroying their internal controls on growth factors or limiting their ability to grow. These drugs include the monoclonal antibodies cetuximab (Erbitux), which targets the epidermal growth factor receptor (EGFR), and bevacizumab (Avastin), which targets vascular endothelial growth factor (VEGF), Recently, a third monoclonal antibody, panitumab (Vectibix), was approved by the U.S. Food and Drug Administration. As with cetuximab, panitumab also targets the EGFR. (See "Common Chemotherapy Drugs for Colorectal Cancer" on pages 42–43.)

Chemotherapy is often given in combinations of medications called regimens, which are more effective than one drug alone (see "Colorectal Cancer Chemotherapy Regimens" on page 47). The combinations and scheduling can be complicated and are tailored to each patient.

Still in the works are new therapies such as immune stimulators, vaccines, and gene-based therapy. Immune stimulators would help the immune system detect cancer cells as invaders and destroy them. Vaccines would make a person immune to cancer. (Recently, a vaccine was approved to prevent cervical cancer.) Gene-based therapies would compensate for the mutations known to cause

NEW RESEARCH

Does Chinese Herbal Medicine Help Reduce Chemotherapy Side Effects?

No—and yes. When put to the test in a double-blind placebo-controlled randomized study, Chinese herbal medicine (CHM) did not reduce the toxic blood-related effects of chemotherapy, such as low white blood cell count and severe anemia. However, it did significantly reduce chemotherapy-induced nausea.

For this study, licensed herbalists with university training and at least 15 years of experience randomly assigned 120 people in China and Hong Kong who had colon or breast cancer to receive either medicinal herbs or nontherapeutic herbs, which were taken daily during chemotherapy.

Both groups experienced moderate to severe reductions in white blood cells and neutrophils. In addition, four patients taking CHM and three on placebo had low neutrophil counts with fevers, requiring admission to the hospital. But significantly fewer patients in the CHM group experienced moderate nausea than did those in the placebo group—16% and 38%, respectively. There was no difference in the effect of CHM on other nonhematologic chemotherapy side effects.

The use of complementary and alternative medications is gaining popularity among cancer patients. Strong clinical research studies such as this one will help clarify their role in the treatment of cancer patients and help increase acceptance among healthcare providers.

ANNALS OF ONCOLOGY
Volume 18, page 768
April 2007

Common Chemotherapy Drugs for Colorectal Cancer

Class of drug	Generic name (brand name)	How it works
Antimetabolite	5-Fluorouracil (5-FU, Adrucil)	Disrupts growth of cancer cells by preventing them from making DNA and RNA by interfering with nucleic acid synthesis.
	capecitabine (Xeloda)	Disrupts growth of cancer cells by preventing them from making DNA and RNA by interfering with nucleic acid synthesis. (Capecitabine is an oral form of 5-fluorouracil.)
Biomodulator	leucovorin (Wellcovorin)	Helps 5-fluorouracil kill cancer cells more effectively by improving its ability to bind to the target enzyme, thymidilate synthase.
Topoisomerase I inhibitor	irinotecan (Camptosar)	Stops cancer cells from growing by inhibiting topoisomerase, an enzyme that uncoils DNA to help cells replicate.
Alkylating agent	oxaliplatin (Eloxatin)	Stops growth of cancer cells by working directly on DNA to prevent cancer cells from reproducing.
Monoclonal antibody	bevacizumab (Avastin)	Prevents growth of new blood vessels, "starving" cancer cells.
	cetuximab (Erbitux)	Stops growth of cancer cells by fitting into receptors on cell surface, blocking epidermal growth factor (EGFR), which is then unable to direct cell division.
	panitumumab (Vectibix)	Works like cetuximab to shrink tumors in patients not responding to other treatments.

Adapted from The American Cancer Society's *Complete Guide to Colon Cancer*, 2006.

cancer, especially those that disrupt the normal regulatory process of cell death. Ultimately, these targeted therapies could have fewer side effects than currently used chemotherapy medicines.

Possible side effects of chemotherapy. Chemotherapy is powerful medicine. Because chemotherapy keeps cancer cells from growing, it also affects normal cells.

The side effects from this depend on the drug and on your individual physiology. The short-term effects generally include fatigue, nausea and vomiting, diarrhea, hair loss, and a low blood count that increases the risk of infection. The drugs also may impair wound healing, bleeding, or clotting. They also can cause a foggy mental state, known as chemobrain (see "It's Not All in Your Head" on pages 52–53). Rashes and mouth sores also are common.

When it's used	Most common side effects
May be used to treat colorectal cancer that has metastasized or used after surgery to prevent recurrence.	Diarrhea, sore mouth. May lower blood counts.
Usually used to treat colorectal cancer that has metastasized or used after surgery to prevent recurrence.	Diarrhea, sore mouth, redness of hands and feet (sometimes peeling skin). May lower blood counts.
Only used with 5-fluorouracil.	Side effects are rare.
Usually used to treat metastasized colorectal cancers. May be used with 5-fluorouracil/leucovorin or cetuximab.	May lower blood counts, cause nausea, vomiting, severe diarrhea.
Used along with 5-fluorouracil and leucovorin or Xeloda to treat metastatic colorectal cancer or for treatment after surgery to prevent recurrence.	May cause nausea, vomiting, numbness and tingling of fingertips or toes.
Used to treat metastasized colorectal cancers.	Hypertension, proteinuria, blood clots. Rarely, allergic reactions or perforation of the intestines.
Used with irinotecan when colorectal cancer no longer responds to irinotecan alone or without it when patient cannot take irinotecan.	Rash, allergic reactions with fever, chills, swelling, shortness of breath.
Used to treat metastasized colorectal cancers.	Skin rash, fatigue, abdominal pain, nausea, diarrhea. Serious adverse effects include lung scarring and severe skin rash.

Long-term effects can include damage to nerves, the reproductive organs, and other organs such as the liver or lungs. Some of these effects can be permanent.

Follow-Up After Treatment

Unfortunately, treatment for colorectal cancer is not foolproof. There are substantial risks that cancer will return or metastasize, although recurrence is not inevitable. Consequently, your medical care will continue after the primary treatment. Regular follow up is crucial not only to allow the doctor to check on how well you are healing but also to identify any recurrences early.

Over the course of your treatment and follow up, you may see experts at many different centers or medical offices. It is helpful to keep a set of medical records and documents for yourself and for your family or caregiver. At the minimum, these should include information about your Medicare or other health insurance policy numbers, your social security number, and the names and contact information of your doctors and other health professionals.

It is also prudent to maintain a record of your tests and results, of every operation and other kinds of procedures, and of all medication you are taking or have taken, with the dosages (including over-the-counter medicines and supplements). You are entitled to have copies of your tests and medical reports. In addition, you are entitled to view and copy your medical records, including all hospital charts and records. (However, you may have to pay a fee for photocopying.)

Treatment of Colon Cancer

The first and most common strategy to treat colon cancer is surgery. If the cancer is in early stages, this may be all the treatment you need. Surgery can vary from a minimally invasive polypectomy or laparoscopic surgery to major abdominal surgery. The type and extent of the procedure depend on where the colon cancer is located and on how much of the colon and the surrounding tissue is involved.

Surgical Procedures for Colon Cancer

If a polyp is cancerous but can be snared and removed (polypectomy) during endoscopy or the cancer is confined to a clearly defined area that has not penetrated the bowel wall, there is usually no need for abdominal surgery.

If abdominal surgery is recommended, the surgeon will usually plan to remove the segment of the colon that contains the tumor and a margin of healthy colon on either side of the tumor. A typical operation for colon cancer removes one fourth to one half of the colon (a section between 1 and 3 feet long).

The nature of the procedure is determined somewhat by the blood supply to the colon. To remove the tumor, surgeons may have to interfere with the main blood supply that comes through a network of vessels to all parts of the colon. When main blood vessels that support a section of colon have to be severed to remove the tumor, the blood supply is cut off from that length of colon. That colon segment must also be removed, because if it were left in place it would deteriorate slowly, ultimately destroying the integrity of the intestinal canal.

In most cases, there is time to discuss different surgical options and other treatments with your doctor before making decisions. Only on rare occasions is there an emergency situation such as an intestinal blockage, internal bleeding, or an abdominal infection (peritonitis) that requires immediate surgery. In such cases, the surgeon takes care of the emergency and schedules further surgeries, as needed.

The basic surgery used for colon cancer is a radical resection: removal of a tumor and a margin of healthy tissue around it. The names of the specific procedures cite the area to be removed. For example, in a transverse colectomy, the surgeon removes the transverse colon; in a radical left hemicolectomy, the surgeon removes the left or descending colon. (See illustrations on pages 38–39.) In a partial colectomy, only the section of the colon with cancer is removed (the most common operation for colon cancer). In a total colectomy, all of the colon, from the cecum to the rectum, is removed.

The surgeon then connects the remaining sections. In some cases, the colon has to be rerouted to make a connection. In rare cases, a colostomy or ileostomy (a surgical opening to allow wastes to pass to the outside) will be temporarily needed to allow the reconnected colon to heal. After six to eight weeks, it usually can be reversed. Occasionally, however, a colostomy or ileostomy will have to remain in place permanently if the muscles of the anal sphincter need to be removed.

Adjuvant Therapies for Colon Cancer

The regimen of adjuvant therapies is determined by the specific situation. Radiation and/or chemotherapy may be used before or after surgery, but in colon cancer these are typically used postsurgery.

Compared with rectal surgery, radiation is rarely given after colon cancer surgery. Chemotherapy is not used at all for stage I colon cancer and its use in stage II colon cancer is still under investigation. It is used in stage III colon cancer, in which the lymph nodes are involved, in advanced cancer, and in cancer that has metastasized. Adjuvant therapies can be used for stage IV or metastasized cancer as palliative therapy to relieve symptoms and to prolong life.

Treatment of Rectal Cancer

Choosing the best treatment for rectal cancer may involve doctors from several specialties, including a urologist or gynecologist. Treatment almost always includes radiation and/or chemotherapy. The risk of recurrence is greater for rectal cancer than for colon cancer.

NEW RESEARCH

Patients Prefer Oral to Intravenous Chemotherapy

All other things being equal, people with stage III colon cancer undergoing chemotherapy prefer using oral chemotherapy medications because they are substantially more convenient than intravenous (I.V.) treatment, a new study shows.

Because oral chemotherapeutic medications are becoming increasingly available, researchers wanted to know patient perceptions about health-related quality of life, therapy side effects, and convenience. They recruited more than 1,600 people with stage II or III colon cancer who had undergone surgery and randomly assigned them to receive either I.V. fluorouracil and leucovorin or uracil/ftorafur (UFT) plus leucovorin given orally. The regimens were equally effective and produced similar adverse effects.

Overall, there were no significant differences between the groups in terms of quality of life. And both regimens were well tolerated. But 60% of people who received oral therapy described treatment as "very convenient" and 70% were "very satisfied" compared with 33% and 57% of those who received I.V. chemotherapy, respectively.

If you need chemotherapy following colorectal cancer surgery but are concerned about the impact of the treatment on your day-to-day activities, ask your doctor whether an oral chemotherapy regimen might be an option.

JOURNAL OF CLINICAL ONCOLOGY
Volume 25, page 424
February 1, 2007

Surgery for Rectal Cancer

As with colon cancer, surgery is the first line of treatment, but it is more technically challenging than colon surgery. Unlike the colon, which is flexible, the rectum is attached and encased deep within the bones of the pelvis, making a tight area in which to operate. There are many organs and systems to work around. These include blood vessels feeding the legs, organs such as the prostate (in men) and the uterus and vagina (in women), the urinary tract and bladder, and nerves that control sexual and urinary functions. There is a possibility that a temporary or permanent colostomy may be required, and nerve damage could result in erectile dysfunction in men or bladder dysfunction in men and women.

The best situation from the surgical point of view is an early-stage tumor that is contained and accessible through the anal canal (see Localized procedures on page 48). If the cancer is confined to polyps that can be snared and removed in a polypectomy or to clearly defined areas that have not penetrated the rectal wall, there is no need for abdominal surgery.

However, abdominal surgery or, in some cases, perineal surgery (performed through the perineum—the area around the anus) is required for cancers that have penetrated the rectal wall or spread to the lymph nodes.

If the tumor is in or very near the anus, a reconnection (anastomosis) may not be possible after removing the cancerous area. Removing the tumor could mean removing the sphincter muscles, making a permanent colostomy unavoidable. This is less likely today than in the past, because the techniques and the philosophy of rectal cancer surgery have changed over the past few decades. Surgical techniques are more precise, and surgeons now believe that it is not necessary to remove as much tissue around the tumor, making it possible to spare the sphincter muscles in many cases. Also, a newer imaging technique called endorectal ultrasound is used to allow surgeons to "see" the tumor precisely and determine the extent to which it has invaded through the rectal wall and whether enlarged lymph nodes are present.

If the cancer is considered to be more advanced (involving growth through the rectal wall or enlarged nodes) but curable, radiation and chemotherapy may be given for about six weeks before surgery, which can often shrink the tumor and thus allow a precise surgical reconnection that avoids a colostomy. However, if the reconnection must be located very low in the pelvis (which happens in a small minority of cases), bowel function may not completely return to normal. If

Colorectal Cancer Chemotherapy Regimens

Regimen name	Drugs in regimen	Mode of administration
AIO	Folic acid, 5-FU,* irinotecan	2-hour infusions of irinotecan and separately of leucovorin on day 1; weekly intravenous (I.V.) infusions of 5-FU via ambulatory pump over 24 hours.
CAPIRI	Irinotecan, capecitabine	Irinotecan infusions on days 1 and 8 every 3 weeks; oral capecitabine twice daily on days 1–14.
CAPOX	Oxaliplatin, capecitabine	Oxaliplatin on days 1 and 8; oral capecitabine twice daily on days 1–14 every 3 weeks.
FOLFIRI	Folic acid, 5-FU, irinotecan	2-hour infusions of irinotecan and leucovorin on day 1; loading dose of 5-FU I.V. bolus on day 1, then 5-FU via ambulatory pump over 46 hours every 2 weeks.
FOLFOX4	Oxaliplatin, leucovorin, 5-FU	2–hour infusion of oxaliplatin on day 1; 2-hour infusions of leucovorin on day 1 and day 2; loading dose of 5-FU I.V. bolus, then 5-FU via ambulatory pump over 22 hours on days 1 and 2 every 2 weeks.
FOLFOX6	Oxaliplatin, leucovorin, 5-FU	2-hour infusion of oxaliplatin and separately of leucovorin on day 1; loading dose of 5-FU I.V. bolus on day 1, then 5-FU via ambulatory pump over 46 hours every 2 weeks.
IFL	Irinotecan, 5-FU, leucovorin	Irinotecan infusion, 5-FU I.V. bolus, and leucovorin I.V. bolus weekly for 4 out of 6 weeks.
Mayo low-dose	5-FU, low-dose leucovorin	Bolus 5-FU plus leucovorin daily for 5 days every 28 days.
Roswell Park	5-FU, high-dose leucovorin	Bolus 5-FU plus leucovorin administered weekly for 6 consecutive weeks every 8 weeks

*FU = fluorouracil.

the cancer is found not to have invaded too far through the bowel wall and no lymph nodes are evident, surgery will be performed immediately.

If surgery has been performed and the tumor has invaded through the rectal wall, or if lymph nodes are involved, radiation and chemotherapy will be given after surgery. If preoperative staging indicates that a patient will need radiation and chemotherapy, many teams of rectal cancer specialists prefer to give the chemotherapy or radiation therapy before surgery. Studies show that side effects, bowel function, and therapeutic results are best with this sequence.

Localized procedures

When the cancer is confined to polyps or to a small area that has not grown through the rectum wall, minimally invasive treatments and therapies can be performed without abdominal surgery. These treatments are done through the anal canal and require special expertise and instruments.

Sigmoidoscopy. Polyps can be removed using a sigmoidoscope, usually at the time of a diagnostic examination.

Transanal endoscopic microsurgery. This procedure, used for larger but still superficial and contained cancers, involves passing specialized instruments through a tube in the anal canal to remove tumors in the middle or upper third of the rectum.

These techniques aren't effective for cancers that have penetrated the rectum wall, and they involve a greater risk of recurrence than abdominal surgery.

Fulguration. Also called electrocoagulation, this technique uses electric current to destroy a tumor by burning it. This is almost always used as a palliative measure when cancer has returned after primary management.

Endocavity radiation therapy. Also called Papillon therapy, endocavity radiation therapy involves passing a radiation source through the anus into the rectum to destroy tumors.

A disadvantage of both fulguration and endocavity radiation therapy is that they destroy the tumors, so there is no tissue for a pathologist to examine. In addition, lymph nodes cannot be removed.

Abdominal surgeries

In most cases, rectal cancer is treated with abdominal surgery, along with adjuvant therapies such as radiation and chemotherapy.

Anterior resection with anastomosis. This is an abdominal procedure in which the cancer is removed (a proctectomy) and the healthy ends are reconnected (anastomosis). There are many levels of this type of surgery. It may remove some or all of the rectum, leaving the sphincter muscles and bowel function intact. In some cases, only a very small stump of rectum—but an important one, containing the sphincter muscles—is reconnected to the colon. Fatty tissues around the rectum and lymph nodes also are removed.

Anterior resection with low anastomosis and temporary colostomy. This procedure does not involve the sphincter muscles but is very close to the anus. Thus there is concern the reconnection may not heal properly or could leak. A temporary colostomy is created and reversed six to eight weeks later in a second operation.

Abdominoperineal resection with permanent colostomy. This type of surgery is used when the sphincter muscles of the anus or all of the rectum and anus must be extracted. There is an incision in the perineum as well as in the abdomen. A permanent colostomy is constructed.

Whatever rectal surgery is performed, it is important that it be done by an experienced colorectal surgeon who will remove all the supporting tissue that holds the rectum in place (mesorectum) in addition to the section of bowel affected by the cancer. Total mesorectal excision (TME) removes lymph nodes and other sites for possible local recurrence. It is one of the major advances in rectal surgery and a good measure of the quality of the surgery performed. You should be sure that TME is part of the planned procedure.

Living With a Colostomy

If the intestines cannot be reconnected to allow for normal bowel function, the surgeon will create a permanent opening in the abdominal wall to allow waste to be expelled into an external pouch. This is called a colostomy when it is connected to the colon or an ileostomy when it is connected to the small intestine.

If you are likely to need a colostomy or ileostomy, your doctors and a specially trained nurse will consult with you before the surgery and work with you afterward to help you learn how to use and change the pouch.

Undoubtedly, living with a colostomy requires an adjustment, but it is often less drastic than most people initially believe. The pouches, when closed, are odorless, flat, and do not show under most clothing, including bathing suits, nor do they interfere with most activities, including sexual intercourse.

Emotional adjustment is often the most difficult part of living with a colostomy. It can be very helpful to speak with others who have been through the procedure. Your cancer treatment center or a branch of the American Cancer Society located nearby will have programs offering information and support. In addition, online chat rooms and other Internet resources are available.

ASK THE DOCTOR

Q. ***I've had a colostomy and I'm having trouble with intestinal gas and odor. Do you have any suggestions that might help?***

A. Intestinal gas is fairly common in the first few weeks or months after colostomy surgery. It generally goes away as you resume your usual diet. However, everybody reacts differently, so gas may persist. Take a look at the foods you've been eating. Foods that often produce gas include beans, beer, carbonated drinks, onions, broccoli, Brussels sprouts, and cabbage. It may take some experimentation to discover which foods are best for you. Try out foods, one at a time, when you will be at home and relaxed.

Other tips: Decrease the amount of air you swallow by avoiding drinking from a straw and chewing gum. Eat slowly, chewing foods well, and avoid eating after 8 P.M. to allow food to digest before going to sleep. If you continue to experience gas, talk with your colostomy nurse or support team. They are specially trained to help you with colostomy issues.

What To Ask Your Doctor About Treatment

There will be many questions you will most likely want to ask about treatment options. It is helpful to make a list and to take someone with you to help you listen to and better understand what the doctor is saying.

If you don't understand an answer, continue exploring the issue until you do. Here are some questions you may want to ask:

- What are my treatment options?
- What is involved in these treatments? Please be specific.
- What are the advantages and disadvantages of these treatments?
- Which treatment option do you recommend, and why?
- What is the best outcome I can expect from this treatment? The worst outcome?
- How long will the treatment take?
- What do you expect will be the outcome? Will it cure the cancer?
- What are the usual side effects of this treatment?
- How much will the treatment impact my quality of life?
- What will be the extent of bowel, bladder, and sexual function?
- Will I need a colostomy?
- What can I do to prevent or lessen adverse affects?
- What is the risk that the cancer might return under this treatment plan?
- Will this treatment be covered by my insurance?
- Can I speak to someone who has had this treatment?

Advanced, Recurrent, or Metastatic Colorectal Cancer

It can be devastating to learn that cancer has recurred or spread. Colorectal cancer that is caught early is the least likely to spread. Less than 5% of localized stage I and about 15–20% of stage II cancers recur. The rate of recurrence increases to 40–60% for stage III cancers. Among newly diagnosed colorectal cancers, by the time they are discovered about 20% are stage IV and have already metastasized.

Colorectal cancer can recur at any time after treatment. Generally, the more time that passes after treatment, the better the chance that cancer will not come back. Recurrence is greatest within the first two years after treatment, and 90% of colorectal cancers that do recur appear within the first four years after treatment.

In colon cancer, the disease tends not to recur at the site of surgery. The risk of recurrence is much higher for rectal surgery because it is more difficult to remove the tumor and all of the cancer cells from the rectal area than from the colon.

Metastasized cancer occurs most often when tumors have penetrated through the wall of the colon or bowel, releasing cells into the bloodstream that are carried to distant sites in the body. The most common site for metastases to occur in colorectal cancer is the liver: About 50% of people with colorectal cancer will be diagnosed with metastasized liver cancer. In fact, in many cases the liver will be the only organ affected. Other sites where cancer may metastasize include the lungs, the skeleton, and the abdominal cavity. The nervous system (including the brain) and other sites can be affected, but this is less common.

Metastasized or recurrent colorectal cancer presents a challenge, but it can usually be treated. It can recur locally at or near the site of surgery and be managed with a second operation.

More often the spread is to other organs and other parts of the body. Surgery may also play a role in some of these situations, but more often chemotherapy and/or radiation therapy are needed. If the recurrent cancer cannot be removed, it will not likely be curable; treatment will be dedicated to extending life and relieving symptoms (see Palliative Care on page 63).

Treating Metastasized or Recurrent Cancer

The treatments for advanced cancer are much the same as for newly diagnosed cancer. However, they are more aggressive. They include:

- Surgery to remove cancer where it has returned or metastasized. Surgery could be localized or could be extensive if there are metastases to the liver or other organs.
- Radiation and/or chemotherapy to control and contain the cancer, especially if it is inoperable.

Other techniques could involve freezing tumors (cryosurgery), burning them away with microwaves, or other methods of treating a well-defined area where a cancer is present.

Surgery

As with newly diagnosed colorectal cancer, successful surgery for a recurrence depends on the location of the cancer, the organs involved, and the extent of cancer that is present in the sites of recurrence.

NEW RESEARCH

Jury Still Out on Value of Sentinel Node Biopsies for Colon Cancer

Checking sentinel nodes—the first lymph nodes reached by cancer cells from a tumor that has spread—for signs of microscopic cancer has been effective in predicting recurrence of melanoma and breast cancers. But the value of this type of biopsy, known as sentinel lymph node biopsy (SLNB), for colon cancer has been equivocal. Now a new study of 268 people with colon cancer found that SLNB identified microscopic evidence of disease spread in more than 20% of those in whom traditionally used methods found no lymph node involvement.

If the value of SLNB is verified in future studies, use of the procedure could help doctors more accurately stage tumors and better determine the best course of treatment. But a number of questions, including the best technique to use, need to be resolved before the technique is ready for use outside a research setting.

ANNALS OF SURGERY
Volume 245, page 858
June 2007

It's Not All in Your Head

Coping with chemotherapy's mental side effects

You were warned: Be prepared for the possibility of nausea, diarrhea, fatigue, and hair loss while undergoing chemotherapy. But you were probably not told about that unsettling state of fuzzy thinking, difficulty focusing, and memory loss that you've been experiencing. Could this also be treatment-related? A growing body of evidence suggests that this may indeed be the case. In fact, researchers now believe that from 40–80% of individuals undergoing chemotherapy experience this phenomenon, dubbed chemobrain.

Some healthcare providers have questioned whether chemobrain actually exists, as it was thought that chemotherapy drugs could not cross the blood-brain barrier that blocks most medications. But surprising new evidence suggests that chemobrain is real and is related to structural changes in the brain caused by these drugs. Although most research to date has been conducted on women with breast cancer, this phenomenon does not appear to be unique to any single type of cancer, and people with colorectal cancer have reported experiencing it as well.

Snapshots of the Brain

Two recent studies that looked at images of the brains of women who had chemotherapy found striking physical changes after treatment.

Researchers in Japan compared MRI (magnetic resonance imaging) scans of the brains of 51 women who had undergone chemotherapy for breast cancer with those from women who had surgery only. One year after treatment, areas of the brain that are crucial for memory and problem solving were significantly smaller in the chemotherapy group. In addition, the greater the reduction in brain size, the worse the women performed on tests of memory and concentration. The good news: Three years later, both groups tested about the same, which suggests that those with chemobrain recovered.

Researchers at the University of California, Los Angeles, reported similar results. The investigators compared PET (positron emission tomography) scans from 21 breast cancer survivors who had undergone chemotherapy five to 10 years previously with scans from women who had not been treated with chemotherapy. When asked to perform simple memory tests, the PET scans of women in the chemotherapy group showed greater blood flow to some areas of the brain than did scans from women who didn't receive chemotherapy, indicating that their brains were working harder.

Although these findings were gleaned from small studies, results from laboratory research provide further evidence that chemotherapy may harm the brain. In one recent study, human brain cells grown in laboratory dishes were destroyed by chemotherapy doses high enough to kill cancer cells. In addition, chemotherapy drugs given to mice killed cells in several regions of the brain and, in some cases, continued killing them weeks after chemotherapy ended.

A Necessary Evil

In spite of the apparent adverse effects of chemotherapy on the brain, for many people the benefits of treatment outweigh the risks. And, as with other chemotherapy side effects, chemobrain doesn't affect everyone equally. You may have no side effects, while others may have a few and still others, many, and they can be short term or last for years. The type and extent of the side effects can be related to the dose of medication given (higher doses tend to have more adverse effects), the drugs used, and your gender. In general, women are more likely to be affected than men, and the effect is greater in females, perhaps

Surgery can be used to remove cancers that recur at the site of anastomosis (where two severed ends of tissue have been joined). The most common use of surgery is removal of metastases to the liver. Use of this approach depends on the number and location of the tumors in the liver and whether cancer has spread to other parts of the body.

because the chemotherapy drugs cause hormonal changes similar to menopause.

Get Help for Your Symptoms

New chemotherapy medications with fewer or less severe side effects (or both) are being developed. In the meantime, treating the symptoms is your best option. So far no medication is approved specifically for the treatment of chemobrain, but some research suggests that dexmethylphenidate (Focalin or d-MPH) could ease your symptoms. This medication is a central nervous system stimulant used to treat attention deficit hyperactivity disorder, and it reduces symptoms, especially fatigue and memory loss, in some people.

A nondrug alternative that may help is cognitive retraining. This type of therapy uses computer programs, puzzles, and games to help improve focus, memory, perception, and problem-solving abilities.

Talk to your healthcare team and be specific about any and all side effects of your chemotherapy, including chemobrain. It doesn't help to "tough it out." You can't be helped unless your health team knows there are problems. Your doctor may be able to change your therapy to reduce unwanted effects.

Tips To Help You Cope

It helps to remember that chemotherapy ends. Even if you have an ongoing chemotherapy schedule, there are periods without treatment, and during these times you're likely to experience fewer symptoms. The passage of time also helps. Many symptoms, including cognitive problems, eventually fade.

Of course, knowing that chemotherapy can extend life and help lower the risk of recurrence makes it easier to cope with the side effects. In a recent study of 150 people treated with chemotherapy for colorectal cancer, 35% would be willing to have the treatment again, even if it only cut the risk of recurrence by 1%.

Here are some other coping strategies that might help:

- **Keep track.** Note your symptoms, and talk with your doctor and healthcare team about changes you notice and ask what can help. Experienced chemotherapy nurses have many tips and suggestions for coping.
- **Ask for referrals.** Consider counseling for emotional stress, cognitive retraining for chemobrain, and support groups.
- **Write it down.** A daily organizer or a notebook to write down "things to do" and completed tasks helps counter chemobrain.
- **Post-it.** Stick-up notes are great reminders.
- **Sleep on it.** Getting enough sleep is important to keep your mind alert. If symptoms keep you from sleeping through the night, consider short naps.
- **Exercise your body.** Physical activity helps with mental functioning and can relieve stress, pain, and other symptoms. Consider yoga and tai chi: The repetitive exercises are good for mind and body.
- **Exercise your mind.** Puzzles and games help improve mental function as well as help distract you from thinking about more stressful concerns.
- **De-stress.** Stress makes most symptoms worse. Deep relaxation and stress reduction courses may help. Films, videos, and music are relaxing for many people.
- **Simplify.** Save energy for the most important tasks. Multitasking may be harder than it used to be, and keeping track of a full schedule may be physically and mentally stressful.

The National Cancer Institute has an excellent brochure with suggestions for dealing with other common chemotherapy side effects. You can order a free printed pamphlet by calling 800-4CANCER (422-6237) or go to www.cancer.gov/cancertopics/coping and click on "Chemotherapy and You." ■

Careful evaluation is needed to be sure that doctors know all of the sites where the cancer has spread before they undertake liver surgery. Improvements in surgical techniques allow experienced surgeons to remove even multiple tumors from the liver (although the results are not as good when multiple tumors are present). The techniques used include removal (resection) of a tumor and destroying some tumors with radiofrequency ablation (RFA), a procedure that can melt away some liver tumors much as a microwave oven can melt butter.

In RFA, an electrode, guided by an imaging process such as ultrasound or CT, is inserted through a small incision into a tumor in the liver. A radiofrequency current then heats the tumor tissue and ablates (vaporizes) it, sealing small blood vessels at the same time. The procedure can be done on an outpatient basis using local anesthetic as well as during major surgery. It is most effective for tumors that are 2 inches or less in diameter. The method is sometimes used for other sites of metastasis, but it is more common to use it for the liver. Generally, use of RFA has supplanted cryosurgery (freezing tumors) for metastatic or recurrent cancer.

In an attempt to improve the results from surgery, chemotherapy may be given either before or after the operation. However, the best way to combine surgery and chemotherapy remains to be determined.

Surgery can also be used to remove lung metastases or tumors in other sites such as the ovaries. Again, this requires careful evaluation to be sure that doctors know the full extent of the cancer's spread. It is seldom helpful to remove cancer from one organ when it is also present elsewhere.

Chemotherapy

For the majority of people with recurrent or metastatic cancer, surgery is not possible and the keystone of treatment will be chemotherapy. Occasionally, chemotherapy can improve the results of surgery, but more often it is the major treatment itself.

In the last few years, chemotherapy of metastatic colorectal cancer has improved significantly, with the availability of a number of new drugs, including the "targeted" antibody therapies like Avastin and Erbitux to other regimens. (Avastin and Erbitux are versions of the same kinds of antibodies that the immune system uses to fight infection, engineered so that they block signals that cause the cancer cells to grow and spread.)

On average, these improvements have doubled the expected survival of people with metastatic colorectal cancer from roughly one year to nearly two years and have increased the number of people who live longer after treatment for colorectal cancer.

This success does not come from using all these drugs together, but rather from having more than one choice available. The choice of initial chemotherapy depends, in large part, on the individuals who are treated and on any medical problems they may have.

One of the choices most commonly recommended is FOLFOX plus Avastin (see page 47). If someone has had a previous problem with blood clots or bleeding, Avastin might not be used. If there is prior nerve damage from a condition like diabetes, then irinotecan might be chosen instead of oxaliplatin (FOLFIRI).

None of these regimens will work forever, because colorectal cancer cells typically develop resistance to chemotherapy drugs over time. When the cancer begins to grow again, the next step would be to switch irinotecan for oxaliplatin, or vice versa.

The third-line treatment currently would be to use Erbitux, either by itself or with irinotecan. These choices need to be made by an oncologist who is familiar with the individual patient. They cannot be easily generalized.

Clinical trials are evaluating other new drugs to see if they have a role in colorectal cancer, as well as whether better results could be achieved by using more drugs together earlier in treatment.

Some chemotherapy techniques can target tumors in the liver directly. This is done by giving the drugs straight into the artery that goes to the liver.

Transarterial chemoembolization (TACE)

This procedure involves inserting a catheter through the artery in the groin up to the artery feeding the liver and injecting small biodegradable beads or oil mixed with chemotherapy. The beads or oil slow the blood flow and allow the chemotherapy to stay in the liver for a longer period. (This is used for other cancers such as hepatoma more often than for colorectal cancer.)

Hepatic artery infusion (HAI)

HAI uses a surgically placed catheter and pump to deliver a drug such as 5-FUdR (a form of 5FU that is more effective in the liver and relatively innocuous to the rest of the body when given in this way) through the artery feeding the liver. Because of possible toxicity to the liver, this needs to be done by medical teams very familiar with the technique. It may be most effective after resection of liver tumors.

Radiation

Radiation is used most often for inoperable tumors, but it may also be a solution when tumors have not responded to chemotherapy. Although it can be administered externally, therapies have become

NEW RESEARCH

New Adjuvant Therapy Not Effective for Stage III Colon Cancer

Adding a powerful drug called irinotecan (Camptosar) to a standard chemotherapy regimen given to people with stage III colon cancer does not improve survival, according to a new report.

Based on findings from a number of studies that showed improvements in survival in people with metastatic cancer when irinotecan was used, researchers randomly assigned more than 1,200 people with stage III colon cancer to receive the standard therapy (fluorouracil plus leucovorin) weekly or standard therapy plus irinotecan.

The investigators found that the toxic effects were significantly higher for those in the irinotecan group than in the standard-therapy group, as was the mortality rate. Nearly 3% of the irinotecan group died within six months compared with 1% of those receiving standard therapy alone.

The results from this study demonstrate the need for and importance of well-designed clinical trials of cancer medications before they are routinely used outside of a research setting. These findings, along with another trial using irinotecan in an adjuvant therapy regimen, suggest it has no benefit.

JOURNAL OF CLINICAL ONCOLOGY
Volume 25, page 3456
August 10, 2007

more refined so that they deliver radiation precisely to a tumor or other small areas to be treated. To achieve this, the radiation source is placed as close as possible to the cancer cells—beamed through catheters or other implants or placed directly into the cancer. This is called internal or interstitial radiation therapy.

Sometimes people receiving internal forms of radiation therapy need to stay in a private room in the hospital to avoid exposing other people to the radiation.

Brachytherapy

Used for rectal cancers, brachytherapy delivers radiation to a targeted area. There are two kinds.

High-dose rate (HDR) brachytherapy. In this procedure, tiny plastic catheters are inserted temporarily into the tumor, and high-dose radiation is beamed though them for a few minutes. This is an outpatient procedure that doesn't expose others to radiation once the treatment is over.

Seed implant brachytherapy. About 100 tiny radioactive "seeds" are planted in the tumor during this form of brachytherapy, where they emit low doses of radiation over weeks or months. This procedure usually requires a hospital stay.

Intensity-modulated radiation therapy (IMRT)

IMRT uses computer programming to deliver a precise three-dimensional dose of radiation to and around a tumor. One version called TomoTherapy combines this with computerized tomography (CT) imaging. The procedure "sculpts" the size and shape of the tumor to be treated, sparing surrounding tissue from radiation.

Intraoperative radiation therapy (IORT)

This treatment focuses a high dose of radiation on the tissue that remains after a tumor has been removed during surgery and while the patient is still in the operating room. Because abdominal surgery is performed, the dose can be delivered just to the areas selected. In some cases, this is the only radiation treatment that is needed.

TheraSphere

In this procedure, a localized internal radiation technique, millions of tiny radioactive glass beads (microspheres) are sent into the bloodstream and guided into the liver through the hepatic artery. The minute microspheres navigate through the large blood vessels that serve healthy tissues to get trapped in the small blood vessels that feed into the tumor, where they beam radiation directly toward it.

Much like the TACE method used for chemotherapy (see page 55), the microspheres are delivered through a catheter that is inserted through the femoral artery in the leg and threaded up to the hepatic artery under fluoroscopy. This procedure is performed in a hospital, but general anesthetic is not usually used.

Cyberknife

This radiation therapy technique delivers high-energy radiation to slice tumors away. The dose administered can be very high because the energy is coming from multiple angles around the tumor, not just from two or three directions. A CT scan identifies the tumor, which is then destroyed by radiation in a four- or five-hour session. The patient is awake during the treatment, which is usually painless.

Alternative and Complementary Therapies

There is no "natural" cure for cancer, and so-called therapies based on that claim have injured many cancer patients—either directly through dangerous "treatments" or indirectly because some individuals turned to unproven therapies in place of treatments validated by solid research.

However, there are several nonmedical therapies that, when used along with conventional therapies, may reduce some of the adverse effects from treatment or may help ease the pain and tension colorectal cancer patients may experience. For example, studies show that practices such as meditation or guided imagery and visualization can be calming. Yoga and tai chi also may be helpful. Acupuncture has been shown to provide relief for some kinds of pain.

Herbs, such as peppermint and ginger, may help ease the nausea and vomiting associated with chemotherapy. However, anything taken by mouth must be used with caution and with your doctor's knowledge. Your prescribed care has been carefully tailored to your situation, and adding herbs, supplements, or other "natural remedies" could interact negatively with these treatments.

Living With Colorectal Cancer

More than a million people living today in the United States have had colon cancer, and that number is expected to increase as detection and treatments improve.

NEW RESEARCH

Socioeconomics Matters More Than Race in Colorectal Cancer Survival

Black Americans have among the highest rates of colorectal cancer in the United States and are much more likely to die of it than whites. This significant disparity has led some to speculate about genetic or racial factors as a cause of the difference in survival rates. But a recent meta-analysis finds that socioeconomic status rather than race is the major reason.

The investigators reviewed 66 medical research articles published from 1966 to 2006 that addressed the association between race/ethnicity and survival in people with colon or colorectal cancer but found only 10 that also considered the impact of socioeconomic status, five of which also factored in the effect of the type of treatment received.

When they analyzed the combined data from those 10 studies, the researchers found that the overall risk of death related to colorectal cancer was only slightly higher for blacks than for whites after adjusting for socioeconomic status and type of treatment. The authors speculate that the marginal disadvantage for blacks is likely to be explained by factors related to low socioeconomic status, which often presents barriers to optimal or even adequate health care.

CANCER
Volume 109, page 2161
June 2007

Food for Thought

Can diet prevent colorectal cancer from coming back?

An unhealthy diet has long been associated with an increased risk of developing colorectal cancer, at times without much evidence other than common sense. Now a growing body of research is backing up these claims with studies showing that people who eat "good" foods may indeed be able to reduce their risk of developing the disease.

While most research has focused on the impact of diet on the initial development of colon cancer (what's known as primary prevention), only a few small studies have examined the effect of diet on colorectal cancer recurrence. But findings from a new, larger study looking at that question suggest that eating "good" foods can reduce your risk of a recurrence as well and improve your odds of survival.

New research also demonstrates the value of certain nutrients in reducing the risk of colorectal polyp recurrence. But when it comes to adding some supplements to your diet to get those nutrients, there can be too much of a good thing.

What's Your Dietary Pattern?

My diet consists primarily of:

A) fruits, vegetables, whole grains, legumes, poultry, and fish

B) red meat, fried foods, full-fat dairy products, refined grains, and desserts.

If you selected B, beware. Investigators who examined the relationship between the dietary patterns of more than 1,000 people who had been treated for stage III colon cancer and their risk of colon cancer recurrence found that those who followed a typical American diet (answer B) were three times more likely to experience a recurrence than their counterparts who followed a more prudent diet (answer A), and they also were more likely to die.

The study, which was reported in the *Journal of the American Medical Association (JAMA)*, is the first to address the effect of diet on recurrence in a population of colon cancer survivors. Since this was an observational study that relied on the participants to remember and report what they ate, the investigators caution that their results do not prove that a typical American diet causes colorectal cancers to recur. However, the results, they say, do strongly suggest that a diet consisting primarily of red and processed meats, french fries, refined grains, and sweets and desserts increases the risk of cancer recurrence and decreases survival.

Preventing Polyp Recurrence

A number of researchers are zeroing in on certain foods and nutrients that may play an important role in preventing the recurrence of adenomas (polyps that have a high likelihood of becoming cancerous).

Dry beans. Findings from the Polyp Prevention Trial, which looked at dietary factors that impacted adenoma recurrence in more than 2,000 men and women, suggest an improved outlook for people with a history of polyps who eat plenty of cooked dry beans. All participants in this study had at least one polyp removed, but none required major surgery for colorectal cancer. Those who reported eating the most cooked dry beans, such as pinto and navy beans, lentils, and bean soups (not green beans or peas), were 65% less likely to experience a recurrence than those who ate the fewest.

According to the researchers, dry beans have a wide range of nutrients that may be protective against cancer. They also have a low glycemic index, meaning that dry beans cause a slower rise in blood sugar compared with white bread. Low-glycemic foods have been associated with a reduced risk of colorectal cancer in a

Most of these individuals call themselves survivors—not a medical term, but one that people with cancer have chosen to describe someone who has overcome a crisis or challenge.

Yet in a very real sense, a person who has had colorectal cancer is always living with cancer. Even when the word "cure" may be used, number of primary prevention studies.

Calcium. According to a recent study in the *Journal of the National Cancer Institute*, use of a calcium supplement for at least four years may protect against recurrent colorectal adenomas for up to five years after you stop using them. These results are from the 11-year Calcium Polyp Prevention Study, which followed more than 800 people who previously had a colorectal adenoma.

In the first phase of the study, participants received either 1,200 mg of elemental calcium daily or placebo for four years. After the treatment phase of the study ended, the investigators followed the participants for an average of seven additional years. In the first five years after treatment ended, people taking calcium were 37% less likely than those in the placebo group to have an adenoma recurrence. Beyond five years, however, previous calcium use had no effect on adenoma risk. Some research suggests that calcium may reduce the risk of colorectal adenomas (and colorectal cancer) by binding to the potentially carcinogenic bile acids in the stomach and preventing them from coming into contact with the lining of the colon.

Although these findings seem promising, the authors caution that it's too early to recommend taking a calcium supplement to reduce the risk of adenoma recurrence. And, they warn, calcium supplementation could be a double-edged sword for men—some evidence suggests it may actually increase the risk of prostate cancer.

Folic acid. A recent study in *JAMA* suggests that not only do folic acid supplements *not* decrease the risk of colorectal tumors, they might actually increase the risk of recurrence in people with a history of colorectal adenomas.

Investigators examined the effect of folic acid on the prevention of new colorectal adenomas in more than 1,000 people with a recent history of this type of polyp. About half of the participants took 1 mg of folic acid daily, and the others took a placebo pill. Colonoscopies were performed three and five years after the start of the study. Surprisingly, more adenomas were seen in the people taking folic acid at both three and five years than in those taking placebo (44% vs. 42% and 42% vs. 37%, respectively).

Why the correlation? One hypothesis is that the study participants may have had undetected early precursor lesions in the lining of their colons and folic acid promoted the growth of those lesions. The investigators caution that more research is needed to confirm their findings, particularly since the differences between the groups were not statistically significant and could have occurred by chance. For now, the best advice is to get your folic acid from foods that naturally contain high amounts—citrus fruits and dark green leafy vegetables, especially spinach—and to avoid folic acid supplements unless directed to take them by your doctor.

Eating To Lower Your Cancer Risk

Unfortunately, there is no special diet that can prevent the recurrence of polyps or colorectal cancer. But based on the evidence available to date, cancer experts suggest this recipe for healthier eating:

- Get most of your foods from plant sources (fresh vegetables and fruits, whole grains, dry beans, and nuts)
- Avoid processed foods, including processed meats and refined grains
- Choose chicken, fish, or beans as your protein foods instead of red meat
- Avoid junk food, including sodas and sugar-laden snacks
- Limit alcoholic drinks to one or fewer a day
- Try to get most of your nutrients from foods rather than supplements. ■

there are no guarantees: The possibility of recurrence is always an issue. While recurrence is not inevitable, the fact is that colorectal cancer can recur, even after several years. Therefore doctors prefer to talk about being "disease free" or "cancer free"—a period of remission during which there are no signs of cancer.

Follow-Up and Surveillance

Vigilant surveillance must continue for several years after colorectal cancer treatment. Early detection of recurrent or metastasized cancer yields the best possibility for cure or containment. For these reasons, at the Sidney Kimmel Comprehensive Cancer Center at Johns Hopkins, most patients come for follow-up every three to six months for the first three years and then every six to 12 months for two years afterwards.

Your doctors will design a follow-up care program for your individual situation. It is crucially important to keep these appointments and to stick faithfully with the follow-up care plan. Your doctors will monitor your recovery progress, look for signs of cancer recurrence or metastases, and check on after effects of treatment. This is also an opportunity to discuss your condition and prognosis with the medical team and to consider lifestyle and other changes to optimize recovery and good health. The usual program for follow-up begins a few weeks after the end of treatment. Your specific follow up schedule and recommended tests depend on your individual situation. However, a typical program includes:

- Blood tests, including tests for cancer markers, such as CEA, every three months for the first two years and then every six months for the next three years
- Liver and lung imaging tests such as x-ray or CT, to screen for cancer spread every six months for three years and then annually for two years
- Colonoscopy after one year, then every one to three years thereafter, depending on the findings.

Patients who were treated for rectal cancer may also have digital rectal examinations, proctoscopies, or sigmoidoscopies in addition to the colonoscopy. The frequency of these tests will depend on the findings and the individual details of the patient.

Dealing With Treatment Aftereffects

The temporary or permanent aftereffects from cancer treatment can range from minor to significant. Short-term problems might involve wound healing from surgery, mouth and skin sores, and digestive problems. Surgeries leave some scar tissue or adhesions that can block the intestinal tract. Chemotherapy and radiation may cause nerve damage, damage to the bladder or vagina, and other problems, including short- or long-term memory loss and "foggy" thinking.

Sexual function can be affected in both men and women: Men may have nerve damage following rectal surgery that makes it difficult to maintain an erection, and women may find that scar tissue following radiation makes intercourse painful. Another possible side effect is numbness or decreased feeling in the arms or legs, a condition known as peripheral neuropathy.

It can be discouraging to face these new challenges along with cancer, especially because it is not always clear whether they are temporary or permanent. It is normal to face some depression and anxiety about these aftereffects, even for someone who has dealt very well with the emotional issues surrounding the cancer itself (see "Surviving the Emotional Aftershock of Colorectal Cancer" on pages 6–7).

There are treatments to manage most aftereffects. Ask your medical team what can be done to ease such problems—especially pain. Research shows that pain can interfere with healing, and optimal recovery demands pain relief. Counseling and medication can relieve depression and anxiety.

It may become difficult to determine which specialist to see for what condition. Your oncologist may be a good place to start, but bear in mind that your oncologist specializes in cancer and that you may need specialists in several other areas. Possibly your best ally at this stage will be your least specialized expert—your primary care doctor. If you can't find appropriate care, contact the patient support program at your cancer treatment center for advice and referrals.

Symptoms of Recurrence

It's a double bind: While it is not productive to worry about recurrent cancer, it is important to be able to begin treating it as soon as possible. Yet signs and symptoms of cancer recurrence or metastases can be vague, especially when you are recovering from major treatment. It may be difficult to sort out new sensations from the ones you had before surgery.

Some symptoms doctors suggest you take seriously include:

- Fatigue, weight loss, loss of appetite, and anorexia. These could be connected to therapy but can also be signs of cancer recurrence
- Abdominal pain and bowel blockage. Cancer can recur in the area of the bowel where it was treated or elsewhere in the colon. This may block normal bowel movements, so do report pain and constipation
- Nausea, vomiting, or yellow discoloration of eyes and skin may be signs of metastases to the liver

ASK THE DOCTOR

Q. ***How soon will I be able to resume my normal activities after having chemotherapy and radiation?***

A. That depends on the specific treatment you receive, the stage of your cancer, the nature of your activities, and how you feel. Some people with cancer can continue with their usual schedule during treatment. But others need more rest and cannot keep up with their normal activities. Your doctor, who knows your specific situation, may have the best answer.

Be sure to ask which side effects you are most likely to have, how serious they might be, and how long they are likely to last. The time it takes to get over treatment side effects depends a great deal on your overall health and on which treatment you will receive.

Many people minimize the impact of chemotherapy and radiation on their usual activities by scheduling their treatment late in the day or before a weekend. Of course, if you become tired, you may need to readjust your schedule. If you are in the workforce, you may be able to arrange to work at home or to work flexible hours. Don't be afraid to ask your employer. Some Federal and state laws require employers to allow patients to work a more flexible schedule while they are undergoing cancer treatment.

- Shortness of breath might indicate lung tumors
- Infrequent urination accompanied by hip or back pain can indicate that the cancer has spread to the urinary system or skeleton.

Making Healthy Choices

So far, there is no guaranteed way to prevent colon cancer or a recurrence. But more and more studies are showing that lifestyle can have a big impact—and much of the new research echoes time-honored common sense: Eat a healthy diet, maintain an appropriate weight, exercise regularly, and avoid unhealthy habits, such as smoking.

Making lifestyle changes is always challenging, and it can be much more difficult when you are coping with cancer treatment and recovery. On the other hand, some people find that having had cancer motivates them to make such changes.

Among the healthy practices shown to lower the risk of new and recurrent cancer are:

- Quitting smoking and limiting intake of alcohol
- Eating a diet that is low in meat and saturated fats and high in vegetables, fruits, and fiber (see "Food for Thought" on pages 58–59)
- Maintaining an appropriate weight for your age and body type
- Exercising regularly

Change is never easy, so ask your healthcare team about support. You might benefit from special programs for smoking cessation and for exercise and weight management. Some people benefit from encouragement from a cancer support group, cancer buddy, or therapist who has experience working with people who have cancer. Your cancer care center and the American Cancer Society also are invaluable sources of information.

Participating in Clinical Trials

Clinical trials are organized medical research studies that evaluate the benefit of treatments in a scientific way. Clinical trials are important at virtually every stage and clinical situation in colorectal cancer.

For example, clinical trials may evaluate what type of treatment is most effective in reducing the risk of recurrence of colorectal cancer after surgery. Many studies are under way to evaluate what chemotherapy program may be most effective in treating people who have metastatic colon cancer.

In some cases the clinical trial might be an evaluation of an unproven new treatment in people who have already been treated with all of the standard drugs known to be effective. Clinical trials can be either the first step in evaluating a new treatment or the final step to establishing a new standard of care for colorectal cancer. Taking part in a clinical trial may give you access to promising new or experimental therapies that are not yet available otherwise. In many (but not all) cases the treatments come at no cost, and you may also receive free related medical care and checkups.

However, there are potential health risks from unproved therapies. It's also possible, if it is a "blinded" study, that neither you nor the researchers will know whether you are in the comparison group receiving a harmless placebo rather than the promising therapy that is the subject of the clinical trial.

Therefore, participation in a clinical trial may not help your individual case, but the knowledge gained could help others. In a very real sense, taking part in a clinical trial is a gift to science and to future cancer survivors. You should ask your doctors if there are clinical trials that are available and appropriate for your situation.

For more information on steps you can take that may help reduce your risk of recurrence, see "Colon Cancer Redux" on pages 64–65.

Palliative Care

There may come a time when cancer treatments are no longer working, and the cancer cannot be stopped. Some people choose to continue treatment even when doctors say there is almost no chance it will be effective.

Others choose to stop aggressive therapies and repeated treatment sessions, in order to concentrate on other priorities that are important. In that case, palliative care may give the best outcome, using therapies that are aimed at maintaining quality of life but are not expected to cure the cancer.

This is not giving up: Palliative care refers to the aspects of care that relieve pain and suffering. It is used at any stage of cancer, alongside treatments that are aimed at curing. However, the term is usually used in the context of advanced disease that no longer responds to treatment. Life with cancer goes on for an indefinable period of time—months or even years in some cases—and palliative care can make it comfortable.

A decision to stop aggressive cancer treatment is a deeply personal

ASK THE DOCTOR

Q. ***Will regular colonics help prevent colon cancer?***

A. While some alternative therapy practitioners promote colonics to cleanse the bowels and remove toxins that they say contribute to cancer and other diseases, this has not been rigorously tested in clinical trials. There is no convincing medical evidence that colonics prevent colon cancer, and the procedure is not without risks.

During a colonic, a flexible tube is inserted into the rectum. Up to 20 gallons of water or other liquid is pumped into the rectum and intestines and then drained. Doctors at Johns Hopkins advise against colonics because of concerns about the potential for infection or perforation of the walls of the rectum or intestines during the procedure. Also, colonics are unnecessary. Your elimination system was designed to clean your bowels.

Because there are no convincing data about the safety or benefits of colonics, it's best to avoid them in favor of practices proven to keep your colon functioning properly and lower cancer risks, such as exercise and a diet of fiber-rich fruits, vegetables, and whole grains.

Colon Cancer Redux

Seven strategies that could help lower your risk of recurrence

If you've had colon cancer, you're understandably likely to be concerned about a recurrence. Indeed, having had colon cancer or a polyp increases your risk of a future bout, usually within the first four years of treatment. The risk of recurrence varies depending on the stage of the cancer and ranges from less than 5% in people with localized early-stage cancer to about 40% in those with advanced disease.

What, if anything, can you do to keep the cancer from coming back? Although there is no magic pill or potion and nothing is guaranteed to prevent your cancer from recurring, research suggests that you can take steps that may reduce your risk.

1. Choose a Colorectal Cancer Specialist

Surgeons who treat large numbers of colorectal cancer patients have more experience using specialized surgical techniques, are more knowledgeable about the current guidelines for treatment and follow-up, and are more likely to be aware of the latest research findings than their counterparts who have less experience in this area.

For example, according to a recent study in the *Journal of the National Cancer Institute* the more lymph nodes removed and examined during surgery, the better the outcome is likely to be. What's the relationship? Cancer cells can spread through the body by traveling through the lymph vessels (tiny thin channels that carry away waste and fluid) to the lymph nodes. Finding and removing lymph nodes that harbor colon cancer cells is crucial since the more lymph nodes that contain those cells, the more likely it is the cancer will return.

While it's not yet known exactly how many lymph nodes should be examined, data suggest that at least 12 nodes be examined to get an accurate staging. Yet, by some estimates, only one third of colon cancer patients in the United States receive an adequate lymph node evaluation. Not surprisingly, other studies show that surgeons with more experience performing colorectal cancer surgery (those who perform 10 or more operations of this kind per year) are more likely to do a thorough job of examining and removing lymph nodes than their less experienced counterparts.

2. Keep Your Follow-Up Appointments

After the cancer is removed, your treatment will no doubt include a prescription for aggressive follow-up, and it is vital to follow that plan. Surprisingly, some people do not, perhaps for fear of hearing bad news. Yet vigilant surveillance can alert doctors to any recurrence when it is in the earliest stages, leading to prompt treatment.

Currently, doctors at Johns Hopkins recommend that people with nonhereditary forms of colorectal cancer get their first follow-up colonoscopy within one year after surgery. That's sound advice. One recent study of more than 1,000 people with colorectal cancer found that 77% of those who had at least one follow-up colonoscopy were alive five years after surgery, compared with only 52% of those who did not.

If your tumor was stage II or higher, follow-up also includes regular blood tests for carcinoembryonic antigen (CEA). An elevated level of this tumor marker can alert your doctor that your cancer has recurred before you start to experience symptoms. And new findings suggest that even a small increase in your CEA level may be significant—even if the level is still within normal limits. Doctors at Johns Hopkins recommend getting a CEA test every three to six months for the first two years following colorectal cancer surgery, then every six months for the next three years. See "Follow-Up and Surveillance" on page 60 for information on additional tests.

3. Ask About Genetic Tests

If you've been diagnosed with colon cancer or polyps, it's important to know whether you have a hereditary form of the disease. Some 15% of all colorectal cancers run in families. And having some types of familial cancer (hereditary nonpolyposis colon cancer, or HNPCC, and APC I1307K) can increase your risk of developing a second primary cancer at another site. Another hereditary syndrome, familial adenomatous polyposis (FAP), is usually diagnosed at a very young age, but it does not recur, as treatment involves removal of the entire colon.

If you haven't been asked about your family history, particularly if you are of Ashkenazi Jewish heritage or have one or more first-degree relatives who had colon cancer (such as a parent, sibling, or child), ask about genetic testing. If you have an inherited form of colon cancer, you'll require even more aggressive treatment and follow-up.

4. Consider NSAID Use—With Caution

Talk with your doctor about the pros and cons of taking aspirin or other nonsteroidal anti-inflammatory drugs (NSAIDs), such as ibuprofen (Advil, Motrin) or celecoxib (Celebrex), a type of NSAID known as a COX-2 inhibitor. Studies show that NSAIDs inhibit the growth of new adenomas (polyps that can become cancerous). But use of NSAIDs to prevent polyps remains controversial.

In one study, known as the Adenoma Prevention with Celebrex (APC) trial, people who previously had a polyp removed who took Celebrex daily had fewer new adenomas than those who took a placebo (dummy pill). However, use of Celebrex in the trial was suspended when it was discovered that users were also more than twice as likely to die of a heart attack or stroke as those taking the placebo pills.

Other studies show that all NSAIDs, with the exception of aspirin, are associated with some degree of cardiovascular risk.

In spite of these findings, for some people with colorectal cancer, the risks of repeated polyp growth or a cancer recurrence are high and may tip the scales in favor of NSAID use. One such group is those with FAP—a rare form of inherited cancer that causes a massive overgrowth of polyps in the colon and rectum. Celebrex remains an approved treatment for this group.

However, for other people with colorectal cancer, troubling cardiovascular side effects coupled with other potentially life-threatening side effects, such as stomach bleeding or kidney damage, appear to rule out NSAIDs as a method of lowering colon cancer risk.

Your doctor can help you decide whether to use NSAIDs to help prevent cancer. Although many NSAIDs are available over the counter, don't begin daily use of these drugs without that advice.

5. Maintain a Healthy Weight

Obesity greatly increases your risk of getting colon cancer: up to 50% for men, 80% for women. Now research suggests the risk of recurrence also may be connected to obesity. According to a new study in the *Journal of the National Cancer Institute*, even after successful treatment for colon cancer, people who were very obese (body mass index [BMI] of 35 or higher) were two thirds more likely to have a colon cancer recurrence than people of normal weight. It's not clear, however, whether losing weight can reduce your risk of recurrence.

6. Exercise Regularly

Colorectal cancer will have a harder time catching you again if you keep moving. Two recent studies in the *Journal of Clinical Oncology* show that regular physical activity in the months following treatment may decrease the risk of colorectal cancer recurrence and death. In the studies, people with early- to later-stage colorectal cancer (but not distant metastases) who engaged in regular activity decreased the likelihood of cancer recurrence and death by 40–50% compared with people who engaged in little or no activity. And the results held true regardless of physical activity levels before cancer. This does not have to be heavy-duty gym time. In one study, walking at a moderate pace (2–3 miles per hour) for six hours each week produced clear benefits. So as soon as you are up to it, start walking, building up to about an hour a day.

7. Ease Off Toxic Habits

If you're a smoker, drink more alcohol than you should, or eat a lot of meats, fats, and sweets, treatment for colorectal cancer may be your wake-up call for a lifestyle change.

Few studies have investigated whether cigarette smoking increases the risk of colon cancer recurrence. Those that have show that cigarette smoking does not increase the risk of recurrent adenomas, but it is linked to an increased risk of developing benign (noncancerous) polyps in people who have been treated for colon cancer.

Several studies show a link between alcohol use and colorectal cancer, and investigators believe that alcohol intake could increase the risk of colorectal cancer recurrence as well. Studies also show that diet plays a role in preventing colon cancer development and recurrence (see "Food for Thought" on pages 58–59).

The best advice: Eat a healthy diet. If you smoke, stop. If you drink alcohol, the American Cancer Society recommends that you limit your intake to one or two drinks per day. It's not easy to change habits, but there are resources to help. Your healthcare team can direct you to counseling programs, nicotine withdrawal products, and other aids that may help. ■

choice. Discussions with family or close friends may help—or such sessions may cause anxiety, especially if those who love you do not agree with your choice.

Counselors trained to assist people with advanced cancer can provide help in exploring these issues. Support groups that include others with colorectal cancer can provide useful perspective while making such decisions.

Palliative treatments

Some palliative treatments are the same as those used to contain cancer, but in advanced cancer their purpose may be to relieve pain and other symptoms.

Palliative radiation therapy may shrink tumors when cancer cannot be removed or contained, relieving pressure, pain, or interference with body functions.

Palliative surgery is rarely used but may be necessary to stop bleeding, to remove an obstruction, or to reduce a tumor's size. Laparoscopic or minimally invasive surgery is preferred.

Colonic stents placed in the colon allow doctors to relieve blockage without surgery. A stent is a mesh tube that can be collapsed, passed through an endoscope to the desired place inside the colon, and then opened up, expanding the colon and relieving a bowel obstruction. It can also be used before surgery, as an emergency treatment for blockage. This is especially useful for elderly and very sick people, who are at particular risk for obstructions but are also poor risks for the stress of major abdominal surgery.

Common problems treated with palliative care

About two thirds of people with advanced cancer have some pain, and one in four people with cancer are clinically depressed. Pain can be relieved with medication, but some people are reluctant to take pain medication, fearing addiction, unpleasant side effects, or loss of mental capacity. But the truth is that people in pain do not become addicted, that many side effects can be relieved, and that pain itself can dull the ability to think and participate in life. Controlling pain is part of treatment and medications can be chosen to address specific situations.

Depression and anxiety can rob life of its pleasure. Yet many people don't recognize the symptoms or tell their doctors, suffering from one disease because of another. Like cancer, depression and anxiety can be relieved with medication. Many people find that counseling also helps.

Hospice Care

The term "hospice" refers to a concept of supportive care at the end of life as well as a place where such care is provided.

The basic tenet underlying this concept is that everyone has a right to die pain free and with dignity. The focus is neither to prolong life nor to hasten death, but rather to make the last stages of life the best they can be.

This can be a difficult concept to accept, but there are many benefits from hospice care for people with cancer and those who love them. It can relieve families of many day-to-day burdens, including medication costs, allowing them to focus on living life fully.

Hospice does not mean immediate death or giving up treatment. A hospice program can help to control symptoms and pain, providing the necessary medications and medical equipment as well as counseling for patients and loved ones, typically available around the clock. A hospice medical team includes a medical director, a nurse, a nurse's aide, a social worker, and a spiritual counselor or chaplain. In most cases the family doctor remains involved as well. Hospice care may be given at home, at a nursing facility or hospital, or, in some cases, at a specialized hospice facility.

Medicare or private insurance covers almost all medical costs for most hospice patients, which can be a significant benefit. Under most insurance reimbursement plans and Medicare, patients are eligible for hospice care when a doctor determines they have six months or less to live.

But many people in hospice care live much longer than expected, some getting a "second wind" partly because of the good care, personal attention, and social and emotional support. Sometimes, people just get better. Whatever the reason, people can choose to withdraw from the hospice-care category at any time.

Most communities have more than one organization that can provide hospice care. See page 70 for more information or ask your doctor for a referral. ■

GLOSSARY

abdominoperineal resection—Surgery that involves cutting through the abdomen and the perineum.

ablation—Destruction of cancer cells or tumors using microwaves or by freezing or burning the tissue.

adenocarcinoma—Cancer in the cells that line the inside layer of the wall of the colon and rectum.

adenoma—See adenomatous polyp.

adenomatous polyp—Also called adenoma. A growth (polyp), usually benign, that protrudes from the mucous membranes and may become cancerous over time.

adjuvant therapy—Treatment, usually chemotherapy or radiation, given in addition to surgery.

anastomosis—Surgical connection or reconnection between two separated parts of the body.

anemia—Having less than the normal number of red blood cells, which lowers the oxygen-carrying capacity of the blood and can be a sign of blood loss.

anus—The opening at the end of the digestive tract through which feces are expelled. A set of sphincter muscles allows the anus to remain closed and to open for a bowel movement.

APC I1307K—An inherited gene mutation (found with noteworthy frequency in descendants of Ashkenazi Jews from eastern Europe but can occur in other individuals) that increases the risk of colorectal cancer.

ascending colon—That portion of colon on the right side of the body that ascends from the small intestine.

barium enema, double-contrast barium enema— An enema with a white, chalky solution that contains barium, given to outline the intestines on a series of x-rays and reveal abnormalities.

biopsy—Removal of a tissue sample to examine for diagnosis.

bolus—The injection of a drug (or drugs) at high doses at once rather than by gradual administration.

bowel—Another term for the lower intestinal tract, the large intestine, or the colorectum, These terms are often used interchangeably

brachytherapy—A radiation treatment that implants or beams radiation directly into or near a tumor.

carcinoembryonic antigen (CEA)—A blood chemical that is measured after treatments as a marker for cancer cells.

CAT (computerized axial tomography) or CT—A computerized imaging method that takes multiple cross-section x-ray images of soft tissues.

cecum—A pouch about 2–3 inches long between the small intestine and the large intestine. The furthest point of a colonoscopy examination.

chemoembolization—Administration of chemotherapy mixed with material to slow blood flow through the liver and allow the drugs to remain longer in the tumor.

colectomy—Surgery to remove part or all of the colon.

colitis—Inflammation of the colon

colon—A term for the large intestine, lower intestinal tract, colorectum, or bowel. These terms are often used interchangeably.

colonic stent—An expandable tube that is placed in the colon with an endoscope to open up a compressed or blocked bowel.

colonoscopy—Internal examination of the entire colon with an endoscope that is passed up through the rectum.

colorectum—A term for the large intestine, lower intestinal tract, bowel, or colon. These terms are often used interchangeably.

colostomy—A procedure in which a portion of the colon is brought through an opening in the abdominal wall to allow waste to pass into a pouch worn on the abdomen.

complementary medicine—Treatments such as herbs or acupuncture that are not accepted as conventional medical practices but that may help with diseases when used along with Western medicine.

Crohn's disease—A chronic inflammation of the bowel that may increase the risk of developing colon cancer.

descending colon—That portion of the colon that descends down the left side, ending in the rectum.

DNA—Deoxyribonucleic acid, the biochemical polymer that encodes genetic information inside a cell. Some new tests can identify DNA from cancerous cells.

DNA fecal test—A new test that can pinpoint DNA from colon cancer cells in a person's feces.

dysplasia—A term that refers to cells that are no longer normal but are not yet cancerous.

endorectal ultrasound—An imaging technique that uses sound waves to visualize and to pinpoint rectal tumors.

endoscope—General term for a tube that is inserted into openings in the body to allow an internal examination without performing surgery.

enterostomal therapist—A healthcare professional, often a nurse, trained to help people with colostomies.

familial adenomatous polyposis (FAP)—A rare hereditary disease that causes massive overgrowth of colon polyps and leads to colon cancer in all who inherit the dominant genes. About 1% of all colorectal cancers are due to FAP.

fecal immunochemical testing (FIT)—A take-home test for hidden intestinal bleeding that is specific for human hemoglobin and does not require diet changes before and during the test.

fecal occult blood test (FOBT)—The most frequently

used take-home test for hidden intestinal bleeding. Requires some diet and drug restrictions before and during the test.

guaiac—A product that reacts to hemoglobin and is used in kits to test for fecal blood.

HAI (hepatic arterial infusion)—Delivering chemotherapy drugs directly into the liver through a main artery.

hemicolectomy—Surgical removal of the right or left side of the colon; a partial colectomy.

hepatic—Referring to the liver.

hereditary nonpolyposis colon cancer (HNPCC)—An inherited genetic predisposition found in 3-6% of people with colorectal cancer. Also called Lynch syndrome.

ileostomy—A procedure in which a portion of the small intestine (ileum) is brought through an opening in the abdominal wall to allow waste to pass into a pouch worn on the abdomen.

inflammatory bowel disease (IBD)—A chronic inflammation of the colon that may increase colorectal cancer risks. Often confused with the spectrum of symptoms known as irritable bowel syndrome (IBS), which does not appear to increase colorectal cancer risk.

interstitial radiation therapy— A radiation treatment in which radioactive material sealed in needles, seeds, wires, or catheters is placed directly into or near a tumor. Also called brachytherapy, internal radiation, or implant radiation.

intraoperative ultrasound—Ultrasound imaging used during surgery to help distinguish cancer from healthy tissue.

laparoscopic surgery—Surgery performed through several small incisions rather than one large opening, with the aid of fiberoptic and other viewing devices.

large intestine—A term to describe the entire colon and rectum, from the cecum at the end of the small intestine to the anus at the end of the rectum. Other terms are colon, bowel, and colorectum.

local excision—Operating through a colonoscope or sigmoidoscope to remove small, early-stage cancers.

lymph nodes—Small bodies of tissue that filter bacteria and foreign particles from lymph fluid.

Lynch syndrome—See hereditary nonpolyposis colorectal cancer (HNPCC).

metastases, metastatic, metastasized—Terms to describe cancer that had spread from its original point and begun to grow in a distant site. The liver is the most common site of metastases in colorectal cancer.

ostomy—A surgically created opening in the abdomen to which part of the bowel is attached so that its contents empty into a pouch attached to the abdomen.

palliative care—Treatment that is not curative but relieves pain and suffering.

pancolitis—Inflammation that involves the entire colon.

peristalsis—The rhythmic contraction of muscles that propels what you ingest from the esophagus through the intestines and down to the rectum.

polyp—A growth that protrudes from the skin or from a mucous membrane. Usually benign, some colon polyps can become cancerous. See adenomatous polyp.

polypectomy—Removal of polyps in the colon and rectum, usually during a colonoscopy or sigmoidoscopy.

proctoscopy—A rectal examination with an endoscope called a proctoscope.

radiofrequency ablation—A procedure in which a special electrode is placed in a tumor and a radiofrequency current heats the tumor tissue to destroy (ablate) it.

rectum—The final 5 inches of the bowel, in which feces are stored before being expelled in a bowel movement.

resection—Surgery in which cancer is removed (resected) along with healthy tissue around it.

sigmoid colectomy—Surgery to remove part of the sigmoid colon.

sigmoid colon—The lower part of the colon right above the rectum. Is curved somewhat like the letter "S," which in Greek is called sigmoid.

sigmoidoscopy—An examination of the lower 25 inches or so of the colon and rectum with a flexible endoscope that is inserted through the anus.

sphincter—A set of muscles at the end of the anus that allow it to remain closed and to open to eliminate feces.

splenic flexure—That portion of the colon that makes a left-hand turn at the top of the ascending colon.

staging—A system developed by surgeons and researchers to assess the extent (or stage) of a cancer and its seriousness. Treatment options are often based on staging.

stoma—The end portion of the bowel that protrudes through the abdominal wall after ostomy surgery.

transverse colon—The middle portion of the colon, which goes horizontally across the body. Removal of this is called a transverse colectomy.

ulcerative colitis—A chronic inflammatory bowel condition that can increase the risk of developing colon cancer.

ultrasound—High-frequency sound waves bounced off soft tissues to create a picture (sonogram) of internal organs.

virtual colonoscopy—A popular term for a developing technology in which the colorectum can be examined with a CT scan.

HEALTH INFORMATION ORGANIZATIONS AND SUPPORT GROUPS

American Cancer Society
1599 Clifton Rd. NE
Atlanta, GA 30329
☎ 800-ACS-2345
www.cancer.org
National, community-based organization that provides accurate, up-to-date information on all aspects of cancer through its toll-free information line, website, and published materials.

Prevent Cancer Foundation
1600 Duke St.
Alexandria, VA 22314
☎ 800-227-2732/703-836-4412
www.preventcancer.org/colorectal/facts
A national health foundation dedicated to the prevention and early detection of cancer through scientific research and education. Provides information and self-help guides for colorectal cancer patients.

Colon Cancer Alliance
5411 N University Dr., Ste. 202
Coral Springs, FL 33067
☎ 877-422-2030
www.ccalliance.org
A national patient advocacy organization dedicated to patient support, education, research and advocacy. Provides information on colon cancer and peer-to-peer support networks.

Colorectal Cancer Network
P.O. Box 182
Kensington, MD 20895-0182
☎ 301-879-1500
www.colorectal-cancer.net
A patient advocacy group that offers support groups, listservs, chat rooms, a matching list that connects newly diagnosed people with long-term survivors, an extensive colorectal cancer library, and a list of resources for patients.

National Cancer Institute
6116 Executive Blvd., Rm. 3036A
Bethesda, MD 20892-8322
☎ 800-4-CANCER
www.cancer.gov
Coordinates the National Cancer Program, which conducts and supports research, training, health information dissemination, and other programs with respect to the cause, diagnosis, prevention, and treatment of cancer, rehabilitation from cancer, and the continuing care of cancer patients and the families of cancer patients. For information specific to colorectal cancer go to www.cancer.gov/cancertopics/types/colon-and-rectal.

National Hospice and Palliative Care Organization
1700 Diagonal Rd., Ste. 625
Alexandria, VA 22314
☎ 703-837-1500/800-658-8898
www.nhpco.org
Provides free consumer information on hospice and end-of-life care. Also provides referrals to hospice programs.

Partnership for Prescription Assistance
950 F St. NW
Washington, D.C. 20004
☎ 888-4PPA-NOW (888-477-2669)
www.pparx.org
A national program sponsored by U.S. pharmaceutical research companies to help patients in need of access to prescription medicines free or at low cost.

LEADING HOSPITALS
for Cancer as Ranked by *U.S. News & World Report*

1. **University of Texas M. D. Anderson Cancer Center**
   Houston, TX
   ☎ 877-MDA-6789
   www.mdanderson.org

2. **Memorial Sloan-Kettering Cancer Center**
   New York, NY
   ☎ 212-639-2000/800-525-2225
   www.mskcc.org

3. **Johns Hopkins Hospital**
   Baltimore, MD
   ☎ 410-502-4003/410-955-5464
   www.hopkinsmedicine.org

4. **Mayo Clinic**
   Rochester, MN
   ☎ 507-284-2511/507-538-3270
   www.mayoclinic.org

5. **Dana–Farber Cancer Institute**
   Boston, MA
   ☎ 617-632-3000
   www.dana-farber.org

6. **University of Washington Medical Center**
   Seattle, WA
   ☎ 206-598-3300
   www.uwmedicine.org

7. **University of Chicago Hospitals**
   Chicago, IL
   ☎ 888-UCH-0200/773-702-1000
   www.uchospitals.edu

8. **University of California, Los Angeles, Medical Center**
   Los Angeles, CA
   ☎ 310-825-9111/800-825-2631
   www.healthcare.ucla.edu

9. **Duke University Medical Center**
   Durham, NC
   ☎ 800-ASK-DUKE/916-684-8111
   www.medschool.duke.edu

10. **Massachusetts General Hospital**
    Boston, MA
    ☎ 617-726-2000
    www.massgeneral.org

INDEX

S

T

U

W

X

NOTES

NOTES

NOTES

Please address inquiries on bulk subscriptions and permission to reproduce selections from this White Paper to Medletter Associates, LLC, 6 Trowbridge Drive, Bethel, CT 06801.
The editors are interested in receiving your comments at whitepapers@johnshopkinshealthalerts.com or the above address but regret that they cannot answer letters of any sort personally.

ISBN 978-1-933087-59-7
1-933087-59-5

Printed in the United States of America

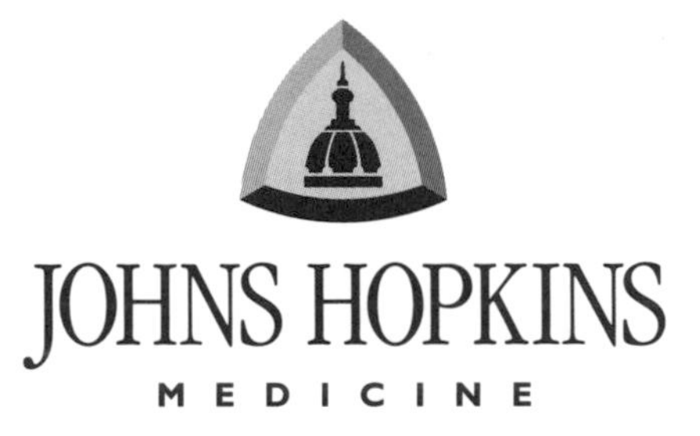

The Johns Hopkins White Papers are published yearly by Medletter Associates, LLC.

CORONARY HEART DISEASE

Gary Gerstenblith, M.D.,

and

Simeon Margolis, M.D., Ph.D.

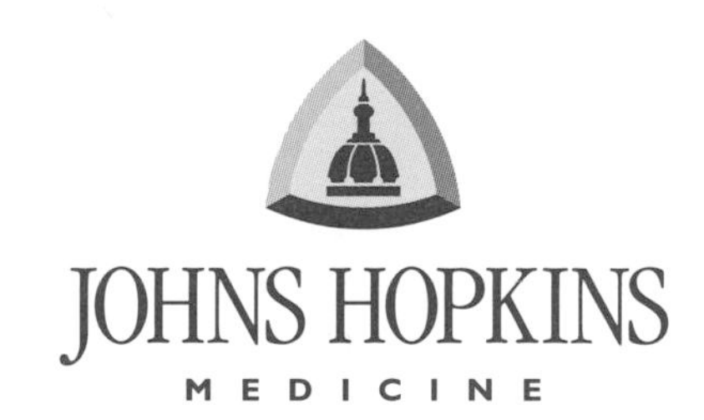

Dear Reader:

Welcome to the 2008 *Coronary Heart Disease White Paper*—your Johns Hopkins guide to managing coronary heart disease and its complications, such as heart attack, heart failure, and arrhythmias.

This year's highlights include:

- How aggressive treatment of **gum disease** may protect your heart. (page 7)
- What to do when **atherosclerosis** strikes in the **legs**. (page 8)
- Find a **heart-friendly painkiller**: The risks of prescription and over-the-counter pain relief. (page 14)
- **Screening tests** that go beyond cholesterol and blood pressure. (page 20)
- The latest **heart-healthy supplements**: Are any worth a try? (page 28)
- How **everyday activities** can give your heart the benefits of exercise. (page 34)
- Having problems **sticking with your medications**? We have some simple solutions. (page 48)
- What the experts are saying about **drug-eluting stents**. (page 58)
- The steps that could **save your life** in the event of a **heart attack**. (page 65)
- The newest treatment for **atrial fibrillation**: A possible cure? (page 80)
- New **driving rules** for people with **implantable defibrillators**. (page 82)

You'll also find a new "Ask the Doctor" column on pages 25, 27, 61, 63, and 77. This year's questions came from my patients, but next year we'd like to answer a few of yours. If you have any heart disease–related queries you want answered in the White Papers, or comments about the White Papers in general, please e-mail the editors at whitepapers@johnshopkinshealthalerts.com.

Wishing you the best of health in 2008,

Gary Gerstenblith, M.D.
Professor of Medicine
Division of Cardiology, Johns Hopkins University School of Medicine

P.S. Please visit www.HopkinsHeart.com for the latest news on heart disease and other information that will complement your Johns Hopkins White Paper.

THE AUTHORS

Gary Gerstenblith, M.D., received his B.A. from New York University and his M.D. from the University of Pennsylvania School of Medicine. He performed his internship and residency at the Hospital of the University of Pennsylvania and received his cardiology training at the National Institutes of Health and the University of Miami School of Medicine. He is Professor of Medicine, Cardiology Division, Department of Medicine at the Johns Hopkins University School of Medicine and is on the full-time staff at Johns Hopkins Hospital.

■ ■ ■

Simeon Margolis, M.D., Ph.D., received his M.D. and Ph.D. from the Johns Hopkins University School of Medicine and performed his internship and residency at Johns Hopkins Hospital. He is currently Professor of Medicine and Biological Chemistry at the Johns Hopkins University School of Medicine and Medical Editor of *The Johns Hopkins Medical Letter: Health After 50.* He has served on various committees for the Department of Health, Education, and Welfare, including the National Diabetes Advisory Board and the Arteriosclerosis Specialized Centers of Research Review Committees. In addition, he has acted as a member of the Endocrinology and Metabolism Panel of the U.S. Food and Drug Administration.

A former weekly columnist for *The Baltimore Sun,* Dr. Margolis lectures to medical students, physicians, and the general public on a wide variety of topics, such as the prevention of coronary heart disease, the control of cholesterol levels, the treatment of diabetes, and the use of alternative medicine.

CONTENTS

CORONARY HEART DISEASE

We do not give much thought to our heart until something goes wrong with it. Weighing a little less than three quarters of a pound, it has the Herculean task of pumping oxygen- and nutrient-rich blood through the 60,000-mile highway of blood vessels to all the tissues of your body. Your heart does this nonstop, decade after decade, for as long as you live.

If your physician has diagnosed you with coronary heart disease (CHD), also called coronary artery disease, you are not alone—some 15.8 million Americans suffer from this health problem. CHD is diagnosed when your coronary arteries—the arteries that carry blood to the heart—become narrowed by the buildup of deposits called plaques within the artery walls. This process, known as atherosclerosis, impairs the ability of the body to pump enough blood through the coronary arteries to provide adequate oxygen and nutrients to the heart. Even worse, formation of a blood clot on top of a plaque can cause a fatal heart attack.

CHD is the number one cause of death in both men and women in the United States. It is responsible for about one in five deaths, and it can lead to serious complications, including angina, heart attacks, heart failure, and arrhythmias. Here's what these terms mean:

Angina. Also called angina pectoris, angina is episodes of chest pain that result from reduced blood flow to the heart. Angina affects about 8.9 million Americans.

Heart attacks. A heart attack, technically known as a myocardial infarction, occurs when complete blockage of a coronary artery interrupts blood flow to a portion of the heart muscle (myocardium), causing death of heart tissue (infarction). Some 865,000 Americans have a heart attack each year.

Heart failure. This medical condition occurs when the heart is unable to pump blood efficiently, and the body's need for circulating blood is not met. Heart failure affects 5.2 million people in the United States.

Arrhythmias. These are disturbances or irregularities in the beating of the heart. Atrial fibrillation—one of the most common arrhythmias—affects more than 2.2 million people in the United States.

Most people have one or more risk factors that increases their chances of developing CHD. But as this White Paper will describe, if you can identify and control your risk factors for CHD, you can help prevent or delay the development and progression of this disease.

Sometimes, however, preventive efforts are not enough, and CHD and its complications occur. Fortunately, thanks to advances in the understanding and treatment of these disorders, you and your doctor can manage them with a combination of lifestyle measures, medications, and revascularization procedures (such as angioplasty and bypass surgery).

This White Paper will provide you with the information you will need to work closely with your physician in your efforts to prevent or manage CHD.

Causes of Coronary Heart Disease

In most people with CHD, the underlying cause of the disease is atherosclerosis—the buildup of deposits called plaques within the walls of the arteries. These plaques decrease the size of the artery's lumen, the channel or space through which blood flows. When atherosclerosis develops in the coronary arteries, it can decrease blood flow to the heart (causing chest pains called angina) or it can completely block blood flow (resulting in a heart attack).

Atherosclerosis doesn't develop overnight; it is a slow process that can take many years. It typically occurs after decades of lifestyle behaviors that lead to the accumulation of cells, fats, and cholesterol on the once-smooth inner lining of the arteries. This process typically starts when the endothelium (the thin layer of cells that lines the arteries) is injured, often because of exposure to toxins (such as cigarette smoke) or because of inflammation. The lining then expresses molecules that attract white blood cells and low-density lipoprotein (LDL) cholesterol. The damaged endothelium becomes permeable to these white blood cells and LDL cholesterol, which then enter the inner surface of the artery.

As these substances (as well as calcium and fibrin) accumulate, they form plaques that increase in size, narrowing the arteries and interfering with normal blood flow. When the plaques grow large enough, they can starve the heart muscle of oxygen, initially causing episodes of short-lived chest pain called angina. If the plaque tears or ruptures, however, the result is a blood clot that can completely block blood flow and cause a heart attack. A heart attack can also occur when a clot breaks loose from a plaque and then travels until it completely obstructs a smaller coronary artery.

Anatomy of the Heart and the Coronary Arteries

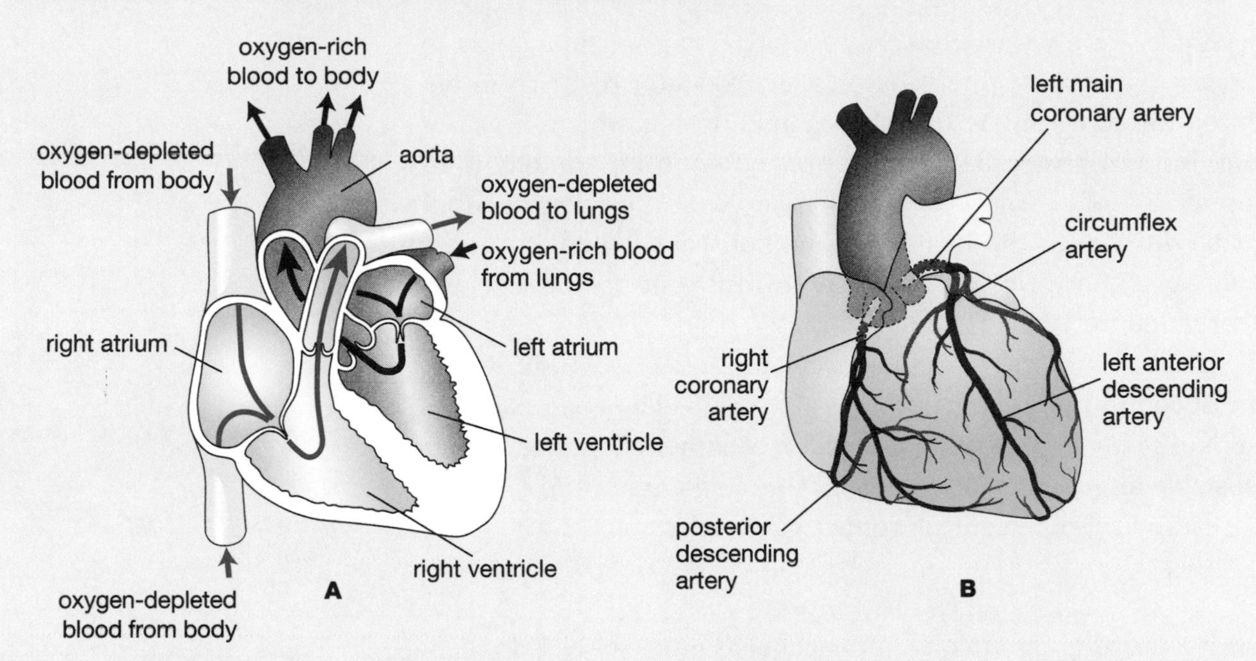

Composed almost entirely of muscle, the heart contains four hollow chambers—the left atrium, the right atrium, the left ventricle, and the right ventricle (see illustration A). Each heartbeat is a muscular contraction that sends blood through the body's circulatory system.

The left ventricle pumps oxygen-rich blood out of the heart via the aorta—the body's largest artery—which branches off into smaller arteries throughout the body. These arteries in turn divide into even smaller blood vessels, called arterioles, and eventually into capillaries, which are microscopic blood vessels that deliver oxygen and nutrients to tissues throughout the body and pick up carbon dioxide and other waste products.

After the blood, now depleted of oxygen and nutrients, passes through the capillaries, it enters tiny veins known as venules and then travels back to the heart through progressively larger veins. When the blood reaches the heart, it enters the right atrium and flows into the right ventricle, which pumps the blood through the pulmonary arteries into the lungs. In the lungs, carbon dioxide is exchanged for fresh oxygen through respiration. The reoxygenated blood passes through the pulmonary veins into the left atrium, and flows into the left ventricle. Then the cycle begins again.

Like other tissues in the body, the heart muscle needs a steady supply of oxygen-rich blood in order to function. However, heart muscle cells do not extract oxygen and nutrients directly from the blood that continually fills the heart's chambers. Instead, the heart receives its blood supply via the coronary arteries, which emerge from the base of the aorta (see illustration B).

The two primary coronary arteries—the left main coronary artery and the right coronary artery—lie on the surface of the heart and branch off into smaller arteries. The left main artery splits into the left anterior descending and the circumflex arteries; a major branch of the right coronary artery is the posterior descending artery. These branches, in turn, split into even smaller arteries (and eventually capillaries) that extend deep into the heart muscle, providing oxygen and nutrients to all portions of the heart and picking up waste products. The blood then passes through the coronary veins and drains directly into the right atrium.

Coronary arteries are susceptible to developing fatty deposits called plaques. If the plaques grow large enough to narrow the space within the artery, the portion of the heart supplied by that artery will suffer from a lack of oxygen (ischemia) that may result in chest pain known as angina. Certain plaques are at increased risk for rupture, which can lead to clot formation, a heart attack, and sudden death. ■

Symptoms of Coronary Heart Disease

Many people are unaware that they have CHD or are susceptible to the disease, particularly if they haven't seen a doctor regularly to undergo routine screening tests such as a lipid profile, which measures the amount of triglycerides and types of cholesterol in the blood. In fact, up to 25% of people with CHD have no symptoms despite insufficient blood flow to the heart—a condition called silent coronary heart disease. That's why it's important to visit your doctor regularly to be screened for CHD.

Eventually, however, symptoms occur in most people with CHD. The most common initial symptom is chest pain. The chest pain can be a sign of stable angina or an indication of something more serious like unstable angina or a heart attack. Unstable angina and heart attacks are also known as acute coronary syndromes.

Stable Angina

Angina is a warning sign that your heart needs more oxygen. In technical terms, the symptoms are the result of myocardial ischemia (a shortage of blood and oxygen to the heart muscle due to partial blockage of a coronary artery by plaque buildup). Stable angina occurs most often during physical activity, when the heart requires more oxygen than at rest but cannot get a sufficient blood supply because of narrowing of one or more of the coronary arteries. Symptoms usually occur when an artery is narrowed by at least 60–70%.

When people feel the discomfort of stable angina, they're often worried they're having a heart attack. However, an episode of angina is not a heart attack; the chest pain subsides quickly with rest or nitroglycerin, and there is usually no lasting damage to the heart muscle.

Types of symptoms

If you have stable angina, the most common symptom is a feeling of pressure beneath the breastbone. Some people experience sensations of tightness, squeezing, burning, aching, heaviness, or choking in the chest area. Angina can also produce pain in the left shoulder that radiates up to the neck and jaw, or pain in the inner part of the left arm that may travel down to the fingers. The intensity of the discomfort usually increases steadily, reaches a plateau, and gradually diminishes with rest—all within a few minutes.

Women do not always experience stable angina in the same way as men. They are more likely to have symptoms when they are at rest or under emotional stress. Women may also feel stable angina as pain in the jaw or as heartburn. Other vague symptoms common in women include breathlessness, nausea, and fatigue.

Because angina is often triggered by physical activity, you might experience symptoms while walking. If you're like most people with stable angina, you'll probably be able to predict what level of exertion will produce symptoms. Stable angina is more likely to occur if you participate in physical activity in the morning, after a meal, during cold weather, or when walking up an incline or into the wind. Some people experience angina with activities that involve the use of the arms—such as shoveling, sweeping, scrubbing, or raking. Sexual activity and bowel movements are other possible triggers. Anger, fear, anxiety, and excitement also can cause episodes of angina or reduce the amount of physical activity needed to produce angina.

To relieve the symptoms, your doctor may recommend rest until the symptoms subside or the use of a nitrate medication. In some cases, your doctor may ask you to take a nitrate medication before participating in an activity that has caused chest pain in the past.

Unstable Angina

This type of angina is a health problem midway in severity between stable angina and a heart attack. If you have unstable angina, an inadequate supply of blood and oxygen is reaching your heart, most likely because a blood clot in or spasm of the coronary artery has narrowed—but not completely blocked—the artery. Like a heart attack, unstable angina is a medical emergency. In fact, it is a sign that a heart attack could occur soon.

Three features distinguish unstable angina from stable angina:

- Chest pain is unexpected and can occur at rest.
- Chest pain is more severe and usually lasts for longer than 20 minutes.
- Chest pain is not relieved by rest or medication.

Call 911 immediately if you think your chest pains are more than just stable angina. You'll be taken to the hospital, where doctors can evaluate your chest pain. If unstable angina is diagnosed, you will likely need to stay in the hospital for about two to five days to receive treatment to prevent a heart attack. For more information on the diagnosis and treatment of unstable angina, see page 64.

Heart Attack

Unlike stable and unstable angina, in which the coronary arteries are partially blocked, a heart attack occurs when a coronary artery becomes completely obstructed. As you've already read, the cause of

NEW RESEARCH

Better Treatment, Lifestyle Cutting Coronary Heart Disease Deaths

The number of Americans dying of coronary heart disease (CHD) fell dramatically in just 20 years, a study reports.

Between 1980 and 2000, the age-adjusted death rate from CHD in the United States dropped by about 50% in both men and women—a total of about 342,000 fewer deaths. The decline was about half due to better treatments and half due to healthier lifestyles and improvements in the control of other heart risk factors.

The biggest treatment lifesavers included emergency treatments for heart attack—such as clot-dissolving medication and artery-clearing procedures like angioplasty—as well as therapies, such as aspirin, statins, and ACE inhibitors, to prevent further heart attacks and other complications.

Lower smoking rates and better control of blood pressure and cholesterol with lifestyle or medication were responsible for much of the benefit from improved control of risk factors.

Still, CHD remains the number one killer of Americans. What's more, this study found that increases in rates of obesity and diabetes undermined some of the gains made in other areas of CHD prevention.

What does this mean for you? Stick with your heart medications, but don't forget the importance of diet, exercise, and weight management in your overall health.

THE NEW ENGLAND JOURNAL OF MEDICINE
Volume 356, page 2388
June 7, 2007

this blockage is often a blood clot that forms where a plaque tears or ruptures. Together, the plaque and blood clot can completely block the artery. Many people who have heart attacks have a history of angina, and some people experience more frequent or severe angina pain in the days leading up to a heart attack. Others may have less distinct warning symptoms, such as increasing fatigue and shortness of breath. In many cases, however, a heart attack strikes suddenly and without any warning. For more information on heart attacks, see pages 65–69.

Risk Factors for Coronary Heart Disease

When your doctor attempts to determine your likelihood of developing CHD, he or she will ask you questions and order tests to assess your health-related traits and habits (risk factors) that may increase your risk. You are probably familiar with many of these risk factors: older age, family history of premature CHD, diabetes, being a man, cigarette smoking, high LDL cholesterol levels, low high-density lipoprotein (HDL) cholesterol levels, and high blood pressure. Some of these risk factors can be changed; others cannot. Having one or more of these risk factors does not mean that you are doomed to develop CHD. However, the more risk factors you have, the greater your chance of CHD.

Risk Factors That Cannot Be Changed

You cannot modify the risk factors described in this section. If you have one or more of them, you need to be conscientious about taking steps to prevent CHD by managing the modifiable risk factors discussed on pages 7–18.

Age

The older you are, the greater your CHD risk. This risk is increased after age 45 in men and after age 55 in women. More than half of the people who have CHD—and four out of five who die of CHD—are over age 65.

Gender

More men than women develop CHD. But a woman's risk starts approaching that of a man's after menopause, when women begin to produce less estrogen, which causes "bad" LDL cholesterol to rise and "good" HDL cholesterol to drop—both of which increase the risk of CHD. In fact, by about age 75, a woman's CHD risk is equal to that of a man.

Family history

If members of your family have been diagnosed with CHD, your own risk of the disease is higher as well. This is particularly true if male members of your immediate family—your father or a brother—have been diagnosed with CHD before age 55 or female members—your mother or a sister—have received a CHD diagnosis before age 65.

Personal history of cardiovascular disease

If you've had a stroke or been diagnosed with peripheral arterial disease, you are also at increased risk for developing CHD. Like CHD, these diseases are caused by the buildup of plaques in the arteries. A stroke is caused by plaque in arteries supplying blood to the brain; peripheral arterial disease is caused by plaque in arteries of the legs (for more details on peripheral arterial disease, see "When Atherosclerosis Strikes in the Legs" on pages 8–9). If you have plaques in these arteries, there is a good chance that you also have plaques in the arteries that carry blood to the heart.

Kidney disease

People with kidney disease have a significantly higher risk of CHD than people in the general population, even when kidney disease is in its early stages. In fact, people with kidney problems are more likely to die of CHD than of the kidney disease itself. One reason for the increased risk is that people with kidney disease are likely to have other risk factors for CHD, including high blood pressure, elevated LDL cholesterol levels, and diabetes. At the same time, kidney disease seems to play a role in CHD independent of these other risk factors, although researchers have not yet been able to explain how.

Risk Factors That Can Be Changed

In this section, we describe the risk factors for CHD that can be controlled—either minimized or eliminated altogether.

Cigarette smoking

Cigarette smoking is a dangerous risk factor not only for lung cancer but also for CHD. Smoking decreases your HDL cholesterol level. It also damages blood vessels and promotes atherosclerosis and blood clot formation. Fortunately, if you stop smoking, you can

NEW RESEARCH

Treating Gum Disease May Improve Health of Coronary Arteries

Aggressively treating periodontitis, a chronic bacterial infection of the gums, may not only save your teeth but also improve the health of your coronary arteries, a study suggests.

The study involved 120 adults with severe periodontitis who were randomly assigned to undergo routine dental cleaning or intensive periodontal therapy. Participants in the latter group received local anesthesia so the dentist could aggressively remove plaque, extract any teeth that couldn't be saved, and inject antibiotics into the infected gums to kill bacteria.

Two months later, endothelial function in the coronary arteries was better in the intensively treated patients than in the comparison group—a difference that was still apparent at the six-month mark. Decreased function of the endothelial cells that line the walls of the coronary arteries is an early sign of the development of coronary heart disease (CHD).

Researchers still need to determine whether such intensive dental treatment helps prevent CHD or heart attacks in people with existing CHD. But the findings add to evidence that taking care of your teeth may be one of many ways to take care of your heart.

THE NEW ENGLAND JOURNAL OF MEDICINE
Volume 356, page 911
March 1, 2007

When Atherosclerosis Strikes in the Legs

The warning signs of peripheral arterial disease and what to do about them

When we hear the word "atherosclerosis," the buildup of plaques in the arteries, we usually think about the heart or the brain. After all, plaques in the arteries of these organs hinder blood flow and can trigger a heart attack or stroke. But when atherosclerosis is present in these parts of the vascular system, chances are it's lurking throughout, including the peripheral arteries that supply blood to the limbs.

Called peripheral arterial disease (PAD), this buildup of plaque in the arteries of the legs affects an estimated eight to 12 million Americans—and up to 20% of those older than age 65. Not surprisingly, PAD is a risk factor for heart attack and stroke. And for some people, the first signs of heart trouble may come from their legs.

But PAD can also cause problems beyond the heart. The lack of blood flow to the legs can make walking difficult. In addition, if PAD becomes severe enough, it can lead to hard-to-heal foot ulcers, infections, or even gangrene requiring amputation.

The good news is that PAD can be diagnosed through simple, noninvasive testing and often managed with lifestyle changes and medication.

How To Recognize PAD

Your body may give you warning signs that you have PAD—typically pain in the buttocks or leg muscles, particularly when you are walking or doing other physical activities. The pain usually subsides once you've stopped moving for a few minutes—a fact that helps differentiate PAD from other causes of leg pain, like spinal stenosis or diabetic nerve damage.

Once PAD progresses, pain and cramps may emerge when you're not exercising. You might, for example, feel pain when you are in bed, but find that it goes away if you hang your leg off the bed and let gravity improve blood flow to your extremities. Other potential signs include sores on your feet or lower leg that are slow to heal and bluish or black discoloration of your toes.

Unfortunately, the majority of PAD sufferers have no clear signs, and so the problem often goes unrecognized. That's why it's important to realize that you are at risk for PAD if you already have coronary heart disease (CHD) or have CHD risk factors. As with CHD, the risk factors for PAD include diabetes, smoking, high blood pressure, high cholesterol levels, being overweight, getting little or no exercise, and having a family history of premature cardiovascular disease.

How To Diagnose PAD

Luckily, a simple test called the ankle-brachial index, or ABI, can be performed during a routine doctor's visit. In an ABI test, your doctor will measure the blood pressure in your arm and in your ankle, and then compare the two measurements. A lower blood pressure in your ankle than in your arm indicates PAD.

From there, your doctor may do additional testing to get more information about your condition. For example, you might undergo a treadmill test to see what level of exercise spurs symptoms and how severe the PAD is. In some cases, angiography is used to spot the precise location of the artery blockages. Angiography allows a doctor to visualize blood flow inside the arteries; after injecting contrast dye into your leg arteries, he or she can trace the flow of the dye using x-rays.

dramatically decrease your CHD risk. Even if you've smoked for many years, your chances of having a CHD event (such as a heart attack) nearly return to those of a nonsmoker within five years of quitting.

Do not forget about secondhand smoke: Even if you are a nonsmoker, inhaling secondhand cigarette smoke makes your blood platelets stickier and more likely to form blood clots—after just 30 minutes of exposure. Some studies show that secondhand smoke

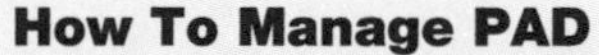

How To Manage PAD

Fortunately, when PAD is caught in its early stages, it can often be treated with lifestyle changes and medications. In fact, you may already be following many of these measures and taking some of these medications to prevent or manage CHD. If PAD worsens, surgical procedures (similar to those that can open or bypass narrowed coronary arteries) may be used to treat narrowed arteries in the legs.

Lifestyle measures. If you smoke, quitting is the single most important lifestyle measure you can pursue. If you have diabetes, strict control of your blood sugar—through medication, diet, and exercise—is essential.

And for everyone, moderate exercise is a cornerstone of treating PAD. The goal is to progressively increase the distance you can walk without pain. Even though it may seem counterintuitive to exercise when physical activity triggers leg pain, moderate walking can help keep PAD from worsening by improving blood circulation in the legs.

For example, research shows that supervised exercise in a PAD rehabilitation program can improve walking ability. There is also some evidence that informal, do-it-yourself exercise is effective, too. One recent study of more than 400 men and women with PAD found that those who walked for exercise at least three times per week maintained a faster walking speed over the next three years, compared with their peers who did not walk for exercise.

Another study found that even everyday activities—walking around or climbing stairs—might be helpful. Of 460 older adults with PAD, those who moved around more in their daily lives were less likely to die over the next five years. For more information on working physical activity into your daily life, see "The Benefits of Incidental Activity" on pages 34–35.

Medications. Besides blood pressure medication and statins to lower cholesterol, you may need an antiplatelet medication, such as ordinary aspirin or the prescription drug clopidogrel (Plavix), to reduce the risk of blood clots. Two other drugs—cilostazol (Pletal) and pentoxifylline (Trental)—can improve blood flow to prevent or decrease pain while walking.

Revascularization. If your PAD is severe, more aggressive treatment may be necessary. One option is angioplasty, in which a doctor snakes a balloon-tipped catheter into the diseased artery, then inflates the balloon to push blockages aside. If the artery disease is more extensive, you may need bypass surgery. Here, your surgeon will take a portion of a vein from another part of your body and sew it onto the diseased artery to reroute blood around the trouble spots. Sometimes, a synthetic vessel is used instead of your own vein.

The Bottom Line

If you have potential symptoms of PAD (for example, leg pain while walking or slow healing wounds on your legs and feet), do not pass them off as a natural part of "getting older." Tell your doctor. Getting diagnosed and treated for PAD in its early stages is the best way to prevent this disease from damaging your legs and increasing your risk of heart attack and stroke.

And even if you do not have symptoms but do have risk factors, ask your physician about PAD. Certain high-risk individuals, such as those with diabetes, should be screened for PAD whether or not they have symptoms. ■

also damages the endothelial cells lining the walls of arteries, which is the first step in the development of atherosclerosis.

High blood pressure

High blood pressure affects nearly one in three adults. It is called a silent disease or silent killer because it usually has no warning symptoms—at least initially—but it can wreak havoc on your body nonetheless, causing damage to your blood vessels and making your heart work harder. For this reason, you need to have your blood pressure checked regularly by your doctor so that high blood pressure can be detected before it causes serious damage to your arteries and heart as well as to other major organs in your body.

Blood pressure is considered normal if it is below 120/80 mm Hg (millimeters of mercury). The upper number (120 mm Hg) is called your systolic blood pressure and is the pressure in your arteries while the heart is pumping blood to the rest of the body. The lower number (80 mm Hg) is your diastolic blood pressure and indicates pressure in your arteries while the heart relaxes between beats.

If your blood pressure is above normal levels, you have a greater risk of developing CHD. There are two types of above-normal blood pressure: prehypertension and hypertension. You have prehypertension if your systolic pressure is between 120 and 139 mm Hg or your diastolic pressure is between 80 and 89 mm Hg. People with prehypertension are more likely to eventually develop high blood pressure. Full-blown hypertension is diagnosed when your systolic blood pressure is 140 mm Hg or more or your diastolic blood pressure is 90 mm Hg or more.

If you have prehypertension or high blood pressure, lowering your blood pressure not only will reduce your likelihood of developing CHD but also can lower your risk of having a heart attack or stroke or developing heart failure. Lowering high blood pressure can also slow the progression of kidney disease.

If you're over age 50, you should pay particular attention to your systolic blood pressure. Research shows that high systolic blood pressure is a significant threat to heart health. Many older people have a condition called isolated systolic hypertension—their systolic blood pressure is elevated but their diastolic blood pressure is normal.

Abnormal levels of blood lipids (fats)

Your doctor has probably measured your blood levels of cholesterol and triglycerides. These substances are lipids (fats) carried through your bloodstream on proteins called lipoproteins. Cholesterol is transported on LDL (low-density lipoprotein) or HDL (high-density lipoprotein); triglycerides are primarily carried on very–low-density lipoprotein (VLDL). If you have high levels of total cholesterol, "bad" LDL cholesterol, or triglycerides or decreased levels of "good" HDL cholesterol, you have an elevated risk of CHD.

To monitor your risk of CHD, the National Cholesterol Education Program (NCEP) recommends that all people over age 20 have a panel of blood tests called a lipid profile at least once every five years. This lipid profile measures the amount of total cholesterol, LDL cholesterol, HDL cholesterol, and triglycerides in the blood.

High total and LDL cholesterol levels. When you have high levels of total and LDL cholesterol in your blood, there is a greater likelihood of cholesterol depositing in the artery walls. Total cholesterol levels should be kept below 200 mg/dL to reduce the risk of CHD.

The LDL cholesterol level you should strive for depends on how many CHD risk factors you have. The fewer of these risk factors, the higher your LDL cholesterol can be without increasing your CHD risk. For example, if you have none or only one CHD risk factor, your LDL cholesterol can be as high as 160 mg/dL. People with many risk factors or who already have CHD need to aim for an LDL cholesterol level of less than 100 mg/dL or, in some cases, less than 70 mg/dL.

Low HDL cholesterol levels. Having an HDL cholesterol level less than 40 mg/dL is another CHD risk factor. In fact, recent research suggests that a total cholesterol level below 200 mg/dL—the level considered desirable—may still be associated with an increased risk of CHD if your HDL cholesterol level is below 40 mg/dL (this is particularly true for women). An elevated HDL cholesterol level (60 mg/dL or higher), however, is considered protective against CHD and will cancel out the effect of one other CHD risk factor when determining your total number of risk factors. HDL protects against CHD by transporting cholesterol to the liver from plaques in the arteries.

High triglyceride levels. Triglyceride levels above 150 mg/dL are considered undesirable. Until recently, researchers were uncertain whether high triglyceride levels directly raise the risk of CHD, since elevated triglycerides are frequently accompanied by low HDL cholesterol levels. The latest research, however, indicates that high triglyceride levels are a risk factor even when HDL cholesterol levels are normal. High triglycerides pose a greater risk in women than in men.

The CHD risk of elevated triglycerides is especially great if you also have low levels of HDL cholesterol and a predominance of small, dense LDL particles (see below). Individuals with abnormally high blood levels of insulin (hyperinsulinemia) also have a greater risk of CHD if they have elevated triglycerides.

How do elevated triglyceride levels increase CHD risk? Excess triglycerides in the blood appear to interfere with the normal widening of coronary arteries that occurs during physical exertion and to increase the risk of blood clots.

Small, dense LDL particles. The size and density of your LDL particles can affect your CHD risk. LDL particles vary in size and density to produce two patterns: A and B. People with pattern A have

NEW RESEARCH

Flu Can Trigger Heart Attacks

A case of the flu can cause you more than misery. It can raise your risk of a fatal heart attack, according to a recent study.

In the study, researchers looked at the relationship between flu outbreaks and autopsy-confirmed deaths from a heart attack or chronic coronary heart disease (CHD) among nearly 35,000 Russian adults who died between 1993 and 2000. Less than 3% of them had received yearly flu shots or taken cholesterol-lowering statin drugs.

The risk of heart attack death was 30% higher during flu-outbreak weeks than other weeks of the year. Each year, heart attack deaths as well as deaths from chronic CHD in general peaked during flu outbreaks.

It's thought that the flu may trigger heart attacks by causing widespread inflammation in the body that either destabilizes or ruptures plaques in the arteries. It's also possible that the stress of the flu increases the workload of the heart and decreases the amount of blood pumped with each heartbeat.

These new findings underscore the importance of getting your flu shot every year, not only to prevent the flu but also to avoid potentially deadly flu complications such as pneumonia and heart attacks.

EUROPEAN HEART JOURNAL
Volume 28, page 1205
May 2007

mostly large LDL particles, while people with pattern B have a predominance of small, dense particles. Pattern B is associated with a higher risk of CHD than pattern A.

High lipoprotein(a) levels. Also known as Lp(a), high levels of this lipoprotein are another risk factor for CHD. Lp(a) has a structure similar to LDL, but on its surface is a protein called apo(a) that resembles another blood protein called plasminogen. Because of this similarity, Lp(a) may interfere with the conversion of plasminogen to plasmin, an enzyme that helps dissolve blood clots in the arteries by breaking down fibrin (a major component of blood clots).

Elevated levels of Lp(a) are of particular concern for individuals who also have high levels of LDL cholesterol. Unfortunately, Lp(a) levels are difficult to lower, although some people are able to achieve modest reductions by taking high doses of niacin. Experts do not recommend that everyone have a blood test to measure their levels of Lp(a). However, the test is sometimes done to get a better idea of CHD risk when other risk factors point to an intermediate risk.

High apolipoprotein B (apo B) levels. This is another risk factor for CHD. Apo B is a protein present on the surface of LDL particles. A recent review of five studies found that high apo B levels are more strongly linked to a risk of heart attacks than high LDL cholesterol levels. But as with Lp(a) testing, current recommendations do not advise testing of apo B in everyone. However, an apo B test may be valuable in people at intermediate risk for CHD.

Obesity

An estimated 65% of adults in the United States are either overweight or obese, and their excess weight translates to an increased risk of CHD. To determine if you're overweight, calculate your body mass index (BMI), a measurement of your weight in relation to your height. Here's how: Multiply your weight in pounds by 703 and then divide the result by the square of your height in inches.

Let's say you weigh 190 lbs, and your height is 5 feet 8 inches. To determine your BMI, you would:

- Multiply 190 by 703 (190 x 703 = 133,570)
- Then divide your answer (133,570) by the square of your height in inches (68 x 68 = 4,624)
- When you divide 133,570 by 4,624, the result is 28.9 (your BMI).

You can also use an online BMI calculator, such as the one on the National Institutes of Health website at www.nhlbisupport.com/bmi.

You are overweight if your BMI is between 25 and 29.9 and obese if it is 30 or more. Therefore, in the example above, you would fall into the "overweight" category.

You can also determine the effect of your weight on your CHD risk by measuring your waist circumference. The adverse effects of obesity depend not only on the total amount of body fat you have but also on how that fat is distributed in your body. Excess weight concentrated in your abdomen is particularly dangerous because it leads to a condition called insulin resistance (a reduced ability of the body to respond to insulin, a hormone secreted by the pancreas that helps the body use glucose, or sugar, as a source of energy). People with insulin resistance tend to also have high triglyceride levels, low levels of HDL cholesterol, high blood pressure, and thus an increased CHD risk. In addition, people with insulin resistance are more likely to develop diabetes, another risk factor for CHD.

To measure your waist circumference, place a tape measure around your waist, level with the top of your hip bones. The tape should feel snug without compressing your skin. Then measure after exhaling normally. A waist circumference of greater than 40 inches in men or 35 inches in women indicates abdominal obesity and a heightened CHD risk.

If you're overweight, you should make efforts to lose those excess pounds. Dropping just a few pounds can make a big difference in your blood pressure and other risk factors for CHD.

Metabolic syndrome

Even if you've never heard of the metabolic syndrome, you may have some of the characteristics associated with it. By definition, you have the metabolic syndrome if you have at least three of the following five findings:

- Excess fat around the abdomen (a waist circumference greater than 40 inches in men or 35 inches in women)
- A high fasting triglyceride level (150 mg/dL or higher)
- A low HDL cholesterol level (less than 40 mg/dL in men or less than 50 mg/dL in women)
- Higher-than-normal blood pressure (130/85 mm Hg or higher) or taking a blood pressure–lowering medication
- An elevated fasting blood glucose level (100 mg/dL or higher).

More than 40% of Americans over age 60 have the metabolic syndrome. The condition increases not only the risk of CHD but also the risk of diabetes and stroke. That's because the metabolic syndrome can damage the walls of blood vessels and raise the likelihood of blood clots. A recent analysis of 37 studies found that people

NEW RESEARCH

Belly Fat Key in Heart Risks

Regardless of the number on the scale, people who carry their weight around their middle may face greater heart risks, two studies confirm. The good news is that exercise may trim both your waistline and your odds of having a heart attack.

In one study of more than 2,700 middle-aged adults, the larger that participants' waistlines were in relation to their hips, the greater their risk of plaque buildup in the arteries. In fact, waist-to-hip ratio was a better predictor of clogged arteries than was body mass index (BMI), a measure of weight in relation to height.

The second study included 169 middle-aged men. In men of the same BMI, those with the lowest cardiovascular fitness had twice as much abdominal fat as their fit counterparts. And that excess belly fat was associated with higher triglyceride levels, increased ratios of total cholesterol to HDL cholesterol, and more insulin resistance (a diabetes risk factor).

Both studies support the notion that too much abdominal fat is harmful to the heart, even if your weight is normal. But the second study also points to a way to keep your waistline trim: regular exercise. As the fittest men had the least belly fat, exercise offers health benefits even when the scale indicates a healthy weight.

JOURNAL OF THE AMERICAN COLLEGE OF CARDIOLOGY
Volume 50, page 752
August 21, 2007

ARCHIVES OF INTERNAL MEDICINE
Volume 167, page 1518
July 23, 2007

The Potential Heart Risks of Painkillers

In pain? Try nondrug options first

Over the past few years, you have no doubt heard news reports that question the safety of some common pain medications, particularly for people with heart disease or with cardiovascular risk factors. If you are confused about which painkiller to reach for when you have painful joints and aching muscles, you are not alone. Doctors haven't been sure either.

But recently published guidelines from the American Heart Association (AHA) aim to cut through the confusion. The latest advice is to consider nondrug options before taking any pain reliever for chronic aches, whether that pain is from osteoarthritis, rheumatoid arthritis, or overuse injuries like tendonitis and bursitis.

Overview of the Guidelines

According to the AHA, people at risk for a heart attack—including those with established coronary heart disease (CHD) or risk factors such as high blood pressure and high cholesterol—should first try pain-relieving tactics like physical therapy, heat and ice packs, and, if necessary, weight loss to reduce stress on the joints. If you fail to find relief with this route, the AHA suggests you talk with your doctor about starting acetaminophen (Tylenol) or aspirin (a nonsteroidal anti-inflammatory drug [NSAID]).

NSAIDs other than aspirin, including over-the-counter drugs like ibuprofen (Motrin, Advil) and naproxen (Aleve), have traditionally been the medication of choice for musculoskeletal pain. But recent research suggests that at least some of these medications carry heart risks similar to those of the prescription NSAIDs known as COX-2 inhibitors. COX-2 inhibitors like rofecoxib (Vioxx), valdecoxib (Bextra), and celecoxib (Celebrex) were highly popular arthritis medications before studies showed that they raise the risk of heart attack and stroke. (Vioxx and Bextra are no longer on the market.)

Ever since the heart risks of COX-2 drugs became clear, researchers have been taking a closer look at all NSAIDs, including the over-the-counter ones. According to the AHA, there's now enough evidence that people with CHD or CHD risk factors should be cautious about using any NSAID. Aspirin is the important exception: Its proven heart benefits separate it from other drugs in this class.

The Trouble With NSAIDs

All NSAIDs work by targeting an enzyme known as cyclooxygenase (COX), which comes in two major forms: COX-1 and COX-2. The COX-1 enzyme is constantly active in most tissues of the body, whereas COX-2 comes into play only when there's inflammation.

Traditional NSAIDs block both of these enzymes. But since COX-1 is required for the formation of prostaglandins, which protect the stomach, traditional NSAIDs can cause stomach upset, ulcers, and gastrointestinal bleeding. The COX-2 drugs were designed to minimize these problems by selectively blocking the inflammation-related COX-2, while leaving the stomach-protecting COX-1 alone.

However, scientists now believe that selective targeting of COX-2 can put the heart at risk, especially if you already have CHD or its risk factors. Blocking only COX-2 appears to create an imbalance in the body's pro- and anticlotting mechanisms, making blood cells more likely to clot. It also changes blood vessel reactivity, increasing the likelihood of constriction of vessels. In addition, COX-2 inhibitors may promote sodium and water retention, which can worsen high blood pressure or heart failure. Experts suspect that these effects explain why people on COX-2 inhibitors have an increased risk of heart attack and stroke.

But what about old-fashioned NSAIDs, like ibuprofen and naproxen, which are considered "nonselective" for COX-2? It turns out these drugs have varying degrees of selectivity for blocking COX-2, with ibuprofen having somewhat more anti-COX-2 activity than naproxen. In line with this, a recent review of studies found that high doses of ibuprofen raise the risk of heart attack and stroke by 50%.

The results were similar when researchers looked at another NSAID called diclofenac (Cataflam, Voltaren). Naproxen, on the other hand, was not clearly linked to heart complications—although the AHA is advising caution with the drug until more research is done.

'Stepped-Care' Approach

The AHA's guidelines are laid out as steps, with the goal of helping you achieve the most pain relief with the least possible heart risks.

Step 1: Non-drug options. Depending on the nature and severity of your pain, you might be able to start with alternatives to medication, such as physical therapy, heat and cold packs, and, if necessary, weight loss. In addition, regular moderate exercise like walking can help with arthritis pain—not to mention aid your heart. In some cases, orthotic shoe inserts are helpful for chronic pain in the feet, legs, or lower back.

Step 2: Acetaminophen or aspirin. If you need medication to relieve your pain, the AHA recommends starting with one of two over-the-counter remedies: acetaminophen or aspirin. Acetaminophen is not an NSAID; aspirin is an NSAID, but its heart-protecting effects are well documented. Another difference: Aspirin can cause gastrointestinal bleeding, while acetaminophen does not.

If you're already taking aspirin for your heart, don't simply take extra aspirin or add acetaminophen without consulting your doctor. Also avoid exceeding the recommended dose on the drug's label, and be sure to call your doctor if pain is not relieved after taking the drug for 10 days straight.

In a controversial recommendation, the AHA also suggests discussing with your doctor the short-term use of a prescription narcotic as a first-choice medication for acute pain. Not all doctors agree with placing these drugs ahead of NSAIDs, because prescription narcotics like codeine, oxycodone, and morphine have side effects and carry the risk of dependency.

Step 3: NSAIDs. If you do need an NSAID other than aspirin, the AHA advises first trying the ones that are least selective for the COX-2 enzyme. Their recommendation is to start with naproxen. See the inset box above for the relative COX-2 specificity of a wide range of NSAIDs.

If you start an NSAID, you may need to also take a low-dose aspirin (if you're not already) to curb the odds of a blood clot, as well as a proton pump inhibitor to lower the risk of gastrointestinal bleeding. Also, ibuprofen can interfere with the heart benefits of immediate-release aspirin (the noncoated variety), so if you start ibuprofen for pain relief, you should take it at least 30 minutes after your daily aspirin or at least eight hours beforehand.

Step 4: COX-2 inhibitors. These newer NSAIDs should be the last resort for pain. If your doctor prescribes one, the AHA recommends that he or she monitor your blood pressure and kidney function—especially if you have existing high blood pressure, kidney problems, or heart failure. Also, a daily aspirin for your heart can undo the reduced chance of gastrointestinal bleeding with a COX-2 inhibitor.

What Is the COX-2 Activity of Your Pain Reliever?

Least COX-2 Activity

aspirin • fenoprofen (Nalfon, Nalfon 200) • flurbiprofen (Ansaid) • ibuprofen (Motrin, Motrin IB, Motrin Migraine Pain, Advil, Advil Liqui-Gels, Advil Migraine Liqui-Gels, Ibu-Tab, Ibu-Tab 200, Medipren, Cap-Profen, Tab-Profen, Profen, Ibuprohm) • indomethacin (Indocin, Indocin SR) • ketoprofen (Oruvail) • ketorolac (Toradol) • nabumetone • naproxen (Aleve, Naprosyn, Anaprox, Anaprox DS, EC-Naprosyn, Naprelan) • oxaprozin (Daypro) • tolmetin (Tolectin, Tolectin DS, Tolectin 600)

Moderate COX-2 Activity

diclofenac (Cataflam, Voltaren, Voltaren-XR) • piroxicam (Feldene) • sulindac (Clinorll)

Highest COX-2 Activity

celecoxib (Celebrex) • meloxicam (Mobic) • etodolac • mefenamic acid (Ponstel)

Some Last Words of Advice

No matter what pain medication you take, the safest route is to take the lowest effective dose, for the shortest possible time. Over-the-counter pain medications (with the exception of aspirin) are intended for short-term use only, and the effects of taking them for months or years are still not fully clear.

The bottom line is to remember that medications are not harmless just because you can purchase them over the counter. Be sure to work with your doctor to find the safest, most effective way to manage your pain. ■

with the metabolic syndrome were 78% more likely than those without the condition to suffer a heart attack or die of cardiovascular disease. Women with the metabolic syndrome were at particular risk, having nearly three times the odds of other women for heart attack or death.

The best therapy for the metabolic syndrome is lifestyle measures, for example, weight loss and increased physical activity. There are also medications to improve cholesterol and triglyceride levels, lower blood pressure, and control blood glucose levels.

Diabetes

About 21 million Americans have diabetes. People with diabetes are two to four times more likely to develop CHD than people without diabetes. One reason is that risk factors for CHD (such as elevated triglycerides, low HDL cholesterol, high blood pressure, and obesity) are more common in people with diabetes. In addition, diabetes itself increases the risk of CHD.

Individuals with prediabetes (blood glucose levels that are higher than normal but not quite in the diabetes range) also have an increased risk of CHD. Prediabetes is diagnosed when glucose levels are between 100 and 125 mg/dL on a fasting blood test. It's estimated that 54 million U.S. adults have prediabetes.

If you have diabetes or prediabetes, it's important to make lifestyle changes to control other CHD risk factors. For example, you should lower your LDL cholesterol level to less than 100 mg/dL (preferably, to less than 70 mg/dL). In addition, you should keep your blood pressure below 130/80 mm Hg.

Physical inactivity

Regular physical activity helps prevent CHD. It can also help prevent heart attacks in individuals who already have CHD.

Regular exercise helps to control weight, lower blood pressure, and improve blood lipid levels. Despite these beneficial effects, too many Americans are content with a sedentary lifestyle. According to the American Heart Association, only about 30% of adult Americans participate in any regular physical activity, and this level of participation tends to decline as people get older. Only 16% of people age 75 and older exercise on a regular basis.

C-reactive protein (CRP)

This protein is produced by the liver in response to tissue inflammation or infection. A high CRP level increases CHD risk, regardless of your age, gender, or presence of other risk factors. A recent study of nearly 4,000 adults with stable CHD found that those with the highest CRP levels (more than 3 mg/L) were 52% more likely than those with the lowest CRP readings (less than 1 mg/L) to suffer a heart attack or stroke or die of cardiovascular disease over five years.

How does CRP contribute to CHD risk? Researchers are unclear. One theory is that CRP injures blood vessels, which in turn contributes to the development of plaque and the formation of blood clots that can lead to a heart attack. Another theory: CRP is simply a marker for blood vessel damage and the events that follow.

Homocysteine

High blood levels of the amino acid homocysteine may increase CHD risk by damaging artery walls and contributing to atherosclerosis. For example, in one study, men who had high blood levels of homocysteine had almost three times the risk of a heart attack as those with low levels of this amino acid.

Researchers are uncertain exactly how homocysteine adversely affects the arteries, but elevated levels may damage the endothelium (the cells lining the artery walls) and may contribute to the development of blood clots that can lead to a heart attack.

Deficiencies in certain B vitamins—particularly vitamins B_6, B_{12}, and folic acid—contribute to high levels of homocysteine, suggesting that taking supplements of these B vitamins might help lower the risk of CHD. While taking these supplements (particularly folic acid) helps lower homocysteine, there is no evidence that these supplements lower the risk of CHD. Therefore, the American Heart Association no longer recommends B vitamin supplements to reduce CHD risk.

Stress

Over the past 30 years, studies have shown a relationship between mental stress and the risk of CHD. When you're under stress, your body responds by releasing epinephrine (adrenaline) and other hormones that speed up heart rate, raise blood pressure, and, possibly, even cause a spasm of the coronary arteries. If the coronary arteries are already narrowed by plaque, a spasm could lead to unstable angina or a heart attack.

Stress is not generally considered a direct risk factor for CHD, partly because it is difficult to quantify the exact amount of stress someone is experiencing. Nevertheless, it is a possible contributing factor to the development of CHD.

NEW RESEARCH

Chronic Anxiety May Raise Heart Attack Odds

Managing coronary heart disease (CHD) can be stressful. But if the occasional worry turns into chronic anxiety, it could raise your risk of a heart attack, a new study suggests.

The study, which followed 516 people with CHD for 3.5 years, found that those whose anxiety escalated over time were more likely to die or suffer a heart attack than their calmer peers. In contrast, patients whose anxiety did not worsen showed declining heart risks, even if their initial anxiety levels were fairly high.

The participants completed an anxiety questionnaire at the study's start and each year during the follow-up. The questions covered anxiety symptoms and feelings like upset stomach, sleep problems, and pessimism about the future.

Researchers also found that men and women with average cumulative anxiety scores in the highest third were twice as likely to suffer a heart attack or die during the study as those with scores in the lowest third. The link still held when the researchers accounted for factors like age, blood pressure, smoking habits, and history of heart attacks.

The physiological effects of chronic anxiety—a revved-up nervous system and elevations in stress-related hormones—may help explain the heart risks. If you are suffering from anxiety, ask your doctor about ways to address it, such as relaxation techniques, talk therapy, and medication.

JOURNAL OF THE AMERICAN COLLEGE OF CARDIOLOGY
Volume 49, page 2021
May 22, 2007

Depression
Many studies have linked depression with an elevated risk of CHD. However, the exact mechanism by which depression contributes to CHD is not clear. Some experts believe the explanation may lie with the reduced attention that people with depression may pay to making lifestyle changes—consuming a low-fat diet, becoming more physically active, stopping smoking—or taking medication to lower their blood lipids or blood pressure. Another possibility is that depression has a more direct effect on CHD risk, by increasing blood pressure and blood cholesterol, promoting blood clot formation, and reducing heart rate variability (the normal changes in heart rate that occur throughout the day).

Like many of the other risk factors for CHD, depression is a treatable condition. The available treatments include psychotherapy and antidepressant drugs. Increased physical activity may also help relieve the symptoms of depression.

Diagnosis of Coronary Heart Disease

If your doctor suspects that you have CHD, he or she will conduct a number of exams and tests that could lead to a diagnosis of the disease. The most common tests are an electrocardiogram (ECG), an exercise stress test, and coronary angiography. These tests help your doctor to determine whether blood flow to your heart is impaired and to identify which coronary arteries are affected and to what degree. Your doctor will also conduct a medical history and physical exam and order some blood tests.

Medical History and Physical Exam

Your doctor will ask whether you have experienced any CHD–related symptoms, such as chest pain, shortness of breath, heart palpitations, nausea, indigestion, or dizziness. The doctor may ask what brings on the symptoms, how often they occur, how long they last, and how they are relieved. You will also be asked about any medications you are taking, whether you exercise regularly or smoke, and whether any of your parents or siblings has CHD. Then your doctor will examine you to listen to your heartbeat and measure your blood pressure.

Blood Tests

Your doctor will order a number of blood tests to evaluate your risk factors for CHD. One important test is a lipid profile to measure the amounts of total cholesterol, LDL cholesterol, HDL cholesterol, and triglycerides in your blood. For accurate results, your physician will ask you to fast for several hours before the test. Adults (age 20 and older) should have a lipid profile at least once every five years.

A test to measure C-reactive protein (CRP) in the blood may also be ordered. CRP levels higher than 3 mg/L are associated with an elevated risk of CHD events such as heart attacks.

Electrocardiogram (ECG)

During an ECG, small metal sensors called electrodes are applied to the skin of your chest, arms, and legs to detect and record patterns of electrical signals from your heart while you lie on an examination table. The test is painless and is used to detect insufficient blood flow to the heart. An ECG can also detect abnormal heart rhythms and new heart attacks. In addition, it may indicate areas of heart muscle damaged by previous heart attacks. Last, an ECG can be used to detect thickening of the wall of the left ventricle and defects in the conduction of electrical impulses within the heart.

A normal resting ECG indicates that your heart is receiving enough blood when you are at rest. However, a normal test does not eliminate the possibility of insufficient blood supply during physical activity. For this reason, your doctor may also recommend an exercise stress test (see page 22), which monitors your heart's electrical activity during exercise.

To detect silent coronary heart disease (insufficient blood flow to the heart that does not produce chest pain), your doctor might recommend a Holter monitor (also called an ambulatory ECG) to record your heart's electrical activity over a 24-hour period. Two or more electrodes are placed on your chest and attached to a small, portable recording device that is worn on a belt around your waist. Afterwards, the tape in the recording device is analyzed using a computer program to detect changes in the electrical signals from your heart as you go about your daily activities. An ambulatory ECG is also useful to evaluate people with unexplained fainting or heart palpitations and to determine the effectiveness of antiarrhythmia drugs.

Echocardiography

Your doctor can also take moving pictures of your heart in motion. This involves the use of a probe (a transducer) that emits ultra–high-frequency sound waves. The probe is passed over your chest while you lie on your side on an examination table. The sound waves bounce off the structures of your heart and blood vessels and are

NEW RESEARCH

Nap Your Way to a Longer Life?

An afternoon nap may do your heart good, according to a new study that links siestas to lower odds of dying of coronary heart disease (CHD).

The study followed close to 24,000 Greek adults who had no history of major disease at the outset. Nearly 17,000 said they took a siesta at least occasionally.

Over the next six years, the midday nappers were one third less likely to die of CHD than their non-napping peers. Moreover, the protective effect was stronger among adults who said they regularly took a siesta—defined as at least three times a week, for a minimum of 30 minutes each time—than in those who napped sporadically.

It's possible that siestas aid heart health by offering stress relief. Supporting this idea, the benefits of siestas in this study were most evident among men who were still working and presumably under more daily stress. So if you tend to feel taxed by your daily routine, a short nap might be a good way to wind down and help keep your heart healthy.

ARCHIVES OF INTERNAL MEDICINE
Volume 167, page 296
February 12, 2007

Screening for Heart Disease

The best tests for people without symptoms

By now, everyone is familiar with the cholesterol and blood pressure measurements that doctors use to gauge heart risks. But a number of newer screening methods—from blood tests to noninvasive imaging techniques—are also available to spot heart trouble ahead.

Studies suggest that some of these newer methods can detect "silent" atherosclerosis and predict heart attack risk in people with no symptoms of coronary heart disease (CHD), such as chest pain and shortness of breath. This is important because, too often, people with CHD have no indication of it until they suffer a heart attack or die suddenly of cardiac arrest.

But with a constant stream of news reports on various new "markers" of CHD risk, it's easy to get confused about which tests you should consider. In fact, in many cases, even experts disagree over the appropriate use of newer CHD screening methods. Here's a breakdown of the traditional ways doctors predict your likelihood of heart problems and which additional tests you might—or might not—want to consider.

Traditional Risk Assessment

For years, doctors have used a measure called the Framingham risk score (FRS) to gauge adults' risks of having a heart attack over the next 10 years. The score, which depends on your age, blood pressure, cholesterol levels, and history of smoking, categorizes you as being low risk (less than a 10% chance of having a heart attack in the next 10 years), intermediate risk (10–20% chance) or high risk (greater than 20% chance). An important exception: People with diabetes or CHD are already considered at high risk regardless of other risk factors.

The FRS is a time-honored predictor of heart attack risk, but there is growing evidence of its limitations, particularly for women, whose risk is often underestimated. A recent Hopkins study found that of more than 2,400 women ages 45 and up who were free of heart disease symptoms, one third had signs of atherosclerosis on coronary calcium scans. But the FRS deemed nearly all of them at low risk for a heart attack, which means they probably would not be started on a statin or aspirin therapy to help protect their hearts.

New Ways of Looking at Risk

The limitations of traditional risk factor assessment, coupled with the fact that CHD is often silent, has researchers looking for ways to improve screening. Here are a few of them.

CRP. Blood C-reactive protein (CRP) is one of the newer CHD screening tests. It is a marker of inflammation in the arteries and is thought to play a role in the accumulation of plaques in the coronary arteries.

A number of studies have found CRP levels to predict a person's risk of heart attack. A 2007 publication in the *Journal of the American Medical Association* concluded that adding a CRP test to the traditional FRS measure may improve heart attack prediction for women. Besides CRP, family history of heart disease (having a parent who had a heart attack before age 60) also helped calculate a woman's odds of heart trouble.

In the study, which included nearly 25,000 women ages 45 and older, adding CRP and family history using a measure called the Reynolds Risk score changed the outlook for nearly half of them; some women were found to have a higher-than-thought heart attack risk, while others were actually at lower risk. To calculate your Reynolds Risk score, visit the website www.reynoldsriskscore.org.

In an editorial published with the study, two Hopkins cardiologists called on doctors to quickly add CRP tests and family history to women's CHD risk assessment. Still the Reynolds Risk score is not ideal since, like the FRS, it only predicts risk in the next 10 years, not over a lifetime. This flaw is important, since the life expectancy of a 50-year-old person is now about 30 years—not 10 years.

Many doctors do not recommend routine CRP testing in women—or in men. Most, however, do order the test for people at intermediate risk or when the risk is unclear (for example, lipid levels and blood pressure are normal but the person has a strong family history of heart disease), to better estimate heart attack risk.

Coronary calcium scans. A coronary calcium scan is another potential CHD screening tool, but its use has been controversial because of uncertainty about its value. In late 2006, however, the

American Heart Association (AHA) released long-awaited guidelines on the test, deeming it a reasonable option for symptom-free people at intermediate risk for CHD.

The test uses high-speed x-ray technology—either electron-beam or multidetector computed tomography—to find calcium deposits in the coronary arteries. Because calcium is frequently a component of the plaques that build up in the arteries, a calcium scan can indicate whether you have atherosclerosis, and how severe it is.

In its guidelines, the AHA concluded that enough studies show that the scans can help predict heart trouble above and beyond traditional risk factor measurements—but just for individuals at intermediate risk for CHD. For instance, if you're at intermediate risk (based on your FRS score, for example) and a calcium scan suggests significant plaques in the arteries, you may need to not only change your lifestyle habits but also start taking a statin, a daily aspirin, or possibly blood pressure medication.

Calcium scans are, however, of little use to people at either high or low risk for CHD. If you're high risk, you're automatically started on more aggressive risk factor management, and if you're low risk, you can work on staying that way by combining a healthy diet with regular exercise.

An obstacle to calcium scans is that insurance companies typically do not cover the cost, which is several hundred dollars.

Exercise stress testing. For individuals with possible symptoms of CHD, such as chest pain, an exercise stress test is often the initial diagnostic test. But the test has also been proposed as a way to screen people who are symptom free but at intermediate risk for CHD.

During an exercise stress test, your heart's electrical activity is monitored by an electrocardiogram (ECG) while you walk on a treadmill or pedal a stationary bike. Because it's simple, relatively inexpensive, and noninvasive, exercise testing could be a good way to predict the likelihood of significant CHD.

However, experts, including those from the American College of Cardiology and AHA, do not recommend the procedure for routine screening in most people, primarily because exercise ECGs are not always reliable. For example, they can yield false positives or fail to detect signs of artery narrowing. Research suggests that inaccurate results are more common in women than in men, because of such factors as hormone differences and generally lower muscle mass and fitness levels in women.

In recommendations laid out in 2005, the U.S. Preventive Services Task Force also advised against routine exercise stress tests to screen for CHD. It did say, however, that the test might be useful for screening adults with diabetes who are about to start a vigorous exercise program. The same may be true for men older than age 45 or woman older than age 55 who want to start a vigorous exercise regimen or who may be at risk for CHD because of diseases like peripheral arterial disease or kidney failure.

Homocysteine. This blood amino acid is linked to a higher CHD risk. Researchers suspect high homocysteine levels may contribute to CHD by damaging the lining of the arteries and promoting blood clots. For now, experts advise against widespread screening of homocysteine levels, because it's unclear whether the information adds anything to standard risk factor measurements. In addition, studies evaluating treatments that lower homocysteine (such as supplements of folic acid and other B vitamins) have demonstrated no improvement in CHD risk.

Ask Your Doctor

It's important to remember that even experts disagree over the value of adding these newer screening tests to traditional risk factor assessment, and there's no one-size-fits-all recommendation for any of them.

For instance, if you're already taking a statin or a daily aspirin, a positive result on one of these tests could prompt your doctor to increase the intensity of measures to lower heart attack risk. But there is also a chance that the test will provide no additional information, simply confirming that you are already taking the appropriate steps.

Another scenario: You are not taking a statin or aspirin but are concerned because your cholesterol isn't optimal and your father had a heart attack at age 45. Then it might be worthwhile to have one of these other screening tests to help clarify your risk. The decision will ultimately come down to a thorough discussion of your CHD risk with your doctor. ■

analyzed by a computer to produce images of your heart that your doctor watches on a video screen.

Echocardiography is commonly performed when your doctor wants to assess your heart function, diagnose heart defects, or find the cause of heart murmurs. The test is painless and takes about 15–20 minutes. Echocardiograms are also sometimes performed in combination with the exercise and pharmacologic stress tests described next.

Exercise Stress Test

Your doctor can collect additional information about blood flow to your heart by asking you to undergo a standard exercise stress test. This test uses an ECG to record the electrical signals from your heart during exercise. In people who are at risk for CHD or are having chest pain, an exercise stress test can be used to detect the presence of CHD. The test can help determine whether there are significant blockages in the coronary arteries that are interfering with blood flow during physical activity. It's also done to determine the safety and appropriate level of activity for people beginning an exercise program after a heart attack or bypass surgery, as well as to evaluate the effectiveness of certain treatments (such as those for arrhythmias).

During the stress test, you'll be asked to walk on a treadmill or to pedal a stationary bicycle. The speed and incline of the treadmill or the resistance of the bicycle are gradually increased until you reach your target heart rate. Your target heart rate is usually about 90% of your maximum heart rate; to calculate your maximum heart rate, subtract your age from 220.

The stress test is stopped early if you become fatigued or experience symptoms such as chest pain, shortness of breath, or dizziness; you develop an irregular heartbeat or very high blood pressure; or the ECG shows evidence of poor blood flow to the heart.

A stress test is not always accurate in detecting CHD. In young women and others at low risk for CHD, the test may be abnormal even though no significant CHD is present. Although the test carries a very small risk of a heart attack or cardiac arrest, you'll be carefully monitored and treated immediately if any serious problems occur.

Pharmacologic Stress Test

Some people—often the elderly and the frail—are not able to walk on a treadmill or pedal a bicycle for an exercise stress test. For these individuals, drugs (such as dobutamine) are used to simulate the effects of physical exercise on the heart. While you remain seated or lying down, the exercise-simulating drug is injected into a vein in your arm. Then the electrical signals from your heart are monitored. Similar to a standard exercise stress test, there is a very small risk of having a heart attack or cardiac arrest while undergoing the test. There is also a possibility of side effects from the dobutamine, which can include shortness of breath and nausea.

Nuclear Medicine Stress Test

A nuclear medicine stress test is sometimes performed when a standard exercise stress test shows no clear abnormalities but symptoms of CHD (for example, chest pain) are present. The test may also be used to pinpoint the areas of the heart that are receiving insufficient blood. In addition, it is sometimes done in people who cannot exercise at a high level of intensity or when ECG results during a standard exercise stress test cannot be interpreted because of abnormalities on the resting ECG.

A nuclear medicine stress test is similar to a standard stress test. However, once a certain heart rate is reached (through exercise or medication), a radioactive substance (typically thallium-201) is injected into a vein in your arm. Once injected, the radioactive substance travels through the bloodstream to your heart, where it can be detected with a special camera.

Heart muscle that receives blood from narrowed coronary arteries will have less radioactive material than heart muscle fed by healthy coronary arteries. To determine more precisely whether or why certain areas of the heart are not getting enough blood, your doctor may request a second measurement of the amount of radioactive material in the heart when you are at rest on the same or next day. If blood flow is normal at rest but not during physical activity, you likely have a partial blockage in one or more of the coronary arteries.

A nuclear medicine stress test is more accurate than a standard exercise stress test. It detects CHD in about 20% of people whose resting ECG and standard exercise stress test are normal despite narrowing of the coronary arteries. As with a regular exercise stress test, there is a very small risk of a heart attack or cardiac arrest.

The amount of radioactivity used in a nuclear medicine stress test is similar to that of an x-ray and is not considered dangerous.

Coronary Angiography

Coronary angiography is the gold standard for assessing blockages in the coronary arteries. It is most often performed when a resting ECG or an exercise stress test indicates insufficient blood flow to the heart. Angiography can identify the affected arteries and determine whether angioplasty or bypass surgery is necessary.

During angiography, the doctor inserts a catheter (a small tube) into an artery through a small incision in the groin or arm. Guided by images projected on a video monitor, the doctor threads the catheter into one of the coronary arteries. Contrast material is then injected into the catheter, making it possible to detect abnormalities in the coronary arteries on x-ray film. This test is usually performed in a hospital catheterization laboratory and takes one to two hours.

Angiography is associated with a small risk of allergic reactions, impaired kidney function, infections, and bleeding. It can also cause a heart attack or death, but this risk is about 1 in 1,000 when performed in a nonemergency situation.

Coronary Calcium Scans

Coronary calcium scans are one of the newest ways to evaluate the health of the coronary arteries. Also known as electron beam computed tomography (EBCT) or multidetector computed tomography (MDCT), these tests measure the amount of calcium in the coronary arteries. Calcium is often a component of plaques but is not present in healthy arteries.

A coronary calcium scan is a painless, noninvasive test that takes less than 10 minutes. It uses a rapid CT imaging system that is 20 times faster than a normal CT scan. During the test, you will lie face up on an examination table while x-rays are passed through your body. Calcium in the artery walls appears as whitish spots or streaks on the x-rays. A computer program is then used to calculate a calcium score that reflects the total calcium buildup in the coronary arteries. Scores of 0–10 indicate arteries essentially free of plaque; scores of 11–400 signify mild to moderate plaque buildup; scores above 400 indicate extensive plaque formation.

People with higher calcium scores have a greater risk of heart attack and stroke than people with lower scores. The American Heart Association considers coronary calcium scanning a reasonable option for people who have no symptoms of CHD but are at intermediate risk for the disease. The association says that the test is unnecessary for people at low or high risk, because test results in these individuals would likely not prompt their doctor to reconsider their risk category.

For those at intermediate risk, however, a coronary calcium scan may be helpful in further defining risk and deciding the intensity of measures taken to reduce the risk of CHD and its complications. For example, someone at intermediate risk who has a high calcium score may be at higher risk for CHD than traditional risk factors indicate and may want to begin taking a lipid-lowering medication to further lower LDL cholesterol levels or start taking aspirin to reduce the risk of a heart attack.

Magnetic Resonance Imaging

Another new method to image the heart and its coronary arteries is magnetic resonance imaging (MRI). Cardiac MRI uses powerful magnets and radiofrequency waves, instead of x-rays, to provide detailed images. The technique can allow doctors to examine the size and thickness of the heart's chambers, determine heart function and the extent of damage from a heart attack or CHD, and detect blockages in the coronary arteries.

During the test, you will lie on an examination table that is slid into a long, tube-like MRI machine. You must lie still and may be asked to hold your breath, while the technician takes pictures of your heart. Depending on how many images are needed, the test may take up to an hour. Because of the magnets involved in MRI, some people with pacemakers or implanted defibrillators cannot have the test.

Lifestyle Measures To Prevent and Treat Coronary Heart Disease

The lifestyle choices you make have a significant impact on your risk of CHD and your ability to manage the disease once it develops.

CHD is a progressive illness. Once it develops, CHD can be controlled but not cured. You'll need to adopt a heart-healthy lifestyle, even if your doctor prescribes medication or you undergo angioplasty or bypass surgery to treat blocked arteries. That is because lifestyle changes can help make your medications more effective and the results of angioplasty or bypass surgery more long lasting. Here are the lifestyle measures for the prevention and treatment of CHD.

Quit Smoking

Smoking is a difficult habit to break. In fact, only 5–10% of people successfully quit on their own, without any kind of aid or reinforcement. But do not let these numbers discourage you. There are several options that can significantly increase your chances of quitting, including nicotine replacement therapy, medication, and counseling. By combining all three, you'll increase the likelihood of quitting to about 35%.

ASK THE DOCTOR

Q. *Is it ever too late to quit smoking?*

A. Research keeps showing that the answer is a resounding "no."

In a recent study of more than 200 smokers hospitalized for a heart attack, severe chest pain, or complications from heart failure, those who quit the habit were less likely to be rehospitalized or die over the next two years. The take-home message: A diagnosis of coronary heart disease (CHD) does not mean it's too late to benefit from smoking cessation.

Quitting does take determination. Study participants were most likely to quit if they received "intensive" counseling—meeting with a counselor once a week for at least three months and using a nicotine replacement product or the prescription drug bupropion (Zyban).

Merely cutting back on cigarettes is not enough. One large study found that cutting smoking in half did not lower the risk of premature death from heart disease.

If you're like most people and can't quit cold turkey, ask your doctor for help. Nicotine replacement gums, patches, and sprays and the prescription drugs Zyban and varenicline (Chantix) are considered safe for people with CHD and can increase your odds of quitting. If you need emotional support, your hospital or local chapter of the American Lung Association or American Cancer Society may have a smoking-cessation program you can join.

What's important is that you don't give up on quitting. Different tactics work for different people, and you may need to make several quit attempts before you find the one that works best for you.

Nicotine replacement therapy minimizes the symptoms of nicotine withdrawal and helps control cravings. Many forms of nicotine replacement therapy are available—gum, skin patch, nasal spray, inhaler, and lozenge. Some of these are sold over the counter; others must be prescribed by your doctor. You should start taking nicotine replacement therapy on your quit date and continue taking it for a minimum of eight to 12 weeks.

Two prescription medications—bupropion (Zyban) and varenicline (Chantix)—also help reduce cravings and withdrawal symptoms. Zyban works by disrupting the pleasurable feelings that smoking typically produces in the brain. Chantix acts on nicotine receptors in the brain. Your doctor may recommend that you begin taking Zyban or Chantix a week or two before your intended quit date and to keep taking the medication for two to three months.

Counseling—either in a group or one-on-one with a therapist—can be helpful as well. During counseling, you'll learn coping skills, ways to prevent a relapse, and stress management. You'll also receive social support and encouragement.

The benefits of quitting smoking are clear. A recent study found that even among smokers who'd been hospitalized for a heart attack, angina, or heart failure, quitting the habit lowered the risk of dying or being hospitalized over the next two years (see the "Ask the Doctor" column on page 25).

Don't forget that secondhand smoke also is bad for your heart. If your local government has not yet banned smoking in public places, sit in the nonsmoking section of restaurants and bars. In addition, don't let people smoke in your home or car.

Eat a Healthy Diet

The food you eat is one of your most potent weapons in reducing your risk of CHD or preventing it from getting worse. By adopting a diet that's low in saturated fat and cholesterol and rich in complex carbohydrates like fruits, vegetables, and whole grains, you can improve your heart health and lower your chances of having a heart attack or other CHD event. However, by making less healthy food choices, you'll increase your likelihood of high LDL cholesterol and triglyceride levels, high blood pressure, and obesity.

Dietary fats

In the average American diet, about 35–40% of calories are from fat. But not all of this fat is bad. In fact, some types of fat (such as monounsaturated fat and omega-3 fat) actually have a beneficial effect on blood lipid levels and may lower your risk of developing or dying of CHD. So you need to choose your fats carefully and emphasize those that are heart friendly.

Saturated fat. The most prevalent type of fat in the American diet is saturated fat, which is a major dietary factor in raising total and LDL cholesterol levels in the blood. Saturated fat is present in most animal and dairy foods and in some oils. To lower your intake of saturated fat, limit your consumption of fatty meats (beef, veal, ham, lamb, and pork), full-fat dairy products (whole milk, cream, cheese, and ice cream), and certain vegetable oils and products (coconut oil, palm oil, palm kernel oil, and vegetable shortening).

According to the American Heart Association, you should limit your saturated fat intake to less than 7% of your total calories. This dietary measure will help reduce your blood cholesterol levels—specifically, your LDL cholesterol—and may also help you maintain an ideal weight (fat contains more than twice as many calories per gram as protein or carbohydrates).

At the same time, you should lower your intake of dietary cholesterol to less than 300 mg per day. This means reducing your consumption of cholesterol-rich foods, such as egg yolks and meat (including beef, pork, poultry, and lamb as well as organ meats like liver and brain). Plant foods (fruits, vegetables, legumes, nuts, and cereals) contain no cholesterol.

Monounsaturated fat. When choosing the fats in your diet, select monounsaturated fats over saturated fats whenever possible. Good sources of monounsaturated fat include olive and canola oils, most nuts (for example, almonds, peanuts, and cashews), and avocados. When substituted for saturated fat in the diet, monounsaturated fats not only lower LDL cholesterol levels but also help maintain—and even raise—HDL cholesterol levels.

Polyunsaturated fat. This type of fat is found in safflower, sunflower, and corn oils. It lowers LDL cholesterol but, when consumed in excess, also reduces HDL cholesterol.

A particular type of polyunsaturated fat known as omega-3 fat lowers triglyceride levels. It may also reduce the risk of dying of CHD by preventing life-threatening arrhythmias. Two specific types of omega-3 fats—eicosapentaenoic acid (EPA) and docosahexaenoic acid (DHA)—have these heart-healthy effects. EPA and DHA are found in fatty fish (such as herring, sardines, salmon, and mackerel), fish oil supplements, and a new prescription medication called Lovaza (omega-3-acid ethyl esters; see page 44).

Omega-3 fats are also present in certain plants (soybeans, walnuts,

ASK THE DOCTOR

Q. ***Butter vs. margarine: Which is better for your heart?***

A. Not long ago, the answer to this question seemed obvious. Butter, made from cream and loaded with saturated fat, was to be avoided in favor of margarine, which is made from vegetable oil. Then trans fats came along to confuse the issue.

Trans fats are created when vegetable oils go through a process called hydrogenation, which is how some margarines are created. The problem is that trans fats are even less healthy than saturated fats; they not only raise blood levels of LDL ("bad") cholesterol but also lower HDL ("good") cholesterol.

So what should you be spreading on your morning toast? The answer is margarine, but you need to be selective. All margarines are lower in saturated fat than butter and—unlike butter—contain no cholesterol, but margarines vary in their trans fat content. In general, the harder the margarine, the more trans fats, so choose a tub or liquid spread rather than a stick version. You should also read product labels and buy those margarines that have the lowest total amount of trans fat and saturated fat. This task is getting easier as more manufacturers are producing trans fat–free margarines with less than 0.5 g of the fat per serving.

You might also want to consider a trans fat–free margarine fortified with plant compounds, called stanol and sterol esters, that can help lower your LDL levels. These include brands like Benecol and Take Control.

Resveratrol: The Latest Heart-Healthy Supplement in Mice

But will it work in humans?

Can you have your cake and a healthy heart, too? Some well-publicized research suggests as much about a substance in red wine called resveratrol. The compound, according to studies in animals, may not only improve cardiovascular health, but also offer the body a general "anti-aging" defense that even counters the effects of a high-fat diet and couch-potato lifestyle.

Though the findings come from mice, not men, resveratrol is already widely available as a dietary supplement. Not surprisingly, some companies have recently come out with higher-dose, "improved" versions they claim could mimic the research results in animals. The question is: Should you head to the health food store now?

The Knowns

Resveratrol is a compound produced by certain plants as part of their defense arsenal against pathogens. It's found primarily in the skins of red grapes (and therefore in red wine), although a handful of other foods, including raspberries, blueberries, and peanuts, contain it as well.

Researchers suspect that the resveratrol in red wine might help explain the famous "French paradox," whereby the French enjoy lower rates of heart disease than their American counterparts without forgoing their high-fat croissants and cheeses. In fact, a growing body of lab research suggests that resveratrol has specific effects on cardiovascular health—from fighting inflammation in the blood vessels to enhancing blood vessel dilation and preventing blood clots.

What's more, recent headline-making studies indicate that resveratrol might mimic the health benefits of a long-term very–low-calorie diet. Scientists have long known that a very–low-calorie diet extends the lifespans of species ranging from yeast to mice (although no one knows if the same is true of humans). The theory is that calorie restriction activates certain genes that defend our body cells from injury. And some researchers suspect that resveratrol pushes these same genes into action.

A recent Harvard study, for example, found that resveratrol allows mice to eat whatever they want yet live long, remarkably healthy lives—despite being obese. Another study published on its heels found that megadoses of resveratrol offset the adverse effects of a high-fat diet by protecting mice from developing the metabolic syndrome—a collection of risk factors for diabetes and coronary heart disease (CHD), including abdominal obesity, low HDL cholesterol, elevated blood triglycerides, impaired blood-glucose metabolism, and high blood pressure. Resveratrol also boosted the animals' endurance, allowing them to run farther than the average mouse and maintain a lower resting heart rate, not unlike a trained athlete.

The Unknowns

Just because resveratrol looks like a wonder drug in mice doesn't mean the same holds true for us. Although human studies report associations between red wine and better heart health, they don't prove that resveratrol, or red wine for that matter, is the reason.

In addition, no one knows how much resveratrol might be necessary to achieve health benefits in people. The researchers used doses akin to 750 bottles of red wine a day in the mouse studies. For a 150-lb man or woman, that's three 500-mg capsules of resveratrol a day at a cost of $15.

Like with all dietary supplements, however, resveratrol is not regulated by the U.S. Food and Drug Administration. As a result, you have no guarantee you are getting the ingredients or the amounts of the ingredients listed on the label.

flaxseeds, and canola), but researchers are still investigating whether omega-3s from these sources are also beneficial to the heart.

The American Heart Association recommends eating fish at least twice a week to receive the heart-protective benefits of omega-3 fat. For people with CHD, it advises consuming 1,000 mg of EPA and DHA from fatty fish, fish oil supplements, or a combination of

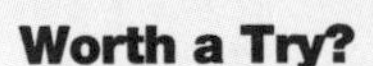

Worth a Try?

The lead Harvard scientist who found resveratrol extended the mouse lifespan publicly admits that he and some of his colleagues take resveratrol supplements. So should you take their lead?

In our opinion it's too early to recommend these supplements, since there's not yet evidence that resveratrol will work in humans like it does in mice. Trials are getting under way to test whether resveratrol improves blood glucose levels, lowers cholesterol, and otherwise fights the common diseases of aging, including CHD. Still, it will be many years before researchers can establish the safety and efficacy of resveratrol in humans. So we advise that you hold off on resveratrol until then.

If you're still tempted to try resveratrol supplements, it's essential that you talk to your doctor first. As with any supplement, resveratrol could interact with medications you're already taking. For example, experiments show that resveratrol can inhibit blood clotting, which could raise your risk of bleeding if you're taking aspirin or another blood-thinning medication.

A last word of caution: Always remember that the word "natural" on a label does not equal "safe," and seemingly benign supplements can be dangerous to your health. ■

The Skinny on Other Heart Supplements

Resveratrol is not the only supplement touted as beneficial for the heart. Here are some other supplements and the research to support or refute them. Always talk to your physician before trying a supplement.

Coenzyme Q10 (CoQ10). The body produces this substance to maintain normal cell function. Some researchers report that CoQ10 supplements lower blood pressure and, in people with heart failure, improve blood vessel function and exercise capacity. However, the body of research on CoQ10 is mixed, and in 2005 an expert panel of the American College of Cardiology concluded that there's insufficient evidence to recommend the supplement.

Policosanol. Although this sugarcane extract is a popular "natural" alternative to statins, several recent studies report it ineffective at lowering cholesterol. One study of 143 adults found that policosanol, even at the highest doses, failed to lower LDL ("bad") cholesterol.

L-arginine. This amino acid helps blood vessels to dilate, and some research suggests that supplements of L-arginine may improve blood flow to the heart. However, a recent Hopkins study showed that L-arginine did nothing to improve heart function or artery stiffness in people who'd suffered a heart attack. In fact, the researchers found that L-arginine might actually raise the risk of death.

Garlic. Garlic has won a reputation as a heart-healthy herb, but research has yielded mixed results. One of the more recent studies, of 90 smokers, found that three months of taking garlic powder supplements did not change participants' levels of cholesterol or several blood proteins that signal inflammation in the arteries.

Fish oil. There's ample evidence that the omega-3 fats found in fish may aid the heart. In fact, the American Heart Association recommends that people with CHD regularly eat fatty fish like salmon, tuna, and mackerel or take fish oil supplements to get the omega-3 fats EPA and DHA. These supplements can also help lower triglyceride levels. But because fish oil supplements can increase the risk of bleeding, take them only under your doctor's supervision.

both. Always check with your doctor before starting to take fish oil supplements.

Trans fat. This type of fat has gained considerable attention in recent years—all of it negative (see the "New Research" column on page 30). Trans fats are found in stick margarines and other prepared foods made with hydrogenated or partially hydrogenated oils. These hydrogenated oils are produced by the food industry when liquid oils are converted into fats that are solid at room temperature and thus more shelf stable.

Studies show that trans fats may be more harmful than saturated fat. They not only raise LDL cholesterol but also lower HDL cholesterol. The American Heart Association recommends that you limit your intake of trans fat to less than 1% of total calories. Be aware that even products labeled "trans fat free" can contain a small amount—0.5 g of trans fat per serving. To truly know how much trans fat you're eating, read ingredient labels: If a product contains partially hydrogenated oil, hydrogenated oil, or shortening, there is some trans fat.

Complex carbohydrates and dietary fiber

There are two types of carbohydrates: simple and complex. While simple carbohydrates are sugars and should be eaten only in small amounts, complex carbohydrates can have a positive effect on your heart. Complex carbohydrates found in vegetables, fruits, and grains help lower blood pressure and total and LDL cholesterol levels.

Foods rich in complex carbohydrates tend to be low in fat and high in fiber, including soluble fiber, which also reduces LDL cholesterol levels. You should try to consume at least 25–30 g of dietary fiber each day. Foods containing soluble fiber (for example, oats, oat bran, barley, legumes, prunes, apples, carrots, and grapefruit) should be included in your diet regularly. Insoluble fiber has also been linked to a lower risk of CHD. It is found in whole grains (like whole wheat, barley, brown rice, and quinoa), seeds, and many vegetables.

As much as possible, you should consume fiber from foods, because high-fiber foods also contain a variety of nutrients. But if you find it difficult to get enough fiber from your diet, regular use of products that contain soluble fiber from psyllium seeds (such as Metamucil) can lower total cholesterol levels by 5–10%. The fiber in psyllium can cause temporary bloating or flatulence, so do not exceed the dose recommended on the label.

It is unclear how soluble fiber reduces cholesterol levels. One theory is that it prevents the intestines from reabsorbing bile acids (substances produced in the liver from cholesterol). When bile acids are not reabsorbed, the liver ends up converting more cholesterol into bile acids, which in turn lowers overall blood cholesterol levels.

Dietary sodium and potassium

Decreasing sodium and increasing potassium intakes can help control your blood pressure levels and lower your likelihood of both

NEW RESEARCH

More Evidence Against Trans Fats

A large study confirms that the trans fats found in some of your favorite snack foods are a threat to your heart health.

Among nearly 33,000 U.S. women in the Nurses Health Study, those with the highest levels of trans fatty acids in their circulating red blood cells were three times more likely to develop coronary heart disease (CHD) over the next six years than those with the lowest levels. The link remained when age, overall diet, and other lifestyle factors were weighed—suggesting that the trans fats themselves contributed to CHD development.

Trans fats are formed when food manufacturers add hydrogen to vegetable oil to make it more solid. Americans get much of their trans fat from the partially hydrogenated oils found in cookies, crackers, pastries, and fried foods. Among dietary fats, trans fats are uniquely hard on the heart, as they raise "bad" LDL cholesterol while lowering "good" HDL cholesterol.

This study bolsters the case against trans fats. Instead of simply relying on reported diet habits, it measured trans fat levels in participants' blood—a more accurate indicator of the intake of trans fat, which the body cannot synthesize.

The bottom line: Instead of processed snack foods, reach for whole foods, like fruits, vegetables, and whole grains. And when it comes to fat, choose the healthy forms found in fish, nuts, and olive oil.

CIRCULATION
Volume 115, page 1858
April 10, 2007

CHD and heart attacks (see the "New Research" column at right).

Sodium. This mineral is essential for life, but most people consume too much. The typical daily intake is 3,000–5,000 mg, yet your body needs only about 200 mg of sodium a day. By cutting back on sodium, you can lower your systolic blood pressure by an average of 2–5 mm Hg and your diastolic blood pressure by 1–3 mm Hg. The benefits of sodium restriction appear to be greatest in older people and in those with high blood pressure.

The American Heart Association recommends that people consume no more than 2,300 mg of sodium a day, which is equivalent to slightly more than 1 tsp of table salt daily. If you have high blood pressure, you should aim for less than 1,500 mg of sodium a day.

One strategy for lowering sodium intake is adding less or no salt to foods during cooking or at the table. Table salt is made up of 40% sodium. However, sodium also occurs naturally in many foods and is used extensively in food processing. For example, cold cuts, canned vegetables, canned soups, cheeses, and many snack foods are all concentrated sources of sodium. Check nutrition labels for the amount of sodium in the foods you buy and eat, and choose low- or no-salt versions of packaged or processed foods whenever possible.

Potassium. A number of studies show that a low potassium intake raises blood pressure, while a high potassium intake lowers blood pressure. You can add more potassium to your diet by increasing your consumption of fresh fruits and vegetables, which are also low in sodium and rich in dietary fiber and antioxidants. Citrus fruits and bananas are particularly good sources of potassium, as are avocados, apricots, potatoes, sardines, and spinach.

The American Heart Association recommends that you consume at least 4.7 g of potassium a day, though this amount may need to be lower if you have kidney dysfunction or severe heart failure. Potassium supplements are not recommended to reach this goal (unless prescribed by your doctor) and may be dangerous for some people with high blood pressure, particularly those who are taking a potassium-sparing diuretic such as spironolactone (Aldactone) or triamterene (Dyrenium).

Stanols and sterols

About a decade ago, the U.S. Food and Drug Administration (FDA) approved the use of cholesterol-lowering food additives called stanols and sterols. Since then, food manufacturers have added stanols and sterols to a wide variety of foods—margarine, orange juice, yogurt, and granola bars, to name just a few.

NEW RESEARCH

More Reason To Go Easy on the Salt Shaker

You know cutting back on salt is good for your blood pressure, but now there's evidence it also prevents heart attacks and deaths from heart disease.

In a multicenter U.S. study that followed more than 3,100 adults with prehypertension, those who cut their sodium intake were 25% less likely to suffer a cardiovascular event (heart attack, stroke, or need for angioplasty or bypass surgery) or die of cardiovascular disease than those who stuck with their regular, often salt-laden, diets.

The findings come from two clinical trials that involved men and women 30–54 years old with high-normal blood pressure. Participants were randomly assigned to either follow their usual diets or learn how to cut salt from their meals; those in the latter group lowered their sodium intake by 25–35%. During the five-year follow-up period, beginning 10–15 years after the trials ended, the salt reducers had fewer heart attacks, strokes, and heart procedures as well as a lower death rate.

These new findings show that the benefits of salt reduction extend beyond lowered blood pressure. So it's even more important to follow experts' advice on sodium: no more than 2,300 mg per day and less than 1,500 mg if you have high blood pressure. Since processed foods are a major sodium source, always read product labels and opt for low-sodium versions whenever possible.

BMJ
Volume 334, page 885
April 28, 2007

Stanols and sterols have a similar structure to cholesterol and thus compete with dietary cholesterol for absorption in the small intestine. As a result, these substances prevent the absorption of some dietary cholesterol in the small intestine.

Studies show that stanol- and sterol-fortified foods reduce LDL cholesterol levels by up to 14% when used regularly in combination with a low-saturated fat, low-cholesterol diet. However, stanols and sterols appear to have no beneficial effect on HDL cholesterol or triglyceride levels. Keep in mind, however, that stanol- and sterol-fortified foods contain calories and thus can cause weight gain when consumed in large quantities. Because they are natural substances, no known side effects are associated with their use.

Soy

Consuming foods rich in soy may help lower your LDL cholesterol level but not for the reason experts once believed. Until recently, researchers thought that estrogen-like compounds called isoflavones were responsible for the beneficial effect of soy on cholesterol levels. But the effect appears to be much less direct: People who consume soy products tend to eat them instead of foods such as meat and dairy that are high in saturated fat and cholesterol. Foods rich in soy include tofu and soymilk.

Antioxidants

Numerous studies show that people who eat a diet rich in fruits and vegetables have a reduced risk of CHD. Some researchers attribute this benefit to antioxidants, substances that are plentiful in fruits and vegetables and help neutralize chemicals called free radicals. These free radicals are natural byproducts of metabolism. But free radicals are also cell-damaging compounds that can lead to CHD, likely by contributing to the development of atherosclerosis.

The most common antioxidants in the diet are vitamin C, vitamin E, and beta-carotene (which is converted to vitamin A in your body). In some studies that measured blood levels of these antioxidants, high levels were associated with a reduced risk of CHD. Researchers had hoped that supplements of these vitamins would slow the development of atherosclerosis in the coronary arteries by preventing LDL oxidation (a process believed to be key in the buildup of plaques in the arteries).

However, large trials that randomly assigned participants to antioxidant therapy or a placebo reported no cardiovascular benefits from taking the supplements. In fact, some studies have found that

NEW RESEARCH

Flavonoid-Rich Foods May Lower Heart Disease Death Risk

Eating foods rich in plant compounds called flavonoids may help lower a woman's risk of dying of heart disease, a study suggests.

The study, which followed nearly 35,000 postmenopausal women in Iowa for 16 years, found that those who reported the highest intakes of flavonoid-rich foods were less likely to die of coronary heart disease during the study, even when a host of other factors—including weight, exercise habits, smoking, and blood pressure—were taken into account. Flavonoid-containing foods that seemed the most beneficial were bran, apples, pears, grapefruit, red wine, strawberries, and dark chocolate.

Flavonoid intake was not associated with a reduced risk of stroke, however.

Flavonoids are a group of antioxidants found in various plant foods, including many fruits and vegetables, tea, nuts, and seeds. Flavonoids may interfere with the oxidation of "bad" LDL cholesterol, a process thought to contribute to the buildup of artery-clogging plaques. They may also inhibit blood clot formation and maintain healthy artery function.

The message here is that you should strive to eat a variety of plant-based foods every day to ensure that you're getting the gamut of flavonoids as well as the vitamins, minerals, and fiber contained in these foods.

AMERICAN JOURNAL OF CLINICAL NUTRITION
Volume 85, page 895
March 2007

high doses of these antioxidant supplements may be harmful to the heart, increasing the risk of heart failure and premature death.

Thus, the American Heart Association does not recommend taking supplements of vitamin C, vitamin E, or beta-carotene to reduce the risk of CHD and its complications. However, you should still get plenty of antioxidants from the food you eat. Fruits and vegetables are excellent sources of antioxidants.

One final note about antioxidants: Moderate alcohol consumption is associated with a decline in the risk of CHD, possibly because alcohol increases HDL cholesterol levels. Although some researchers believe that antioxidants found in red wine and dark grapes may be the reason for these alcohol-related improvements in HDL levels, all types of alcoholic drinks are equally effective in raising HDL cholesterol and lowering the risk of CHD. But moderation is the key: Men should drink no more than two drinks a day, and women no more than one drink a day. Drinking more than this amount is associated with a greater risk of CHD—as well as a higher risk of liver disease and accidents.

Increase Physical Activity

Regular exercise has many advantages. It helps control body weight, raises levels of HDL cholesterol, reduces blood pressure, and relieves stress. Exercise also makes your heart more efficient in pumping blood and enhances your body's responsiveness to insulin, which reduces the risk of type 2 diabetes. Exercise can also lower your risk of osteoporosis and possibly even dementia.

You might think that you must engage in strenuous physical activity for exercise to have any benefit, but this isn't the case. For example, brisk walking can be a healthy form of exercise when performed regularly. If you're ready to start an exercise program, walking is one of your best choices; it does not require any special equipment and is associated with a lower risk of injury than jogging and other high-impact activities.

The recommendations. The Centers for Disease Control and Prevention and the American College of Sports Medicine recommend that adults get 30 minutes or more of physical activity on most, and preferably all, days of the week. This activity should be performed at a moderate intensity—equivalent to walking at a pace of three to four miles per hour.

If exercising for 30 minutes sounds daunting, you don't need to do it all at one time. Short bursts of activity for 8–10 minutes, three times a day, are enough to reduce the risk of CHD, as long as the

NEW RESEARCH

Pumping Iron for Your Heart

A light workout with weights is not only safe if you have coronary heart disease (CHD) but should be part of your regular exercise routine, according to new recommendations from the American Heart Association (AHA).

Though strength training was once considered ill advised for people with CHD, recent research has changed that thinking. By building your muscle mass and strength, light weight training enhances the heart benefits of aerobic exercises like walking. Greater muscle mass also boosts your metabolism, which aids in weight control. And increased strength makes daily tasks, like carrying groceries, a little easier.

According to the AHA, you should strive to do strength training two or three days each week, aiming to strengthen the major muscles of your upper and lower body—chest, shoulders, triceps, biceps, upper and lower back, abdominals, quadriceps, hamstrings, and calves. But you should forgo any idea of becoming a bodybuilder: Use only light weights and lift slowly, never straining or holding your breath. Also, limit yourself to only one set of 10–15 repetitions for each exercise.

As always, talk to your doctor before launching a new exercise regimen. Strength training is not for everyone, including those with uncontrolled blood pressure above 180/110 mm Hg and those with unstable angina, severe heart failure, or uncontrolled arrhythmias.

CIRCULATION
Volume 116, page 572
July 31, 2007

The Benefits of Incidental Activity

Even everyday moves count as exercise

You know you're supposed to exercise. But the idea of joining a gym, signing up for a yoga class, or investing in a treadmill may seem not quite you. Luckily, all is not lost. Recent studies are broadening the definition of exercise, and it need not involve gym equipment, a running track, or workout clothes.

Indeed, we burn calories simply by standing instead of sitting, walking around instead of standing, and even fidgeting instead of being still. Simply put, the mundane, incidental activities of daily life—doing laundry, pulling weeds, carrying groceries—count as exercise.

Unfortunately, desk jobs, suburban living, and modern conveniences are chipping away at the physical activity that was once an integral part of daily life. And some experts believe this is contributing to the growing problems of obesity and the health consequences that often come with it—including coronary heart disease.

Benefits of Everyday Moves

For those of us who manage to keep moving throughout the day, research suggests that the rewards may include not only a trimmer middle but also a longer life, lower blood pressure, improved cholesterol levels, and a reduced risk of heart attack.

A longer life. In one recent study, researchers at the National Institute on Aging found that older adults who burned the most calories through everyday activities lived the longest. All of the study participants were 70 years of age or older and in similarly good health at the beginning of the six-year study.

The researchers found no differences in the levels of formal exercise between the high calorie-burners and the lower ones. Instead, the longer-lived group expended more calories through incidental exercise like climbing stairs, doing housework, and grocery shopping.

Better blood-pressure and cholesterol control. The National Institute on Aging study did not examine the reasons for the longevity benefit. But preliminary research suggests that daily activities might help lower blood pressure and improve blood cholesterol levels, both of which can reduce the likelihood of heart attack and stroke.

For example, one small study of adults with high blood pressure found that participants' systolic blood pressure (the top number in a reading) dropped by several points after they added incidental activity to their daily routines—including raking leaves, gardening, or walking around the neighborhood. Another recent study reported that four short walks, spaced out throughout the day, might be more effective at lowering blood pressure than one 40-minute walk—at least among people with borderline-high blood pressure.

When it comes to cholesterol, a small study from England reported that women who walked up stairs, six times a day for two minutes at a time, lowered their total cholesterol level from an average of 190 mg/dL to 175 mg/dL and increased their average high-density lipoprotein (HDL) cholesterol level from 48 mg/dL to 57 mg/dL. Cholesterol levels did not change in the women who shunned the stairs.

Reduced heart attack risk. Researchers have also examined whether incidental activity can decrease your risk of a heart attack.

In a recent study of more than 41,000 people from Finland, walking or cycling to and from work was associated with a reduced heart-attack risk in the subsequent 10 years in women—but not in men. However, high levels of either leisure-time or work-related physical activity were associated with about a

activity is performed at moderate intensity. Examples of such moderate-intensity activities include walking up stairs, walking short distances instead of driving, and doing calisthenics or pedaling a stationary bicycle while watching television. Gardening, housework, dancing, and playing with your grandchildren also count as part of

40% reduced heart attack risk in both men and women.

A leaner physique. Still other research reports that a "fidgety" nature may help separate the heavy from the lean. In a well-publicized study published in the journal *Science*, researchers found that normal-weight adults typically moved around much more throughout the day than did their obese peers—even though all of the study participants were self-professed couch potatoes who avoided formal exercise.

But it wasn't just a matter of heavier people having a harder time moving around. Even after the researchers put the obese adults on a diet that helped them lose weight, they were no more likely to get moving.

This suggests, according to the researchers, that some of us are programmed to be restless and fidgety, while some are made to be still—and, more important, that it makes a difference in our weight over time.

Being an Everyday Mover

So how does a seemingly natural-born sitter overcome this tendency? Since most of us are unlikely to hop straight from the couch to the gym, focusing on incidental activity may be the ideal way to make exercise a part of your life and an important part of your heart-disease management plan.

Think about the ways that your environment—where you live, where you work, how you travel—keeps you from moving, and then make changes. No matter how small each individual change may seem, they do add up. To get you started, here are some small changes you can make today.

On the road. You can incorporate incidental activity into your daily travels.

- Become less reliant on your car. This can be a challenge in the suburbs, where some neighborhoods don't have sidewalks. But whenever possible, walk or bike to the store or to work.
- If public transportation is an option, take it. That walk to the bus stop or train certainly counts as exercise.
- Even if you have to drive everywhere, try parking farther from your destination.

At work. Your office offers a number of opportunities for incidental activity.

- Don't eat at your desk. Instead, take your lunch to the park or some other destination that forces you to walk or climb stairs.
- Don't e-mail or call a colleague when you can walk to his or her desk instead.
- Stand or fidget (discreetly) at meetings. Try swinging your legs under the table or tapping your toes.

At home. This is one of the best places to incorporate incidental activity into your daily life.

- Many household chores are a great form of moderate exercise. Mop the floor, scrub the bathtub, or dust the living room.
- Wash your car by hand instead of going to the car wash.
- When carrying groceries from the car, take one bag at a time so you make extra trips. Similarly, when putting laundry on the line to dry, carry one article at a time.
- Try to use old-fashioned chore tools. Water your lawn with a hose instead of using a sprinkler. Reach for a broom or a rake instead of a leaf blower. Be careful, however, about heavier duties like shoveling snow or lifting large loads of leaves. These activities are akin to a workout at the gym, and people with heart disease should consult with their physician before performing these physically stressful activities.
- Take advantage of your cordless phone, and walk around while you talk.
- Hide your remote control, so you have to get up to change the channel. ■

the 30-minute total—if they are performed at an intensity that corresponds to brisk walking. If you engage in lower-intensity activities, they should be performed more often and for longer periods of time. For tips on increasing your day-to-day activity levels, see "The Benefits of Incidental Activity" on this page.

A number of other exercise recommendations have come out in the past couple of years. For example, the U.S. government's Dietary Guidelines for Americans released in 2005 recommends 60–90 minutes of moderate to vigorous activity on most days of the week to help prevent weight gain and achieve and maintain weight loss. If you can comfortably exercise for 30 minutes on most days, you might want to try to gradually increase your exercise time to 60 minutes.

If you already have CHD or other chronic health problems or if you are middle-aged or older and have been sedentary for a while, ask your doctor about how to safely begin an exercise routine.

Control Your Weight

If you combine a reduced-calorie, low-fat diet with regular physical activity, you have an excellent chance of losing weight and maintaining that weight loss over the long term. When it comes to your heart, weight loss is the most effective way to lower triglyceride levels and raise HDL cholesterol. In addition, weight loss is an important way to prevent and treat type 2 diabetes and to lower blood pressure.

To lose weight, you need to expend more calories than you consume. A healthy weight loss is 0.5–2 lbs a week. To achieve this goal, you need to eat 250–1,000 fewer calories a day. But if you increase your level of physical activity, this calorie restriction does not need to be as drastic.

Reduce Stress

Virtually everyone feels stress from time to time, whether they're caught in a traffic jam or anxious about a pressing deadline. People can cope effectively with stress in a variety of ways. Regular aerobic exercise—even a daily walk after dinner—can ease stress, as can a supportive network of family and friends. Relaxation techniques such as yoga, tai chi, and meditation can be useful as well. In addition, some people benefit from behavior modification techniques, such as biofeedback, anxiety management training, and stress inoculation therapy, which can be learned from a mental health professional.

Medications To Prevent and Treat Coronary Heart Disease

For some people, lifestyle changes are all that are needed to control risk factors for CHD. However, when these measures don't produce the desired results, medications can be added. Drugs can not only control blood lipid levels but also help lower blood pressure as well as decrease the risk of blood clots and episodes of angina. Remember that continuing your lifestyle changes will help make these medications more effective and may allow you to take a lower dose, reducing your likelihood of experiencing side effects.

Lipid-Lowering Medications

When it comes to managing your blood lipid levels, you and your doctor have many drugs to choose from. Before prescribing any of these medications, however, your doctor may first recommend trying lifestyle measures for three months to see if these changes can sufficiently lower blood cholesterol and triglycerides. If lifestyle measures do not produce the desired effects, your doctor will choose one or more medications from the following six classes of lipid-lowering drugs: statins, bile acid sequestrants, cholesterol absorption inhibitors, niacin, fibrates, and omega-3-acid ethyl esters.

Statins

Statins are the most effective drugs for lowering total and LDL cholesterol levels. They produce a 25–55% reduction in LDL cholesterol, a 5–15% increase in HDL cholesterol, and a 10–25% reduction in triglycerides. These drugs block the action of an enzyme that is required for the liver to manufacture cholesterol. As a result, the liver makes less cholesterol and more LDL receptors. These receptors help remove LDL from the blood.

The statins include atorvastatin (Lipitor), fluvastatin (Lescol), lovastatin (Mevacor), pravastatin (Pravachol), rosuvastatin (Crestor), and simvastatin (Zocor). Your doctor will consider a number of factors when selecting a statin drug for you, including your risk of a heart attack; the drug's side effects, costs, and interactions with other medications; and the time of day that the drug should be taken.

Some doctors prescribe a statin in combination with another lipid-lowering drug that works to lower cholesterol in a different way than statins—for example, a statin plus gemfibrozil (Lopid) or niacin (Niacor, Niaspan). Some of these combinations are available in a single pill: lovastatin plus Niaspan (brand name: Advicor) and simvastatin plus Zetia (brand name: Vytorin). In addition, Lipitor is available with the blood pressure drug amlodipine (Norvasc) in a formulation called Caduet; it's prescribed for people with elevated cholesterol who have high blood pressure or angina. These drug cocktails may be more effective than a single medication.

Statins have benefits other than their effects on blood lipids. For

NEW RESEARCH

High-Dose Statin May Benefit Elderly People, Too

A clinical trial suggests that aggressive cholesterol lowering with a high-dose statin may prevent more heart attacks and deaths than lower-dose therapy in older adults with coronary heart disease (CHD)—just like it does in relatively younger patients.

In the trial, high-dose atorvastatin (Lipitor; 80 mg a day) was compared with moderate-dose pravastatin (Pravachol; 40 mg a day) among 893 adults ages 65–85 with CHD.

Over a one-year period, participants randomly assigned to receive high-dose Lipitor had a greater drop in "bad" LDL cholesterol than the moderate-dose Pravachol group. The high-dose group also had a lower rate of major complications like heart attacks and hospitalization for severe chest pain—although this difference was not statistically significant, meaning it could have been a chance finding.

There was, however, a meaningful difference in the death rates between the two groups. Those on high-dose Lipitor were 77% less likely to die of any cause.

If you're on a statin and following a heart-healthy lifestyle but still have less-than-optimal LDL cholesterol levels, consider talking with your doctor about a higher dose or adding a second cholesterol-lowering drug that acts via a different mechanism, such as ezetimibe (Zetia) or colesevelam (Welchol).

CIRCULATION
Volume 115, page 700
February 13, 2007

example, they appear to improve the function of the endothelium (the cells lining the artery walls). Specifically, they help arteries regain some of their ability to widen and thus permit increased blood flow during exercise. Statins also reduce the risk of plaque rupture by decreasing inflammation within the walls of arteries. In fact, people who take statins can reduce their blood levels of C-reactive protein (CRP), a marker of inflammation in the body. All of these beneficial effects mean that taking a statin lowers your risk of a heart attack, of having to undergo angioplasty or bypass surgery, and of dying of CHD. Taking a statin also decreases your risk of a stroke.

Side effects of statins are uncommon, occurring in only 1–2% of people. The most frequent side effect is muscle aches, although other side effects can occur, including bloating, gas, heartburn, nausea, allergic reactions, stomach pain, and increases in liver enzymes. In rare cases, the kidneys can become damaged by severe muscle inflammation. Call your doctor immediately if you experience unusual or unexplained muscle aches while taking a statin.

Bile acid sequestrants

These cholesterol-lowering medications—which include cholestyramine (Questran), colesevelam (Welchol), and colestipol (Colestid)—are safe and effective for reducing total and LDL cholesterol levels. They are often taken alone but are more effective in combination with a statin or niacin. In a number of studies, such combinations have slowed the progression—and sometimes even caused the shrinkage—of plaques. There's a potential negative effect, however: Bile acid sequestrants can moderately raise triglyceride levels.

Bile acid sequestrants are available in powder or pill form. These drugs work by binding bile acids in the intestine and eliminating them in your stool. Bile acids are made in the liver from cholesterol and are released from the gallbladder into the intestine during meals. Normally, bile acids are reabsorbed from the intestine and returned to the liver for reprocessing. But when bile acid sequestrants remove bile acids from the body, the liver must make more. The liver does this by removing more LDL particles from the blood and using the cholesterol in these particles to make new bile acids.

Common side effects of bile acid sequestrants include constipation, upset stomach, and gas. Although intestinal obstruction is a rare side effect, you should stop taking the medication and contact your doctor if you experience severe abdominal pain. Taking a bile acid sequestrant at the proper times is important to avoid interfering with the absorption of folic acid and certain drugs.

Cholesterol absorption inhibitors

Cholesterol absorption inhibitors work by blocking the absorption of cholesterol from the small intestine. This includes cholesterol from your diet as well as cholesterol in bile acids.

Ezetimibe (Zetia) is the only drug approved in this class. Studies show that Zetia lowers total cholesterol and LDL cholesterol by about 15–25%. The combination of Zetia and a statin reduces LDL cholesterol even more. A pill containing both simvastatin and Zetia (brand name: Vytorin) is available and can lower LDL cholesterol levels by up to 60%.

The side effects of Zetia are infrequent but include dizziness, headache, diarrhea, and back pain.

Niacin

Large doses of this B vitamin (also called nicotinic acid) are the most effective medication for raising HDL cholesterol levels. Niacin raises HDL cholesterol by 15–30%. It also can lower triglyceride levels by 20–30% and reduce LDL cholesterol by 10–20%.

Niacin lowers triglycerides by decreasing the production of VLDL in the liver. VLDL is the major carrier of triglycerides in the blood.

The major drawback of niacin is frequent side effects such as skin flushing and itching. These side effects, while uncomfortable, are not dangerous and tend to lessen with time. More serious (and less common) side effects include liver damage, peptic ulcers (ulcers in the stomach or upper intestine), gout, and a rise in blood glucose levels. You should not take niacin if you have a history of peptic ulcers or if you have liver disease or gout. If you have diabetes or prediabetes, you should take no more than 2 g of niacin a day.

Two prescription forms of niacin are commonly prescribed: immediate release (Niacor) and extended release (Niaspan). Niaspan is used more often because it is associated with less flushing and needs to be taken only once a day. Even though some niacin preparations are available without a prescription, all preparations should be used only under a doctor's supervision.

Fibrates

The fibrates—gemfibrozil (Lopid) and fenofibrate (Lofibra, Tricor, Triglide)—are the lipid-lowering medication of choice for people with extremely elevated blood triglyceride levels (500 mg/dL or more). Fibrates stimulate the activity of an enzyme called lipoprotein lipase that breaks down triglycerides.

Although fibrates decrease triglyceride levels, they can cause total

Drugs for Lowering Lipid Levels 2008

Drug type: Brand (generic)	Typical daily dosages*	How to take†	Monthly cost‡: Brand (generic)
Statins			
Crestor (rosuvastatin)	5–40 mg	One 5-, 10-, 20-, or 40-mg tablet 1x/day at any time with or without food.	$95–98
Lescol (fluvastatin)	20–80 mg	One 20- or 40-mg capsule 1x/day in the evening or one 40-mg capsule 2x/day in the morning and evening with or without food. Swallow whole (do not open capsule).	$75–162
Lescol XL (fluvastatin, extended-release)	80 mg	One 80-mg tablet 1x/day with or without food, preferably in the evening. Swallow whole (do not break, crush, or chew).	$95
Lipitor (atorvastatin)	10–80 mg	One 10-, 20-, 40-, or 80-mg tablet 1x/day at any time with or without food.	$82–111
Mevacor (lovastatin)	10–80 mg	One 10-, 20-, or 40-mg tablet 1x/day with dinner or one 40-mg tablet 2x/day with breakfast and dinner.	$41–246 ($23–70)
Pravachol (pravastatin)	10–80 mg	One 10-, 20-, 40-, or 80-mg tablet 1x/day with or without food, preferably in the evening.	$93–162 ($18–133)
Zocor (simvastatin)	5–80 mg	One 5-, 10-, 20-, 40-, or 80-mg tablet 1x/day in the evening with or without food.	$64–147 ($28–50)
Cholesterol absorption inhibitor			
Zetia (ezetimibe)	10 mg	One 10-mg tablet 1x/day with or without food.	$93
Bile acid sequestrants			
Colestid (colestipol)	*Pill:* 2–16 g *Powder:* 5–30 g	*Pill:* Two or more 1-g tablets 1–2x/day. Swallow each tablet whole (do not crush or chew) one at a time with a full glass of water. *Powder:* One or more packets or level scoopfuls (each packet or level scoopful contains 5 g colestipol) mixed with 3 oz or more of liquid 1–2x/day.	*Pill:* $41–311 *Powder:* $34–362
Questran, Questran Light (cholestyramine)	8–24 g	One to three packets or level scoopfuls (each packet or level scoopful contains 4 g of cholestyramine) mixed with 2–6 oz of liquid 2x/day before meals.	$65–631 ($23–236)
Welchol (colesevelam)	3.75–4.375 g	Six or seven 625-mg tablets 1x/day with a meal and a large glass of liquid or three 625-mg tablets 2x/day with meals and a large glass of liquid.	$182–213

Precautions	Most common side effects	Call your doctor if...
Because statins may cause liver damage, your doctor may perform blood tests to measure liver function before you start a statin and periodically while you are on it. If you take the bile acid sequestrants Colestid or Questran, take your statin at least 1 hour before or 4 hours afterward. If you consume large quantities of grapefruit or grapefruit juice, wait at least 4 hours before taking a statin; these foods can increase the amount of some statins in your blood.	Muscle aches.	You experience unexplained muscle pain, tenderness, or weakness, fever, dark urine, nausea, vomiting.
If you're taking the bile acid sequestrants Colestid or Questran, take Zetia 2 hours before or 4 hours afterward. Don't take with a statin if you have liver problems.	Dizziness, headache, diarrhea, back pain.	You are also taking a statin and experience muscle pain, tenderness, or weakness, fever, dark urine, nausea, vomiting.
To prevent constipation, drink plenty of fluids throughout the day and increase your fiber intake or ask your doctor if you can take a fiber supplement or a stool softener. *Colestid and Questran only:* Take other medications at least 1 hour before or 4 hours afterward, because these bile acid sequestrants can interfere with the absorption of other medications. Can discolor your teeth and promote tooth decay if the mixture is not swallowed quickly.	Constipation, upset stomach, gas.	Constipation persists or worsens. You experience severe abdominal pain.

* These dosages represent the usual daily dosages for the treatment of abnormal lipid levels. The precise effective dosage varies from person to person and depends on many factors. Do not make any changes to your medication without consulting your doctor.

† These instructions represent the typical way to take the medication. Your doctor's instructions may differ. Always follow your doctor's recommendations.

‡ Prices per drugstore.com.

continued on the next page

Drugs for Lowering Lipid Levels 2008 (continued)

Drug type: Brand (generic)	Typical daily dosages*	How to take†	Monthly cost‡: Brand (generic)
Fibrates			
Lofibra, Tricor, Triglide (fenofibrate)	*Lofibra:* 67–200 mg	*Lofibra:* One 67-, 134-, or 200-mg capsule 1x/day with food.	*Lofibra:* $29–81
	Tricor: 48–145 mg	*Tricor:* One or two 48-mg tablets or one 145-mg tablet 1x/day with or without food.	*Tricor:* $38–113
	Triglide: 50–160 mg	*Triglide:* One or two 50-mg tablets or one 160-mg tablet 1x/day with or without food.	*Triglide:* Not available
Lopid (gemfibrozil)	1,200 mg	One 600-mg tablet 2x/day 30 minutes before breakfast and dinner.	$117 ($16)
Omega-3-acid ethyl esters			
Lovaza (omega-3-acid ethyl esters)	4 g	Four 1-g capsules 1x/day with or without food or two 1-g capsules 2x/day with or without food.	$150
Niacin (nicotinic acid)			
Niacor (niacin)	2–6 g	Two to four 0.5-g capsules 2–3x/day with food.	($9–25)
Niaspan (niacin, extended-release)	1–2 g	One or two 0.75- or 1-g tablets 1x/day at bedtime after a low-fat snack. Swallow whole (do not break, crush, or chew).	$114–228
Combination drugs			
Advicor (Niaspan/lovastatin)	500–2,000 mg Niaspan/20–40 mg lovastatin	One or two 500/20-, 750/20-, 1,000/20-, or 1,000/40-mg tablets at bedtime with a low-fat snack. Swallow whole (do not break, crush, or chew).	$92–213
Vytorin (Zetia/simvastatin)	10 mg Zetia/ 10–80 mg simvastatin	One 10/10-, 10/20-, 10/40-, or 10/80-mg tablet 1x/day in the evening with or without food.	$93–98

* These dosages represent the usual daily dosages for the treatment of abnormal lipid levels. The precise effective dosage varies from person to person and depends on many factors. Do not make any changes to your medication without consulting your doctor.

† These instructions represent the typical way to take the medication. Your doctor's instructions may differ. Always follow your doctor's recommendations.

‡ Prices per drugstore.com.

and LDL cholesterol levels to rise. When this occurs, your physician may prescribe a statin to take with the fibrate.

A fibrate is often added to statin therapy when triglyceride levels remain above normal (150 mg/dL or higher) while taking a statin. This drug combination causes muscle inflammation in about 1% of

Precautions	Possible side effects	Call your doctor if...
If you are taking warfarin (Coumadin), you may need more frequent blood clotting tests. If you take the bile acid sequestrants Colestid or Questran, take fenofibrate at least 1 hour before or 4 hours afterward.	Stomach upset or pain, constipation.	You experience persistent nausea or vomiting, severe stomach pain, dark urine, yellowing of eyes or skin. You are also taking a statin and experience unexplained muscle pain, tenderness, or weakness, fever, dark urine, nausea, vomiting.
Use with caution if you have an allergy or sensitivity to fish. If you are taking warfarin (Coumadin), you may need more frequent blood clotting tests.	Upset stomach, burping, strange taste in your mouth.	You experience easy bleeding or bruising, black or tarry stools, vomit that looks like coffee grounds.
Take with food to decrease flushing and upset stomach. To minimize flushing, also avoid alcohol and hot beverages around the time you take niacin. With your doctor's permission, taking aspirin or another nonsteroidal anti-inflammatory drug (such as ibuprofen) 30 minutes beforehand may also help with flushing. If you take the bile acid sequestrants Colestid or Questran, take niacin at least 1 hour before or 4 hours afterward.	Skin flushing, upset stomach.	You experience dizziness. You have diabetes and experience changes in your blood glucose levels.
See separate entries for Niaspan and lovastatin.	See separate entries for Niaspan and lovastatin.	See separate entries for Niaspan and lovastatin.
See separate entries for Zetia and simvastatin.	See separate entries for Zetia and simvastatin.	See separate entries for Zetia and simvastatin.

people; it's more of a problem with gemfibrozil than with fenofibrate. The muscle inflammation is reversible when both drugs are discontinued, but if the drugs are not promptly stopped, the muscle inflammation can cause kidney damage. Call your doctor immediately if you notice unusual or unexplained muscle aches while taking a fibrate.

Other possible adverse effects of fibrates include stomach upset, stomach pain, and constipation.

Omega-3-acid ethyl esters

Lovaza (formerly called Omacor) is the only medication in this new class of lipid-lowering drugs. Like the fibrates, it is approved for lowering triglycerides in people with very high levels (500 mg/dL or greater). Lovaza contains two omega-3 fats, eicosapentaenoic acid (EPA) and docosahexaenoic acid (DHA), which are also in fatty fish and nonprescription fish oil supplements. The difference: Lovaza is a more concentrated source of omega-3 fats than fish or supplements.

Research shows that Lovaza can reduce triglycerides by as much as 45% and raise HDL cholesterol by 9%. The drug likely works by reducing production of triglycerides in the liver. It may also lower the liver's manufacture of VLDL, the major carrier of triglycerides in the blood.

Side effects are uncommon but can include burping, upset stomach, and changes in sense of taste. Lovaza can also cause LDL cholesterol levels to rise. If this happens, you doctor may prescribe a statin. People taking warfarin (Coumadin) should use Lovaza with caution, as both these medications increase the risk of bleeding.

Blood Pressure–Lowering Medications

When your blood pressure is high and lifestyle measures have not lowered it to the desired level, your doctor will likely prescribe medication. This usually happens when your blood pressure is higher than 140/90 mm Hg—or above 130/80 mm Hg if you have diabetes or kidney disease.

Five classes of medications are commonly used to lower blood pressure: diuretics, beta-blockers, ACE inhibitors, angiotensin II receptor blockers, and calcium channel blockers. These drugs can be prescribed individually or in combination, although most people need at least two blood pressure medications to reduce their blood pressure readings to normal levels.

Diuretics

These drugs (often called water pills) reduce blood pressure by increasing the amount of sodium and water excreted in the urine. This water loss reduces blood volume, and as a result less pressure is exerted on the walls of blood vessels as blood flows through them. Diuretics also reduce blood pressure by widening small blood vessels, which facilitates blood flow.

Thiazide diuretics are the most commonly used diuretics and are often the first medication prescribed to lower blood pressure. That's because along with their blood pressure–lowering effects, thiazide diuretics also reduce the risk of heart failure. What's more, they're inexpensive and need to be taken only once a day.

Possible side effects of diuretics include weakness; fatigue; erectile dysfunction; a rise in blood glucose, uric acid, and triglyceride levels; a lowering of HDL cholesterol levels; and an excessive loss of potassium in the urine. To prevent this last side effect, your doctor may prescribe a potassium-sparing diuretic such as triamterene (Dyrenium) or recommend that you take a potassium supplement.

Beta-blockers

These drugs block the actions of the hormone epinephrine (adrenaline). This effect lowers blood pressure by slowing heart rate and decreasing the amount of blood the heart pumps with each beat. Beta-blockers not only lower blood pressure but can also alleviate symptoms of angina, treat heart failure, and reduce the risk of death and future heart attacks in people who have had a heart attack. That's why many people with CHD are taking a beta-blocker to reduce their blood pressure.

Possible adverse effects of beta-blockers include dizziness, lightheadedness, drowsiness, diarrhea, unusual dreams, vision problems, and trouble sleeping. Beta-blockers may mask the warning symptoms of hypoglycemia (low blood sugar) in people with diabetes who are taking insulin or certain oral diabetes drugs.

ACE inhibitors

"ACE" stands for angiotensin-converting enzyme. One way ACE inhibitors lower blood pressure is by inhibiting the formation of angiotensin II, a substance that constricts blood vessels and stimulates the adrenal glands to release aldosterone (a hormone that promotes sodium retention). By reducing angiotensin II and relaxing blood vessels, blood can move through the vessels at a lower pressure.

Besides lowering blood pressure, ACE inhibitors help reduce the risk of CHD events in some people with CHD and in those with diabetes who have one or more CHD risk factors. ACE inhibitors may also reduce the risk of diabetes, kidney disease, and stroke. In addition, they are effective for the prevention of heart failure in people with impaired heart function and for the treatment of heart failure.

ACE inhibitors cause fewer side effects than diuretics or beta-blockers. A dry cough is the most frequent side effect. People who

NEW RESEARCH

Dark Chocolate May Relax Your Blood Vessels

A little dark chocolate can be a soothing indulgence—one that might even help your blood vessels relax, researchers report.

In a small study, 44 adults (ages 56–73) with mildly elevated blood pressure levels were randomly assigned to eat a 0.25-oz piece of either dark or white chocolate every day.

Over 18 weeks, those given the dark chocolate saw their systolic and diastolic blood pressures dip slightly—by 2–3 mm Hg on average—while the white-chocolate group experienced no change in their blood pressure levels. Eating these small amounts of chocolate did not cause weight gain or harmful increases in blood cholesterol or blood glucose.

Unlike white and milk chocolates, dark chocolate is rich in polyphenols, plant compounds that increase nitric oxide production. Nitric oxide helps blood vessels relax and dilate to facilitate blood flow. In fact, during the study, the formation of nitric oxide appeared to increase in the blood vessel linings of the dark-chocolate eaters but remained constant in the white-chocolate group.

These results are not a chocolate lover's dream. The daily allotment amounted to 30 calories—akin to a Hershey's Kiss rather than a Hershey bar. Remember that overindulgence can lead to weight gain, which can send your blood pressure on the rise.

JOURNAL OF THE AMERICAN MEDICAL ASSOCIATION
Volume 298, page 49
July 4, 2007

develop a cough while using an ACE inhibitor may be able to take an angiotensin II receptor blocker (see below) instead. Uncommon side effects of ACE inhibitors include an increase in blood potassium levels and impaired kidney function. Women who are pregnant or planning to become pregnant should not take ACE inhibitors.

Angiotensin II receptor blockers

These drugs (also known as ARBs) lower blood pressure by interfering with the ability of angiotensin II to constrict blood vessels. They may also halt the growth of smooth muscle cells in vessel walls.

Like ACE inhibitors, ARBs can benefit the heart and kidneys. There's evidence that ARBs are helpful in treating heart failure and in preventing diabetes, kidney disease in people with diabetes, and strokes in people with high blood pressure and a thickened heart muscle (called left ventricular hypertrophy).

Side effects of ARBs include dizziness, back pain, and sore throat. Like ACE inhibitors, ARBs should not be used by pregnant women or women planning a pregnancy.

Calcium channel blockers

These drugs lower blood pressure by dilating arteries and decreasing the amount of blood the heart pumps with each heartbeat. Calcium channel blockers also help relieve symptoms of angina and are sometimes used to reduce the risk of stroke and kidney disease.

Long-acting calcium channel blockers are used because they are safer and more effective than the short-acting versions. The long-acting medications need to be taken only once a day.

The side effects of calcium channel blockers are usually mild and include headache, flushing, dizziness, nausea, and constipation.

Antiplatelet Medications

When your doctor wants to reduce your risk of blood clots, he or she may prescribe an antiplatelet drug. These drugs work by preventing blood cells called platelets from clumping together to form a blood clot that could rapidly trigger a heart attack. Antiplatelet medications include aspirin, clopidogrel (Plavix), and glycoprotein IIB-IIIA inhibitors, such as abciximab (ReoPro), eptifibatide (Integrilin), and tirofiban (Aggrastat).

Aspirin

You've probably taken an aspirin to ease the pain of a toothache or to reduce the inflammation of a sprained ankle, but aspirin also has a role to play in the prevention and treatment of CHD. For example, by taking aspirin over the long term, you can reduce your risk of a heart attack, stroke, or cardiovascular-related death. In fact, a daily aspirin is routinely prescribed to people who have already had a heart attack, with the goal of preventing a second one. In addition, chewing a regular-dose aspirin immediately after the onset of heart attack symptoms can increase your chances of survival.

Aspirin is also sometimes recommended for people who have no signs of CHD or other cardiovascular disease but have one or more risk factors for a heart attack. You should talk to your doctor about taking aspirin for preventing a first heart attack if you fall into one or more of these categories: You are a man age 45 and older or a woman age 55 and older; you are a smoker; or you have high blood pressure, diabetes, high total or LDL cholesterol levels, low HDL cholesterol levels, or a family history of premature heart attacks (before age 55 in a father or brother or age 65 in a mother or sister).

Aspirin is also prescribed to reduce the risk of stroke in some people with atrial fibrillation (an abnormal heart rhythm that can occur in people with CHD), usually in those who cannot use the anticoagulant warfarin (Coumadin).

Despite the many benefits of aspirin, the drug increases the risk of gastrointestinal bleeding and hemorrhagic (bleeding) stroke. People who have poorly controlled high blood pressure or who regularly take other anticlotting medications like warfarin have the greatest chance of experiencing these serious side effects. Because of these dangers, you should talk to your doctor before starting to take a daily aspirin to reduce your heart attack risk.

Plavix

This drug is another type of antiplatelet medication. It is more potent than aspirin and is used over the short term (up to a year) to prevent the formation of blood clots in people at high risk, including those with unstable angina, those who have had a heart attack, and those who have undergone angioplasty followed by implantation of a drug-eluting stent (see pages 56–59).

Common side effects of Plavix include nausea, upset stomach, stomach pain, diarrhea, rash, and itchy skin. Like aspirin, Plavix can increase the risk of bleeding, and the same precautions apply.

Glycoprotein IIB-IIIA inhibitors

These antiplatelet drugs, which include ReoPro, Integrilin, and Aggrastat, are usually used before and during angioplasty to prevent

NEW RESEARCH

Most Can Skip Antibiotics Before Dental Work

People with certain heart abnormalities may no longer require antibiotics before dental work.

For years, the American Heart Association recommended use of antibiotics before dental and medical procedures in people with structural heart disease to prevent endocarditis, a potentially lethal infection of the heart's inner lining. But based on an analysis of recent research, the group now says this practice is unnecessary for those with mitral valve prolapse, rheumatic heart disease, bicuspid aortic valve disease, or aortic stenosis.

That's because no solid evidence exists that preventive antibiotics lower the risk of endocarditis in these individuals, and thus the risks of antibiotic resistance or the small chance of a fatal allergic reaction outweigh the benefits.

However, people with heart conditions that put them at very high risk for endocarditis—those with artificial heart valves, a history of infective endocarditis, congenital heart defects other than hypertrophic cardiomyopathy or atrial or ventricular septal defect, and heart transplant patients with valve problems—should still receive antibiotics before extensive dental work (such as tooth extractions) or procedures on the respiratory tract, skin, or musculoskeletal tissue.

It's not necessary—no matter the risk of endocarditis—to take antibiotics before procedures on the gastrointestinal tract (such as colonoscopy) or the urinary tract.

CIRCULATION
Volume 116, page 1736
October 9, 2007

Sticking With Your Medications

It just might lengthen your life

Have you ever thought of skipping your medication when you're feeling good? How about when you're feeling bad and think it's a drug side effect? Do you ever skip doses because you think the medication isn't working? What about skipping doses not by choice, but because you have trouble remembering to take them all?

You probably answered "yes" to at least one of these questions, if recent surveys of people with coronary heart disease (CHD) are any indication. But even though skipping medication is common, research clearly shows that this practice can sabotage your health.

Importance of Compliance

If taking your heart medications seems like more trouble than it's worth, consider the findings of these two studies:

- A 2007 study in the *Journal of the American Medical Association* reported that in more than 31,000 heart attack survivors, those who were most compliant with their statin and beta-blocker drugs had a lower risk of dying over two years. For example, participants who were most compliant with their statins had a death rate of 16%, compared with 24% in those who were least compliant.
- Another study, in the *Archives of Internal Medicine*, revealed that 12% of heart attack survivors stopped taking all three of their prescriptions—aspirin, a statin, and a beta-blocker—within a month of being hospitalized for the attack. Another 22% stopped taking at least one of their drugs. There were consequences for those who discontinued their medication altogether: Over the next year, their survival rate was 89% vs. 98% in study patients who stayed with at least one of their medications.

Overcoming the Obstacles

There are obviously obstacles to sticking with your medications, but as these two studies show these hurdles are well worth overcoming. Here are some tips to help you do just that.

Obstacle #1: "Why am I taking all these drugs?" When you're taking multiple pills a day for your heart and possibly other health issues, you might be wondering whether all of these medications are truly necessary. Here's some advice.

- Knowing exactly why you need a given drug should motivate you to take it. So whenever your doctor prescribes a new medication, don't be afraid to ask questions so you understand what it does, how and how long you're supposed to take it (many heart drugs need to be taken for a lifetime), and what side effects you may expect. If you're uncertain about any medications you're already on, don't be shy to ask about those as well.
- If you typically forget what the doctor said about your medication by the time you get home or pick up the prescription at the pharmacy, take notes or ask your doctor to write down the details for you.
- If you have trouble understanding all of your medication information, have your spouse or another family member accompany you when you talk to your doctor or pharmacist. That person can ask questions, too.

Obstacle #2: "Is this medication really working?" The effects of drugs you take for high blood pressure or high cholesterol, for instance, are basically "silent." That is, you might not feel any better whether you take them or you don't, so it can be easy to rationalize skipping them from time to time. To overcome this thinking:

- Ask your doctor to recommend a home blood pressure monitor. By checking your blood pressure at home between doctor visits, you'll have an opportunity to see your blood pressure decline in real time.
- The next time your doctor orders a lipid profile, ask for the specific numbers, and keep a record of them so you can see how the numbers change over time.

Obstacle #3: "I can't keep track of all my medications." If you're using several medications, it can be hard to keep track. First, ask your doctor to simplify your regimen—for example, switching to a medication that needs to be taken only once a day, taking as many of your medications as possible at the same time of day, or using combination pills that contain two or more drugs in a single tablet. Here are a few other suggestions:

- A simple pill box, divided into sections for each day of the week, is a good start to getting organized. Fill the box with your medications (and any vitamins you're taking) at the beginning of every week. Then keep the pill box somewhere you won't miss it—right by your place at the kitchen table, or next to something you use every day, like your reading glasses. You can buy a pill box at your local drug store.

• Take advantage of bells and whistles. You can use the alarm on your watch or cell phone to remind you it's time to take a pill. Some pill boxes come with built-in alarms. There are even automated medication dispensers, which can cost anywhere from $30–800, that announce when it's time to take your medicine, then dole out the appropriate pill. You can buy these online from sites like Amazon.com or epill.com.

• Keep a medication chart. This can be a simple dry-erase board on the refrigerator door; put a check next to each medication after you take it. You can also create a more detailed medication calendar, with the names of your medications and the doses listed vertically down one side (list the morning ones first, then afternoon and evening), and the dates of the month (numbers 1–31) listed across the top. Alternatively, ask your pharmacist if he or she has similar charts you can use, or download a medication calendar from the American Heart Association website (www.americanheart.org/presenter.jhtml?identifier=92).

• Ask your pharmacist whether special packaging is available to help you take your medications. For example, blister packs contain individual tablets with the days listed on the card, and pill bottles with timer caps beep when it's time to take your medication.

Obstacle #4: "I can't stand the side effects." If side effects are bothersome, don't stop taking your medication on your own. Tell your doctor about them, and he or she will help you figure out what to do. Here's some more advice:

• Before you start taking a new medication or a new dosage, discuss the possible side effects with your doctor. You might be able to prevent some of them from happening in the first place. For example, if you know that constipation is a potential problem (as with certain medications for cholesterol, angina, or heart failure), you can help prevent it by drinking more water and eating enough high-fiber foods. Similarly, dizziness is an manageable side effect of many blood pressure drugs and other heart medications; simple measures like avoiding alcohol and being careful not to stand up too quickly can help minimize the problem.

• When side effects do arise, remember that many of them are only temporary—lasting for several weeks until your body becomes accustomed to the medication. But if a side effect is long lasting, you and your doctor can take steps. For example, stomach upset caused by aspirin can often be minimized by taking the medication with food or taking a second medication that suppresses stomach acid production. Drowsiness can be dealt with by taking your medication at bedtime. If these strategies don't help, your doctor may recommend that you try a lower dose or switch to another medication.

• If it's hard for you to swallow your medication, you can get a pill cutter at the drug store. But first check with your doctor or pharmacist; some drugs must be swallowed whole.

Obstacle #5: "I keep running out of my medication." Here's some help in getting timely refills.

• Plan to get your refills about a week before you are going to run out of pills. Mark the day on your calendar or write yourself a note and put it in a prominent place, such as the fridge door. You can also ask whether your pharmacy will give you a refill reminder by mail or phone.

• If money causes you to delay refills, ways exist to reduce your drug costs. First, ask your pharmacist if there are generic versions of the drugs you're taking. Second, ask your doctor about "pill splitting"; in some cases you can get a higher dose of your medication at the same price, then split the pills so you have twice as many. Third, if you have prescription drug coverage but it doesn't cover your particular medication, find out whether a comparable alternative is covered; if not, ask your doctor for help in getting an "exception" from your insurance plan. Fourth, many drug companies have assistance programs to help low-income people afford their medications (for more information, visit www.rxassist.org or www.pparx.org).

The Bottom Line

There are ways to surmount obstacles you may have to sticking with your drug therapy. Try out a number of the above suggestions and don't hesitate to talk to your doctor or pharmacist; it just might mean a longer, healthier life. ■

blood clots. They may cause bleeding, especially when combined with anticoagulant drugs and aspirin.

Anticoagulant Medications

Anticoagulant medications work by interfering with the formation of fibrin (a protein involved in blood clotting). These medications include warfarin, heparin, and low-molecular-weight heparin.

These drugs are often given to heart attack patients who have a blood clot inside their heart or whose heart is functioning poorly. Warfarin is also used to treat atrial fibrillation, especially when other stroke risk factors are present—for example, high blood pressure, previous stroke or transient ischemic attack (TIA; also known as a ministroke), or age 75 and over. Heparin is often given in the hospital to prevent blood clots during bypass surgery. The risk of bleeding is high with these anticoagulant medications. To minimize the risk, you will need periodic blood tests to check how quickly your blood clots.

Antiangina Medications

The chest pain associated with angina can be frightening but is treatable. The medications used to relieve chest pain work by decreasing the heart's demand for oxygen and increasing its blood supply. Nitrates, beta-blockers, and calcium channel blockers are the three main types of drugs used to treat angina. A combination of these drugs may be needed to sufficiently relieve chest pain. When a nitrate, beta-blocker, or calcium channel blocker is not enough, a new drug called ranolazine (Ranexa) may be tried.

Nitrates

These drugs dilate arteries and veins. By dilating the coronary arteries, blood flow to the heart increases; by dilating peripheral veins, blood pools in the extremities. When this pooling occurs, the heart has less blood to pump and its workload and need for oxygen are reduced.

There are two types of nitrates: fast acting and longer acting. The fast-acting nitrates help relieve acute episodes of angina and can also be taken shortly before physical activity to prevent an acute attack. On the other hand, the longer-acting nitrates offer more long-term, day-to-day protection against angina symptoms.

Fast-acting nitrates. The most common treatment to relieve an acute bout of angina is Nitrostat or Nitroquick, a nitroglycerin tablet placed under the tongue. Other options include Nitrolingual and

Nitromist (sprayed on or under the tongue) and isosorbide dinitrate sublingual tablets (Isordil), which are placed under the tongue like Nitrostat.

These nitrate formulations generally bring relief within two to three minutes. If symptoms are not relieved in five minutes, a second dose may be taken. If symptoms persist for another five minutes, some doctors recommend a third dose. But if symptoms continue for more than 15 minutes, you may be having a heart attack and should call 911 immediately and chew a regular-dose aspirin.

If you're prone to angina and are about to engage in an activity that has provoked chest pain in the past, your doctor may recommend that you take a fast-acting nitrate shortly before the activity. Follow your doctor's instructions as to when to take your nitrates.

Longer-acting nitrates. These nitrates provide protection against angina symptoms for longer periods of time. Some examples are controlled-release nitroglycerin capsules, nitroglycerin patches (Deponit, Minitran, Nitro-Dur) that are applied to the skin, and nitroglycerin ointment (Nitro-Bid) that is spread on the skin. Other options include isosorbide dinitrate (Isordil Titradose, Dilatrate-SR) and isosorbide mononitrate (ISMO, Monoket, Imdur).

Because you can develop a tolerance to these longer-acting nitrates, you may need to take higher dosages over time to achieve the same effect. To prevent tolerance, your doctor may advise you to stop taking your longer-acting nitrate for a period of time each day—usually overnight. For example, you can remove your nitroglycerin patch while you are sleeping.

Many people experience headaches when they first start taking a nitrate. This side effect, however, tends to become less of a problem after a week or two. Other caveats: People who use nitrates should not take the erectile dysfunction drugs sildenafil (Viagra), tadalafil (Cialis), or vardenafil (Levitra), because the combination can cause a potentially fatal drop in blood pressure. In addition, you should sit or lie down the first time you take a nitrate, in case you experience a drop in blood pressure that could cause you to faint.

Beta-blockers

These drugs help control angina by slowing heart rate and reducing the force of the heart's contractions, thus decreasing the heart's workload and amount of oxygen the heart needs to function. The slower heart rate also prolongs the time between contractions, which allows more blood to flow to the heart. Beta-blockers are often prescribed in combination with a nitrate.

Drugs for Angina 2008

Drug type: Brand (generic)	Typical daily dosages*	How to take†	Monthly cost‡: Brand (generic)
Nitrates			
Fast-acting nitroglycerin Nitroquick, Nitrostat (sublingual nitroglycerin)	As needed	Dissolve a 0.3-, 0,4-, or 0.6-mg tablet under your tongue or between your cheek and gum every 5 minutes for up to three tablets to relieve an acute attack of angina. You can also take one tablet 5–10 minutes before an activity that may cause an angina attack.	100 tablets: $9–18 ($16)
Nitrolingual, Nitromist (translingual nitroglycerin)	As needed	One or two sprays (0.4–0.8 mg) onto or under your tongue every 5 minutes for up to 3 sets of sprays to relieve an acute attack of angina. You can also use one or two sprays 5–10 minutes before an activity that may cause an angina attack.	12-g bottle (0.4-mg/spray): $126
Longer-acting nitroglycerin (nitroglycerin, controlled-release)	2.5–9 mg	One 2.5-, 6.5-, or 9-mg capsule 1x/day in the morning without food. Swallow whole with 4 oz of water.	($8–13)
Nitro-Bid (nitroglycerin ointment)	2–4 inches (30–60 mg)	Spread 1–2 inches (15–30 mg) of ointment onto the skin of your chest or back 2x/day 6–7 hours apart. Remove at bedtime.	$0.27–0.54
Deponit, Minitran, Nitro-Dur (transdermal nitroglycerin)	1.2–11.2 mg	Apply one 0.1-, 0.2-, 0.3-, 0.4-, 0.6-, or 0.8-mg/hour patch to the skin of your upper arm or upper chest and leave on all day. Remove at bedtime.	$51–95 ($26–40)
Other nitrates ISMO, Monoket (isosorbide mononitrate)	20–80 mg	One or two 10- or 20-mg tablets 2x/day once on awakening and again 7 hours later.	$49–204 ($15–38)
Imdur (isosorbide mononitrate, extended-release)	30–240 mg	One or two 30-, 60-, or 120-mg tablets 1x/day in the morning with or without food. Swallow whole with 4 oz of water.	$67–154 ($16–30)
Isordil (isosorbide dinitrate sublingual tablets)	As needed	Dissolve a 2.5- or 5-mg tablet under your tongue or between your check and gum 15 minutes before an activity that may cause an angina attack.	100 tablets: $31–33 ($19–39)
Isordil Titradose (isosorbide dinitrate)	20–120 mg	A 10-, 20-, 30-, or 40-mg tablet 2–3x/day.	$22–78 ($18–20)
Dilatrate-SR (isosorbide dinitrate, extended-release)	40–160 mg	One to four 40-mg capsules 1x/day.	($22–86)
Other antiangina drug			
Ranexa (ranolazine)	1,000–2,000 mg	One or two 500-mg tablets 2x/day with or without food. Swallow whole (do not crush, break, or chew).	$201–404

* These dosages represent the usual daily dosages for the treatment of angina. The precise effective dosage varies from person to person and depends on many factors. Do not make any changes to your medication without consulting your doctor.

† These instructions represent the typical way to take the medication. Your doctor's instructions may differ. Always follow your doctor's recommendations.

‡ Monthly cost (unless specified otherwise) per drugstore.com.

Precautions	Most common side effects	Call your doctor if...
Sit or lie down when taking nitroglycerin to prevent falls; the medication can make you lightheaded, dizzy, or faint. Limiting alcohol and getting up slowly from a seated or lying position help minimize lightheadedness and dizziness. Call 911 and chew a regular-dose aspirin if chest pain is not relieved within 15 minutes. Do not take while using the erectile dysfunction drugs sildenafil (Viagra), tadalafil (Cialis), or vardenafil (Levitra). *Fast-acting nitroglycerin:* To prevent tolerance, do not overuse. *Longer-acting nitroglycerin:* To prevent tolerance, remove the ointment or patch at bedtime.	Headache, lightheadedness, flushing, dizziness. Headache can be treated with an over-the-counter pain reliever such as acetaminophen (Tylenol).	The number of your angina attacks increases, you need more nitroglycerin than usual to relieve the attacks, or the side effects listed at left persist or worsen.
Because Ranexa can cause dangerous changes in the heart's electrical activity, it should be used only when other medications do not offer significant relief from chest pain. You should have an electrocardiogram (ECG) before starting Ranexa and periodically while you are on it. Avoid grapefruit and grapefruit juice to prevent high blood levels of Ranexa. To minimize dizziness, avoid alcohol and get up slowly from a seated or lying position.	Dizziness, headache, lightheadedness, nausea, tiredness, constipation.	You experience heart palpitations or fainting spells.

continued on the next page

Drugs for Angina 2008 (continued)

Drug type: Brand (generic)	Typical daily dosages*	How to take†	Monthly cost‡: Brand (generic)
Beta-blockers			
Corgard (nadolol)	40–240 mg	One or two 40-, 80-, 120-, or 160-mg tablets 1x/day with or without food.	$75–200 ($13–34)
Inderal (propranolol)	80–320 mg	One 40-, 60-, or 80-mg tablet 2–4x/day.	$57–152 ($9–50)
Inderal LA (propranolol, extended-release)	80–320 mg	One or two 80-, 120-, or 160-mg capsules 1x/day. Swallow whole (do not crush or chew).	$51–165 ($35–110)
Lopressor (metoprolol)	100–400 mg	One or two 50- or 100-mg tablets 2x/day with or immediately following meals.	$73–226 ($12–20)
Tenormin (atenolol)	50–200 mg	One or two 50- or 100-mg tablets 1x/day.	$49–137 ($8–11)
Toprol XL (metoprolol, extended-release)	100–400 mg	One or two 100- or 200-mg tablets 1x/day with or immediately following a meal. Swallow whole (do not crush or chew).	$40–131
Calcium channel blockers			
Calan (verapamil)	240–360 mg	One 80- or 120-mg tablet 3x/day with or without food. Swallow whole (do not crush or chew).	$77–97 ($15–17)
Cardizem (diltiazem)	90–360 mg	One 30-, 60-, 90-mg, or 120-mg tablet 3–4x/day before meals and at bedtime.	$51–141 ($10–26)
Cardizem CD, Cartia XT, Dilacor XR, Diltia-XT, Tiazac (diltiazem, extended-release)	120–360 mg	One 120-, 180-, 240-, 300-, or 360-mg capsule 1x/day at bedtime with or without food. Swallow whole (do not crush or chew).	$24–117 ($24–59)
Cardizem LA (diltiazem, extended-release)	120–360 mg	One 120-, 180-, 240-, 300-, or 360-mg tablet 1x/day in the evening or morning. Swallow whole (do not crush or chew).	$60–113
Norvasc (amlodipine)	5–10 mg	One 5- or 10-mg tablet 1x/day in the morning with or without food. Swallow whole.	$54–74 ($47-64)
Procardia XL (nifedipine, extended-release)	30–90 mg	One 30- or 90-mg tablet 1x/day on an empty stomach. Swallow whole (do not crush or chew).	$51–100 ($34-68)

* These dosages represent the usual daily dosages for the treatment of angina. The precise effective dosage varies from person to person and depends on many factors. Do not make any changes to your medication without consulting your doctor.

† These instructions represent the typical way to take the medication. Your doctor's instructions may differ. Always follow your doctor's recommendations.

‡ Monthly cost (unless specified otherwise) per drugstore.com.

Calcium channel blockers

Calcium channel blockers reduce the heart's workload, which allows more blood to flow through the coronary arteries. These drugs also decrease the oxygen requirements of heart muscle. Calcium channel blockers can also alleviate angina caused by a coronary artery spasm.

Precautions	Most common side effects	Call your doctor if...
Do not stop taking or change the dose without consulting your doctor. Abruptly stopping a beta-blocker may worsen angina. To minimize dizziness, get up slowly from a seated or lying position and avoid alcohol. Beta-blockers may make your hands and feet cold because of reduced blood flow to the extremities; dress warmly and avoid smoking. May mask symptoms of hypoglycemia (fast, pounding heartbeat, nervousness, shakiness) in people with diabetes who are taking insulin.	Dizziness, lightheadedness, drowsiness, tiredness, diarrhea, unusual dreams, vision problems, trouble sleeping.	You experience any of the side effects listed at left. You experience symptoms of a very slow heartbeat: persistent dizziness, faintness, unusual fatigue. You experience signs of high blood glucose levels: increased thirst or urination.
Do not stop taking or change the dose without consulting your doctor. Abruptly stopping a calcium channel blocker may worsen angina. To minimize dizziness, get up slowly from a seated or lying position and avoid alcohol. To prevent constipation, eat a high-fiber diet, drink plenty of water, and exercise. If you become constipated while using this drug, ask your doctor if you can take a stool softener. *Calan and Procardia XL only:* Avoid eating grapefruit or drinking grapefruit juice to prevent excessive amounts of these medications in your blood.	Headache, dizziness, flushing, nausea.	You experience chest pain that is more severe or occurs more often; swelling of the ankles or feet; shortness of breath; persistent fatigue; a fast, irregular, or very slow heartbeat; fainting.

Ranexa

This drug is different from the other antiangina medications, because it does not increase blood flow to the heart or slow heart rate. In addition, it's not a first-line treatment for angina and is prescribed only when other medications are not enough to control angina symptoms. That's because Ranexa (particularly when used at high doses) can cause potentially dangerous changes in the electrical activity of the heart.

Revascularization Treatments

When medication does not control angina pain or when the buildup of plaque in your coronary arteries is so severe that you are at high risk for a heart attack, your doctor may recommend angioplasty or bypass surgery, which are revascularization procedures. These procedures are not a cure for atherosclerosis, so you will need to follow them up by adopting or continuing with the dietary and other preventive lifestyle measures described on pages 25–36. You will also need to take medication to improve lipid levels, lower blood pressure, and prevent blood clots.

Angioplasty

About 1.2 million Americans a year undergo angioplasty (also called percutaneous coronary intervention, or PCI). Angioplasty does not remove plaque from the coronary arteries. Instead, it widens the channel (lumen) through which blood flows by one or more of the following mechanisms: squeezing the plaque against the artery wall; cracking the hard part of the plaque; or stretching the artery. About 90% of individuals notice an immediate improvement in symptoms when the lumen of the artery is at least 50% open after angioplasty.

Angioplasty, which takes about one to two hours, is performed in a cardiac catheterization laboratory. The procedure does not require general anesthesia and usually involves no more than a night's stay in the hospital. After the patient receives a sedative and a local anesthetic in the groin area, a tiny catheter (flexible tube) with a deflated balloon at its tip is inserted through a small incision into the femoral artery in the groin. Guided by x-ray images on a monitor, the cardiologist threads the catheter toward the heart and positions the balloon at the site of the plaque obstruction in the coronary artery. The cardiologist then inflates the balloon repeatedly for 30 seconds to several minutes to compress the plaque and open the artery.

Angioplasty with stenting

In about 85% of cases, a small, scaffold-like device called a stent is permanently placed in the artery during angioplasty to help keep it open over the longer term. Without a stent, the rate of restenosis (narrowing of the artery after angioplasty) ranges from 30–40%. Stent use reduces this rate to 10–20%.

But problems remain with the use of stents. These problems include blood clots and tissue growth on the stent itself. Your doctor will take steps to lower the risk of these problems. For example, you will receive powerful anticlotting drugs called glycoprotein IIB-IIIA inhibitors to prevent blood clots after the procedure. These drugs are usually given intravenously for 12–24 hours. You will also take the antiplatelet drug Plavix for one month or longer to reduce the risk of blood clots.

Tissue growth on the stent can be minimized with drug-eluting stents. These stents are coated with one of two medications: the antibiotic sirolimus or the anticancer drug paclitaxel. These drugs are slowly released from the stent over time, inhibiting the growth of cells that can lead to restenosis. Studies show that these stents are more effective than traditional, noncoated stents in preventing restenosis.

But these drug-eluting stents also carry an increased risk of blood clots at the stent site, particularly after antiplatelet therapy is stopped—for example, before undergoing surgical procedures, including dental procedures, to prevent excessive bleeding. If you are taking antiplatelet medication to prevent blood clots after implantation of a drug-eluting stent, always consult your cardiologist before discontinuing the therapy, even temporarily. To reduce the risk of blood clots with drug-eluting stents, it's now recommended that, when possible, people take two antiplatelet drugs: aspirin for an indefinite time and Plavix for one year after the procedure. For more information on drug-eluting stents, see "Are Drug-Eluting Stents a Help or Hazard?" on pages 58–59.

Complications

A serious complication during angioplasty with or without stenting is total closure of the artery due to a clot, spasm, or tear in the artery wall. Closure of the artery can cause a heart attack (this occurs in about 2–4% of patients) or require emergency bypass surgery (this happens in 1–2% of patients). Because of this risk, if you require angioplasty in several vessels, you will probably need to recover for at least a day after angioplasty on the first artery before the procedure is repeated on another vessel.

Overall, few major risks are associated with angioplasty. Less than 1% of individuals die during the procedure. Complication rates are lower when angioplasty is performed by an experienced doctor. But

NEW RESEARCH

Drugs As Good As Angioplasty for Stable Coronary Heart Disease

Angioplasty may offer little advantage over drug therapy alone for people with stable coronary heart disease (CHD), according to a major clinical trial.

In findings that came as a surprise to many heart experts, the study found that of 2,287 patients with stable CHD, those who received angioplasty and stents to prop open clogged arteries generally fared no better than those given medication alone. Over five years, both groups had similar rates of heart attack, hospitalization, and death.

During the study period, 19% of both the medication-only and angioplasty group suffered a nonfatal heart attack or died of any cause. Although angioplasty patients initially had better blood flow to the heart and less chest pain, this advantage waned as more medication patients became free of chest pain over time.

These findings do not apply to people who are having an acute heart attack or have unstable angina (chest pain at rest or frequent or increasing episodes of chest pain that are associated with an increased risk of a heart attack). For these individuals, angioplasty can be lifesaving.

However, for many people with stable CHD, angioplasty can be deferred until medications are tried first. If medications are not successful, angioplasty should then be considered.

THE NEW ENGLAND JOURNAL OF MEDICINE
Volume 356, page 1503
April 12, 2007

Are Drug-Eluting Stents a Help or Hazard?
What the experts are saying

If you've had angioplasty within the past few years to clear blockages from your coronary arteries, it's more than likely you had at least one drug-eluting stent implanted to help keep your arteries open. When these devices were introduced in 2003, doctors quickly adopted them because they helped avert the key problem with traditional, bare-metal stents: the tendency of scar tissue to form around the stent and renarrow the artery, a process called restenosis.

Indeed, studies show that drug-eluting stents cut the odds of restenosis by about 50% compared with their bare-metal counterparts, minimizing the need for repeat angioplasty. But, as you've no doubt heard, the newer stents carry a problem of their own.

In 2006, studies began to show that a small number of people with the devices suffered blood clots months or years after having the stents implanted, particularly after discontinuing antiplatelet medications. The risk of this complication, known as late thrombosis, appears small but is nonetheless concerning since such blood clots can lead to a heart attack or sudden death.

In December 2006, the FDA convened an expert panel to examine the safety of drug-eluting stents. The panel came up with as many questions as answers, but some key facts emerged, along with some recommendations.

The Stent Backstory

Stents are small, scaffold-like devices that help prop open arteries following angioplasty. While stents do help keep arteries open, restenosis is a common problem with bare-metal stents, occurring about 20% of the time. Drug-eluting stents were created to prevent this renarrowing, by gradually releasing a medication (sirolimus or paclitaxel) that inhibits the growth of scar tissue into the stent.

FDA approval. When the FDA approved drug-eluting stents, the devices were given the go-ahead for specific patients—those with less-extensive heart disease who had small, new plaques, were not at imminent risk for a heart attack, and had no other major medical conditions like diabetes or kidney disease. However, in a practice called off-label use, doctors are free to use therapies for people who fall outside the FDA's approved indications.

Because drug-eluting stents were heralded as a breakthrough when they hit the market, they largely supplanted bare-metal stents. In 2006, an estimated 60% of patients receiving drug-eluting stents fell into the off-label category. These individuals had more extensive heart disease—longer blockages, blockages in two or more coronary arteries, or a previous heart attack—or suffered from diabetes or kidney disease.

Troubling findings. Experts knew from early on that drug-eluting stents carried a small risk of blood clots (bare-metal stents do, too, but only in the short term). To lower the risk, patients typically used anticlotting medication, aspirin and clopidogrel (Plavix), for several months after the procedure. But then studies began to suggest that drug-eluting stents carried a higher risk of late blood clots, often forming after patients stopped taking Plavix.

In 2006, Swiss researchers found that in 746 people who'd received stents, those with drug-eluting ones were more likely than those with bare-metal stents to have a heart attack or die in the year after they stopped taking Plavix. In all, 5% of patients with drug-eluting stents had a nonfatal heart attack or died of a heart-related cause, compared with 1% of those with bare-metal stents. The researchers concluded that the reason might have been higher rates of late blood clots with the drug-eluting stents.

Two subsequent studies indicated that drug-eluting stents raise the odds of blood clots a year or more after implantation. But one of those studies, an analysis of 17 clinical trials, found no evidence that people with drug-eluting stents actually had a higher risk of dying.

FDA re-evaluation. Amid confusion over the real risk of drug-eluting stents, in December 2006, the FDA convened an expert advisory panel to hear the available, and often conflicting, research data.

On the one hand, there were reassuring findings from research that continues to follow people in the stent manufacturers' original trials. One study that analyzed data from nine of these trials found that those with drug-eluting stents had a higher rate of blood clots after one year: 14 cases vs. two in people with bare-metal stents. However, there was no difference in heart attacks or deaths between the two groups over four years.

But the FDA panel also heard sobering statistics, in particular from a Swedish study based on a national patient registry—meaning "real-world" patients treated outside of a clinical trial, including those with more severe heart disease who received drug-eluting stents off-label. Between six months and three years after angioplasty, drug-eluting stent patients were one third more likely to die than their counterparts with bare-metal stents.

The Current State of Stents

At the end of the FDA meeting, the panel summed up what's known and what remains to be learned about drug-eluting stents.

FDA-approved use. When used as directed, the risks of suffering a blood clot are less than 2% in the three years after implantation of drug-eluting stents. Fortunately, this risk does not appear to result in a higher risk of heart attacks and death, most likely because the reduced chance of restenosis with drug-eluting stents offsets the clot risks. So, if you meet the criteria for on-label use, drug-eluting stents are likely a safe and beneficial choice.

Off-label use. The risks with off-label use are less clear, in part because data are lacking for people with more extensive heart disease or with other chronic illnesses. In these individuals, drug-eluting stents lead to a higher risk of clots than bare-metal stents, as well as an increased risk of heart attacks and deaths. But it's not certain that drug-eluting stents are the reason, nor is there research on whether bare-metal stents are a safer alternative. So, if you fit into the off-label category, consider bypass surgery as an alternative to angioplasty.

Anticlotting therapy. The FDA as well as the American Heart Association now recommend that people with drug-eluting stents take two anticlotting medications: aspirin for an indefinite period of time and Plavix for at least one year (up from the three to six months recommended on the stents' labels). This recommendation is based on expert opinion, not on hard evidence. Thus, more research is needed to determine when, if ever, the excess risk of blood clots with drug-eluting stents disappears or whether the use of Plavix continues to prevent these clots over the long term.

What Should You Do?

Experts agree that we shouldn't return to the bare-metal era. Drug-eluting stents are an important advance that benefits many people.

You already have drug-eluting stents. It's vital that you follow your doctor's directions on anticlotting therapy if you have drug-eluting stents. Terminating therapy too early will increase your risk of a potentially life-threatening blood clot at the stent. Thus, never stop your anticlotting medication without talking to your cardiologist, even if another doctor or a dentist tells you to, for example, before a surgical procedure. In addition, you should postpone any elective surgery while on anticlotting therapy.

If you've already stopped taking Plavix, ask your doctor whether it is worthwhile to restart it. The answer will depend on how long you've been off Plavix, how many heart attack risk factors you have, what other health problems you have, and the anatomy of your coronary arteries.

You are considering drug-eluting stents. If you meet the on-label criteria, drug-eluting stents are a viable option, but only if you are committed to taking anticlotting medication for the long term and are not at high bleeding risk.

Don't forget that stenting is not the only way to relieve angina pain and reduce heart attack risk. For example, some people with mild coronary heart disease can safely manage the illness with medication alone, without fear of putting themselves at risk for a heart attack or death (see the "New Research" column on page 57).

The other alternative is bypass surgery. Though it's a major invasive procedure, surgery is highly effective at relieving angina for the long term, and it can lower heart-attack risk. Bypass surgery may be your best option if you have multiple obstructions in a coronary artery, narrowing in several coronary arteries, or diabetes.

The Last Word...for Now

Clearly there are many unknowns about drug-eluting stents. Ongoing studies will hopefully shed more light on who should get the stents and how best to lower the long-term risk of blood clots. Improvements in stents could also change things. For example, researchers are working on drug-eluting stents that dissolve after they've helped prevent restenosis.

For now, the best thing you can do is carefully discuss with your doctor the pros and cons of all the treatment options. You might also want to get a second opinion. ■

the complication rate depends on many other factors as well, and doctors who perform fewer angioplasties can still have low complication rates if they perform the procedure only on patients at low risk for complications.

Bypass Surgery

Each year, more than 400,000 people in the United States undergo coronary artery bypass graft surgery (often called CABG or, simply, bypass surgery) to improve blood flow to the heart. During the surgery, a blood vessel from elsewhere in the body (usually an artery from the chest or a vein from the leg or arm) is sewn into the aorta of the heart and used to reroute blood around a section of a coronary artery narrowed by atherosclerosis. When needed, five or more of these bypass grafts can be performed during a single operation. Cardiologists often recommend bypass surgery when there are blockages in all three of the major coronary arteries.

In most cases, at least one of the bypass grafts is constructed using a blood vessel called the left internal mammary artery (LIMA), which provides blood to the left side of the chest wall. The surgeon surgically detaches one end of the LIMA from the chest wall and sews it into the coronary artery at a point beyond the blockage. A LIMA graft usually lasts 20–30 years, compared with only about 10 years for a vein graft. A major reason for the better results with LIMA grafts is that they are less susceptible to the formation of new blockages.

How successful is bypass surgery? It is very effective, even in people who require several bypass grafts, have extensive heart disease, or are elderly. For example, about 90% of people who undergo bypass surgery experience relief of angina symptoms.

Despite the success of bypass surgery, and its ability to decrease the risk of having a heart attack, it is a major surgical procedure. It takes three to six hours to perform and requires general anesthesia, four to six days of hospitalization, and an additional six to 12 weeks for a full recovery.

Complications after surgery include heart attack (in 2–5% of patients); stroke, memory loss, or confusion (in 6% of patients); and infection (in 1–2% of patients). Deaths due to the procedure occur in less than 5% of operations, although the risk rises sharply when the patient's overall health is poor.

Off-pump bypass surgery

In traditional bypass surgery, the heart is stopped and the patient is placed on a heart-lung machine that maintains blood circulation until the heartbeat is restarted. Many of the complications of bypass surgery result from this stoppage of the heart. But there is an alternative: beating-heart or off-pump bypass surgery. In this procedure, surgeons use suction or compression to immobilize only a small portion of the heart during the surgery, which eliminates the need to stop the heart from beating.

Studies suggest that the off-pump procedure is at least as effective as traditional bypass surgery and is associated with fewer immediate complications, such as blood loss and short-term cognitive (thinking) problems. However, off-pump bypass surgery may carry a higher risk of new blockages over the long term.

Bypass Surgery vs. Angioplasty

Angioplasty has several advantages over bypass surgery. It is a relatively simple procedure, there's no need for general anesthesia, and the risks of open heart surgery are avoided. In addition, after only a one-night hospital stay, you can resume your normal activities almost immediately. Angioplasty is also less expensive.

As we've already described, restenosis is a possibility with angioplasty. Thus, if you undergo this procedure, you must accept the possibility of needing another angioplasty procedure, or ultimately bypass surgery, to treat the restenosis. In comparison, bypass surgery keeps coronary arteries open longer and may produce better blood flow through these arteries. Bypass surgery generally provides good relief of angina for at least five years. Bypass surgery is usually favored over angioplasty for people with one or more of the following:

• **Narrowing of the left main coronary artery.** This blood vessel is the main artery supplying blood to the heart. Even a brief period of blockage of blood flow through this artery could damage the heart muscle and be fatal.

• **Narrowing of three or more vessels.** Bypass surgery is a better option than angioplasty when the buildup of plaque has caused multiple obstructions in an artery or has narrowed several arteries. This is because angioplasty is a more complex procedure to perform when the affected area is large and requires implanting several stents.

• **Narrowing at an arterial branch.** An arterial branch is where one artery meets another artery. Because angioplasty to remove plaque at this site may shift the plaque into an adjacent artery, which could cause a new blockage, bypass surgery is sometimes preferred.

• **Diabetes.** In a study conducted in the mid-1990s—the Bypass Angioplasty Revascularization Investigation (BARI)—the seven-year survival for people with diabetes was significantly better in those who

ASK THE DOCTOR

Q. ***How do I know if I'm having heart surgery at a top-notch hospital?***

A. Until recently it has been easier to shop for a high-quality car than for high-quality healthcare. Fortunately, a number of organizations are making performance records of hospitals available to consumers.

One of these is the Department of Health and Human Services, whose site www.hospitalcompare.hhs.gov ranks hospitals based on their adherence to treatment guidelines for certain conditions, including heart attacks and heart failure. The site also gives each hospital's death rates for these diseases.

The Joint Commission, which accredits hospitals, offers quality reports at www.qualitycheck.org that show how a hospital stacks up against others in its state and nationwide. Some websites focus on hospitals within a certain state: mhcc.maryland.gov/consumerinfo/hospitalguide/index.htm details Maryland hospitals; data on New York hospitals can be found at www.myhealthfinder.com.

Companies such as Health Grades (www.healthgrades.com) also offer reports rating hospitals according to various criteria, such as the ratio of nurses to patients.

But the data offered by all of these sites needs to be taken with a grain of salt. A higher death rate may simply be a sign that a hospital treats sicker patients—not that it offers subpar care. So what should you focus on? One of the most important factors is procedure volume. You want to choose a hospital in your area that performs heart surgery most often. If you can't find this information online, call local hospitals or ask your doctor.

underwent bypass surgery (76%) than in those who had angioplasty (56%). Subsequent research confirms this finding: A 2007 report from the BARI study found that among people with diabetes who had narrowing in multiple coronary arteries, 10-year survival was better with bypass surgery than with angioplasty.

Drawbacks of bypass surgery include longer hospital stays and longer rehabilitation times than with angioplasty. In addition, a study of 261 bypass surgery patients found that about 40% had a decline in their mental abilities that persisted five years after surgery. It's possible, however, that this decline was caused by underlying cardiovascular disease rather than the surgery itself.

Except in an emergency situation, you have time to get a second opinion when deciding between angioplasty and bypass surgery. Getting that second opinion will help you feel more confident that you have made the right decision. Your doctor will not be offended if you seek a second opinion. When it comes to major surgery, most doctors expect their patients to seek another assessment of their disease and the best way to treat it.

Other Revascularization Procedures

Besides bypass surgery and angioplasty, other, newer procedures such as atherectomy, laser ablation, and enhanced external counterpulsation (EECP) are sometimes used to improve blood flow through the coronary arteries to the heart.

Atherectomy

This procedure removes plaque from the inside of arteries. It involves a high-speed rotary blade or drill that shaves away portions of plaque that are narrowing a coronary artery. Using a catheter, the blade or drill is delivered to the site of the blockage.

Atherectomy is often done before angioplasty to remove some of the plaque. The procedure works best on large, straight arteries. The blade is preferred when plaque is limited to one side of the artery; the drill typically produces better results for very long obstructions.

Serious complications with atherectomy are rare but may include unexpected vessel closure or a heart attack.

Laser ablation

This procedure is similar to angioplasty, but instead of a balloon at the tip of the catheter there is a probe. The probe is heated with a beam of laser light that cuts through the plaque and burns it away. The greatest risk is accidentally making a hole in the artery wall.

At present, laser ablation is rarely used to treat blockages in the coronary arteries. It may one day, however, prove useful in reopening completely blocked arteries or in destroying plaques that cannot be treated with angioplasty because the plaques are too long or too hardened by calcium deposits.

Enhanced external counterpulsation (EECP)

Some people with angina do not get sufficient pain relief from medication or angioplasty, and they cannot undergo bypass surgery because of poor health. For these individuals, a noninvasive procedure called EECP may improve angina symptoms and quality of life.

In EECP, you lie on a table and inflatable cuffs are placed around your calves, lower thighs, and upper thighs. While your heart activity is monitored by ECG, the cuffs are rapidly inflated in sequential order beginning with the ones at the calves. Cuff inflation is timed so that it occurs when the heart is at rest (when the heart muscle is receiving oxygen-rich blood from the coronary arteries). Then the cuffs are deflated to coincide with the heart's contractions (when oxygenated blood is pumped to the rest of the body).

EECP is an outpatient procedure and typically requires 35 sessions over six to seven weeks. Each session takes one to two hours. Some people require a second round of treatments. Researchers are uncertain why EECP helps decrease angina. One possibility is that it stimulates the growth of tiny coronary blood vessels, creating a natural bypass around the narrowed vessels that are causing angina pain.

People with uncontrolled heart failure, very high blood pressure, a heart rate faster than 120 beats per minute at rest, lung disease, or a history of phlebitis (vein inflammation) should not undergo EECP. Possible side effects include flushing or chafing of the skin. Five-year follow-up studies show that EECP has long-lasting benefits.

Complications of Coronary Heart Disease

Even if you make changes in your lifestyle, take the medication your doctor recommends, and possibly undergo revascularization treatments to improve blood flow through your coronary arteries, CHD complications may develop. This section describes some of the most common complications and how they are diagnosed and treated. These complications are acute coronary syndromes, heart failure, and arrhythmias (irregular heart rhythms).

ASK THE DOCTOR

Q. ***What's the latest on stem cells for treating coronary heart disease?***

A. The use of stem cells to regenerate damaged heart tissue remains far from prime time, but some progress has been made.

Most of the studies have used stem cells taken from patients' own bone marrow. Such "adult" stem cells do not have the same capacity that embryonic stem cells do for developing into any tissue in the body, but they do have the advantage of coming from the patient's own body, which eliminates the risk of immune system rejection. Adult stem cells also skirt the ethical issues surrounding the use of stem cells from human embryos.

In one recent German trial of 204 people, bone marrow stem cells or a placebo were infused directly into participants' coronary arteries within seven days of a heart attack. The stem cell infusion improved the pumping ability of the left ventricle and lowered the risk of dying or suffering another heart attack over the next year.

When a similar procedure was carried out in 100 Norwegian patients, however, no benefits were detected in those receiving the bone marrow stem cells. Also, researchers are uncertain whether stem cells are morphing into heart muscle cells or having some other effect on the heart.

Researchers are also investigating other sources of cells. At Johns Hopkins, doctors are taking human stem cells from the heart, growing them in the lab, and injecting them into the injured hearts of mice. The result: an increase in the regeneration of the mice's heart tissue.

Acute Coronary Syndromes

Unstable angina and heart attacks are known as acute coronary syndromes.

Unstable angina

Unstable angina is chest pain resulting from a blood clot or a coronary artery spasm that interferes with the flow of blood and oxygen to the heart. The chest pain is more severe than that of regular angina, occurs more frequently (sometimes at rest), and cannot be relieved easily by rest or medication. It may persist for more than 20 minutes and limits ordinary activity. Because unstable angina can lead to a heart attack, you should treat it as an emergency. Call 911 and contact your doctor at once if you experience this type of chest pain.

Diagnosis. To diagnose unstable angina, a doctor will take a complete medical history, including questions about your chest pain: When did it start? Did it occur at rest? Were you able to do anything to relieve the pain? Have you experienced similar pain in the past? A number of tests may be conducted, including an electrocardiogram (ECG), blood tests, and angiography. Echocardiography may also be performed to evaluate changes in the heart's functioning associated with reduced blood flow to the heart. Blood tests may include measurements of substances like creatine kinase and troponin, which are proteins released into the bloodstream when heart damage occurs.

Treatment. An episode of unstable angina often requires hospitalization. At the hospital, an anticoagulant drug called heparin is given intravenously along with aspirin to reduce the risk of blood clots. Intravenous nitroglycerin is also administered to help dilate the coronary arteries and reduce chest pain. Drugs like calcium channel blockers or beta-blockers may be given to decrease episodes of reduced blood flow to the heart.

After unstable angina is brought under control at the hospital, long-term management of the condition may involve regular use of aspirin and, sometimes, Plavix. Both aspirin and Plavix help prevent blood clots that can cause a heart attack. Longer-acting nitrates should be taken to widen blood vessels, and beta-blockers may be prescribed to decrease the workload of the heart. Angioplasty or bypass surgery may be needed when these medications fail to prevent subsequent episodes of unstable angina. However, many patients undergo angiography and angioplasty shortly after being admitted to the hospital with unstable angina.

Be Prepared for a Heart Attack

The steps that could save your life

Many people who are having a heart attack—even those who have had one before—wait too long to seek help. This delay may increase the extent of permanent damage to the heart and thus the chance of heart failure or death. Seek treatment immediately, even if your symptoms subside or you are not sure whether you are having a heart attack.

You can save time during a cardiac emergency by planning ahead. Here are some ways to prepare for a heart attack and possibly increase your chances of survival.

Know the Warning Signs

Not everyone who has a heart attack experiences the same symptoms. In fact, although some people have no symptoms, the most common ones are:

- chest discomfort (pressure, squeezing, fullness, or pain)
- pain radiating to the arms, back, neck, jaw, or stomach
- shortness of breath
- other symptoms, for example, sweating, nausea, vomiting, or lightheadedness.

Know What To Do

If you experience symptoms of a heart attack:

- Call 911 immediately. Because emergency medical personnel can begin treatment before you reach the hospital, transport to the hospital in an ambulance is the best way to receive prompt care. If calling 911 is not possible, have someone drive you to the hospital. Never drive yourself unless you have no other alternative.
- While waiting for help to arrive, chew a regular-dose aspirin to help prevent blood clots. Wash the aspirin down with a glass of water.
- If you've been prescribed nitroglycerin tablets or spray for angina, take one to three doses to see whether symptoms are relieved.
- Lie down, breathe deeply and slowly, and try to stay calm.

Consider Developing an Action Plan

If you are at high risk for a heart attack, consider some of the following suggestions:

- Think through what you would do if you had a heart attack in various situations, such as at home or while driving.
- Decide who would take care of any dependents. Make sure these back-up people are willing to help out in an emergency.
- Write down a list of medications you are currently taking, medications you are allergic to, your doctors' phone numbers (both during and after office hours), and contact information for a friend or relative. Keep copies of this information in several places, such as at home, at work, in your car, and in your wallet or purse.
- Give instructions to your family and friends. Tell them the warning signs of a heart attack and what to do if you experience these signs. Encourage them to take a cardiopulmonary resuscitation (CPR) class so that they can provide assistance if your breathing or heartbeat stops before the ambulance arrives.
- Keep a bottle of aspirin in your home, car, office, and toiletry bag. A cell phone may also be a good idea in case you need to call for help. ■

Heart attack

A heart attack typically occurs when a blood clot in a coronary artery completely blocks blood flow to a segment of the heart. When this blockage takes place, portions of the heart muscle are deprived of oxygen and become permanently damaged. Damage to the heart muscle can impair the ability of the heart to pump blood efficiently, which can lead to heart failure. The impaired blood flow can also damage the electrical system of the heart and lead to arrhythmias.

Symptoms. The most frequent signs of a heart attack include:

- Uncomfortable pressure, fullness, squeezing, or pain in the

center of the chest that lasts longer than 10 minutes
- Pain spreading to the jaw, neck, shoulders, arms (especially the left arm), back, or upper abdomen
- Chest discomfort accompanied by lightheadedness, intense sweating, nausea, shortness of breath, or fainting.

Not everyone experiences the same heart attack symptoms. Men are more likely to feel severe pain and pressure in the chest, while women typically have pain in the shoulders, upper back, neck, and jaw. Women are also more likely to have vague symptoms, such as mild chest pain, shortness of breath, dizziness, heartburn, or nausea. Many men and women experience no pain at all.

What to do. If you think that you might be having a heart attack, you need to get immediate medical help by dialing 911 to call for an ambulance. Up to a half of all deaths from heart attacks occur within the first hour, but your chances of survival are greatly improved with prompt medical attention. If an ambulance cannot arrive within 20–30 minutes, someone should drive you to the nearest emergency room. You should never drive yourself to the hospital, unless there is absolutely no other alternative. While waiting for the ambulance, chew a regular-dose aspirin to reduce the risk of blood clotting; don't forget to tell the paramedics that you've taken an aspirin.

In the ambulance. On the way to the hospital, the paramedics will evaluate you and begin treating your symptoms. They may administer oxygen, give nitrates and aspirin, begin cardiopulmonary resuscitation (CPR) in the event of cardiac arrest, and treat arrhythmias.

At the hospital. If an ECG indicates complete blockage of a large coronary artery, you may be taken directly to the catheterization laboratory. Most often, however, you will be taken to the coronary care unit. Morphine is usually given to relieve pain, provide sedation, and reduce the heart's need for oxygen. You will be attached to an ECG monitor to detect arrhythmias that may require treatment.

Meanwhile, a series of tests will be performed to confirm whether you are having a heart attack. Blood tests will be conducted, looking for enzymes (creatine kinase-MB and troponin) that enter the bloodstream when damage occurs to the heart muscle. Depending on the levels of these enzymes, doctors may be able to determine when the heart attack began. An echocardiogram may be performed to evaluate damage to the heart muscle, and an angiogram may be done to identify any narrowing of the coronary arteries.

Treatment. The treatment options for a heart attack include:

Thrombolytic therapy. When a heart attack is diagnosed early, usually within 12 hours of the onset of symptoms, a thrombolytic (clot-dissolving) drug will be administered intravenously. This medication helps open the blocked coronary artery by dissolving the clot impeding blood flow. Studies show that thrombolytic therapy can restore blood flow through the blocked artery, reduce the amount of damage to the heart muscle, and improve survival after a heart attack.

However, there are drawbacks to thrombolytic therapy, including failure to open the artery in about 20% of patients as well as potentially serious side effects such as bleeding (especially in the brain) in up to 5% of people. If thrombolytic therapy is given and fails to open the blocked artery, then emergency angioplasty or bypass surgery may be performed (see below).

Intravenous heparin is usually administered with or after thrombolytic therapy to reduce the likelihood of further clot formation. Heparin is generally continued for 24–48 hours, and a daily aspirin is taken indefinitely thereafter.

Emergency angioplasty/bypass surgery. In some patients, doctors choose to perform an emergency angioplasty if the obstructed artery needs to be opened as rapidly as possible. Several recent studies show that blocked arteries are more likely to remain open in people who undergo emergency angioplasty than in those who receive thrombolytic therapy immediately following a heart attack.

Both angioplasty and thrombolytic therapy are similarly effective at preventing heart muscle damage if the artery is opened. However, angioplasty can be done much faster in an emergency setting and is better at preventing recurrent ischemia (insufficient blood supply to the heart), future heart attacks, and heart-related deaths. Emergency angioplasty also appears preferable to thrombolytic therapy for people who have the highest risk of death—for example, those older than age 75, those who have damage to the front portion of the heart, or those who have sustained low blood pressure.

Not all hospitals are equipped to carry out emergency angioplasty. While it's advisable for an ambulance to take you to a hospital that can perform angioplasty, the emergency medical technicians will weigh this against the extra time it may take to reach that hospital. In fact, in some states, the ambulance is required by law to take you to the nearest hospital—whether or not that hospital can carry out emergency angioplasty.

Doctors will consider performing emergency bypass surgery when thrombolytic treatment does not dissolve the clot and angiography shows that blockages cannot be treated effectively with angioplasty—for example, in patients with multiple blockages, most physicians will recommend bypass surgery rather than angioplasty.

NEW RESEARCH

Diabetes Drug May Boost Heart Attack Risk

The widely prescribed diabetes drug rosiglitazone (Avandia) may increase the risk of heart attacks and, possibly, death from heart disease, according to an analysis of 42 clinical trials.

Avandia users were 43% more likely to suffer a heart attack than those not taking the drug. There was also a higher risk of death from any cardiovascular cause, although the numbers were small: 39 deaths in more than 15,000 Avandia users and 22 in 12,000-plus people not taking the drug.

These findings are controversial, since not all studies have shown an increased heart attack risk with Avandia. An advisory panel for the FDA reviewed the studies and recommended that the drug remain on the market but with a stronger warning about heart attack risk.

The advisory panel's review revealed that the risk of heart attacks with Avandia appears to be greatest in people with diabetes who have heart failure or other cardiovascular diseases or who are taking insulin or nitrates (for chest pain). The other thiazolidinedione diabetes drug pioglitazone (Actos) does not appear to be associated with an increased risk of heart attacks, according to the panel.

If you are concerned about your use of Avandia, do not stop taking it unless your doctor determines that the risks outweigh the benefits in your case.

THE NEW ENGLAND JOURNAL OF MEDICINE
Volume 356, page 2457
June 14, 2007

Risk stratification. Early in your hospital stay, you will be risk stratified, which means that you will undergo tests to assess your risk of future CHD events. The results of these tests help your doctor determine whether angioplasty or bypass surgery (if it hasn't already been performed) is needed before you leave the hospital.

Coronary angiography is an important part of the risk stratification process. In addition, your left ventricular function will be assessed, either during angiography or by echocardiography. In some cases of mild heart attacks or when angiography is not appropriate, a low-level exercise stress test will be carried out five to seven days after a heart attack. Risk stratification also takes into account your likelihood of developing serious complications associated with heart attacks, such as heart failure and arrhythmias.

Not everyone will benefit from having an invasive procedure after a heart attack. One recent clinical trial found that for certain patients, angioplasty performed three or more days after a heart attack offered no advantage over drug therapy. These patients had a complete blockage in a major coronary artery but were in stable condition and not suffering any chest pain at the time of angioplasty. People with continuing chest pain after a heart attack, however, may need angioplasty or bypass surgery.

Cardiac rehabilitation. For years, the popular belief was that a heart attack signaled the end of an active, healthy life. Today, however, cardiac rehabilitation is an important component of recovery after a heart attack (as well as after undergoing bypass surgery or angioplasty). Indeed, many people who follow a rehabilitation plan prescribed by their doctor are healthier and more active than they were before the heart attack.

In-hospital rehabilitation. Typically, rehabilitation begins while you're still in the hospital. You'll be encouraged to begin moving around within a day or two of the heart attack. You'll be instructed to do this slowly: first, sitting up in bed; then, sitting in a chair; next, performing simple range-of-motion exercises; and finally, taking short walks around the room or down the hallway. During these activities, the function of your heart will be closely monitored.

You'll also be given information on improving your diet, quitting smoking, and other lifestyle measures to help decrease the risk of future heart attacks. Psychological counseling may be available to help cope with the emotional stresses of a heart attack.

Outpatient rehabilitation. If your recovery is uneventful and angioplasty or bypass surgery was not necessary, you'll probably be discharged from the hospital in less than a week. (A longer stay may be needed if you've undergone bypass surgery or developed complications such as arrhythmias, heart failure, or recurrent chest pain.) Before leaving the hospital, your doctor will recommend an outpatient rehabilitation program.

In an outpatient rehabilitation program, you will work on improving your physical strength and endurance, minimizing the risk of future angina episodes or heart attacks, managing your weight, easing back into your daily routines, and improving your quality of life and understanding of your heart condition.

The main component of all rehabilitation programs is supervised exercise. With the help of a nurse or physical therapist you will gradually work up to a standard aerobic workout—five to 10 minutes of warm-up, 20–30 minutes of aerobic activity (such as walking, jogging, or swimming), and five minutes of cool-down—at least three times a week. The pace and type of workout will be personally tailored to you, taking into consideration the condition of your heart and any other illnesses you may have. Light weight training may be included.

The major advantage of an outpatient rehabilitation program is continual encouragement to improve your lifestyle habits. In addition, most people find it helpful to share their experiences with the other heart attack survivors in the program. If possible, you should participate in an outpatient program for at least two months. To increase your chances of keeping your new habits over the long term, some programs offer a maintenance phase (usually six to 12 months long) that continues even after participants have recuperated enough to return to work and other normal activities.

Heart Failure

Heart failure is caused by a weakening of the heart's ability to pump blood. Between 500,000 and 900,000 new cases are diagnosed each year in the United States. The most common cause of heart failure is heart damage due to CHD or high blood pressure. Less often, heart failure is caused by heart valve abnormalities or infection of the heart valves or heart muscle. Sometimes, the cause of heart failure cannot be pinpointed.

Symptoms

If you have heart failure, you may experience fatigue, shortness of breath, fluid retention, and excessive urination at night. Initially, the symptoms are mild—for example, feeling overly tired after physical exertion—but eventually even slight activity becomes exhausting.

NEW RESEARCH

Chest Compressions Alone Better for Cardiac Arrest?

Victims of cardiac arrest stand a better chance of surviving if a bystander performs only chest compressions and forgoes mouth-to-mouth ventilation, a study suggests.

Japanese researchers found that of 4,068 adults who had a cardiac arrest outside the hospital, those who received chest compressions alone were twice as likely to survive with good brain function 30 days later as those who received standard CPR (22% vs. 10%).

The findings go against the long-held principles of CPR, which combine chest compressions and "rescue breaths." But they also support what a number of experts have said for years: Mouth-to-mouth resuscitation does little for cardiac arrest victims and may actually dim their already low odds of survival. What's more, mouth-to-mouth ventilation is often a barrier to bystanders initiating CPR.

Chest compressions are vital to keep blood flowing to and from the heart until medical help arrives; stopping to deliver rescue breaths may impede this blood flow.

Though these study results have spurred calls for revamped CPR recommendations, guidelines from the American Heart Association still advise rescue breaths (two breaths after every 30 chest compressions) for all cardiac arrest victims. We advise that you follow the AHA recommendations.

THE LANCET
Volume 369, page 920
March 17, 2007

As fluid accumulates in the lower extremities, swelling of the feet, ankles, legs, and, sometimes, the abdomen may occur.

Fluid may also settle in the lungs, particularly when you are lying down. This causes extreme shortness of breath that may awaken you at night; sitting up may relieve this symptom. Severe shortness of breath, accompanied by wheezing, coughing, and blood-tinged phlegm, is a sign of pulmonary edema (marked buildup of fluid in the lungs) and requires immediate medical treatment. Older people with heart failure may also experience lightheadedness or confusion.

Your doctor may use the following system, developed by the New York Heart Association, to classify the severity of your heart failure:

- **Class I:** No symptoms and no limitation in ordinary physical activity.
- **Class II:** Mild symptoms and slight limitation in ordinary physical activity. Comfortable at rest.
- **Class III:** Marked limitation of ordinary physical activity. Comfortable only at rest.
- **Class IV:** Discomfort occurs with any physical activity, and symptoms of heart failure may occur at rest.

Diagnosis

There is no specific test to diagnose heart failure. Your doctor will begin with a medical history and physical examination, looking for the characteristic symptoms—swollen ankles, shortness of breath, fatigue, and weight gain associated with fluid buildup. The doctor will use a stethoscope to listen to the heart and lungs (to detect any abnormal sounds that may indicate fluid accumulation in the lungs). Blood and urine tests will also be performed, such as a test to measure the hormone B-type natriuretic peptide (BNP). Blood levels of BNP are increased in people with heart failure. An ECG and an exercise stress test may be performed, as well as an echocardiogram to get images of the heart's function.

Treatment

You and your doctor have many options for managing heart failure. In the early stages, lifestyle measures and medications are usually all that are needed to keep symptoms under control. But as the disease becomes more severe, you may need more advanced treatments, such as implantable devices, to improve heart function.

Lifestyle measures. The first steps in the treatment of heart failure may include limits on the amount of fluids consumed (including alcohol) and reductions in dietary sodium (no more than 2,000 mg a day). In addition, follow your doctor's instructions on getting regular exercise, which can help prevent symptoms from worsening.

Medications. A variety of drugs may be used to manage heart failure. The medications your doctor prescribes will depend on your specific condition, including the severity of your heart failure, its cause, and the presence of other health problems. Here's a look at the key drugs for heart failure patients:

ACE inhibitors. These drugs—such as enalapril (Vasotec) and lisinopril (Prinivil, Zestril)—are the cornerstone of drug treatment for people with heart failure. ACE inhibitors promote dilation of the blood vessels and thus improve blood flow and slow the progression of CHD. They can also reduce blood pressure and lighten the workload on the heart.

Diuretics and digoxin. Your physician may prescribe diuretics to reduce fluid buildup and digoxin (Lanoxin) to strengthen the heartbeat. Thiazide diuretics are effective for mild heart failure, but more potent drugs such as the loop diuretic furosemide (Lasix) are used for severe fluid retention. People whose heart failure does not respond to a single diuretic may require a combination of several types of diuretic drugs, each with a different mechanism of action.

Beta-blockers. These drugs—such as carvedilol (Coreg) and metoprolol (Toprol XL)—can also decrease the workload of the heart. In an analysis of data from 17 separate studies, researchers concluded that the risk of death from all causes was 31% lower in heart failure patients treated with beta-blockers than in those not receiving such medications. In three other large trials, Coreg reduced deaths and total hospitalizations by 19–49% when added to standard treatment for heart failure.

Eplerenone (Inspra). This newer drug option for people with heart failure blocks the activity of aldosterone (an adrenal hormone associated with sodium retention). Inspra is prescribed to people who develop heart failure after a heart attack; it can reduce the risk of hospitalization and death from cardiovascular disease.

Implantable devices. A special cardiac pacemaker—called a biventricular pacemaker—is sometimes used in patients with moderate to severe heart failure who have not responded to medication and have delays in the conduction of electrical impulses in their heart. Implanted in the chest, this device delivers electrical impulses to the heart to improve its pumping capacity, primarily by maintaining coordinated contractions of the ventricles.

Heart transplants. In individuals with class IV heart failure, a heart transplant may be needed if other treatments fail. Transplant

NEW RESEARCH

Untreated Sleep Apnea Tied to Heart Failure Death

Left untreated, sleep apnea—the nighttime breathing disorder—may hasten death from heart failure, a small Canadian study suggests.

Obstructive sleep apnea (OSA) occurs when the temporary collapse of soft tissues in the throat causes repeated stops and starts in breathing during sleep. Up to half of people with heart failure have OSA.

The study enrolled 164 people with heart failure: 37 had OSA but declined treatment; 14 with OSA were treated with continuous positive airway pressure (CPAP); and 113 were OSA free. Over three years, the death rate among those with untreated OSA was twice that of those without the disorder (24% vs. 12%).

In comparison, no deaths occurred among OSA patients treated with CPAP—though, given the small number of subjects in this group, it's not possible to conclude that CPAP prolongs the lives of people with heart failure.

Still, the findings provide further evidence of the toll OSA can take on the heart. The disorder is known to stress the cardiovascular system; it can raise blood pressure, trigger abnormal heart rhythms, and reduce the amount of blood pumped with each heartbeat. If you have OSA symptoms, such as chronic, loud snoring and daytime sleepiness, talk to your doctor about an evaluation for the disorder.

JOURNAL OF THE AMERICAN COLLEGE OF CARDIOLOGY
Volume 49, page 1625
April 17, 2007

Drugs for Heart Failure 2008

Drug type: Brand (generic)	Typical daily dosages*	How to take†	Monthly cost‡: Brand (generic)
ACE inhibitors			
Accupril (quinapril)	20–40 mg	One 10- or 20-mg tablet 2x/day on an empty stomach, 1 hour before or 2 hours after a meal or with a light, low-fat meal.	($44)
Altace (ramipril)	10 mg	One 5-mg capsule 2x/day with or without food. Swallow capsule whole.	$106
Capoten (captopril)	75–300 mg	One 25-, 50-, or 100-mg tablet 3x/day on an empty stomach 1 hour before meals.	$361 ($13–25)
Mavik (trandolapril)	4 mg	One 4-mg tablet 1x/day with or without food.	$39 ($34)
Monopril (fosinopril)	20–40 mg	One 20- or 40-mg tablet 1x/day with or without food.	$37–42 ($30–31)
Prinivil, Zestril (lisinopril)	5–20 mg	One 5-, 10-, or 20-mg tablet 1x/day with or without food.	$29–40 ($11–19)
Vasotec (enalapril)	5–40 mg	One 2.5-, 5-, 10-, or 20-mg tablet 2x/day with or without food.	$56–107 ($14–22)
Angiotensin II receptor blockers (ARBs)			
Atacand (candesartan)	4–32 mg	One 4-, 8-, 16-, or 32-mg tablet 1x/day with or without food.	$50–66
Diovan (valsartan)	160–320 mg	One 80- or 160-mg tablet 2x/day with or without food.	$127–128
Beta-blockers			
Coreg (carvedilol)	6.25–50 mg	One 3.125-, 6.25-, 12.5-, or 25-mg tablet 2x/day with food.	$116–118
Coreg CR (carvedilol, extended-release)	10–80 mg	One 10-, 20-, 40-, or 80-mg tablet 1x/day in morning with food. Swallow whole (do not crush or chew).	$118
Toprol XL (metoprolol, extended-release)	25–200 mg	One 25-, 50-, 100-, or 200-mg tablet 1x/day with or immediately after a meal. Swallow whole (do not crush or chew).	$28–65 ($23–182)

* These dosages represent the usual daily dosages for the treatment of heart failure. The precise effective dosage varies from person to person and depends on many factors. Do not make any changes to your medication without consulting your doctor.

† These instructions represent the typical way to take the medication. Your doctor's instructions may differ. Always follow your doctor's recommendations.

‡ Prices per drugstore.com.

Precautions	Most common side effects	Call your doctor if...
ACE inhibitors can raise potassium levels; do not take potassium supplements or use salt substitutes containing potassium without your doctor's knowledge. Do not take if you are pregnant or planning to become pregnant. To minimize dizziness, get up slowly from a seated or lying position and avoid dehydration.	Dry cough, dizziness, sore throat.	You experience a dry cough or symptoms of angioedema: swelling of your face, eyes, lips, or tongue, difficulty swallowing or breathing.
Same as for ACE inhibitors (see above).	Back pain, dizziness, cold-like symptoms such as sore throat and stuffy nose.	You experience symptoms of kidney problems: sudden weight gain and swelling of your arms, hands, legs, and feet.
Do not stop taking without consulting your doctor. To minimize dizziness, get up slowly from a seated or lying position and avoid alcohol. May reduce blood flow to the hands and feet, making them cold; to prevent this, dress warmly and avoid smoking. May mask symptoms of hypoglycemia (low blood sugar) in people with diabetes who are taking insulin or certain oral diabetes drugs.	Dizziness, drowsiness, diarrhea, trouble sleeping, dry eyes.	You experience symptoms of worsening heart failure: weight gain or worsening shortness of breath; symptoms of a very slow heart rate: persistent dizziness, faintness, unusual fatigue; changes in your blood glucose levels if you have diabetes.

continued on the next page

Drugs for Heart Failure 2008 (continued)

Drug type: Brand (generic)	Typical daily dosages*	How to take†	Monthly cost‡: Brand (generic)
Aldosterone blockers			
Aldactone (spironolactone)	25–200 mg	One 25-, 50-, or 100-mg tablet 1–2x/day. If the medication upsets your stomach, take it with milk or food. Take before 6 P.M. to prevent nighttime urination.	$25–129 ($13–70)
Inspra (eplerenone)	50 mg	One 50-mg tablet 1x/day with or without food.	$110
Vasodilator			
BiDil (isosorbide dinitrate/hydralazine)	60–120 mg isosorbide dinitrate/112.5–225 mg hydralazine	One or two 20-mg/37.5-mg tablets 3x/day. Can be taken with food if it upsets your stomach.	$176–352
Loop diuretics			
Bumex (bumetanide)	0.5–2 mg	One 0.5-, 1-, or 2-mg tablet 1x/day. If stomach upset occurs, take with food or milk. Take before 6 P.M. to prevent nighttime urination.	$21–49 ($9–19)
Demadex (torsemide)	10–200 mg	One or two 10-, 20-, or 100-mg tablets 1x/day with or without food. Take before 6 P.M. to prevent nighttime urination.	$32–241 ($20–152)
Lasix (furosemide)	20–600 mg	One or more 20-, 40-, or 80-mg tablets 1–2x/day with or without food. Take before 6 P.M. to prevent nighttime urination.	$12–124 ($9–18)
Digitalis glycoside			
Lanoxin (digoxin)	0.125–0.25 mg	One 0.125- or 0.25-mg tablet 1x/day with or without food.	$9–10 ($9)

* These dosages represent the usual daily dosages for the treatment of heart failure. The precise effective dosage varies from person to person and depends on many factors. Do not make any changes to your medication without consulting your doctor.

† These instructions represent the typical way to take the medication. Your doctor's instructions may differ. Always follow your doctor's recommendations.

‡ Prices per drugstore.com.

Precautions	Most common side effects	Call your doctor if...
Can raise blood potassium levels; do not take potassium supplements, use salt substitutes containing potassium, or eat large amounts of potassium-containing foods such as bananas and orange juice without your doctor's consent. Your doctor may monitor your blood potassium levels before you start an aldosterone blocker and periodically while you are on it. To minimize lightheadedness, get up slowly from a seated or lying position and avoid alcohol.	Drowsiness, lightheadedness, dizziness, stomach upset, diarrhea, nausea, vomiting, headache.	You experience any of the side effects listed at left.
Do not take with oral erectile dysfunction drugs such as sildenafil (Viagra), tadalafil (Cialis), or vardenafil (Levitra). Doing so can cause a potentially dangerous drop in blood pressure. To minimize lightheadedness, get up slowly from a seated or lying position, drink plenty of liquids (to prevent dehydration), and avoid alcohol.	Headache, lightheadedness. You can take acetaminophen (Tylenol) for headache.	You experience fainting, a fast irregular heartbeat, chest pain.
May increase blood glucose levels; if you have diabetes, check your blood glucose regularly. Your doctor may recommend that you take potassium supplements or eat foods high in potassium (such as bananas and orange juice) to prevent low blood potassium levels. To minimize dizziness and lightheadedness, get up slowly from a seated or lying position, drink plenty of liquids (to prevent dehydration), and avoid alcohol. *Lasix and Demadex only:* The bile acid sequestrants cholestyramine (Questran) and colestipol (Colestid) can decrease the absorption of Lasix and Demadex. If you are taking a bile acid sequestrant, take it 2 hours before or 2 hours after Lasix or Demadex.	Dizziness, lightheadedness, headache, blurred vision, loss of appetite, stomach upset, diarrhea, constipation.	You experience signs of dehydration or mineral loss: muscle cramps, weakness, confusion, severe dizziness, drowsiness, unusual dry mouth or thirst, persistent nausea or vomiting, fast or irregular heartbeat, unusual decrease in urine, fainting, numbness or tingling of the arms or legs, seizures.
Certain foods and medications should be avoided for at least 2 hours before and 2 hours after taking digoxin, because these foods and medications reduce absorption of digoxin. These include high-fiber foods, such as bran, and medications such as cholestyramine (Questran), colesevelam (Welchol), colestipol (Colestid), and psyllium (for example, Metamucil).	Nausea, vomiting, headache, loss of appetite, diarrhea.	You experience any of the side effects at left.

recipients should be younger than 60 years old and have no other major diseases like cancer or kidney disease that could shorten their lifespan.

Donor hearts are in short supply, and a mechanical pump called a left ventricular assist device (LVAD) can help the heart work more effectively until a donor heart becomes available. This device, which helps pump blood through the heart, was recently approved as a permanent therapy in people with class IV heart failure who are not candidates for a transplant and have an estimated one-year survival of less than 50%.

The success of heart transplants has improved significantly over the past decade: About 85% of transplant patients are alive after one year, and about 70% survive for at least five years. These improvements in survival are primarily the result of advances in the prevention and early detection of tissue rejection, which occurs when the immune system recognizes the donated heart as foreign and attempts to destroy it.

If you've undergone a heart transplant, your doctor will prescribe medications to suppress your immune system. These immunosuppressive drugs include cyclosporine (Neoral, Sandimmune), azathioprine (Imuran), and prednisone. You will also need to undergo biopsies of your heart on a regular basis to identify early rejection. In a biopsy, a small piece of tissue is removed from the heart and examined under the microscope. The biopsy is done under local anesthesia. It involves inserting a small tube into a vein in the groin or arm and advancing the tube to the heart.

Many people with a donor heart develop plaques in the coronary arteries of the new heart. This risk can be reduced by adopting the same lifestyle changes and taking the same medications that help prevent CHD in nontransplant patients. To monitor for CHD, heart transplant patients often undergo coronary angiography once a year.

Artificial hearts. In 2004, the FDA approved the first implantable artificial heart. It weighs about 2 lbs, is surgically implanted in the chest, and is powered by electricity that passes through intact skin from an external battery. The artificial heart mimics the activity of the heart by pumping blood throughout the body.

The artificial heart is for people with class IV heart failure who are waiting for a donor heart. The FDA approval was based on a study in which 81 patients with class IV heart failure had the artificial heart implanted. Of these patients, 79% survived until they were able to have a transplant, compared with 46% of 35 patients who did not receive the temporary artificial heart.

In 2006, a second artificial heart won a limited FDA approval known as humanitarian device exemption. The device, called the AbioCor implantable replacement heart, is approved for class IV heart failure patients who are ineligible for a heart transplant and are unlikely to live more than a month without intervention. Unlike the temporary artificial heart, which replaces the failing heart's ventricles and valves, the AbioCor heart is a permanent replacement for the entire heart.

Arrhythmias

Under normal circumstances, the heart beats about 60–80 times per minute, with coordinated electrical surges that keep the heart beating in a steady rhythm. But sometimes the heart beats irregularly—either too fast, too slow, or in an erratic rhythm. These abnormalities called arrhythmias can cause disruptive and frightening symptoms; in the worst case scenario, they can trigger cardiac arrest and death.

A normal heartbeat begins with an electrical signal generated by cells in the upper right part of the heart—a region called the sinus node. The sinus node is the heart's natural pacemaker, initiating the heartbeat. Arrhythmias occur when these signals or their transmission go awry.

The various types of arrhythmias are categorized according to two features: their site of origin and their effect on heart rate. Arrhythmias can originate in the atria (the upper chambers of the heart, which receive blood from the body); the atrioventricular (AV) node (a cluster of cells in the center of the heart that conducts electrical impulses from the atria to the ventricles); or the ventricles (the pumping chambers in the lower part of the heart). They can produce a heart rate that is too slow (bradycardia—under 60 beats a minute) or too fast (tachycardia—over 100 beats a minute at rest).

Common types

Atrial fibrillation, ventricular tachycardia, and ventricular fibrillation are common arrhythmias.

Atrial fibrillation. About one in four adults age 40 and older develop atrial fibrillation, a form of tachycardia. In atrial fibrillation the atria quiver (fibrillate) chaotically, instead of contracting normally, which causes the ventricles to contract irregularly and often rapidly. As a result, blood is not circulated efficiently throughout the body. The risk of atrial fibrillation increases with age. People with CHD, heart valve abnormalities, or an overactive thyroid (hyperthyroidism) also are at higher risk.

ASK THE DOCTOR

Q. ***Does having depression make heart failure worse?***

A. Your outlook after a diagnosis of heart failure does not depend just on your heart. Depression, which often accompanies heart failure, can worsen this heart condition.

One recent study of about 1,000 heart failure patients found that even those with mild depression had a higher risk of dying over the next 2.5 years than their nondepressed counterparts. Another trial found that depressed heart failure patients were more likely to be hospitalized or die over a three-year period, even when the severity of heart failure was factored in.

How might depression worsen heart failure? It can promote blood clots. It affects nervous system activity, which regulates blood pressure and heart rate. Also, depressed people tend to neglect their health—not exercising, eating well, taking medications, or seeing doctors as often as they should.

Depression can be difficult to recognize in people with heart failure because the two share symptoms like fatigue and appetite loss. But if you're feeling persistently sad or pessimistic about the future, talk to your doctor.

Depression is treatable. One recent study found that 12 weeks of antidepressant therapy improved depression and quality of life in heart failure patients, compared with a placebo. Nondrug options, like talk therapy, relaxation techniques, and exercise, also can improve quality of life. It's not known, however, whether successful treatment of depression improves the outcome of heart failure.

Common symptoms of atrial fibrillation include weakness, shortness of breath, lightheadedness, palpitations, and chest pain. However, some people have no symptoms. Atrial fibrillation can lead to blood clots in the atria. If these clots loosen and travel through the circulatory system, they can block arteries supplying blood to vital organs such as the brain.

Ventricular tachycardia and ventricular fibrillation. These arrhythmias are much more serious than atrial fibrillation. Both are caused by abnormal electrical signals that originate within the ventricles. These rhythm disturbances can occur during a heart attack or in the weeks or months afterward. This happens because damaged heart muscle releases substances that interfere with the normal conduction of electrical impulses in the heart.

In ventricular tachycardia, the heart beats at a rate of 100 beats a minute or more. This rapid heartbeat can cause symptoms such as palpitations, lightheadedness, dizziness, weakness, fainting, and dangerous drops in blood pressure, because the amount of blood pumped with each beat is significantly decreased. Depending on how fast the heart rate is, people with ventricular tachycardia can survive for hours without treatment. But ventricular tachycardia can progress to ventricular fibrillation, which is fatal if not treated promptly.

In ventricular fibrillation, the ventricles twitch rapidly and chaotically and thus are unable to pump blood throughout the body. As a result, ventricular fibrillation leads to unconsciousness within seconds. The person collapses, and cardiac arrest (sudden cessation of an effective heartbeat) can occur quickly, leading to death within a few minutes without treatment. More than 350,000 Americans die each year of sudden cardiac death associated with ventricular fibrillation.

Diagnosis

If your physician suspects that you have an arrhythmia, he or she will first take a medical history to find out whether you have any medical conditions or are taking any medications that could be causing the problem. The doctor will also listen to your heart with a stethoscope. The definitive test for diagnosing an arrhythmia is an electrocardiogram (ECG) obtained at the time of the arrhythmia. The ECG records the electrical pattern of the heart while you are lying down on an examination table at your physician's office. Your doctor might also check your heart rhythms with a Holter monitor, which records your ECG for 24 hours as you go about your daily activities.

Electrophysiological studies are also used to assess arrhythmias. Performed in a cardiac catheterization laboratory, these tests provide information about the electrical activity of the heart and allow the doctor to evaluate where the arrhythmia originates as well as its severity. In this procedure, a catheter is inserted into a vein in the groin and threaded into the heart. Local anesthesia is used to numb the area where the catheter is inserted. The catheter contains electrodes to record the heart's electrical activity. The electrodes can also be used to transmit electrical signals to the heart to reproduce arrhythmias. Medications are then administered intravenously and orally to determine which ones are the most effective at preventing or suppressing the arrhythmias.

Treatment

Arrhythmias can be treated in a number of ways. In many people, medication is helpful, although the drugs used can have serious side effects. Some types of arrhythmias require the administration of an electrical stimulus to the heart to return the heart to its normal rhythm—a technique called electrical cardioversion. In addition, an increasing number of arrhythmias are treated with radiofrequency catheter ablation or an implanted electrical device such as a pacemaker or cardioverter-defibrillator.

Medication. Drugs are used to suppress abnormal activity where the arrhythmia originates or to block the conduction of abnormal electrical impulses.

For example, beta-blockers and calcium channel blockers are frequently used to treat atrial fibrillation. These drugs slow the conduction of electrical impulses through the AV node (the relay station between the atria and ventricles) and reduce the response of the ventricles to the rapid rhythm of the atria. Another useful drug is ibutilide (Corvert), which may quickly return the heart to its normal rhythm. Antiarrhythmic drugs such as procainamide (Pronestyl and other brands), sotalol (Betapace, Sorine), amiodarone (Cordarone, Pacerone), flecainide (Tambocor), and propafenone (Rythmol) may be used to control atrial fibrillation.

Be aware that these antiarrhythmic medications have potentially serious adverse effects—for example, bradycardia (slowed heart rate) and hypothyroidism (a deficiency in the body's thyroid hormone production). Aspirin or warfarin also is prescribed to people with atrial fibrillation to reduce the risk of blood clots in the heart that could lead to a stroke.

The most effective drug for controlling ventricular arrhythmias

NEW RESEARCH

Blood Pressure Numbers Signal Atrial Fibrillation Risk

The difference between the two numbers in your blood pressure reading may predict your odds of developing atrial fibrillation (AF), research suggests.

In a study that followed more than 5,300 adults from the Framingham Heart Study for two decades, the odds of developing AF rose in tandem with pulse pressure—the difference between the numbers for systolic and diastolic blood pressures.

Normal pulse pressure is about 40, as in the case of someone who has a blood pressure reading of 120/80 mm Hg. Pulse pressure is an indirect way to gauge stiffness in the aorta, the main artery supplying blood to the body. The higher the pulse pressure, the greater the arterial stiffness—and, as the new findings suggest, the greater the risk of AF.

For every 20-point increase in pulse pressure, the odds of developing the heart arrhythmia went up by one quarter. That was after adjusting for other factors that influence AF risk, including age, smoking, and diabetes.

The results suggest that pulse pressure is an important risk factor for AF. Because a high pulse pressure typically results from a rise in systolic blood pressure (the upper number), controlling your systolic pressure through diet, exercise, and medication (if necessary) may also reduce your pulse pressure.

JOURNAL OF THE AMERICAN MEDICAL ASSOCIATION
Volume 297, page 709
February 21, 2007

Zapping Abnormal Heart Rhythms

Catheter ablation gaining ground as a treatment for atrial fibrillation

For people with the heart rhythm disorder atrial fibrillation (AF), the traditional treatment route is to try various medications first and opt for invasive procedures such as open-heart surgery as a last resort. Now a middle-of-the-road option, a minimally invasive procedure known as catheter ablation, is growing in popularity.

In fact, in their latest guidelines for AF, the American College of Cardiology (ACC) and the American Heart Association (AHA) list catheter ablation as a "second-tier" therapy—meaning physicians can consider it after just one antiarrhythmic drug has not controlled heart rhythm, rather than exhausting all medication options. In fact, catheter ablation may allow people with AF to stop taking antiarrhythmic drugs altogether.

Traditional Route

Traditionally, when medications to slow heart rate, such as beta-blockers, calcium channel blockers, and digoxin (Lanoxin, Lanoxicaps), and drugs to regulate heart rhythm, such as amiodarone (Cordarone, Pacerone), flecainide (Tambocor), and sotalol (Betapace, Sorine), did not control AF or caused intolerable or dangerous side effects, an operation known as the Maze procedure was considered.

In this procedure, a surgeon makes small incisions on the heart to create scar tissue that interferes with the abnormal electrical signals. The technique is highly successful in suppressing AF but is not widely used because it requires open-heart surgery.

Catheter Ablation Procedure

Like the Maze procedure, catheter ablation aims to correct the abnormal electrical signals but does so without major surgery. During the procedure, an electrophysiologist (a doctor who specializes in heart rhythm disturbances) inserts a catheter (a long, flexible tube) into a vein, typically in the groin, and threads it up to the heart. A special x-ray technique called fluoroscopy is used to visualize the catheter on a video screen.

Once positioned in the left atrium, electrodes at the catheter's tip gather data that allow the doctor to pinpoint the pathway that generates and maintains the abnormal electrical activity. After these "hot spots" are mapped, radiofrequency waves, delivered through a separate catheter, are used to heat and destroy tiny areas of tissue. The result: scar tissue that blocks the aberrant electrical signals.

The procedure is performed in an electrophysiology lab in a hospital. Patients generally receive a sedative as well as a local anesthetic to numb the area where the catheters will be inserted. The procedure is usually not painful, but some people experience chest discomfort while the radiofrequency energy is applied. In all, the process typically takes several hours.

Afterward, patients are required to lie still for a few hours and then spend the night in the hospital for monitoring of their heart rhythm and rate. Most people can resume their normal activities a couple of days after returning home.

Because it takes time for scar tissue to form after the ablation, people often take antiarrhythmic drugs for a few months to suppress any AF episodes. In some individuals, continued medication or a repeat ablation is necessary to become fully AF free.

Catheter Ablation Studies

When catheter ablation was first introduced for AF in the mid-1990s, it had limited effectiveness. But in 1998, researchers discovered that many of the aberrant electrical signals originate around the pulmonary veins, which drain blood from the lungs back to the heart. Since then, researchers have been modifying the catheter ablation technique to make it both safer and more effective.

The latest research suggests that AF episodes are safely suppressed in 75–80% of patients one year after the procedure. In contrast, only about half of people on antiarrhythmic medications remain AF free for a year, and they often experience drug side effects.

One 2006 study, in *The New England Journal of Medicine*, reported on 146 adults with chronic AF. Half (the control group) were randomly assigned to treatment with the rhythm-regulating drug amiodarone plus two cardioversions if necessary. The rest also had catheter ablation. One year later, 75% of the ablation patients were free of AF and did not need antiarrhythmic medication. Ablation had to be repeated, however, in one third of the ablation group. In contrast, three quarters of the patients in the control group had recurrent AF and opted to have the ablation procedure.

In another study, researchers focused on ablation for people with paroxysmal (periodic) AF. All 198 patients had been suffering an average of three AF episodes a month for six years and had failed to improve with antiarrhythmic drugs. Patients were assigned to undergo catheter ablation or to try a different medication. After a year, 93% of ablation patients had maintained a normal heart rhythm vs. 35% of those given a new drug.

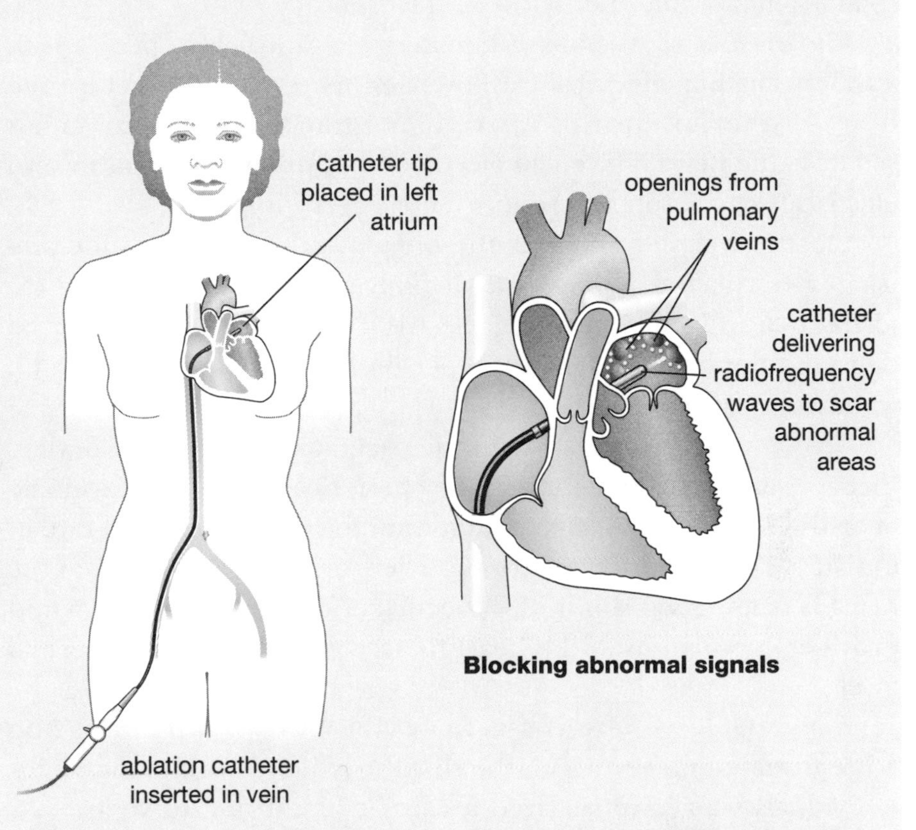

Blocking abnormal signals

Risks and Long-Term Benefits
Major complications from catheter ablation are uncommon, but there is a small risk of a blood clot traveling from the heart to the brain or elsewhere in the body. There's also a small chance that the catheter will puncture the heart wall or the radiofrequency energy will damage the esophagus, which lies behind the left atrium.

Long-term benefits of catheter ablation are unclear—including whether the procedure prevents strokes, lowers the risk of death, or allows people to go off antiarrhythmic medication indefinitely. Also unclear is whether you can safely stop taking blood-thinning medication. Current recommendations are to remain on warfarin (Coumadin) for at least two months after the procedure—and for the long term if you have risk factors for stroke besides AF.

Is It for You?
According to the new ACC/AHA guidelines, an antiarrhythmic drug should be your first choice. But if medication fails to suppress your AF episodes or if the side effects are intolerable, you and your doctor can consider catheter ablation.

The procedure can be safely and effectively performed in people of almost any age, with either periodic or chronic AF, as long as the left atrium is not significantly enlarged and no blood clots are detected in the left atrium. That said, the risk of complications does rise with age, and the outcome is better in people with only periodic AF symptoms.

Many people mistakenly believe they'll be able to discontinue anticoagulant therapy, such as warfarin, after the procedure. But this is true only for those at very low stroke risk. People at high risk—those over age 75, those with a prior stroke or transient ischemic attack, and those with heart failure, high blood pressure, or diabetes—must continue warfarin indefinitely, even if the procedure is successful. Thus, a desire to discontinue warfarin is not a valid reason for undergoing catheter ablation.

What the Future Holds
The catheter ablation procedure is still evolving, and the safety and efficacy of the procedure will likely continue to improve. But if you decide to have catheter ablation today, be sure to choose a doctor who is highly experienced in the procedure—an electrophysiologist who performs at least 20–40 procedures a year. The experience of the hospital is important, too. Look for one that has performed more than 100 catheter ablations. ■

varies from person to person. These drugs include procainamide, sotalol, amiodarone, Tambocor, and Rythmol.

Electrical cardioversion. When drug therapy fails in people with atrial fibrillation, electrical cardioversion may be tried to return the heart rhythm to normal. After administration of an intravenous sedative, the heart is given an electrical shock that interrupts its own electrical activity and may restore a normal rhythm.

Electrical cardioversion is the only effective treatment for ventricular fibrillation. With the availability of portable automated external defibrillators, life-saving electrical cardioversion can now be delivered not only by emergency personnel but also by anyone who witnesses a cardiac arrest.

Artificial pacemakers. Artificial pacemakers are small devices that are surgically implanted in the chest. Leads from the pacemaker to the heart provide electrical stimuli to control the heart rate in individuals with bradycardia or disorders of the AV node. When the heart is beating too slowly, the pacemaker detects the problem and provides stimulation to the heart to accelerate its rate to a normal level.

Implantable cardioverter-defibrillator (ICD). An ICD can stop a life-threatening ventricular arrhythmia. It is recommended for individuals who have survived a cardiac arrest due to ventricular fibrillation, experienced other life-threatening ventricular arrhythmias, or are at high risk for ventricular arrhythmias (because they have had a heart attack that severely affected the function of the heart's left ventricle).

The ICD constantly monitors the heart's rhythm. When it detects a dangerous rhythm, it delivers an electrical shock that returns the heart to its normal rhythm. The shocks can be startling and even painful, but the discomfort lasts only for a short time.

Implantation of an ICD is a surgical procedure performed under local anesthesia. It generally requires a stay in the hospital of two to three days so doctors can test the device. Most ICDs also have a pacemaker component so that a single device can be used to treat people who have more than one type of arrhythmia.

Radiofrequency catheter ablation. This is an increasingly popular method to suppress tachycardias that originate in the atria, such as atrial fibrillation (see "Zapping Abnormal Heart Rhythms" on pages 80–81), and a similar but less common condition called atrial flutter. Ablation can also be used for ventricular tachycardias, although this is less common.

The procedure requires an electrophysiological study to detect

NEW RESEARCH

Shorter Driving Limits for Some Users of Implantable Defibrillators

If you receive an implantable cardioverter-defibrillator (ICD), you may be back to driving in less time than you think.

Updated guidelines from the American Heart Association (AHA) now say that people who receive an ICD for purely preventive reasons can start driving again one week after surgery. This recommendation refers to individuals who have an ICD implanted because they have risk factors for, but have not yet suffered, the dangerous heart rhythm disturbances ventricular fibrillation (VF) or ventricular tachycardia (VT), which can lead to loss of consciousness and death.

The recommendation differs substantially from the long-standing (and unchanged) guideline for people who receive an ICD for "secondary prevention"—meaning they've already suffered VF or VT and thus are at higher risk for cardiac arrest. They are advised to wait six months before driving.

When the AHA originally published its ICD and driving guidelines in 1996, most people were receiving ICDs for secondary prevention. Now the devices are often implanted in people who have not yet suffered VF or VT. If you fall into this category, a one-week healing period after ICD implantation is generally sufficient. Should you suffer an episode of VF or VT thereafter, you should follow the six-month driving restriction and not get behind the wheel until you are VF or VT free for half a year.

CIRCULATION
Volume 115, page 1170
March 6, 2007

the area of the heart responsible for generating the abnormal rhythm. Then with the patient mildly sedated, the doctor inserts a catheter (often into a vein in the groin) and guides it to the site in the heart where the rhythm disturbance is occurring. The abnormal tissue is then destroyed (ablated) using radiofrequency energy delivered through a heated electrode at the tip of the catheter. The effectiveness of this technique is high (up to a 90% success rate) in people with certain types of tachycardia. The risks are minimal, although bleeding or infections sometimes occur. ■

aneurysm—Ballooning or bulging of the wall of the heart, an artery, or a vein caused by weakening of the wall.

angina—Pain, pressure, or tightness in the chest that arises when the heart muscle receives less oxygen than it needs.

angiography—An imaging technique in which a catheter is threaded through an artery to the heart to evaluate the presence of plaque. It is the best method for detecting blockages in the coronary arteries.

angioplasty—A procedure in which a catheter with a balloon at its tip is directed to a site where a coronary artery is narrowed by plaque. The balloon is inflated to compress the plaque against the walls of the artery and to stretch the artery.

anticoagulants—Drugs that decrease the formation of blood clots by inhibiting the production of fibrin, a major protein component of clots. Examples are heparin and warfarin (Coumadin).

antioxidants—Substances that help the body neutralize free radicals. Beta-carotene, vitamin E, and vitamin C are naturally occurring antioxidants.

antiplatelets—Drugs that decrease the formation of blood clots by inhibiting the aggregation, or clumping together, of blood platelets. One example is aspirin.

aorta—The body's main artery. It transports oxygenated blood from the left ventricle of the heart to the arteries that supply the rest of the body.

arrhythmia—An abnormal heart rhythm.

atherectomy—A method of removing plaque from the inside of an artery using a rotary blade or drill.

atherosclerosis—An accumulation of deposits of fat and fibrous tissue, called plaques, within the walls of arteries. This process narrows the arteries and reduces blood flow through them.

atria—The two upper chambers of the heart.

atrial fibrillation—A common heart rhythm abnormality in which the atria contract at a rapid, chaotic rate and cause rapid and irregular contractions of the ventricles.

body mass index (BMI)—A measurement of weight in relation to height.

bradycardia—A slow heart rate, usually defined as less than 60 beats per minute in an adult.

bypass surgery—A surgical procedure that uses an artery from the chest or a portion of a vein from the leg to channel blood around a narrowed segment of a coronary artery.

cardiac arrest—A sudden, abrupt loss of the heart's ability to pump blood, most often as a result of ventricular fibrillation.

cardiovascular disease—Disease affecting the arteries supplying blood to the heart and other organs. Coronary heart disease, stroke, and peripheral arterial disease are the most common cardiovascular diseases.

cerebrovascular disease—Disease that affects arteries supplying blood to the brain.

cholesterol—A soft, waxy substance present in cells throughout the body. Deposits of cholesterol within the walls of arteries can lead to the formation of plaques.

coronary calcium scan—A noninvasive imaging technique that reveals calcium deposits in the coronary arteries. Calcium indicates atherosclerosis.

coronary heart disease (CHD)—A narrowing of the coronary arteries by atherosclerosis. It can reduce or completely block blood flow to the heart.

coronary heart disease (CHD) event—Often defined as a heart attack, episode of unstable angina, or CHD-related death.

c-reactive protein—A protein produced by the liver in response to inflammation. High CRP levels in the blood are associated with a higher CHD risk.

defibrillation—Use of an electric shock to re-establish a normal rhythm in a heart that is beating ineffectively as a result of ventricular fibrillation.

diastolic blood pressure—The lower number in a blood pressure reading. The pressure in the arteries when the heart relaxes between beats.

drug-eluting stents—Stents that are coated with a medication that reduces the risk of artery re-narrowing.

echocardiography—A diagnostic test that uses ultrasound waves to visualize the heart, its valves, and the flow of blood within the heart.

electrocardiogram (ECG)—A graphical record of the heart's electrical activity obtained by applying small metal sensors to the skin.

endothelium—The layer of cells that line the walls of arteries. Injury to these cells is an important first step in the development of atherosclerosis.

free radicals—Chemical compounds formed during normal metabolism. They can damage cells and oxidize low-density lipoproteins, which can then be deposited in the walls of arteries.

heart attack—Tissue death caused by the complete blockage of blood flow to a portion of the heart muscle. Technically known as a myocardial infarction.

heart failure—A condition in which the heart is unable to pump enough blood to meet the body's needs.

high-density lipoprotein (HDL)—A lipoprotein that protects against atherosclerosis by removing cholesterol deposited in artery walls and returning this cholesterol to the liver.

Holter monitor—A portable device worn to monitor the heart's rhythm, usually for 24 hours.

homocysteine—High blood levels of this amino acid may promote atherosclerosis by damaging the endothelium and stimulating the formation of blood clots.

hypertension—Chronic high blood pressure that can increase the workload of the heart and lead to CHD.

ischemia—An inadequate supply of blood to any part of the body. Ischemia to the heart may cause chest pain.

laser ablation—A method of removing plaque from the inside of an artery using heat from a laser.

lipids—Fats, like cholesterol, that can travel through the bloodstream and accumulate within artery walls.

lipoprotein—A protein that transports cholesterol and other fats in the blood.

lipoprotein(a)—A lipoprotein with a structure similar to low-density lipoprotein but containing another protein called apo(a). High levels of lipoprotein(a) are a risk factor for CHD. Also called Lp(a).

low-density lipoprotein (LDL)—A lipoprotein that transports cholesterol in the bloodstream. A major contributor to atherosclerosis.

monounsaturated fat—A type of fat found in avocados, almonds, and olive and canola oils. Can raise HDL cholesterol and, when substituted for saturated fat in the diet, can lower LDL cholesterol.

myocardium—The muscle of the heart.

omega-3 fats—Polyunsaturated fats found in fish and some plant foods that have beneficial effects on the heart.

pacemaker—An implanted, battery-operated device that can take the place of the heart's normal pacemaker when it is not functioning properly.

peripheral arterial disease—A narrowing of the arteries in the extremities, usually the legs. Commonly due to atherosclerosis.

plaque—An accumulation of cholesterol-laden cells, smooth muscle cells, fibrous proteins, and calcium in the inner walls of arteries.

platelets—Small, irregularly shaped blood components that play a key role in the clotting process.

polyunsaturated fat—A type of fat found in safflower, sunflower, and corn oils. Can lower LDL cholesterol when substituted for saturated fat in the diet.

radiofrequency catheter ablation—A technique for treating arrhythmias that uses radio waves to suppress or destroy the site producing an abnormal electrical circuit within the heart.

restenosis—Renarrowing of an artery that has been opened during angioplasty.

revascularization—A procedure to improve blood flow to the heart. Usually refers to bypass surgery or angioplasty.

saturated fat—A type of fat found in most animal and dairy fats and some oils, such as palm and coconut oils. A major dietary factor in raising total and LDL cholesterol.

stable angina—An episode of angina triggered by a predictable amount of activity or stress. The characteristics of the pain are similar in each attack, and the pain is usually relieved by rest or a nitrate drug.

statins—The most popular class of lipid-lowering drugs. The most effective medications for lowering total and LDL cholesterol levels.

stent—A wire mesh tube that is permanently inserted into a coronary artery during angioplasty to help keep it open.

systolic blood pressure—The upper number in a blood pressure reading. The pressure in the arteries when the heart is contracting.

tachycardia—A heart rhythm abnormality characterized by a heart rate higher than 100 beats per minute at rest.

trans fats—Fats formed when food manufacturers add hydrogen atoms to unsaturated fats to make them more saturated, solid, and shelf stable. Found in stick margarines, store-bought baked goods, and other processed foods. Trans fats raise LDL cholesterol more than saturated fats and lower HDL cholesterol.

triglycerides—A type of lipid (fat) that is a storage form of energy. High levels of triglycerides in the blood contribute to atherosclerosis.

unstable angina—A condition intermediate in severity between stable angina and a heart attack. Caused by a blood clot or spasm in a coronary artery.

ventricles—The two chambers in the lower part of the heart.

ventricular fibrillation—A heart rhythm abnormality in which the pumping action of the ventricles is completely lost. Death occurs within a few minutes unless the heart's rhythm is returned to normal by administering an electrical shock to the heart.

ventricular tachycardia—A heart rhythm abnormality that originates in the ventricles and produces a heart rate faster than 100 beats per minute. Can be fatal if not treated.

very-low-density lipoprotein (VLDL)—A lipoprotein that is the major carrier of triglycerides in the blood.

HEALTH INFORMATION ORGANIZATIONS AND SUPPORT GROUPS

American College of Cardiology
2400 N St. NW
Washington, D.C. 20037
☎ 800-253-4636/202-375-6000
www.acc.org
Professional medical society and teaching institution that provides professional education, promotes research, offers leadership in the development of standards and guidelines, and forms healthcare policy.

American Dietetic Association
120 S. Riverside Plaza, Ste. 2000
Chicago, IL 60606-6995
☎ 800-877-1600
www.eatright.org
Provides recorded nutrition messages, helps consumers locate registered dietitians for counseling, and provides answers to food and nutrition questions related to heart-healthy eating.

American Heart Association
7272 Greenville Ave.
Dallas, TX 75231
☎ 800-242-8721
www.americanheart.org
National health organization that provides information and public education programs on all aspects of heart disease. Check for local chapters.

Mended Hearts, Inc.
7272 Greenville Ave.
Dallas, TX 75231
☎ 888-HEART-99/214-360-6149
www.mendedhearts.org
Support group for people with heart disease and their families. Call, write, or visit the website for information and to get in touch with other people with heart disease in your area.

National Heart, Lung, and Blood Institute Information Center
P.O. Box 30105
Bethesda, MD 20824-0105
☎ 301-592-8573
www.nhlbi.nih.gov/health
Branch of the National Institutes of Health that provides written information on all heart-related issues.

National Rehabilitation Information Center
8201 Corporate Dr., Ste. 600
Landover, MD 20785
☎ 800-346-2742/301-459-5900
301-459-5984 (TTY)
www.naric.com
Information center with database of literature and information on thousands of products and devices devoted to rehabilitation, including cardiac rehabilitation.

LEADING HOSPITALS
for Heart Disease and Heart Surgery as Ranked by *U.S. News & World Report*

1. **Cleveland Clinic**
   Cleveland, OH
   ☎ 800-223-2273/216-444-2200
   www.clevelandclinic.org

2. **Mayo Clinic**
   Rochester, MN
   ☎ 507-284-2511/507-538-3270
   www.mayoclinic.org

3. **Brigham and Women's Hospital**
   Boston, MA
   ☎ 617-732-5500
   www.brighamandwomens.org

4. **Johns Hopkins Hospital**
   Baltimore, MD
   ☎ 410-502-4003/410-955-5464
   www.hopkinsmedicine.org

5. **Massachusetts General Hospital**
   Boston, MA
   ☎ 617-726-2000
   www.massgeneral.org

6. **New York-Presbyterian University Hospital of Columbia and Cornell**
   New York, NY
   ☎ 877-NYP-WELL
   www.nyp.org

7. **St. Luke's Episcopal Hospital, Texas Heart Institute**
   Houston, TX
   ☎ 832-355-1000
   www.sleh.com

8. **Duke University Medical Center**
   Durham, NC
   ☎ 888-ASK-DUKE/919-684-8111
   www.mc.duke.edu

9. **Stanford Hospital and Clinics, Stanford, California**
   Palo Alto, CA
   ☎ 650-723-4000
   www.stanfordhospital.com

10. **Barnes-Jewish Hospital/ Washington University**
    St. Louis, MO
    ☎ 314-747-3000/314-TOP-DOCS
    www.barnesjewish.org

INDEX

ISBN 978-1-933087-60-3
1-933087-60-9

Printed in the United States of America

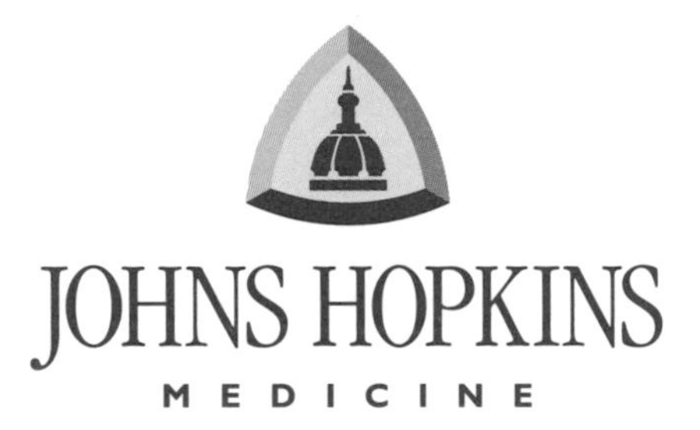

The Johns Hopkins White Papers are published yearly by Medletter Associates, LLC.

Visit our website for information on Johns Hopkins Health Publications, which include White Papers on specific disorders, home medical encyclopedias, consumer reference guides to drugs and medical tests, and our monthly newsletter *The Johns Hopkins Medical Letter: Health After 50*.
www.JohnsHopkinsHealthAlerts.com

DEPRESSION AND ANXIETY

Karen L. Swartz, M.D.

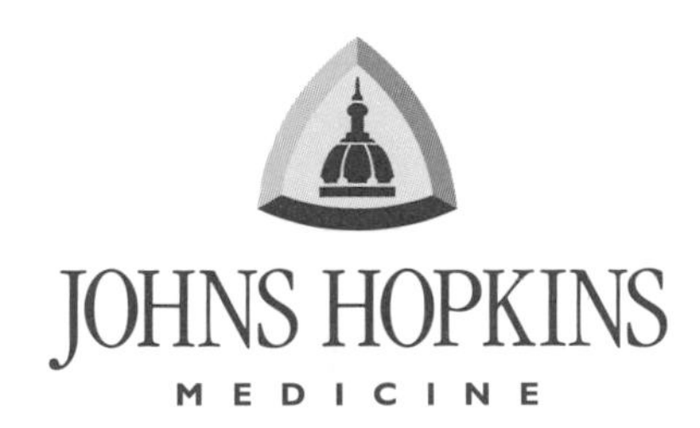

Dear Reader:

Welcome to the 2008 *Depression and Anxiety White Paper*—your Johns Hopkins guide to understanding the causes, symptoms, and management of mood and anxiety disorders in older adults.

This year's highlights include:

- Recognizing the danger signs of **depression in men**. (page 6)
- Why you're never too old to have an **eating disorder**. (page 10)
- What you can expect during the **grieving** process, and when it is considered a **problem**. (page 12)
- Managing **chronic pain** to improve your **mood**—and vice versa. (page 14)
- Preventing **weight gain** from psychiatric **medications**. (page 28)
- Which **medications** can **worsen** your depression and anxiety. (page 34)
- Recognizing and treating **alcohol** or **drug abuse** after age 60. (page 48)
- Discover a **natural way** to ease anxiety and depression. (page 51)
- New research on the link between **anxiety** and your **physical health**. (page 53)
- Conquering anxiety with **cognitive-behavioral therapy**. (page 58)
- Determining the best drug for **obsessive-compulsive disorder**. (page 67)

You'll also find a new "Ask the Doctor" column on pages 27, 33, 45, 50, and 63. This year's questions came from my patients, but next year we'd like to answer some of yours. If you have any depression- or anxiety-related queries you want answered in the White Papers, or comments about the White Papers in general, please e-mail the editors at whitepapers@johnshopkinshealthalerts.com.

Wishing you the best of health in 2008,

Karen L. Swartz, M.D.
Director of Clinical Programs, Johns Hopkins Mood Disorders Center
Assistant Professor of Psychiatry, Johns Hopkins University School of Medicine

P. S. Please visit www.HopkinsDepression.com for the latest news on depression and anxiety and other information to complement your Johns Hopkins White Paper.

THE AUTHOR

Karen L. Swartz, M.D., is Director of Clinical Programs at the Johns Hopkins Mood Disorders Center and Assistant Professor of Psychiatry at the Johns Hopkins University School of Medicine. She is also Co-Director of the Women's Mood Disorders Center, founder of the Adolescent Depression Awareness Program, and an attending psychiatrist at Johns Hopkins, with extensive clinical expertise in mood disorders, anxiety disorders, and eating disorders.

CONTENTS

DEPRESSION AND ANXIETY

Elation, sadness, anxiety, grief—we all feel these emotions at various times in our lives. Sadness may be caused by a setback or a loss, while anxiety may be triggered by a threat or a challenge. It is perfectly natural for our emotions to wax and wane with the ups and downs of our lives. The difficulty comes when these feelings persist—or when they seem to occur out of the blue—and begin to interfere with our functioning. When that's the case, a mood disorder (which includes depression and bipolar disorder) or an anxiety disorder may be present.

In any given year, about one in four Americans develops at least one mental health disorder, according to a national assessment. Nearly one in two Americans develops a mental health disorder at some point in their lives. Luckily, effective treatments are available. Proper diagnosis and treatment of mood disorders lead to a remission of symptoms in about 80% of cases. This White Paper describes the causes, symptoms, diagnoses, and treatments of depression, bipolar disorder, and anxiety disorders.

MOOD DISORDERS

Depression and bipolar disorder are referred to as mood (or affective) disorders. Major hallmarks of depression include a persistent low or sad mood, decreased or absent interest in almost all activities, loss of self-confidence, and a sense of worthlessness. Most people with bipolar disorder (formerly known as manic-depressive illness) experience alternating episodes of both depression and mania. Mania, which can be thought of as the opposite of depression, is characterized by an elated or elevated mood, increased activity, an overblown self-image, and exaggerated self-confidence. Usually, both depression and bipolar disorder are episodic—that is, bouts of illness are separated by periods of no symptoms and feelings of relative well-being.

Causes of Mood Disorders

The exact causes of depression and bipolar disorder are not well understood, but some combination of genetic predisposition and psychological and medical factors appears to play a role in these disorders.

Changes in the Brain

When people get depressed, chemical changes occur in the brain, and researchers believe that these changes are linked to the symptoms of mood disorders, especially depression.

The brain is composed of distinct regions, each made up of networks of nerve cells called neurons that transmit messages throughout the nervous system. Individual neurons are separated by small gaps at each end called synaptic clefts. Chemicals called neurotransmitters bridge the synaptic clefts and pass messages from one neuron to the next. Imbalances in three particular neurotransmitters—serotonin, norepinephrine, and dopamine—appear to contribute to depression and bipolar disorder, although less is known about changes in the brain that occur during the manic phase of bipolar disorder.

One specific brain region thought to be involved in depression is the limbic system, which affects our emotional behavior. An area within this system, the hypothalamus, regulates the pituitary gland, which in turn regulates key hormones and may be involved in the hormonal imbalances sometimes associated with depression.

Genetic Factors

Depression is often a family affair. Scientists, for example, have identified a gene that may be linked to bipolar disorder. In addition, they have found that a common genetic mutation can predict whether a person will become clinically depressed when faced with traumatic events in his or her life.

Research also shows that when one identical twin has a mood disorder, there is about a 50% chance that the other twin, who shares the same genes, will develop the illness at some point in life. One study found that if one twin developed depression, the other twin also suffered from depression in 46% of identical twins, compared with 20% of fraternal twins (who share half of their genes, like any full siblings).

Studies have also found that adopted children whose biological parents had a mood disorder had a three times greater incidence of depressive illness than the biological children of the same adoptive parents. Finally, children whose parents and grandparents experienced moderate to severe depression are at much greater risk for developing psychiatric problems than those whose relatives were not affected, according to a three-generation study.

Genetics also plays a role in treatment, influencing an individual's response to a particular drug, for example. There is evidence that

The Biology of Depression and Anxiety

Although a comprehensive understanding of the causes of depression and anxiety has not been reached, scientists have identified certain biological changes that may predispose a person to these disorders. The following is a summary of some of the theories that are currently under exploration.

Neurotransmitters

One area of study is the role of neurotransmitters—chemical messengers that carry information between neurons (nerve cells) in the brain. Decreased availability of certain neurotransmitters (such as norepinephrine, serotonin, and dopamine) may result in depression. Anxiety is thought to result from problems with the neurotransmitter gamma-aminobutyric acid (GABA), which normally suppresses the action of neurons.

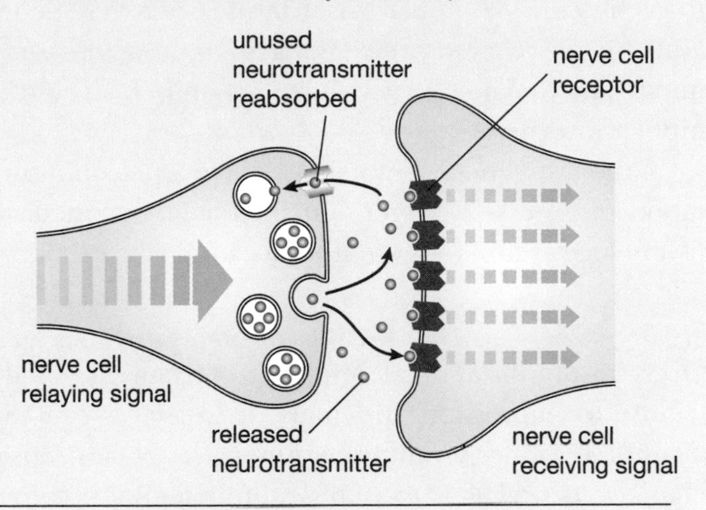

Structures of the Brain

Much current research also focuses on particular structures in the brain that may be responsible for depression and anxiety. In general, it is believed that depression and anxiety may largely result from chemical imbalances affecting the brain's limbic system—a ring of structures (including the cerebral cortex, thalamus, hypothalamus, and hippocampus) that appears to be the seat of human emotions such as depression, fear, and rage.

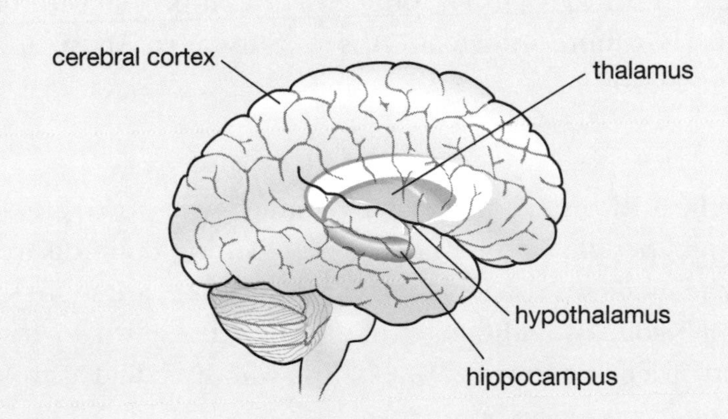

The Endocrine System

Depression can also affect the endocrine system—the network of glands that regulates body functions by releasing various hormones into the bloodstream. However, these changes seem to be effects rather than causes of depression. On the other hand, some endocrine disorders can directly cause depression or mania. An example is Cushing's disease, in which the adrenal glands produce too much of the hormone cortisol. And some experts believe seasonal affective disorder (SAD) may stem from disordered release of the hormone melatonin by the pineal gland during winter.

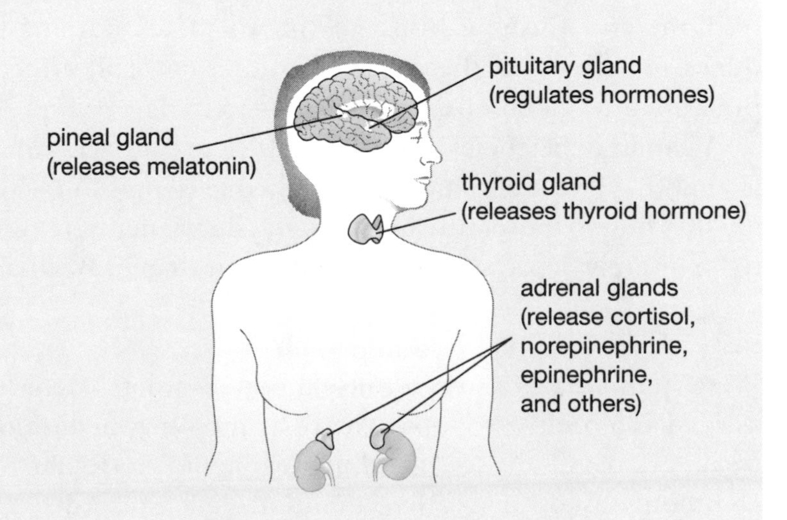

people may do better if prescribed the same antidepressant medication that has been effective for a depressed first-degree relative (a parent, sibling, or child).

Because researchers are not sure exactly which genes are linked to depression or bipolar disorder, specific genetic tests will not be available for years to come. But as with heart disease and cancer, it is important to know if you have a family history of depression or bipolar disorder.

Although genetic factors may make a person more susceptible to mood disorders, a trigger—such as a serious medical condition or psychological stress—is often what causes a mood disorder to emerge.

Drugs and Alcohol

Overconsumption of alcohol and certain illegal drugs can contribute to depression and make it worse, as can withdrawal from alcohol, cocaine, or amphetamines. Drugs can cause other mental changes as well. For example, amphetamines, cocaine, and phencyclidine (PCP) can all induce mania in people with bipolar disorder. (For more information, see "Substance Abuse and Aging" on pages 48–49.)

Medical Conditions

Medical disorders can make people prone to depression. For example, people who have dementia-causing brain disorders, such as Alzheimer's disease or Huntington's disease, are more susceptible to depression. In addition, stroke has been known to trigger depression, affecting about 25% of those who have had a stroke in the left frontal area of the brain.

Hormonal disorders, such as an underactive thyroid (hypothyroidism) and Cushing's disease (in which the adrenal gland produces too much of the stress hormone cortisol, affecting blood pressure and metabolism) also can lead to depression.

Vitamin deficiencies, such as insufficient folic acid, vitamin B_6, or vitamin B_{12} levels, also have been linked to depression. (In one study of 700 women, those with a vitamin B_{12} deficiency were twice as likely to be severely depressed as those without a vitamin B_{12} deficiency.)

Medication

Prescription drugs also can cause mood disorders. Medications such as corticosteroids, levodopa (Parcopa and other medications used to treat Parkinson's disease), and methylphenidate (Ritalin and others, commonly used for treating attention deficit disorder) can trigger mania in bipolar disorder. Other drugs, including some used to treat high blood pressure and cancer, have been known to cause depression (see "Medications That Can Worsen Depression and Anxiety" on pages 34–35).

Brain Trauma

Neurological disorders or injury to the brain from trauma or tumors also can cause behavioral changes, anxiety, and/or mood disorders.

Symptoms and Diagnosis of Mood Disorders

Although many mood disorders are readily recognized, it can be difficult to distinguish milder forms of depression or anxiety from the emotional changes that are part of everyday life. Unlike most medical disorders, mood disorders cannot be detected by blood and other laboratory tests.

Rather, a doctor must rely on a person's medical history to diagnose a mood disorder. The American Psychiatric Association has established various classification systems to help doctors make consistent diagnoses of major depression, bipolar disorder, and various forms of anxiety. These criteria are defined in the *Diagnostic and Statistical Manual of Mental Disorders*, a reference guide used by psychiatrists and psychologists. The manual is periodically revised to keep up with the latest research; the current edition is referred to as the *DSM-IV-TR*.

Major Depression

According to the *DSM-IV-TR*, a person is suffering from a major depressive episode if he or she experiences items 1 or 2 from the list of symptoms below, along with any four others, continuously for more than two weeks:

1. Depressed mood with overwhelming feelings of sadness and grief
2. Apathy—loss of interest and pleasure in activities formerly enjoyed
3. Sleep problems—insomnia, early-morning waking, or oversleeping nearly every day
4. Decreased energy or fatigue
5. Noticeable changes in appetite and weight (significant weight loss or gain)

NEW RESEARCH

Depression and Anxiety Often Coexist

It has been believed that generalized anxiety disorder (GAD) typically precedes the development of depression. However, researchers now assert that depression occurs before anxiety as frequently as anxiety manifests before depression, and that the two disorders often develop at the same time.

The observations are from a long-term New Zealand study that followed 1,037 people and examined them for anxiety and depression at seven intervals between ages 11–32.

In 37% of those diagnosed with depression, anxiety surfaced before or at the same time as depression, while in those diagnosed with anxiety, depression began before or concurrently with anxiety in 32%. Seventy-two percent of lifetime anxiety cases had a history of depression, while 48% of lifetime depression cases had anxiety. As adults, 12% of the participants had been diagnosed with both GAD and major depressive disorder; of these people, 66% had recurrent depression, 47% had recurrent anxiety, 64% had used mental health services, 47% had taken psychiatric medication, 8% had been hospitalized, and 11% had attempted suicide.

The authors suggested that the lifetime prevalence of coexisting anxiety and depression is probably higher than typically estimated, and that the two conditions could be classified in one category of distress disorders.

ARCHIVES OF GENERAL PSYCHIATRY
Volume 64, page 651
June 2007

Men and the Blues

Depression looks different in men than in women

Is depression really less common in men than in women? Researchers are beginning to wonder. In fact, some experts believe that depression may actually be just as common in men as in women but is often overlooked because of its different signs and symptoms. Rather than feeling sad, weepy, worthless, or guilty, as women usually do, men are more inclined to get angry and irritable, feel an increasing loss of control over their lives, take greater risks, become more aggressive, and complain about problems at work.

But the consequences of depression in men—and of not being diagnosed and treated—can be even more dangerous than for women. Tragically, men are four times more likely than women to commit suicide. And while depression is associated with a greater risk of coronary heart disease in both genders, a study in the *Archives of Internal Medicine* shows that only depressed men, not depressed women, suffer a higher death rate from heart disease.

Roughly six million of the 18 million Americans who experience depression each year are men—many famous "manly men" among them, too, including the late writer William Styron (author of *Sophie's Choice*), *60 Minutes* correspondent Mike Wallace, and baseball hitter Mark McGwire.

Researchers believe that men are more vulnerable than women to stressful life changes that can trigger depression, such as divorce, loss of a spouse, unemployment, or retirement. This may be a result of their having a different genetic makeup that makes their susceptibility to depression different from that of women. In a study published in the *American Journal of Medical Genetics*, researchers found 19 chromosomal regions connected to major depression—but men and women shared only three of these regions; the rest were linked to one gender or the other.

The Strong, Silent Type

All too often, men fail to get treatment because they may not recognize the symptoms of depression or, even if they notice something is wrong, they can't admit they have a problem for fear of being perceived as "weak" or "dependent." They may see themselves as independent or rugged and believe there is shame attached to being diagnosed with depression. Older men are especially apt to adopt a "John Wayne" attitude; they're also more prone to depression and suicide than younger men.

And healthcare providers may overlook depression in older men because their symptoms can be more physical than psychological, they could have other medical illnesses that mask depression, or they may be using medications that can cause depression. Naturally declining testosterone levels may also contribute to the onset of the blues in older men.

Typically, when men try to cope with depression on their own, they often become argumentative and combative, withdraw from relationships, engage in dangerous sports or unprotected sex with multiple partners, and self-medicate with alcohol or drugs. Ultimately, these risky

6. Inability to concentrate or think, or indecisiveness

7. Physical symptoms of restlessness or being physically slowed down

8. Feelings of guilt, worthlessness, and helplessness

9. Recurrent thoughts of death or suicide, or a suicide attempt.

The diagnosis is more certain when a person also has a family history of depression; a previous episode of depression or bipolar disorder; a general medical problem likely to trigger depression, such as a recent stroke or heart attack; or if the person is taking a medication known to cause mood disorders.

behaviors only make the condition much worse.

Getting Help

The stigma surrounding depression is lessening in this country, even for men, as researchers are learning about the physical basis for depression—it's not a sign of weakness, but rather a brain disorder that can be treated. Because of the change in thinking, men are slowly coming around to the idea that it's okay to get help for a mental illness.

So if you've noticed that you're feeling more irritable or withdrawn than usual, be sure to tell your primary care doctor about it. He or she can perform tests to check for illnesses that could be causing depression, assess whether your medications are a contributing factor, and evaluate the need for antidepressant medication or psychotherapy.

If you'd rather not discuss the way you're feeling with your regular doctor, you can also seek help from:

- Mental health specialists (psychiatrists, psychologists, social workers, mental health counselors)
- Religious leaders or counselors
- Health maintenance organizations
- Community mental health centers
- Hospitals (psychiatry departments or outpatient mental health clinics)
- Social service agencies
- Private clinics and facilities
- Employee assistance programs
- Local medical and psychiatric societies.

The point: Assistance is readily available in a variety of treatments that can help manage depression and make you feel better. The good news is that men who receive treatment respond as well as women do to medication and psychotherapy, although they, too, may have to try a few different medications to find the one that works best.

There is no disgrace in seeking help—and no one except you and your doctor needs to know you're doing so. The only shame is in letting outdated notions about depression and masculinity stop you from taking advantage of the support that is available. Now all you need to do is take the first step. ■

Common Symptoms of Depression in Men

- Irritability
- Anger
- Withdrawal from relationships
- Loss of interest in work or hobbies
- Increased alcohol and substance use
- Greater risk taking and reckless behavior
- Aggression
- Suicidal thoughts
- Sexual problems (loss of interest, erectile difficulties)
- Sleep disturbances

Other symptoms of depression may include disorganized thinking and delusions. In addition to these disturbances in mood and cognition (thinking), people with major depression may experience physical changes such as constipation or decreased sexual drive.

Episodes of major depression range from mild to severe. In mild episodes, symptoms barely meet the requirements for a diagnosis and the person is able to get through the day without too much trouble. Severe episodes are characterized by several debilitating symptoms, including worsening mood that markedly interferes with daily life. People who are struggling with severe depression have difficulty with almost every activity—going to work, socializing, and even getting up in the morning. They may be unable to feed and dress themselves or to maintain personal hygiene.

Major depression affects about 15 million adults each year. It is believed to be twice as common in women as in men, although that statistic is now being questioned; in fact, depression symptoms may be different in men and women, as well as in older vs. younger people (see the feature "Men and the Blues" on pages 6–7).

Dysthymia

Dysthymia is a chronic form of depression that is milder than major depression. It is characterized by the presence of depressed mood for most of the day for more days than not, over a period of at least two years. It may be intermittent and interspersed with periods of feeling normal, but these periods of improvement last for no more than two months.

Dysthymia is believed to be twice as common in women as in men. People who have dysthymia before age 21 tend to have a higher incidence of personality disorders. Because the onset of symptoms is insidious, dysthymia often goes unnoticed. And because of its chronic nature, the person may come to believe, "I've always been this way." In addition to depressed mood, symptoms include two or more of the following:

- Poor appetite or overeating
- Insomnia or hypersomnia (excessive sleeping)
- Low energy or fatigue
- Low self-esteem
- Poor concentration or difficulty making decisions
- Feelings of hopelessness.

It is far better to treat dysthymia than to think of it as a minor condition, according to a recent seven-year prospective study of more than 1,000 young people in New Zealand. Bypassing treatment places people at increased risk for subsequently developing major depression. In fact, about 10% of people with dysthymia also have recurrent episodes of major depression, a condition known as double depression.

Biological causes

Some medical conditions, including neurological disorders (such as multiple sclerosis and stroke), hypothyroidism, fibromyalgia, and chronic fatigue syndrome, are associated with dysthymia. Investigators believe that developing dysthymia is not a psychological reaction to being ill in these cases but rather is connected biologically with these disorders. There are many reasons for this connection—it may be that these medical conditions interfere with the action of neurotransmitters, or that medications (such as corticosteroids or beta-blockers) taken for a medical illness may trigger the dysthymia, or that both dysthymia and the medical illness are related in some other way, reinforcing each other in a complicated manner.

Dysthymia can also follow severe psychological stress, such as the death of a spouse or caring for a chronically ill loved one. Older people who have been free from psychiatric disorders are particularly susceptible to developing dysthymia after significant life stresses.

Atypical Depression

Atypical depression, despite its name, is not unusual and occurs in 25–40% of depressed patients seen by doctors. It derives its name from the fact that it is different from typical depression in certain key respects. For example, sufferers do manage to find pleasure in certain activities at certain times, and, rather than having insomnia and loss of appetite, many people with atypical depression overeat and oversleep.

Other symptoms include:

- General sadness that can be broken by enjoyment of pleasurable experiences or circumstances
- Strong feelings of rejection
- A sensation of heaviness, especially in the arms
- A strong preference to overeat carbohydrate-rich foods because ingestion of carbohydrates causes an increase in serotonin in the brain, which can boost mood.

The disorder is just as debilitating as major depression despite the apparent lack of sadness. People with atypical depression often have shorter but more frequent episodes of depression.

Seasonal Affective Disorder (SAD)

As seasons change, so does the amount of sunlight each day, which in turn causes changes in people's internal biological clocks (also called circadian rhythm). This rhythm is a 24-hour cycle that affects things such as our eating and sleeping patterns, brain wave activity, hormone production, cell regeneration, and other biological activities. In some individuals, less daily sunlight and changes in circadian rhythm can induce depression, which usually peaks in January and February when there is the least

Eating Disorders: Not Just for the Young

The compulsion to be slim doesn't always fade with age

Body dissatisfaction is not only a signature problem of youth, as an increasing number of middle-age and older women are developing eating disorders. Our cultural obsession with thinness as well as looking and feeling young may be contributing factors, leading women to fixate on dieting and exercise as a way to combat the signs of aging.

Traumatic life events also may be a cause. The death of a spouse, the onset of menopause, a divorce, and children leaving home may lead midlife and older women to feel like they're losing control of their lives, sparking them to focus too much on things they can control, such as their eating habits and weight. Stress, in fact, is known to exacerbate eating disorder problems, and many older women may use bingeing, purging, and restricting food intake as a way to cope with anxiety, anger, or depression. Others may develop eating disorders to get attention from family members, because they can't afford to eat well, or to protest being placed in a nursing home.

Even older men aren't immune to eating disorders, albeit in very small numbers. Only 10% of younger patients with eating disorders are male, usually from high-risk groups like dancers and athletes for whom excessive exercise is part of daily life. However, changes in eating habits with marked weight loss can be associated with depression and numerous medical problems in both older men and women.

Eating disorders in older women may often go undiagnosed by doctors, not only because they're unexpected but because weight loss and changes in appetite can also occur as a complication of another illness or medication use. Fortunately, researchers are starting to shed light on this overlooked health issue.

Never Good Enough

A recent Austrian study is among the first to investigate poor body image and eating disorders in older women. Investigators surveyed a random sample of 475 women ages 60–70 about their eating behaviors, weight history, and attitudes toward their bodies. Around 90% of the women said they felt very or moderately fat, and 60% reported being dissatisfied with their bodies. The majority of women had a body mass index (BMI) of 25, which is considered just slightly overweight, and wanted to have a normal-weight BMI of 23. Over 80% of the women made efforts to manage their weight.

Four percent of the women (18 total) met the diagnostic criteria for an eating disorder: One had anorexia nervosa, two had bulimia nervosa, and 15 had symptoms of an unspecified eating disorder that did not meet the criteria for anorexia or bulimia (see the inset box at right for definitions of these disorders). In addition, another 4% of the women (21 overall) reported a single symptom of an eating disorder, such as using laxatives, diuretics, or vomiting to lose weight, or binge eating.

Typically, it's been assumed that as women age, these problems become less common—but this study suggests that the desire to be thin never fades. In fact, some of the women may actually be experiencing recurrences of eating disorders they suffered from in their teens, 20s, or 30s. Others may have had continuous problems throughout their lifetimes, and still others

sunlight. Researchers believe that the lack of sunlight during these times may alter brain levels of certain mood-controlling substances—for example, the hormone melatonin, which may increase.

People with SAD often eat and sleep excessively, crave sugary or starchy foods, and have a full remission in the spring and summer when more daily sunlight is available.

may have developed the problems anew in their later years.

Not Too Late for Help

Whether the problem is a new or an old one, the good news is that better treatments for eating disorders have been devised over the past three decades. Cognitive behavioral therapy, which focuses on changing distorted thinking patterns and behaviors that lead to eating disorders, is often beneficial, as is nutritional counseling.

Effective medications also have been developed to combat some eating disorder behaviors, most notably the selective serotonin reuptake inhibitors (SSRIs), including citalopram (Celexa), escitalopram (Lexapro), fluoxetine (Prozac), sertraline (Zoloft), and paroxetine (Paxil). These drugs can also treat the depression and anxiety that may often accompany eating disorders.

The important thing is to seek help for an eating problem, either from your physician, an eating disorder specialist, a psychotherapist, or another qualified mental health professional, before it starts to threaten your health. (The National Eating Disorders Association can provide referrals to specialists; visit www.edap.org.) Treatment may need to be long term, but the problem is unlikely to go away on its own. If left unchecked, it will undoubtedly affect the quality of all areas of your existence—and may even shorten your lifespan. ■

Eating Disorders Defined

Anorexia nervosa is a condition in which individuals starve themselves as a result of misperceptions about the way their bodies look. Symptoms include a refusal to eat, an abnormal fear of weight gain, and an altered body image. Health consequences can include fatigue, depression, an irregular heart rate, growth of baby-fine hair all over the body (known as lanugo), anemia (iron-poor blood), constipation, bloating, brittle nails and hair, and low blood pressure. This insidious disease is difficult to treat and can be life threatening if the individual's weight drops too low. It can also lead to heart disease, bone loss, and nerve damage.

Bulimia nervosa is characterized by a pattern of eating copious amounts and then purging the food by vomiting or abuse of laxatives to prevent weight gain. Many people with this eating disorder are of normal weight. Like anorexia, bulimia can cause serious health consequences, including fatigue; depression; dehydration; electrolyte abnormalities; constipation; damage to teeth, gums, and cheeks (from exposure to stomach acid during vomiting); and an irregular heartbeat.

Binge eating, which is not officially categorized as an eating disorder but may be more common than anorexia and bulimia combined, is diagnosed when someone repeatedly and excessively overeats at one sitting. Binge eaters typically feel like they can't stop eating, then they're ashamed or feel guilty afterwards. They may suffer from fatigue and joint pain and can develop high blood pressure and cholesterol levels, heart disease, type 2 diabetes, or gallbladder disease. They are usually overweight or obese and have a history of weight fluctuations.

Grief vs. Depression

Sometimes we experience huge changes in our lives. These events can cause intense emotional anguish, and grieving during such life changes is a normal and healthy, if painful, process. Grief can be the result of a major change in our lives such as:

- The death of a loved one (a person, a pet)
- A move to a new and unfamiliar community

- An opportunity or life goal that becomes closed to us
- A loved one contracting a life-threatening illness.

Occasionally, however, this anguish triggers a major depressive episode, although few people in mourning experience true clinical depression.

Even just a serious illness can increase the risk of stress and, potentially, depression in a partner: A recent study of 518,000 couples over age 65 found that when one spouse was hospitalized for a serious illness, the other spouse had a greater risk of dying within the next year. The probable reasons: increased stress and withdrawal of social, emotional, economic, and other support.

Grieving often produces a wide range of feelings. The psychological process itself is a means for the mind to adjust, over time, to the acute sorrow of a loss. Grieving also allows us to accept the finality of the loss, to experience a full range of feelings as a result of the loss, and to adjust to our changed lives. The end of grieving does not entail forgetting; rather, it usually comes with the acceptance of our loss.

A good sign that mourning is successful is a gradual shift from sad thoughts and feelings to thoughts of positive and realistic plans for the future. As this shift occurs over time and the mourner begins to enjoy life more than feeling weighed down by it, the process of grieving moves forward.

Although grief and depression may both entail sadness and feeling "blue," they are different. The sadness of grief usually comes in "waves," with varying degrees of intensity and bouts of crying, and feeling intensely sad, guilty, angry, irritable, or lonely. A person experiencing grief, however, can enjoy some of life's activities. Grief is generally time limited and resolves without specific treatment.

Depression is a more persistent and unremitting sadness and is notable for a consistent inability to enjoy pleasurable life activities. Muted or "deadened" feelings are often a sign of depression. If such symptoms persist following a life change that produces grief, mourning may have been unsuccessful and the help of a physician or other health professional is warranted. Check for the following symptoms, especially over a prolonged period or if they arise months or even years after the loss:

- Physical symptoms that mimic the illness or injury of the person who died
- Overuse of alcohol, illegal drugs, or prescription drugs
- Persistent depression (see pages 5–6 for symptoms)
- Chronic sleep disturbances

NEW RESEARCH

Grief Characterized By Acceptance, Not Disbelief

A new study says that the dominant emotional responses for most people after the death of a loved one are acceptance and yearning for the deceased—not disbelief, as proposed by the traditional stage theory of grief. While the predominant initial reaction is disbelief for those whose loss is due to a sudden, traumatic death, the same is not true for those who lose someone after an extended illness.

Investigators analyzed data on 233 people participating in the Yale Bereavement Study who had lost a spouse (84%) or an adult child, parent, or sibling (16%). They found that disbelief peaked at one month post-loss and then declined. Yearning peaked at four months post-loss, anger at five months post-loss, and depression at six months post-loss. Acceptance of the loss increased throughout the three-year observation period. At all stages, acceptance was greater than disbelief, yearning, anger, or depression. Likewise, yearning was greater than disbelief, anger, or depression, while depression was greater than anger.

Individuals who continue to have negative emotions beyond six months after their loss may be having a difficult time adjusting and could benefit from further psychological evaluation.

JOURNAL OF THE AMERICAN MEDICAL ASSOCIATION
Volume 297, page 716
February 21, 2007

- Thoughts of or attempts at suicide (see a health professional immediately)
- Inability to carry out normal daily routines.

It is important to seek medical help for physical symptoms that arise during mourning and to attend to any medical or psychiatric conditions that existed before the death occurred. Some evidence suggests that acute mourning may suppress the immune system and make people more susceptible to illness.

Depression in Older Adults

Depression and aging do not necessarily go hand in hand. A survey of Californians ages 50–95 found that factors such as chronic illness, physical disabilities, and social isolation—which often coincide with increasing age—were stronger predictors of depression than age itself. That said, the incidence of depression is clearly higher in older adults. The National Institute of Mental Health's Epidemiologic Catchment Area Study, which focuses on several major geographical areas, estimated that at least one million of the nation's 31 million people age 65 and older suffer from major depression, and an additional five million have depressive symptoms that are severe enough to require treatment. Unfortunately, the disease is often undiagnosed, misdiagnosed, or left untreated in the elderly and can increase the risk of early death and repeated hospitalization. There is also reason to believe that late-life depression can be more serious than depression in younger people.

One reason depression may be left undiagnosed is because of life circumstances that are common as we age, such as loss of a spouse, family members, or friends (by death or geographic relocation); retirement, which may be accompanied by a loss of status and self-identity; financial concerns; fears of death or loss of independence and self-sufficiency; social isolation; and medical problems. Any of these factors may trigger symptoms of depression that are mistakenly attributed to life stresses and are not recognized as a true depressive illness.

Many older people who live alone do not have adequate support networks; some also do not know where to find help or are overwhelmed by the many resources that provide medical care, social services, and financial assistance for their medical needs. Older adults also tend to be embarrassed or reluctant to seek professional help for emotional problems, partly because the stigma of psychiatric illness is especially strong among people in this age group, and/or because they remember the days when less effective treatments were

NEW RESEARCH

Specialty Care Extends Life in Older People With Depression

According to a new study, older adults who are depressed are considerably less likely to die within five years if they are treated by primary care physicians who team with depression-care managers than if treated by primary care doctors alone.

In a randomized, controlled study, 1,226 individuals ages 60–75 were screened for depression: 396 were diagnosed with major depression, 203 with minor depression, and 627 with no depression. Twenty primary care practices in New York and Pennsylvania were then designated to treat the depressed participants with usual care by a primary doctor or usual care plus depression care with a social worker, nurse, or psychologist. All participants with depression also received the antidepressant citalopram (Celexa).

Of the 223 participants who died during the follow-up period, which averaged 4.5 years, those with major depression had a 45% reduced risk of death if they received specialty depression care compared with the usual-care-only group; however, the same benefit did not apply to those with minor depression.

The reduced risk of dying also seemed to be limited to deaths due to cancer, though the researchers remained unclear why and say it warrants further investigation.

ANNALS OF INTERNAL MEDICINE
Volume 146, page 689
May 2007

The Pain-Mood Connection

Chronic physical discomfort can cause depression and anxiety—and vice versa

Pain is ubiquitous in America: One in four adults say they've had pain that lasted 24 hours within the past month (acute pain) and one in 10 say their pain has lasted a year or more (chronic pain), according to data released by the Centers for Disease Control and Prevention.

Older persons are often the hardest hit by pain: One fifth of people over age 65 report that they've experienced acute pain in the past month and three fifths say they have chronic pain. More women than men report pain, especially as they age. The most common types are lower back pain, migraine or severe headache, and joint pain, aching, or stiffness.

Although we like to think of ourselves as stoic, physical pain can wear down even the most robust of spirits and eventually lead to depression or anxiety. For those who have a family history of mood disorders or have had prior episodes, the stress of pain can trigger a new episode. So if you're struggling with persistent pain and find your mood is becoming affected, it's important not to ignore it and to seek treatment.

Pain Pathways

When your nerve endings detect damage to a part of the body, they send messages through the nerve pathways to the brain which interprets these signals as pain. It's the brain's way of telling the body that it needs to take steps to protect itself from physical harm—for instance, move away from a candle that is burning the skin. Pain is part of the body's defense system and important for our survival. That's the upside of pain.

The downside of pain, of course, is that it can be debilitating, unpleasant, and bring on a wide range of negative emotions from anger to despair and fear. Because it stirs up uncomfortable feelings and may be associated with a loss of function and the ability to interact with others and enjoy life, it's no surprise that chronic pain can cause depression and anxiety. Chronic pain is stressful, both physically and psychologically, and may alter your brain chemistry in a way that makes you vulnerable to such mood disorders.

In addition, the more pain you feel, the more severe your mood symptoms tend to be, and the longer your pain persists, the more likely you are to feel depressed (30–80% of people with chronic pain suffer from clinical depression).

On the other hand, pain is one of the most common symptoms people with depression complain about, and people who are depressed experience more impairment from their pain than those who are not depressed. Often, the depression-pain scenario plays out in a vicious cycle, and to find relief from one, you must treat the other.

Pain and anxiety are also closely linked: Anxiety about pain can intensify its severity—if you fear that you'll have pain after surgery, it's likely you will, according to one study. Previous experiences with pain can also increase your anxiety about it in the future: If you've thrown your back out in

available. In addition, friends and family often fail to perceive signs of distress. Older depressed people are more likely to tell their primary care physician about physical complaints than about subjective feelings of depressed mood. For example, they may report loss of appetite, insomnia, or lack of energy but not a loss of interest or enjoyment in daily activities. Unfortunately, doctors and patients alike often consider these symptoms a normal part of aging.

In addition, because older people often have other medical illnesses and take more prescription drugs, it can take some medical sleuthing to accurately pin down a diagnosis of depression. The

the past, doing so again in the future may bring on the same or more intense pain. Finally, anxiety about pain may inhibit you from getting exercise or cause you to stiffen up in anticipation of painful sensations, which can lead to even more pain. (Doctors now say that in the face of conditions such as back pain, a little exercise is a good thing.)

Managing Pain and Your Mood

Chronic pain can be difficult to cure, but it almost always can be managed. The first thing to do is to see a healthcare provider, your primary care doctor, or perhaps even a psychiatrist or pain specialist who can treat both your pain and the accompanying depression or anxiety. This clinician can help you set realistic goals for how much pain relief you can likely expect and at the same time help you improve your physical functioning, psychological outlook, and overall quality of life.

Medication. In the arena of medications, both the selective serotonin reuptake inhibitors (SSRIs)—such as fluoxetine (Prozac), paroxetine (Paxil), sertraline (Zoloft), and the like—and the serotonin and norepinephrine reuptake inhibitors (SNRIs)—such as duloxetine (Cymbalta), trazodone, and venlafaxine (Effexor)—affect brain chemicals that are responsible for both mood and pain and are therefore often very effective.

Psychotherapy. Beyond medications, cognitive-behavioral therapy and interpersonal therapy can help you deal with depression by teaching you how to change your mindset and attitudes toward life and uncover emotional conflicts that could be increasing your pain. For instance, it's been found that people who are prone to catastrophizing—focusing on the worst that could happen in any situation—have more pain than people who are more realistic or optimistic.

Stress management. Stress-management techniques such as relaxation exercises, listening to music, hypnosis, and biofeedback also can help in distracting you and teaching you to reduce both pain and stressful feelings. However, such non-medication approaches require you to be an active participant in their use in order for them to work—that means you have to be motivated to practice them on a regular basis.

Combination therapy. Finally, like all forms of depression, it's important to be aware that the first treatment strategy you try may not work immediately or completely. Doctors have noticed that there are differences in the way that men and women experience pain (women feel more of an emotional component, while men tend to perceive it in a more cerebral or analytic manner) and react to pain treatments (women may not respond as well or to the same medications as men). There are also natural individual variations in the response to various pain medications.

So you may have to experiment to find the right combination and doses of medications and psychotherapy that will offer the most relief for your physical and psychological distress. But don't give up—given the many different treatments available today, help can be found. ■

depression might be the primary disorder or it might result from an underlying condition such as cancer, stroke, or a reaction to a prescription drug. It also might be a psychological reaction to a diagnosis of a serious illness or debilitating chronic pain or impairment. Finally, it could be a direct or indirect biological effect of an illness on the brain.

The possibility of dementia adds further difficulties: Symptoms of major depression can mimic symptoms of a dementia-causing condition such as Alzheimer's disease (disorientation, distractibility, and memory loss, for example). Doctors need to evaluate an individual's mental status, medical history, and current physical health status carefully to find the primary cause of the psychological symptoms.

Effects of Depression on Physical Health

Depression clearly has a harmful effect on physical health, although the biological reasons for the link between body and mind are unclear. It may be that depression affects health because people develop a fatalistic attitude and stop taking care of themselves. Whatever the reasons, over the past 20 years, it has become evident that a depressed mood after a heart attack is much more than an "understandable emotional reaction" to a stressful, life-changing event—it is profoundly dangerous, raising a person's chances of having a second, fatal heart attack.

More recently, researchers have studied the flip side of the equation—the question of whether someone who is depressed is at increased risk for developing coronary heart disease (CHD) down the line. Indeed, prospective studies show that people who had no CHD but were depressed when the studies began were more likely to develop or die of heart disease.

Depression also aggravates chronic illnesses such as diabetes, arthritis, back problems, and asthma, leading to more work absences, disability, and doctor visits.

Bipolar Disorder

Bipolar disorder strikes men and women equally and affects about 4% of American adults during some point in their lives. A person with bipolar disorder typically has alternating periods of major depression and mania. In rare cases, mania can occur on its own.

Manic episodes are characterized by a distinct period of abnormally and persistently elevated, expansive, or irritable mood. The episodes, with their restless energy and volatile mood swings, are severe enough to cause trouble at work, home, or both. Episodes of milder manic symptoms are termed hypomania. Men with bipolar disorder tend to have more manic episodes; women are more likely to experience depressive episodes. The time between cycles can vary greatly (see Natural History and Prognosis of Mood Disorders on page 18).

The illness can begin with a bout of either depression or mania, but about two thirds of cases start with a manic episode, and mania tends to predominate. A manic episode is accompanied by at least three of the following seven symptoms:

- Feelings of grandiosity or inflated self-esteem
- Diminished need for sleep
- Being extremely talkative
- A sense that thoughts and ideas are racing
- Being easily distracted
- Increased productivity and/or activity at work, at school, or in social situations
- Excessive involvement in high-risk activities that are likely to have serious consequences.

Because manic episodes can cause impaired judgment, people must be protected from engaging in self-destructive actions, such as making unwise investments, going on large spending or gambling sprees, driving recklessly, or impulsively starting intense and unwise romantic or sexual relationships.

Certain medications and health conditions can cause significant mood swings that mimic the symptoms of bipolar disorder. These include corticosteroids, antidepressant or antianxiety drugs, drugs for Parkinson's disease such as tolcapone (Tasmar), abuse of alcohol or other drugs, an underactive or overactive thyroid gland, a neurological or adrenal disorder, vitamin B_{12} deficiency, and other mental health conditions such as schizophrenia. These potential causes of mood swings should be taken into account when a person is suspected of having bipolar disorder or is not responding to treatment.

Suicide

Suicide—the 11th leading cause of death in the United States—is a major complication of depression. About one in 16 people diagnosed with depression die by suicide, and approximately two thirds of people who die by suicide are depressed.

In the United States, suicide risk is highest in older white males and in those who live alone, have made prior suicide attempts, refuse psychiatric evaluation, or abuse alcohol or other drugs. Although women attempt suicide three to four times more often than men, men are three to four times more likely to die by suicide. In addition, a study found that older people with a serious physical illness were six times more likely to die by suicide than those without an illness. In a U.K. study, interpersonal problems and bereavement, along with chronic physical illness (pain, breathlessness, and functional limitation) were commonly associated with suicide in older people.

The risk of suicide is particularly high in people with untreated bipolar disorder. About 25–50% of those with the condition attempt

NEW RESEARCH

Depression Increases Risk of Death From Multiple Causes

It's long been known that depression increases the risk of death from heart disease and suicide, but a large Norwegian study suggests that it also contributes to death from most other major diseases, including stroke, respiratory illnesses, cancer, multiple sclerosis, and Parkinson's disease. It is also associated with accidental deaths.

Researchers gathered baseline information on physical and mental health for 61,349 Norwegian men and women, average age 48, and then noted the number of deaths and their causes during an average follow-up of nearly 4.5 years. Participants who had significant depression (2,866) had a higher risk of dying of most major causes of death, even after adjusting for age, medical conditions, and physical complaints at the study's outset. In contrast, a diagnosis of anxiety did not increase the risk of death. However, coexisting anxiety-depression appeared to raise the risk of accidental death and suicide.

The researchers theorize that depression may increase the risk of death by directly affecting the cardiovascular and nervous systems. In addition, the mood disorder may lead to poor health habits, such as smoking, alcohol abuse, and a sedentary lifestyle, and may affect people's ability to follow treatment regimens.

PSYCHOSOMATIC MEDICINE
Volume 69, page 323
May 2007

suicide at least once. Moreover, suicide is a major concern among adolescents and young adults—it is the third leading cause of death among younger people ages 15–24.

Up to three quarters of people who die by suicide have visited their medical doctor in the prior month. This suggests that they were aware that something was wrong but that neither they nor their doctor identified depression as the problem. Although it is impossible to predict accurately who will attempt suicide, there are warning signs that a severely depressed person may make an attempt. All too often, friends and family of people who die by suicide are unaware of these red flags until it is too late.

The most important steps to prevent suicide are to recognize the risk factors and warning signs and to facilitate appropriate treatment of the underlying psychiatric illness. Typical warning signs are listed below. However, not all people who die by suicide have these risk factors, and most people who do have them are not suicidal. Signs include the following:

- Social isolation that may be self-imposed
- Drastic mood swings or overall personality changes
- Neglecting home, finances, or pets
- Recent psychological trauma, such as a divorce, death of a loved one, or job loss (which may trigger suicidal thinking in an already depressed person)
- Exaggerated complaints of aches or pains
- Giving away cherished belongings to loved ones or putting one's affairs in order
- Sudden calm or cheerfulness after a period of depression
- Frequent use of alcohol or other drugs
- Buying a gun
- Verbal threats of suicide or statements that suggest a desire to die
- Family history of suicide or previous suicide attempts.

Natural History and Prognosis of Mood Disorders

Mood disorders most often surface between ages 20 and 30 but they can occur at any age. There is often a delay in accurate diagnosis because symptoms are typically not recognized as being related to an illness but, rather, are thought to be a reaction to life circumstances.

Depression

An untreated episode of major depression usually lasts eight to nine months. This period can be shortened considerably with proper diagnosis and treatment. Most people with depression have their first episode before age 40, and most will have more than one episode in their lifetime. Relapse rates are lower in people who continue with treatment when they are feeling well. Approximately 10% of depressed people have a chronic form of depression that is resistant to current treatments.

Alcoholism or other drug use can make recovery from depression (and bipolar disorder) more difficult. A recent study compared 176 men and women who fit the criteria for both alcoholism and major depression with 412 people who had major depression alone. Those who had never been alcoholics or who no longer drank were twice as likely to recover from an episode of major depression than those who were still drinking. Unfortunately, many depressed people slow their recovery by attempting to self-medicate with alcohol.

Bipolar Disorder

Bipolar disorder usually begins at an earlier age than depression and can even occur in childhood. But it is also an unpredictable disease that can emerge later in life. In one large study of people treated at Veterans Affairs hospitals, 25% of the more than 65,000 people with bipolar disorder treated during one year were age 60 or older. And in this over-60 age group, approximately 6% had new-onset disease.

In a second study, 9.8% of 1,157 people between the ages of 18 and 70 treated in an urban primary care clinic screened positive for bipolar disorder. Of those, 41% reported first being affected at age 40 or older.

Overall, men are more likely than women to suffer from bipolar disorder, but women may be more likely to experience the late-onset form. A study of 48 older adults with bipolar disorder showed that women were 2.8 times more likely to be in the late-onset group.

About two thirds of people with bipolar disorder who recover completely from an acute episode have recurrent bouts of either depression or mania. Half of these recurrences tend to be manic, even when the first episode is depression. Although the average number of recurrences is four, this number can vary significantly from person to person. The episodes can be separated by weeks, months, or years. Over time, recurrences tend to happen more frequently, and they may become more severe.

NEW RESEARCH

Anxiety and Depression Rise and Fall With Cognitive Decline

It's well known that people with dementia often suffer from anxiety and depression, but a new study shows that symptoms actually wax and wane as cognitive dysfunction increases.

The researchers compared four groups in various stages of cognitive decline from a community-based sample and a clinical sample of older people diagnosed with Alzheimer's. The prevalence of anxiety and depression symptoms among people in various stages of cognitive decline was established, then analyses were conducted to determine differences between the levels of cognitive functioning.

Anxiety symptoms were noted in 8.6% of people with good cognitive functioning, rising to 11.8% in those with moderate functioning and dropping to 10.7% in those with poor functioning. Similarly, depressive symptoms were found in 8.9% of those with good functioning, 22.1% of those with moderate functioning, and 21.1% of those with poor functioning. Of those diagnosed with Alzheimer's disease, only 6% had anxiety and 16.7% suffered from depression.

The increase in depression and anxiety symptoms earlier in the course of cognitive decline may be attributed to individuals noticing the decrease in functioning, while in later cognitive decline (and Alzheimer's) anxiety and depression may appear to decrease due to lack of awareness.

DEMENTIA AND GERIATRIC COGNITIVE DISORDERS
Volume 24, page 213
August 2007

Antidepressant Drugs 2008*

Drug type: Brand (generic)	Typical daily dosage†	How they appear to work
Selective serotonin reuptake inhibitors (SSRIs)		
Celexa (citalopram[‡])	20–60 mg	Block the reabsorption and inactivation of the neurotransmitter serotonin. This increases the availability of serotonin to carry messages between nerve cells.
(fluvoxamine[§])	50–300 mg	
Lexapro (escitalopram[‖])	10–20 mg	
Paxil (paroxetine[‡])	20–50 mg	
Paxil CR (paroxetine, controlled-release[‖])	12.5–62.5 mg	
Prozac (fluoxetine[‡])	20–80 mg	
Prozac Weekly (fluoxetine)	90 mg	
Zoloft (sertraline[‡])	50–200 mg	
Serotonin and norepinephrine reuptake inhibitors (SNRIs)		
Cymbalta (duloxetine)	40–60 mg	Block the reabsorption of serotonin and norepinephrine, increasing the availability of these neurotransmitters in the brain.
(trazodone[§])	150–400 mg	
Effexor (venlafaxine[‡])	75–375 mg	
Effexor XR (venlafaxine, extended-release)	37.5–225 mg	
Dopamine reuptake inhibitors		
Wellbutrin (bupropion[‡])	200–450 mg	Block the reabsorption of the neurotransmitter dopamine, increasing its availability in the brain.
Wellbutrin SR (bupropion, sustained-release)	150–400 mg	
Wellbutrin XL (bupropion, extended-release)	150–450 mg	
Tricyclics		
(amitriptyline[§])	50–200 mg	Block the reabsorption of the neurotransmitters serotonin, norepinephrine, and, to a lesser extent, dopamine, increasing their availability in the brain.
Aventyl (nortriptyline[‡])	75–150 mg	
Norpramin (desipramine[‡])	100–300 mg	
Pamelor (nortriptyline[‡])	75–150 mg	
Sinequan (doxepin[‡])	25–300 mg	
Surmontil (trimipramine[‡])	50–200 mg	
Tofranil (imipramine[‡])	75–200 mg	
Vivactil (protriptyline[‡])	15–60 mg	

Precautions	Common side effects
Do not take with MAO inhibitors, triptans, or St. John's wort. If discontinuing use, reduce dosage gradually to prevent withdrawal symptoms. The development of a skin rash can be the sign of a serious medical problem; see a doctor immediately.	Anxiety, nervousness, insomnia, drowsiness, weakness, headache, diarrhea, increased sweating, nausea, impaired sexual function, weight gain. Side effects appear to be lesser with escitalopram.
Do not take with MAO inhibitors or triptans. If discontinuing use, reduce dosage gradually to prevent withdrawal symptoms. Venlafaxine may increase blood pressure and/or cholesterol levels in some people, especially at high doses; regular blood pressure and cholesterol monitoring is advised.	Nausea, weakness, sweating, insomnia, drowsiness, dry mouth, dizziness, constipation, nervousness, impaired sexual function, appetite loss.
Do not take if you have seizures or an eating disorder, are using MAO inhibitors, or are using another product that contains bupropion (such as the smoking-cessation drug, Zyban).	Loss of appetite, weight loss, dry mouth, skin rash, sweating, ringing in the ears, shakiness, stomach pain, agitation, anxiety, dizziness, trouble sleeping, muscle pain, nausea, fast heart beat, sore throat, increased urination. Higher doses are associated with a greater risk of seizures. Low risk of sexual side effects and weight gain.
Do not take with MAO inhibitors. Do not stop treatment abruptly. It is not advisable to take most tricyclic antidepressants if you have seizures, a heart disorder, glaucoma, or use alcohol excessively.	Dizziness on standing, drowsiness, weakness, headache, dry mouth, blurred vision, constipation, nausea, difficulty urinating, increased appetite (which may include a craving for sweets), impaired sexual function, increased heart rate. Skin is more sensitive to sunlight and may result in itching, redness, discoloration of skin.

* This list represents the most commonly prescribed antidepressants.

† These dosages represent an average range for the treatment of depression and may differ from the dosage prescribed by your doctor. The precise effective dosage varies from person to person and depends on many factors. Do not make any change to your medication without consulting your doctor. *Starting dosages tend to be lower for older adults.*

‡ Generic version available at lower cost.

§ Generic only available.

|| Generic version approved as of press time.

continued on the next page

Antidepressant Drugs 2008* (continued)

Drug type: Brand (generic)	Typical daily dosage†	How they appear to work
Tetracyclics		
(maprotiline§)	75–200 mg	Block the reabsorption of serotonin and norepinephrine, increasing the availability of these neurotransmitters.
Remeron (mirtazapine‡)	15–45 mg	
Remeron SolTab (mirtazapine‡)	15–45 mg	
Monoamine oxidase (MAO) inhibitors		
Emsam skin patch (selegiline)	6–12 mg	Block the action of MAO, which is an enzyme that inactivates the neurotransmitters serotonin, norepinephrine, and dopamine. MAO inhibitors thereby increase levels of these neurotransmitters, increasing their availability for carrying messages between neurons.
Marplan (isocarboxazid‡)	10–60 mg	
Nardil (phenelzine‡)	45–90 mg	
Parnate (tranylcypromine‡)	10–30 mg	

* This list represents the most commonly prescribed antidepressants.

† These dosages represent an average range for the treatment of depression and may differ from the dosage prescribed by your doctor. The precise effective dosage varies from patient to patient and depends on many factors. Do not make any change to your medication without consulting your doctor. *Starting dosages tend to be lower for older adults.*

‡ Generic version available at lower cost.

§ Generic only available.

Some people with bipolar disorder can cycle between depressive and manic episodes as often as four times a year (this is known as rapid cycling). There is tremendous variability in the course of the condition, with some people experiencing full recovery between episodes and others experiencing chronic (ongoing) symptoms.

Treatment of Mood Disorders

In treating depression, doctors have three goals. The first is to relieve the symptoms of depression, the second is to restore the person's ability to function socially and in the workplace, and the final goal is to reduce the likelihood of a recurrence.

The goals for bipolar disorder are somewhat different because it is usually more challenging to treat. Doctors primarily strive to reduce the frequency and severity—and the social and psychological impact—of episodes. Improving social and mental functioning between episodes is the other major goal of treatment.

When a person seeks treatment for a mood disorder, the first

Precautions	Common side effects
Do not take with MAO inhibitors. Caution advised with use of mirtazapine in the elderly because of delayed metabolism and clearance of the drug, which may increase the risk of adverse events.	Sleepiness, nausea, increased appetite, weight gain, dizziness, blurred vision, weakness, dry mouth, headache, constipation, shakiness, nervousness.
Foods containing tyramine (see page 36) should be avoided because they may cause a sudden, severe rise in blood pressure (hypertensive crisis), which can be fatal. There are no dietary restrictions with the 6-mg Emsam skin patch, however, as it does not interfere with the breakdown of tyramine in the digestive tract. (Restrictions do apply for the higher-dose patches.) MAO inhibitors may interact dangerously with numerous drugs, including other antidepressants and cold medications.	Dizziness, lightheadedness (especially in older persons), drowsiness, headache, dry mouth, constipation, nausea, insomnia, decreased sexual function, weight gain. Patch can cause skin irritation.

step is a complete evaluation, which includes a detailed psychiatric and medical history, and a mental status examination. Because treatment varies considerably based on the diagnosis, it is crucial to have this comprehensive assessment.

Treatment goals for depression and bipolar disorder are accomplished over three stages—acute, continuation, and maintenance. During *acute treatment,* the focus is on immediately relieving symptoms and restoring the person's ability to function. Once symptoms respond to acute treatment, *continuation treatment* begins; the focus here is on preventing a relapse. If a person has no symptoms for four to nine months after an episode, he or she is considered recovered. At this point, *maintenance treatment* begins, with the goal of preventing a new episode. Maintenance treatment can last from one year to a lifetime, depending on the individual.

Depression recurs in about half of cases within two years of stopping treatment, so timing must be considered carefully when stopping medications. The longer a person remains on treatment, the smaller the likelihood of relapse. The decision to try tapering off medications for bipolar disorder is more complicated because it involves the risk of recurrent manic and depressive episodes and, especially, the risk of suicide.

The main treatment options for dealing with depression and bipolar disorder are medications, psychotherapy, electroconvulsive therapy (sometimes informally referred to as shock therapy), or any combination of these. Light therapy is often used to treat SAD. In addition, exercise, getting enough sleep, and eating a healthy diet play a role in improving mood and self-image.

These days, medications are the most common form of therapy for depression. Any given antidepressant has up to a 70% chance of working in a particular person. It is important to start treatment as early as possible, however, as these disorders become more difficult to treat the longer they last. Because response to any particular treatment varies from one person to another, an individual who does not improve with the initial treatment may respond to a different one.

In fact, that's the important lesson to be learned from a large, six-year multi-center study called the Sequenced Treatment Alternatives to Relieve Depression Trial, or STAR*D, which looked at the use of popular antidepressants in people with chronic depression (lasting, in some cases, 15–16 years). This study found that systematically trying different doses of antidepressant medications, maintaining a longer duration of therapy, trying a different drug altogether, or combining medications can lead to a remission in symptoms for many severely depressed, treatment-resistant patients.

Like antidepressant medications, psychotherapy alone also can work to relieve depression—with fewer side effects. While it requires more time than antidepressant therapy to reduce symptoms, its positive effects may last longer than medication.

Severe cases of depression are best treated with medication. In the most extreme cases, electroconvulsive therapy may be recommended. Up to 90% of extremely depressed people improve with electroconvulsive therapy when it is used as a first-line treatment. However, the therapy is usually used only after other therapies have failed. When used as a last resort, the response rate drops to 50–60%.

Combination therapy (medication plus psychotherapy) has been shown in some research studies to be more effective than either therapy alone for mild to moderate depression. This option may be beneficial if either treatment alone produces only partial results, if depression is chronic, or if the person is facing multiple challenges that are best treated by different means, such as medication for depressive symptoms and psychotherapy for job-related problems.

NEW RESEARCH

Factors Affecting Treatment-Resistant Depression

Despite the wide variety of antidepressants available, 30–40% of depressive episodes are deemed "treatment resistant," failing to respond to either of two consecutive medications. A new study offers insights into why that may be.

A European multicenter trial analyzed 702 participants diagnosed with major depressive disorder. Using data from the 356 individuals considered treatment resistant, researchers examined the link between individual variables and depression that doesn't respond to medication.

Co-occurring anxiety—in particular panic disorder and social phobia—had the strongest link with treatment-resistant depression, as current or lifetime anxiety was found in 40% of the treatment-resistant participants. The researchers identified eight other factors linked with treatment resistance: personality disorder, suicide risk, severe depression prior to treatment, melancholia (nonspecific depression marked by lack of pleasure in anything), repeated hospitalizations for depression, recurrent depressive episodes, onset of depression before age 18, and a lack of response to the first antidepressant tried for depression.

The hope is that more research into genetic, demographic, and other factors, as well as early recognition of the newly identified variables, will lead to better strategies for treatment-resistant depression.

JOURNAL OF CLINICAL PSYCHIATRY
Volume 68, page 1062
July 2007

Recent research suggests that combination therapy may prevent or delay relapses and recurrences of depression.

Treatment of Depression With Medications

Today, physicians can choose from a wide range of antidepressant medications (see the drug chart on pages 20–23). These include selective serotonin reuptake inhibitors (SSRIs), tricyclics, tetracyclics, dopamine reuptake inhibitors, serotonin and norepinephrine reuptake inhibitors, and monoamine oxidase (MAO) inhibitors.

There are several advantages to treating depression with antidepressant medications:

- They are effective against mild, moderate, and severe forms of major depression.
- People usually respond more quickly to medications than to psychotherapy.
- They are easy to administer.
- They are not addictive and, when properly used, are usually quite safe.
- They can be used in combination with psychotherapy.

The disadvantages are:

- Medication therapy can cause unwanted side effects.
- It requires strict adherence to a medication schedule and repeated visits to your doctor to monitor response.
- It may take some time—and some tinkering—to find the right medication at the right dose.

Because of these factors, many people do not have an adequate trial of a therapeutic dose for a sufficient period of time. Older people and those with chronic illnesses are more susceptible to the adverse effects of antidepressants.

Researchers believe that antidepressants work by affecting levels of neurotransmitters—chemical messengers in the brain that facilitate communication between nerve cells. However, physicians cannot predetermine which medication will be the most effective in any particular individual. Drug selection relies largely on a process of educated guesses, although most people do have some positive response to the first antidepressant they try.

Choosing a medication

For a person with a first-time episode of moderate to severe depression and no other psychological symptoms or medical conditions, the choice of medication is generally based on avoidance of side effects. For example, the tricyclic antidepressant amitriptyline can

NEW RESEARCH

Success With First Antidepressant Affects Next Treatment Choice

The effectiveness of the first antidepressant one tries greatly influences the choice of subsequent treatments for depression, according to a new analysis of data from the landmark Sequenced Treatment Alternatives to Relieve Depression (STAR*D) trial.

A group of 1,439 people who didn't respond fully to their treatment with citalopram (Celexa) went on to a second stage where they indicated whether it was acceptable to add a second medication to their regimen, switch to a different medication, and/or try cognitive therapy in addition to adding or switching medications.

Only 1% of the individuals were willing to be randomized to try all options. Three percent accepted a switch to cognitive therapy without medication, while 26% would undergo being randomly assigned to cognitive therapy while also switching medications or adding a second antidepressant to treatment with Celexa. Participants who experienced more side effects or lower symptom reduction on Celexa typically opted to switch to a new medication instead of adding another one.

Individuals most willing to undergo cognitive therapy had a higher education level, a family history of depression or bipolar disorder, or had spent a longer time in first-step treatment with Celexa, while those with panic disorder were the most unlikely to accept cognitive therapy as an option.

AMERICAN JOURNAL OF PSYCHIATRY
Volume 164, page 753
May 2007

lower blood pressure and cause drowsiness and confusion—side effects that are especially troublesome for older people. The drug nortriptyline (Aventyl, Pamelor) is less likely to cause these side effects.

Family history can also help predict which drugs are most likely to be effective, as well as which ones are most likely to cause side effects. In addition, older people are typically started on lower doses than younger people to reduce the risk of side effects.

By themselves, antidepressant medications usually produce a significant improvement by four to six weeks, although it may take up to 12 weeks on a therapeutic dose to see the full benefit. If a person's depression responds fully to medication after this period, treatment moves on to the continuation phase, which lasts for six months to one year at the same dosage level and then to the maintenance phase. Those who have improved somewhat but still have a few symptoms after six weeks should be reassessed six weeks later (many are likely to improve further during this time). At the reassessment, the physician may adjust the dosage to improve response.

When a drug does not work, a doctor may prescribe an antidepressant from a different class of medications, because drugs in the same class tend to work similarly. When a drug from one class is producing good results but causes unacceptable side effects, switching to a different medication within the same class can often help.

In 20–50% of people, adding the drug lithium can help boost the action of an antidepressant. However, the addition of lithium increases the risk of side effects and adverse drug interactions, requiring close monitoring by a physician.

If maintenance treatment is no longer needed, drugs are discontinued slowly over a period of one to three weeks to avoid withdrawal symptoms. Relapses are most common during the first two months after a person stops taking an antidepressant. It is therefore important for individuals to remain in contact with their physicians during this period. Should a relapse occur, the same drug that was used successfully the first time often proves effective again.

Suicide and medication

All antidepressants must be used with caution if a person is suicidal. When this is the case, the person will need to see his or her doctor for frequent follow-up visits and will receive a prescription for a relatively small number of pills at a time. Suicide attempts or suicidal thoughts are common symptoms of depression, and the risk of suicide may increase as depression begins to respond to treatment because the person might regain just enough energy and motivation to follow through on a suicidal urge.

In 2004, a federal panel of drug experts said that antidepressants could increase the risk of children and teenagers becoming suicidal. Later that year, the U.S. Food and Drug Administration (FDA) required the makers of antidepressants to add a "black box" warning to that effect to the drug labels of these medications. In 2005, the agency issued a public health advisory stating that suicidal thoughts and behaviors may also be increased among adults on antidepressants. The risk of suicide is higher at the start of drug therapy and when the dosage is changed, according to the FDA (see the "Ask the Doctor" column at right).

Antidepressants are the fourth leading cause of drug overdose and the third leading cause of drug-related death when taken improperly. (Tricyclics such as amitriptyline are the most common cause of death from an antidepressant overdose.) In addition, when a person with latent bipolar disorder starts taking antidepressants, manic symptoms may develop and require treatment.

Although up to 70% of people with depression respond positively to antidepressants—and some studies suggest that use of antidepressants, particularly newer SSRIs, decreases the risk of suicide—it is true that some people might have responded just as well to a placebo. But whether a person responds to an antidepressant because of the action of the medication or the placebo effect, or possibly a combination of both, the fact remains that antidepressants provide real relief to many people. Moreover, because studies of the placebo effect have only followed people for a limited period of time, there are no data showing whether or not the placebo effect can be sustained in the long term; by contrast, there are data showing that the positive effects of medication are sustained long term.

When it comes to the length of treatment for depression, there is no "one size fits all." However, recent evidence shows that many people require a year or more of antidepressant therapy to treat a major depressive episode adequately. (This includes roughly three months of acute treatment to significantly improve depressive symptoms and an additional six months to a year of continuation/maintenance treatment.) People with severe or recurring depression and older adults may require much longer maintenance therapy.

Selective serotonin reuptake inhibitors (SSRIs)

Low amounts of the neurotransmitter serotonin have been linked to depression. SSRIs such as citalopram (Celexa), escitalopram

ASK THE DOCTOR

Q. ***Can taking an antidepressant make me suicidal?***

A. Whether antidepressants raise suicide risk has been a hotly contested issue since the U.S. Food and Drug Administration (FDA) issued black-box warnings that they could increase suicide risk in children and teenagers, then extended the risk to adults. On the other hand, suicide remains a risk of untreated depression, and research suggests that SSRIs decrease suicide risk by improving symptoms, while the increased use of fluoxetine (Prozac) in the United States has been linked with a lower suicide rate.

The risk of antidepressants increasing suicidal thoughts in those with severe depression appears to occur during the first few treatment weeks or when changing the dose. At this time, when the medications might not yet be having an effect, depression and suicidal thoughts may worsen. Also, when some individuals begin to respond to the medication, they may have just enough energy and motivation to commit suicide. In addition, people with bipolar disorder who have been misdiagnosed with depression and given antidepressants may be at greater risk for suicide.

A good strategy is to stay in close contact with your healthcare provider, family, and friends when you start on an antidepressant or if your dose is adjusted so that they will notice any warning signs if your symptoms worsen. It's always a good idea, too, to engage in some form of talk therapy, which has been shown to enhance the effectiveness of antidepressants.

Psychiatric Medications and Weight Gain

Fending off unwanted pounds

While recovery from mental illnesses such as anxiety and depression can be lifesaving, weight gain often can be an unwanted side effect of treatment for many people. Psychiatric medications including antidepressants, mood stabilizers, and antipsychotics may increase weight by stimulating the appetite or slowing the body's metabolism, and that gain can range from minimal (a few pounds) to significant (up to 50 lbs).

Such rapid weight gain may increase the risk of many health conditions associated with being overweight, such as high blood pressure, diabetes, heart disease, arthritis, and some types of cancer. That's why it's so important to discuss all the potential benefits and risks of taking psychiatric medication with your doctor before you start treatment.

Strategies should be put in place to prevent weight gain and, if it does occur, to manage it before it jeopardizes your health.

Medication Alert

Many types of medications are used to treat mental health problems. The following are the most commonly prescribed medications grouped according to type, highlighting the ones that are most likely to cause weight gain and the alternatives less associated with weight gain.

- **Monoamine oxidase inhibitors (MAOIs):** Antidepressant drugs such as isocarboxazid (Marplan), phenelzine (Nardil), selegiline (Emsam), and tranylcypromine (Parnate) are likely to cause weight gain both in the short term (less than six months) and long term (over one year).
- **Tricyclic antidepressants:** These agents (amitriptyline, doxepin [Sinequan], imipramine [Tofranil], and nortriptyline [Aventyl and Pamelor]) stimulate appetite—particularly cravings for sweets—and are linked to both short- and long-term weight gain.
- **Tetracyclic antidepressant mirtazapine (Remeron):** This drug causes weight gain in as little as four weeks of treatment, according to an analysis of four studies, as well as over the long term. In these studies it does appear less likely to cause weight gain than tricyclic antidepressants, although doctors at Johns Hopkins have found it to be equal to tricyclics.
- **Selective serotonin reuptake inhibitors (SSRIs):** Paroxetine (Paxil, a popular drug for depression and anxiety) often causes weight gain, especially when used for six months or more. Escitalopram (Lexapro) can cause weight gain, too. One study found that 26% of Paxil users gained a significant amount of weight over six months, compared with 7% of people using fluoxetine (Prozac) and 4% using sertraline (Zoloft). These other SSRIs, as well as citalopram (Celexa) and fluvoxamine, are generally considered "weight neutral."
- **Serotonin and norepinephrine reuptake inhibitors (SNRIs):** Duloxetine (Cymbalta) and venlafaxine (Effexor), commonly prescribed for depression and anxiety, are believed to have little effect on weight.
- **Dopamine reuptake inhibitor bupropion (Wellbutrin):** This antidepressant, also commonly prescribed as an anti-smoking aid, is less likely to cause weight gain than SSRIs and may, in fact, cause weight loss.
- **Atypical antipsychotics:** These drugs, which are prescribed to treat bipolar disorder, schizophrenia, and other mental illnesses, can cause significant weight gain. They can even continue to increase weight one year after the initiation of treatment. Drugs in this class that are most associated with weight-related side effects include clozapine

(Lexapro), fluoxetine (Prozac), fluvoxamine, paroxetine (Paxil), and sertraline (Zoloft) increase levels of serotonin in the brain. All of the SSRIs are equally effective and have similar rates and types of side effects, although it is possible that an individual might respond better or experience fewer side effects with a particular SSRI. Side

(Clozaril), olanzapine (Zyprexa), quetiapine (Seroquel), and risperidone (Risperdal). Weight-neutral alternatives include aripiprazole (Abilify) and ziprasidone (Geodon).

• **Mood stabilizers:** Divalproex (Depakote) and lithium (Eskalith, Lithobid), the primary medications for bipolar disorder, have also been found to cause both short- and long-term weight gain.

Can Drug Combinations Manage Weight?

Recently, doctors have been looking into whether adding other drugs to a psychiatric medication that is causing weight gain might be helpful. Although little scientific data supports their use, stimulants such as methylphenidate (Ritalin) or amphetamines (Benzedrine, Dexedrine); famotidine (Pepcid, an ulcer drug); triiodothyronine (Cytomel, a thyroid hormone replacement medication); topiramate (Topamax, an antiseizure and migraine drug); and the antidepressant bupropion (Wellbutrin) have been found to prevent weight gain in some people when combined in low doses with psychiatric medications.

For some overweight people, the weight-loss drugs orlistat (Xenical) or sibutramine (Meridia) also may curb medication-related weight gain.

Managing Your Weight

Despite the fact that many psychiatric medications have weight gain as a side effect, that does not mean it's a *fait accompli*. Be aware of the potential for weight gain and follow these strategies to head off extra pounds:

• Weigh yourself weekly and keep a diary of your weight so you can notice small increases quickly and take steps to counter further gains. Also keep a food diary for an accurate gauge of how much you're really eating on a daily basis.

• Avoid or limit high-calorie, high-fat foods.

• Eat smaller portions—and smaller meals and snacks overall.

• Don't keep large quantities of junk foods in your home. If you need to snack, choose healthy foods such as fresh fruit or vegetables or unbuttered popcorn.

• Eat slowly. Many people eat too quickly—the brain needs about 20 minutes to recognize that the stomach is full, so if you eat too fast, you'll be apt to consume more calories than you need to satisfy your hunger.

• Don't skip meals. Going for long periods of time without food only serves to make you hungrier in the long term and more likely to overeat once you do eat.

• Exercise every day to counteract any extra calories you're consuming and give a boost to your metabolism. Try resistance training and aerobic exercise. To get your heart pumping, buy a pedometer (a small, inexpensive device that tracks how many steps you walk) and shoot to walk 10,000 steps a day. To build muscle, lift weights or use resistance machines three times a week.

• Drink frequently. Hunger is one of the symptoms of dehydration, so quench your thirst with calorie-free beverages such as water, seltzer, diet soda, and decaffeinated coffee and tea.

• If all else fails, talk to your healthcare provider about switching to a medication that is less likely to cause weight gain or adding another one that might help avoid weight gain (see the inset box above). Don't stop taking your medication without discussing it with your doctor, as your depression or anxiety may return or you may experience withdrawal side effects. ■

effects are not always a reason to change medications. For example, paroxetine can produce a sedative effect in some people, but this may be beneficial to people who suffer from both anxiety and depression.

Because side effects of SSRIs are more mild than most other

antidepressants, most doctors now consider them the first-line drug treatment for depression. Studies have demonstrated that SSRIs are as effective as tricyclics; about half of those who take an SSRI see their symptoms of depression lift completely. Advantages of SSRIs over other antidepressants such as tricyclics include a lower risk of fatal overdoses and serious heart rhythm disturbances in people with cardiac disease. SSRIs are also effective against chronic low-grade depression (dysthymia).

Side effects. SSRIs can produce side effects such as anxiety, nervousness, insomnia, drowsiness, and nausea. Another troublesome side effect is sexual dysfunction—diminished sexual desire, changes in the sensations of arousal, or disturbances in the ability to achieve orgasm—which may occur in about 37% of both men and women taking these drugs. Sexual side effects usually develop within the first week of starting an SSRI, though they may arise more slowly as blood levels of the medication build up. Strategies to alleviate sexual dysfunction include switching to a medication with a low rate of sexual side effects (such as the dopamine reuptake inhibitor bupropion [Wellbutrin]), waiting to see if sexual side effects abate, changing the time you take the medication (possibly to nighttime), reducing the dosage, taking drug holidays (for example, not taking the medication on the weekend), or adding another medication such as the erectile dysfunction drug sildenafil (Viagra). If you experience worrisome symptoms, do not make any changes in your drug regimen on your own—be sure to consult your doctor first.

Recently, it was recognized that SSRIs may produce neurological side effects—symptoms like those of Parkinson's disease, such as impaired muscle tone, tremors, and spasms or feelings of restlessness. These symptoms can become so severe that sitting still becomes impossible. Fortunately, they are rare: In one study, they occurred in only 0.27% of people. By comparison, the most common side effects of Prozac—agitation and anxiety—occurred in twice as many people, although they were still relatively uncommon. If you experience any of these symptoms, contact your doctor before you stop taking your medication.

In addition, people taking a combination of drugs that raise the level of serotonin in the body can develop a disorder called serotonin syndrome. The most common causes are taking an SSRI at the same time as an MAO (monoamine oxidase) inhibitor or a triptan migraine drug (frovatriptan [Frova], rizatriptan [Maxalt], sumatriptan [Imitrex], and others). The syndrome is characterized by altered mental status, neuromuscular abnormalities, and dysfunction of the autonomic nervous system, which controls involuntary reflexes that affect breathing, heart rate, blood pressure, and the digestive tract. Tricyclic antidepressants may also contribute to serotonin syndrome.

SSRIs can increase the risk of gastrointestinal bleeding, particularly when taken with nonsteroidal anti-inflammatory drugs (NSAIDs), such as aspirin, according to a recent Danish study. This increased risk of bleeding means blood is less likely to clot, an effect that may be beneficial to certain people at risk for heart attacks and ischemic strokes—conditions caused by blood clotting. Another study found that depressed heart patients treated with the SSRI Zoloft showed significant reductions in the level of clotting factors in their blood, compared with those receiving a placebo.

Although the side effects tend to be similar among the SSRIs, fluvoxamine and Paxil may be more likely to cause nausea, and diarrhea is more common with Zoloft. Because Prozac may take several days to clear from the body, interactions with other drugs are more likely to occur. One advantage of Prozac is that it is now available in a once-a-week capsule.

SSRI withdrawal. SSRIs are not addictive in the conventional medical use of the word, but suddenly discontinuing their use after taking them for more than six weeks is known to produce both physical and mental withdrawal symptoms.

About 25% of people who abruptly stop taking an SSRI experience withdrawal symptoms, most commonly dizziness, nausea, lethargy, and headache. Other symptoms include irritability, nervousness, crying spells, flu-like symptoms (body aches, chills, and fatigue), and shooting pains in and around the head.

SSRI withdrawal—also called SSRI discontinuation syndrome—is not dangerous, but it can be distressing. Fortunately, it is usually mild, commences within one week of stopping treatment, and resolves within three weeks.

To minimize SSRI discontinuation syndrome, doses of SSRIs (like other antidepressants) should be reduced gradually.

Tricyclics

Tricyclics—such as amitriptyline, desipramine (Norpramin), doxepin (Sinequan), imipramine (Tofranil), nortriptyline (Aventyl, Pamelor), protriptyline (Vivactil), and trimipramine (Surmontil)—are named for their chemical structure: a chain of three rings. These drugs raise brain concentrations of the neurotransmitters norepinephrine, serotonin, and, to a lesser extent, dopamine by blocking reabsorption of these chemical messengers by the nerve

NEW RESEARCH

SSRIs May Increase Fracture Risk in Older Adults

Taking the selective serotonin reuptake inhibitors (SSRIs) citalopram (Celexa), fluoxetine (Prozac), fluvoxamine, paroxetine (Paxil), and sertraline (Zoloft) can double the risk of fractures in older adults, according to a Canadian study.

Researchers followed 5,008 adults age 50 and older for five years for the incidence of clinical fragility fractures. They found that 137 people who were using SSRIs on a daily basis had twice the risk of breaking a bone during the study as those who were not using SSRIs, even after adjusting for potential contributing factors. SSRI users also had an increased risk of falling (the larger the dose, the greater the risk) as well as lower bone mineral density at the hip and often at the spine.

The investigators suggested that SSRIs may raise the risk of fractures by compromising bone quality and strength as well as by increasing the chance of falling. Since older adults are at risk for both osteoporotic fractures and depression, the risk of using SSRIs must be balanced against the benefits to be gained by the treatment of depression. Further studies are needed to confirm these findings and clarify the risks.

ARCHIVES OF INTERNAL MEDICINE
Volume 167, page 188
January 2007

cells that release them. Tricyclics are used mainly to treat moderate to severe depression and have proven less effective for chronic low-grade depression. About 60% of people who take tricyclics experience significant improvement within four to six weeks. Each of the tricyclics is believed to be equally effective, but side effects may differ.

When a person begins tricyclic therapy, he or she will be given a small dose and will be carefully monitored for side effects. The dose is often raised over several weeks because a gradual increase may be less likely to lead to side effects. Side effects also tend to diminish with continued use. For older people, dosages are usually 30–50% lower than those indicated in the chart on pages 20–23. When the proper dosage is established, tricyclics can be taken by a person at bedtime to help bring on sleep rather than cause daytime drowsiness.

Although a positive response to tricyclics typically appears within four to six weeks, doctors recommend giving the medication six to eight weeks at a full dosage to assess the effects. During this time, blood tests may be ordered to make sure that the drug level is high enough to exert a therapeutic effect but not so high as to be toxic (nortriptyline's optimal blood level is the one most accurately known). If a person's depression does not improve while taking a tricyclic, it may be that the drug is not effective for that person or that he or she is not taking the drug as prescribed. About one-third of people stop taking tricyclics because of side effects, and about two-thirds of older people miss 25–50% of their doses. Poor compliance leads to fluctuating blood levels of the drug and, consequently, a poor response. Therefore, it is important to tell your doctor about unpleasant side effects instead of just stopping your medication.

Side effects. The most prominent side effects of tricyclics are postural hypotension (dizziness on standing due to a drop in blood pressure), drowsiness, weakness, headache, dry mouth, blurred vision, constipation, nausea, and difficulty urinating. Many of these side effects can be managed, however. Drowsiness can be remedied by taking the dose before bedtime (if your doctor approves). Postural hypotension, which can lead to falls and broken bones in older people, can be reduced by standing up slowly after sitting or lying down, and waiting 30 seconds before trying to walk. Pilocarpine (Pilocar) eyedrops may alleviate blurred vision. Chewing sugar-free gum or candy will help dry mouth. (Be sure to mention dry mouth to your dentist—a lack of saliva can lead to an increase in cavities and oral infections.) Bethanechol (Duvoid, Urabeth, Urecholine) may be prescribed to counteract problems with urination. And constipation can be managed by consuming foods high in fiber and drinking at least eight glasses of water or juice a day. Amitriptyline and Tofranil are more likely than other tricyclics to cause side effects in older people.

People who should not take tricyclics. Tricyclics are not given to people with closed-angle glaucoma (a form of glaucoma characterized by a rapid increase in pressure within the eye) and should be used with caution in men who have symptoms of benign prostatic hyperplasia (an enlarged prostate), as they may develop an inability to urinate. This medical emergency must be treated with catheterization. Tricyclics can also magnify the depressive effects of alcohol and benzodiazepines. The combination of tricyclics with antihistamines can lead to severe constipation, impacted stools, or difficulty urinating, particularly in older adults. In addition, tricyclics (and SSRIs) should not be mixed with the drug selegiline (Eldepryl), which is used to treat Parkinson's disease. Although rare, an interaction between these drugs may cause high fever, tremors, agitation, restlessness, or, in some cases, death. Other symptoms resulting from such drug combinations may include fainting, profuse sweating, seizures, behavioral changes, and stiffened muscles.

Tricyclics are not currently recommended for use in most people with coronary heart disease (CHD) because they can cause life-threatening ventricular fibrillation (abnormal rhythm in the heart's lower chambers) in these individuals. Despite the cardiac risks of tricyclics, they are still used to treat depression because they are sometimes the only effective antidepressants for severely depressed older people.

An older person with mild to moderate depression and severe CHD may first be given a medication from another drug class (SSRIs, such as fluvoxamine, Celexa, Lexapro, Prozac, Paxil, and Zoloft, or the dopamine reuptake inhibitor Wellbutrin). If the individual does not respond to these drugs, a tricyclic would then be tried. Because the risk of ventricular fibrillation from tricyclics increases with the severity of CHD, the doctor must weigh the severity of the depression against the potential cardiac danger.

Tetracyclics

The action, efficacy, and side effects of drugs like maprotiline and mirtazapine (Remeron) are similar to those of the tricyclics. However, maprotiline is more likely to cause seizures than most other antidepressants. A version of Remeron is available that dissolves on the tongue and does not need to be chewed or swallowed whole.

ASK THE DOCTOR

Q. ***If your depression is triggered by stress, should it be treated with medication?***

A. The relationship between mood disorders and stress is complicated, but we do know they're closely interconnected. Stressful events can potentially cause changes in brain chemistry that predispose people to depression and anxiety. It's also possible that certain individuals' brain chemistry is already vulnerable to depression and a trauma such as the death of a loved one, moving to a new town, or losing a job triggers a depressive episode. Stressful events or even chronic stress may spark depression by prompting feelings of helplessness and negative self-talk—especially if you've experienced major depression in the past.

The issue of whether medication is needed for stress-induced depression is also complex. No one should automatically be prescribed antidepressants for any problem. Your doctor should perform a physical examination and ask about your symptoms and medical history before recommending a course of treatment. In many cases, antidepressants have a crucial role in treating depression triggered by stress.

Cognitive-behavioral therapy (CBT) may also help in cases of stress-induced depression: A Canadian study showed that people who recovered from a major depressive episode through medication were more likely to fall back into negative thought patterns than people who had treated depression with CBT. The ability to recognize dysfunctional thinking and disengage from such thoughts can be a valuable tool.

Medications That Can Worsen Depression and Anxiety

Some common treatments are associated with mood disorders

Your antihypertensive medication is doing a great job of lowering your blood pressure—but you suspect that it may be at the sake of your mood. And you just might be right.

In fact, many commonly used prescription medications, especially those used by older people, have been recognized as having negative effects on mental health (see the inset box at right). Even medications designed to relieve depression and anxiety may worsen mental health—at first.

Lowering Blood Pressure—and Mood

The link between blood-pressure treatments and depression has been known for more than 40 years. Research shows that, by affecting the central nervous system, methyldopa, clonidine (Catapres), and reserpine (Serpalan) may present risks for worsening or even causing depression. Other heart-related medications like beta-blockers, including atenolol (Tenormin) and propranolol (Inderal), may also prompt depression as a side effect.

Even over-the-counter remedies can put your mental health at risk. For instance, cold medications like Sudafed that contain the decongestant pseudoephedrine and headache remedies such as Excedrin that list caffeine as an ingredient can induce or worsen anxiety. In addition, drinking alcohol with these medications, or even by itself, can cause chemical changes in the brain that worsen the symptoms of depression or anxiety.

Psychiatric Medication Backfires

At times, treatments intended to lessen anxiety or depression may actually increase the symptoms they're meant to quell, at least temporarily. This is known as a paradoxical effect. For instance, some people report initially feeling more, instead of less, anxious when placed on the anti-anxiety medication escitalopram (Lexapro); after a few weeks, however, most begin to feel positive, beneficial effects.

It's also well known that people may continue to feel sad and even suicidal during the first few weeks of using an antidepressant. That's because it can take up to 12 weeks for the medication to reach therapeutic levels in the blood. It is also possible to be one of the people who don't respond to a certain medication.

A large, six-year government study called the Sequenced Treatment Alternatives to Relieve Depression (STAR*D) trial found that 70% of people with chronic major depression may not recover completely with the first medication that they try and may need to experiment with another type or combination. And many people may benefit from talk therapy as well, which has been found to be as beneficial as pharmacological treatments in some studies for mild or moderate depression.

Dopamine reuptake inhibitors

Wellbutrin decreases the reuptake of dopamine, a neurotransmitter and a precursor of other neurotransmitters. This drug causes less drowsiness and fewer side effects than the tricyclics (especially fewer sexual side effects), but on rare occasions it can cause seizures, particularly at higher doses. Wellbutrin XL is the first drug approved to prevent major depressive episodes in people with seasonal affective disorder (SAD).

Serotonin and norepinephrine reuptake inhibitors

Medications like trazodone, venlafaxine (Effexor), and duloxetine

It's also possible to develop a tolerance to antidepressant and anti-anxiety medications over the long term so that symptoms rebound, although this phenomenon hasn't been well studied.

Finally, people with bipolar disorder who receive an antidepressant alone (without a mood stabilizer such as lithium) may have more manic episodes and rapid cycling between depression and mania than they did before being treated (see pages 39–42 for information).

Work With Your Doctor

Because there are so many medications available now to treat common ailments like hypertension, be sure to let your doctor know if you notice a change in your mood or anxiety level when you're taking a certain drug. He or she may be able to switch you to a different medication that is less likely to cause or worsen depression or anxiety. For instance, antihypertensive agents such as diuretics, calcium channel blockers, and ACE inhibitors are less likely than other drugs to cause depression.

Medications To Watch

Antihypertensives and other heart medications
- Methyldopa
- Beta-blockers propranolol (Inderal), atenolol (Tenormin), and others
- Clonidine (Catapres)
- Digoxin (Lanoxin)
- Reserpine (Serpalan)

Arthritis medications
- Indomethacin (Indocin)

Asthma medications
- Albuterol (Proventil and others)
- Theophylline

Cancer medications
- Cycloserine (Seromycin)
- Tamoxifen (Nolvadex, Soltamox)
- Vinblastine
- Vincristine

Corticosteroids
- Cortisol
- Prednisone

Decongestants
- Pseudoephedrine

Hormones
- Estrogen
- Progesterone

Pain medications
- Codeine
- Propoxyphene (Darvon, Darvocet, Wygesic)

Parkinson's disease drugs
- Bromocriptine (Parlodel)
- Carbidopa/levodopa (Carbilev, Parcopa, Sinemet)

Stimulants
- Amphetamine/dextroamphetamine (Adderall)
- Dextroamphetamine (Dexedrine, Dextrostat)
- Methylphenidate (Daytrana, Ritalin, and others)

Tranquilizers/antianxiety medications
- Diazepam (Diastat, Valium)
- Triazolam (Halcion)

Also be sure to let your doctor know if you have a history of depression or anxiety so that you can be prescribed a treatment from the outset that poses little risk of influencing your mental well-being. ■

(Cymbalta) are serotonin and norepinephrine reuptake inhibitors (SNRIs). These medications work by raising brain concentrations of the neurotransmitters serotonin and norepinephrine. SNRIs are often the most effective drugs for older people. Possible side effects include nausea, weakness, sweating, insomnia, drowsiness, dry mouth, dizziness, and constipation. Effexor may increase blood pressure and cholesterol levels in some people, so monitoring blood pressure and cholesterol is important for anyone taking this drug. Cymbalta and Effexor in combination with triptan migraine medications may result in serotonin syndrome.

Monoamine oxidase (MAO) inhibitors

MAO inhibitors such as phenelzine (Nardil) and tranylcypromine (Parnate) increase brain levels of norepinephrine, serotonin, and dopamine by blocking the action of the enzyme MAO, which normally inactivates these three neurotransmitters. MAO inhibitors are effective in many depressed people, especially those whose depression is accompanied by marked anxiety, panic attacks, heightened appetite, or excessive sleeping.

People who should not take MAO inhibitors. MAO inhibitors can cause some of the same side effects as the tricyclics; side effects can be reduced in similar ways (see "Side effects" on page 32). But there are some individuals for whom MAO inhibitors pose greater risks. If you are a heavy drinker, have heart failure or severely impaired liver or kidney function, or take multiple medications for high blood pressure, you should not take an MAO inhibitor. In addition, MAO inhibitors can cause a sudden, extreme elevation in blood pressure (known as a hypertensive crisis) when people using them take certain drugs or consume foods or beverages containing tyramine. (Tyramine is found in nasal decongestants, cold or allergy medicines, very ripe bananas, beer, and aged or smoked meats, among other things.) People taking an MAO inhibitor must get a complete list of restricted foods and drugs from their doctor.

Normally, the enzyme MAO breaks down any tyramine consumed in the diet, preventing its hypertensive effect. This protective mechanism is disabled by MAO inhibitors, which block the action of MAO in the liver and intestine, allowing tyramine levels to rise and increase blood pressure. Symptoms of a hypertensive crisis include severe chest pain, excruciating headache, sweating, clammy skin, nausea, and vomiting. Immediate treatment with blood-pressure–lowering drugs is essential. Because of this risk and the dietary restrictions, MAO inhibitors are now only used as second-line drugs for the treatment of depression, despite their proven efficacy.

A skin patch of the MAO inhibitor Emsam is now available. At the lowest dose, Emsam does not interfere with the breakdown of tyramine in the digestive tract and can therefore be used without dietary restrictions.

Treatment in older adults

Older people are more susceptible to adverse effects than younger people, so drug therapy must be approached carefully. Smaller dosages as well as closer monitoring for toxic reactions are often required, and ensuring that the medications are being taken as prescribed may be an issue. Drug interactions are a concern, as the elderly use prescription drugs more than the general population. Treatment can also be difficult in reluctant individuals and in those lacking a social support system to help them with practical considerations, such as costs and transportation for visits to a doctor.

Despite all of these obstacles, older people usually respond well to treatment for depression; even partial success can lead to improved quality of life and productivity. Some studies even suggest that treatment with medications is more effective in older individuals than in younger ones.

Alternative treatments

Many people are curious about alternative treatments for depression, either because they hope to avoid drug-related side effects or because they are reluctant to see a doctor for their depression. Such self-treatment can put people at risk, however. For one thing, a person who self-medicates may not realize the depth of his or her depression or recognize worsening symptoms. For another, herbal and other alternative remedies are not benign and have potential side effects of their own, including the risk of drug-herb interactions.

St. John's wort, an extract from a yellow flowering plant called *Hypericum perforatum,* is the best known of the "natural antidepressants." The American College of Physicians and the American Society of Internal Medicine have included it in their guidelines as a short-term treatment option for mild depression, but a recently published overview of research on the herb notes that studies conducted to date have produced "inconsistent and confusing" results.

Until there is clear evidence that the supplement is effective, people with major depression should avoid using St. John's wort, and those with mild to moderate depression should use caution and be sure to consult their doctors before using it. In addition, anyone who uses St. John's wort needs to be aware of potential side effects. Research shows that St. John's wort interferes with a range of medications, including those prescribed to treat depression, heart disease, seizures, and some cancers. The supplement may also cause increased sensitivity to the sun.

Another supplement widely touted for treating depression is S-adenosylmethionine (also called SAM-e, pronounced "sammy"). But results of the published studies that purport to show the benefits of

NEW RESEARCH

Augmentation Therapy Effective in Older Adults

Major depression can be difficult to treat in older adults since they generally tend not to respond as well to antidepressants as younger people. In fact, some older individuals who receive adequate medication don't recover fully or respond and quickly relapse during the first six to 12 weeks of therapy. A new study suggests that, in these cases, adding to the treatment regimen may be beneficial.

Researchers monitored depression levels in 195 participants over age 75 during open-label treatment with paroxetine (Paxil) and interpersonal psychotherapy, then selected those that required augmentation with bupropion (Wellbutrin), nortriptyline (Aventyl, Pamelor), or lithium (Eskalith, Lithobid).

Of the 69 participants on augmentation, recovery occurred in 50% of those who had an initial inadequate response and 67% of those who had a relapse after initial treatment. In comparison, 87% of those who didn't require augmentation recovered. In addition to lower recovery rates, participants receiving augmentation were slower to recover and had slightly more side effects than those who didn't require augmentation. Those with coexisting anxiety and/or medical conditions were most likely to have a slower treatment response.

Despite these drawbacks, augmentation can still be a helpful treatment option for older people when one medication alone is not effective.

AMERICAN JOURNAL OF PSYCHIATRY
Volume 164, page 892
June 2007

SAM-e are not at all convincing, and there are troubling hints that it may trigger mania in susceptible people.

Researchers have studied melatonin for SAD, but there is limited information on the optimal dose and timing. In addition, melatonin is a hormone (in the body, it is produced by the pineal gland) and thus should be taken only with your doctor's knowledge.

Treatment of Bipolar Disorder With Medications

The goal of treatment of bipolar disorder is to prevent both manic and depressive episodes, controlling the extreme highs and lows to create a stable mood. (For more information on the drugs used to treat bipolar disorder and their side effects, see the chart on pages 40–43.)

The core treatment is mood-stabilizing medication. Lithium (Eskalith, Lithobid) was the first medication to be approved for treating mania, and it remains the mainstay of treatment today. (Blood levels of lithium are measured regularly to ensure adequate doses and to avoid the dangerous effects of toxic levels.) Because lithium can take over a week to have an effect, a neuroleptic (an antipsychotic drug) or a benzodiazepine (an antianxiety drug) may be added to treat symptoms of acute mania. Benzodiazepines should be used with caution, however, because of the risk of dependency and abuse. They can also disinhibit some manic patients, escalating inappropriate behavior.

Instead of lithium, psychiatrists may choose to use other mood-stabilizing medications—carbamazepine (Equetro), valproic acid (Depakene, Depakote), or lamotrigine (Lamictal)—in combination with one another or with neuroleptics or benzodiazepines to treat acute mania. The neuroleptic drugs aripiprazole (Abilify), olanzapine (Zyprexa), quetiapine (Seroquel), risperidone (Risperdal), and ziprasidone (Geodon) have also been approved for treating manic episodes. Valproic acid and neuroleptics are also good options for people who have what's known as mixed states—simultaneous symptoms of mania and depression.

A neuroleptic drug is prescribed in combination with a mood-stabilizing drug when manic episodes are severe or involve hallucinations or delusional ideas. Neuroleptics are usually taken only for short periods because of their neurological side effects, which include repetitive, involuntary, purposeless movements or twitches (called tardive dyskinesia) that may not go away even if medication is stopped. These side effects occur less often with some newer (or atypical) neuroleptics, such as Zyprexa and Risperdal.

A new episode of mild or moderate depression in people with bipolar disorder is typically treated with a mood stabilizer such as lithium. If the depression is severe, only then would an antidepressant drug be added to the mood stabilizer. (Lithium has been shown to be effective in preventing suicide, and antidepressants must be used with caution in people with bipolar disorder.) If the depression involves psychotic symptoms, the person may need to take neuroleptic medication in addition to the mood stabilizer and antidepressant.

The reason antidepressants must be used with extreme care in people with bipolar disorder is that they can stimulate a manic episode or cause rapid cycling between depression and mania. This is particularly true for tricyclic antidepressants. A recent study published in the *The New England Journal of Medicine* suggests that they offer no clear benefit but were also associated with no significant increase in manic symptoms when prescribed in combination with a mood-stabilizing medication during the 26 weeks of study. Despite the presumed risk and lack of proven benefit, it's estimated that 50–70% of people with bipolar disorder are prescribed antidepressants. Each individual's situation must be assessed, since some clinical situations such as prominent coexisting anxiety symptoms may be the reason for including an antidepressant in the treatment.

SSRIs and other relatively new antidepressants, such as Wellbutrin or Effexor, are the most likely drugs to be used. In addition, Symbyax—a combination of an atypical neuroleptic (olanzapine) and an SSRI (fluoxetine)—has been approved by the FDA to treat depressive episodes in people with bipolar disorder.

Despite the risk of mania, according to a study in the *American Journal of Psychiatry*, people with bipolar disorder whose depression responded to treatment with antidepressant medication (in addition to their other medications) had a low incidence of relapse into depression or mania during the first year after the depression eased if they remained on antidepressant medication during that time.

Long-term treatment of bipolar disorder

People who have had at least two episodes in five years (that is, at least two manic episodes, two depressive episodes, or one manic and one depressive episode) or three serious lifetime episodes will need to take medication over the long term, even when they experience no symptoms. This can be difficult for people to accept once they stabilize and begin to feel well again. However, the research

NEW RESEARCH

Psychotherapy Improves Recovery From Bipolar Disorder Depression

Adding intensive psychotherapy to medication treatment for bipolar disorder significantly hastens and improves recovery from a depressive episode, according to a new study.

In 293 people with bipolar disorder, researchers compared the benefits of four types of psychotherapies used with a mood stabilizer (lithium [Eskalith, Lithobid], valproate [Depacon], or carbamazepine [Equetro]) plus the antidepressants bupropion (Wellbutrin) or paroxetine (Paxil). Of these, 163 participants received one of three intensive psychotherapies for up to 30 times over nine months: family-focused therapy, cognitive behavioral therapy, and interpersonal and social rhythm therapy (which focuses on stabilizing routines). The rest received collaborative care, a brief psychoeducational intervention of three sessions over six weeks.

Those who received intensive psychotherapies had a 64% recovery rate in an average time of 113 days compared with 52% of the collaborative-care group, whose average recovery time was 146 days. Those receiving intensive psychotherapy were also 1.6 times more likely to be classified clinically well during the study than the collaborative-care group.

No significant differences were found among the different intensive psychotherapies, suggesting that all can be beneficial additions for treating bipolar disorder.

ARCHIVES OF GENERAL PSYCHIATRY
Volume 64, page 419
April 2007

Drugs for the Treatment of Bipolar Disorder 2008*

Drug type: Brand (generic)	Typical daily dosage†	How they appear to work
Mood stabilizers		
Equetro (carbamazepine§)‡	400–1,600 mg	Mechanism of action is unknown.
Eskalith, Lithobid (lithium§)ǁ	600–1,800 mg	
Depakene (valproic acid§)‡ǁ Depakote (divalproex)‡ ǁ	250–2,000 mg	
Anticonvulsants		
Lamictal (lamotrigine§)ǁ	200–400 mg	Suppress excessive and abnormal firing of neurons, but their exact mechanism in treating bipolar disorder is not established.
Neurontin (gabapentin§)	300–1,800 mg	
Topamax (topiramate§)	200–1,000 mg	
Atypical neuroleptics		
Abilify (aripiprazole)	15–30 mg	Symptoms of bipolar disorder may be produced by overactivity of dopamine. By blocking dopamine receptors, neuroleptics reduce the activity of dopamine, produce antipsychotic and tranquilizing effects by preventing overstimulation of nerve cells.
Clozaril, FazaClo ODT (clozapine§)	12.5–450 mg	
Geodon (ziprasidone)ǁ	40–160 mg	
Risperdal (risperidone)ǁ	2–6 mg	
Seroquel (quetiapine)ǁ	100–800 mg	
Zyprexa (olanzapine)ǁ	5–20 mg	
Neuroleptics (typical)¥		
Haldol (haloperidol§)	2–18 mg	Produce antipsychotic and tranquilizing effects by blocking dopamine receptors and preventing overstimulation of nerve cells.
(fluphenazine§)	2.5–20 mg	
Atypical neuroleptic/selective serotonin reuptake inhibitor		
Symbyax (olanzapine/fluoxetine)ǁ	3/25–12/50 mg	Increases the availability of the neurotransmitters serotonin, norepinephrine, and dopamine to treat depression associated with bipolar disorder.

* This list represents the most commonly prescribed drugs for bipolar disorder. Depressive episodes in bipolar disorder are often treated with a combination of mood stabilizers and antidepressant medications. Manic episodes are often treated with a combination of mood stabilizers and neuroleptic medications (either typical or atypical). Anticonvulsants are potential mood stabilizers. Benzodiazepines are often used to treat agitation and related symptoms.

† These dosages represent an average range for the treatment of bipolar disorder and may differ from the dosage prescribed by your doctor. The precise effective dosage varies from person to person and depends on many factors. Do not make any change to your medication without consulting your doctor. *Starting dosages tend to be lower for older patients.*

Common side effects

Carbamazepine may cause drowsiness, weakness, blurred or double vision, dizziness, unsteadiness, nausea, sun sensitivity.

Lithium may cause gastrointestinal discomfort, nausea, vertigo, muscle weakness, a dazed feeling, tremor, fatigue, thirst.

Valproic acid and divalproex can cause drowsiness, dizziness, nausea and other gastrointestinal symptoms, appetite loss, weight gain or loss, transient hair loss, hand tremor.

Dizziness, fatigue, poor coordination, altered vision, nausea, vomiting, headache, difficulty concentrating, impaired memory, sleepiness, insomnia. Lamotrigine may cause serious rashes, especially when used with valproic acid without dosage adjustment, requiring hospitalization and termination of treatment.

Drowsiness, headache, dizziness, constipation, weight gain or loss, nausea, abdominal pain, tremor or twitches, restlessness, salivation, dry mouth. Atypical neuroleptics increase the risk of death in elderly patients with dementia. Clozapine has more potential side effects than the other drugs in this class. It may increase the risk of elevated blood glucose and diabetes. It also can put you at risk for serious illnesses such as agranulocytosis (a decrease in the number of white blood cells that increases the risk of infected lesions of the throat and gastrointestinal tract) and myocarditis (inflammation of the walls of the heart), seizures, and low blood pressure. See a doctor immediately if you experience signs of neuroleptic malignant syndrome (characterized by muscle stiffness or spasms, high fever, and confusion or disorientation) or infection (fever, chills, sweating, and fatigue).

Blurred vision, stiffness, drowsiness, tremor, dry mouth, decreased sweating, sensitivity to cold and sun, persistent restlessness, loss of coordination, involuntary twitches and muscle spasms (risk highest in elderly women taking high doses). Patients taking neuroleptics experience, in rare instances, neuroleptic malignant syndrome (see atypical neuroleptic side effects).

Weight gain, sleepiness, increased appetite, weakness, swelling in legs and arms, tremors, sore throat, difficulty concentrating.

continued on the next page

‡ Carbamazepine and valproic acid are anticonvulsants as well as mood stabilizers.

§ Generic version available at lower cost.

|| Lithium, divalproex, lamotrigine, olanzapine/fluoxetine, olanzapine, quetiapine, risperidone, and ziprasidone are the only drugs approved by the U.S. Food and Drug Administration for the treatment of bipolar disorder. Although the remaining drugs in this chart do not have FDA approval for treating bipolar disorder specifically, they are nonetheless commonly prescribed for this use.

¥ These are the highest potency neuroleptics. Many other neuroleptics can be used to treat bipolar disorder.

Drugs for the Treatment of Bipolar Disorder 2008* (continued)

Drug type: Brand (generic)	Typical daily dosage†	How they appear to work
Antidepressants		
All types of antidepressants can be used (with caution) to treat depression in people with bipolar disorder. See the chart on pages 20–23 for more information on these medications.		
Benzodiazepines¶		
Ativan (lorazepam§)	2–6 mg	Increase activity of gamma-aminobutyric acid (GABA), a neurotransmitter that inhibits the excessive firing of certain neurons.
Klonopin (clonazepam§)	0.5–4 mg	

* This list represents the most commonly prescribed drugs for bipolar disorder. Depressive episodes in bipolar disorder are often treated with a combination of mood stabilizers and antidepressant medications. Manic episodes are often treated with a combination of mood stabilizers and neuroleptic medications (either typical or atypical). Anticonvulsants are potential mood stabilizers. Benzodiazepines are often used to treat agitation and related symptoms.

† These dosages represent an average range for the treatment of bipolar disorder and may differ from the dosage prescribed by your doctor. The precise effective dosage varies from person to person and depends on many factors. Do not make any change to your medication without consulting your doctor. *Starting dosages tend to be lower for older patients.*

clearly shows that bipolar disorder is a chronic, cyclic disease and that the consequences of going off medication can be tragic. Treatment usually involves a mood stabilizer; other medications may be added on a short-term basis if depression or mania worsens or if symptoms such as impulsivity, irritability, or poor concentration develop. A person on long-term treatment for bipolar disorder will need periodic blood tests; these allow his or her physician to monitor blood levels of the medication and check for any serious side effects, such as liver, kidney, or thyroid problems.

Sleeping problems are common in people with bipolar disorder because mania can cause a reduced need for sleep and depression can cause insomnia. Benzodiazepines and certain neuroleptics may help promote sleep but are given only for short periods.

Sometimes a depressive episode occurs in someone who has been doing well with long-term treatment (known as breakthrough depression). When this happens, there are a number of treatment options. Those who experience mild to moderate depression may be given a higher dosage of their mood stabilizer. (In some instances, however, the mood stabilizer may actually induce mild depression, and the doctor may therefore choose to lower the drug dosage.) If depression is severe, the person may be given an SSRI or a second mood stabilizer. Rapid cycling between mania and depression despite long-term treatment precludes use of antidepressants.

Common side effects

Dizziness, loss of coordination, drowsiness, lightheadedness, slurred speech, unsteady gait. See a doctor immediately if you experience symptoms of infection (fever, chills, sweating, and fatigue) or problems with behavior (anger, depression, hallucinations, or difficulty concentrating) or memory.

¶ Many benzodiazepines can be used to treat people with bipolar disorder. Lorazepam and clonazepam are the most frequently used. See the chart on pages 64–65 for a more complete list of benzodiazepines.

§ Generic version available at lower cost.

Psychotherapy

Most people think of psychotherapy simply as counseling. In fact, the term *psychotherapy* is used to describe a variety of different talk therapies that treat emotional, behavioral, personality, and psychiatric disorders. It involves a commitment to a series of appointments with a licensed mental health professional, enabling a relationship to form between the therapist and the individual. This relationship focuses on helping the person to cope with or avoid factors contributing to his or her condition, with the overall goals being personal development and self-understanding. Like any medical treatment, it has advantages and disadvantages.

Psychotherapy is commonly used to treat people with depression. It has proven effective in treating mild and moderate forms and can be combined with drug therapy to treat all degrees of depression.

Advantages

A major advantage over treatment with medication is that psychotherapy has few physiological side effects—an especially important consideration for older adults who are often taking more than one type of medication. In addition, it offers the possibility of effective treatment for those who have not responded to medications.

Disadvantages

A disadvantage is that psychotherapy typically takes longer than drug therapy to produce benefits that are noticeable to the person receiving treatment—six to eight weeks or longer for psychotherapy, compared with four to six weeks for medication. Also, psychotherapy alone is not effective in people with severe depression or bipolar disorder.

Depending on the severity of the depression and other factors specific to each individual, a therapist selects a combination of techniques from the range of psychotherapeutic approaches. Regardless of the particular approach, the essential foundation of all psychotherapy is the establishment of a trusting relationship with the therapist. This allows the patient to share confidences, life experiences, and problems. If psychotherapy alone leads to no improvement by six weeks, or if a person has only a partial or weak response by 12 weeks, medication should be strongly considered.

Although people with bipolar disorder should be on medication, they can also benefit from psychotherapy. Environmental factors such as stress may trigger episodes of mania or depression, and counseling can help a person identify and deal with these triggers. It can also help the person gain insight into his or her condition, confront the dysfunctional thinking often associated with bipolar disorder, and improve his or her ability to handle work, family, and financial challenges. Furthermore, counseling that involves the individual's family can help to educate relatives about the disorder.

Unfortunately, a person who is in an acute manic state would likely be unable to attend or benefit from therapy. For those with mania or severe depression who do not respond to drug treatments or psychotherapy, electroconvulsive therapy may be needed (see page 47).

Interpersonal therapy

Also known as crisis intervention, interpersonal therapy is most effective when depression is the result of a major life event, such as the death of a spouse, the loss of a job, divorce, or another difficult life transition. Because the depressive symptoms stem from an immediate problem, the goal is to help the person cope with the stressor by improving self-awareness, resolving emotional conflicts, and possibly making some behavioral changes. Interpersonal therapy can be extremely effective at helping individuals restore balance to their lives.

Psychodynamic therapy

This form of psychotherapy focuses on an individual's past experiences in an attempt to understand present-day conflicts and feelings about recent life changes, such as retirement or grief. This therapy attempts to treat the "whole person" rather than just the symptoms of depression. A crucial component of the therapy is transference—the transfer of feelings about important childhood figures from the patient on to the therapist, who then works to help the patient resolve residual past conflicts. This therapy can be effective in helping a person overcome destructive personality patterns.

Supportive therapy

Supportive therapy teaches individuals about their illness, with the idea that a better understanding of the mood disorder will enable the person to set more realistic and tangible goals. In supportive therapy, the person is encouraged to focus on current challenges and relationships and develop strategies for dealing with them. The therapy is goal oriented, and the individual works with the therapist to set goals. The person's family members or close friends may be included in counseling or education sessions.

Behavioral therapy

This type of therapy is based on the premise that depressed people have learned destructive patterns of thinking and acting, and these patterns cause and/or prolong their depression. Counseling is provided to improve social skills, problem solving, and self-control and to change how a person reacts to problems. Behavioral therapy emphasizes step-by-step improvements in behavior and is most often effective when the problem is clearly defined. Although less studied in the treatment of depression, behavioral therapy has been useful in relieving some types of anxiety states, such as obsessive-compulsive disorder and phobias.

Cognitive therapy

The aim of cognitive therapy is to reverse a person's destructive and exaggerated belief that his or her weaknesses and inadequacies doom him or her to future failure. The therapist not only encourages the individual to recognize that these views are distorted—by listing positive attributes or past and present successes, for example—but also attempts to bolster confidence by demonstrating that the person can successfully complete increasingly challenging "assignments." The treatment generally requires a series of sessions over several

ASK THE DOCTOR

Q. ***Are there some people, especially those with mild depression, who may be better off forgoing medication in favor of psychotherapy?***

A. Everyone is different, and it's true that medication isn't necessary for all people with depression. It's important for a doctor to assess how depressed a person is and the surrounding circumstances.

For instance, someone who is mourning the recent loss of a spouse typically doesn't need medication unless an intense, disabling level of grief persists for many months. Other individuals with depression may not want to take medication or are unable to tolerate it. And many with seasonal affective disorder, who get depressed in winter months, may do just as well with bright light therapy as with medication.

Studies have found that many types of psychotherapy are as effective as medication for milder depressive episodes, allowing people to successfully deal with their sense of loss, anxiety, or distress. Talk therapy takes longer than medication to show results, but it usually has fewer side effects and its benefits may last longer than those of medication.

Getting more physical exercise, adequate rest, and following a good diet may also boost your mood.

months. It is often combined with behavioral therapy, known as cognitive-behavioral therapy (CBT). (For more on CBT, see "The Power of Positive Thinking" on pages 58–59.)

Psychoanalytic therapy

The psychoanalytic theory of depression derives from the Freudian concept that altered mood develops because of anger directed toward oneself. The theory asserts that curing depression requires exposing the cause of anger and confronting it in a constructive and realistic manner. The patient meets with the therapist three to five times a week in a stream-of-consciousness, free-associative atmosphere that involves minimal feedback from the therapist. Because classic psychoanalysis requires years of treatment, it is not suitable for managing acute depression. It is used infrequently in its classic form today, although aspects of the Freudian approach have survived under psychodynamic therapy.

Group therapy

In this method, a small group of people with similar problems meet regularly to discuss their troubles under the guidance of a therapist. Participants can share personal feelings, experiences, and solutions in a supportive atmosphere. The resulting interaction often reduces feelings of isolation and can heighten awareness and understanding of personal problems. It is useful for people who benefit from feedback from peers.

Finding a therapist

If you think you have depression or bipolar disorder, you do not necessarily have to see a psychiatrist. Many people with mood disorders are treated by their primary care physician, who can identify other medical conditions that could be responsible for the symptoms. If the diagnosis does turn out to be a mood disorder, your primary care physician can initiate drug therapy, coordinate care from other specialists, or both.

Many different kinds of mental health professionals are available—psychiatrists, psychologists, psychiatric nurses, and social workers. Which therapist is best for you? That depends on several factors, including how severe your symptoms are and the cost of treatment. No matter what type of therapy you select, keep in mind that it may take some time and research to find the right therapist. A family physician will be able to provide some recommendations, but other resources are available. Local medical societies, university medical centers, and national mental health organizations may be able to provide assistance. Also check community mental health clinics, local schools, and religious organizations, which sometimes offer inexpensive or even free counseling programs.

Compatibility is extremely important, and it may take more than one referral to find a comfortable counseling relationship. It is also important to ask about a therapist's education and professional licenses, either before making an appointment or during the first appointment. You can get a sense of a therapist by describing your condition and asking the therapist how he or she would treat it. Reputable practitioners will not object to requests for information about their background and will understand your desire to interview other therapists.

Electroconvulsive Therapy

Many people think electroconvulsive therapy (ECT) is a thing of the past, but it is still being used today, given its effectiveness in treating major depression. In recent years, the National Institute of Mental Health, the American Psychiatric Association, and the U.S. Surgeon General have all concluded that ECT is a valuable tool in the treatment of certain mental disorders, particularly depression.

Before ECT, a person with depression typically first receives psychotherapy, antidepressant medication, or a combination of the two. While these treatments are often effective, they take time to work. This delay can be dangerous for people whose depression is accompanied by intense suicidal thoughts or delusions. For these individuals, who are at immediate risk for self-injury or suicide, ECT can work much more quickly than antidepressants and is therefore a good option.

ECT can help other people as well. It may be recommended when antidepressant medications do not work. It can also be useful for older people who cannot tolerate antidepressants and for pregnant women (if there is concern that medication might affect the health of the fetus). People suffering from bipolar disorder or schizophrenia may also benefit from ECT.

ECT can be performed in an inpatient or outpatient setting. After the patient is given general anesthesia and a muscle relaxant, electrodes are placed on two areas of the scalp. A short, controlled set of electrical pulses is then administered for about a minute. The electrical pulses must produce generalized seizures to be effective. (Because patients are under anesthesia and have taken muscle relaxants, they do not convulse or feel the current.)

NEW RESEARCH

Loss of Memory With ECT Affected By Technique

Electroconvulsive therapy (ECT) can be extremely effective for severe depression that doesn't respond to medication and psychotherapy, but it can also lead to memory loss. Now comes research suggesting that the technique used to perform ECT may be a factor in memory loss.

In the first large-scale, prospective study of the cognitive effects of ECT, investigators at New York State Psychiatric Institute enrolled 347 patients with major depression and gave them memory and psychological tests before and after they received ECT.

They found that participants who received bilateral ECT with electrodes placed on both sides of the head had more severe and persistent memory problems than those who received unilateral ECT with electrodes placed just on the right side of the head. Immediately after ECT, those in the bilateral group had 3.4 times more memory loss than healthy controls, and six months after ECT, they had 2.8 times more memory loss. The researchers also reported that another type of ECT known as sine-wave stimulation led to a pronounced slowing of reaction time, both immediately and six months after ECT.

In addition, older people, those with lower cognitive function prior to the onset of depression, and women were more prone to memory problems after ECT.

NEUROPSYCHOPHARMACOLOGY
Volume 32, page 244
January 2007

Substance Abuse and Aging

Alcohol and drug use is on the rise, but help is readily available

Current guidelines suggest that one alcoholic drink a day for women and two drinks a day for men may be beneficial for health. If you drink more than that, you could have a drinking problem... and you're not alone.

Researchers are beginning to acknowledge the prevalence of alcohol and drug abuse among people over age 60, saying that it affects as many as 17% of older adults. Recent government statistics reveal that 12% of adults over age 50 report binge alcohol drinking over the past month and 3% say that they drink heavily on a frequent basis.

In addition, 2% of older adults report using illicit drugs such as marijuana, prescription drugs like painkillers for nonmedical purposes, and cocaine. Men are much more likely than women to report substance use.

A Dangerous Habit

Many older individuals may be self-medicating with alcohol and drugs as a way of managing depression or anxiety symptoms, coping with loneliness or loss, or dealing with pain. While these substances may temporarily ease a person's discomfort, many negative health consequences can develop from continually relying on them as a mental-health crutch. For instance, excessive drinking can lead to liver damage and failure, especially when combined with certain common medications such as acetaminophen (Tylenol). Use of aspirin by heavy drinkers can also cause bleeding in the gastrointestinal tract.

Taking antihistamines and alcohol together can dangerously lower blood pressure and cause problems with balance as well as confusion. The combination can also depress the central nervous system, slowing breathing and heart rate, which can be deadly. Taking large doses of prescription benzodiazepines such as diazepam (Valium) with alcohol also can be lethal. And alcohol and drug use can blunt the positive effects of medications for health problems such as diabetes and heart disease.

Finally, these substances may have deleterious effects on the ability to drive safely, to work effectively, and to interact with friends and family. It even appears that substance abuse in older men with depression increases the risk of suicide.

Finding Support

Substance abuse often goes undiagnosed in older people for a myriad of reasons. Older adults are more likely to hide their substance abuse and refrain from seeking professional help. If they do seek support, healthcare providers may overlook the problem by mistaking the symptoms for dementia or depression. Also, many relatives may be embarrassed by the problem and choose to ignore it. The result is, unfortunately, that thousands of older people who need help remain untreated.

If you suspect that substance abuse is an issue for yourself (see the inset box at right) or someone you love, don't be ashamed to speak up and reach out for support. There are a variety of treatment options today, from once-a-week counseling sessions and group meetings, to daily outpatient services, to residential or hospital-based programs where doctors can prescribe medications to ease withdrawal symptoms while patients learn how to manage their addiction in therapy.

Patients awaken about five to 10 minutes after the end of the treatment. Most are oriented and alert within 30 minutes. If done as an oupatient procedure, a family member or friend must drive the patient home after the procedure (driving is not allowed in the 24 hours following an ECT session) and stay until he or she goes to sleep that night.

Typically, ECT is given two to three times a week for a total of six to 12 sessions. These sessions typically improve depression in 50–60%

The first step is to be honest about the problem. The next, as a substance abuser, is to talk openly with your primary care provider about your drinking or drug use—if asked if you drink heavily or overuse prescription drugs, reply truthfully. If your doctor doesn't ask you, bring up the topic yourself. He or she can counsel you on how best to tackle the problem, address physical and mental health problems such as depression that may be causing it, and assist you in drawing up a plan to quit.

Your physician can also refer you to trained counselors and other mental health professionals as well as age-appropriate treatment groups where you can obtain further support to help control the urge to drink or use drugs. It may also be helpful to join a group such as Alcoholics Anonymous or Narcotics Anonymous, where you can interact with other people who share your problem.

Some older people who drink very heavily, have been drinking for a long time, or are addicted to drugs may need an intensive intervention like a detoxification program to prevent medical problems (such as seizures or delirium) while overcoming their habit. Patients receive ongoing medical care in a safe environment, which can be helpful for people who live alone and don't have a good support system as well as for those who are depressed or suicidal, who have uncontrolled medical conditions such as kidney disease or diabetes, who don't respond to outpatient treatments, or who have multiple addictions.

Do You Have a Problem?

One way to tell if you have a drinking or drug problem is to ask yourself the following questions, which are part of The Cage Questionnaire, a screening test used by doctors to determine if a substance is being overused:

1. Have you ever felt you should **c**ut down on your drinking or drug use?
2. Have people **a**nnoyed you by criticizing your drinking or drug use?
3. Have you ever felt bad or **g**uilty about your drinking or drug use?
4. Have you ever had a drink first thing in the morning to steady your nerves or get rid of a hangover (an "**e**ye opener")?

Score 1 point for each yes answer. A score of 2 or more suggests you have a substance-use problem and should seek help.

Clean and Sober

Despite the fact that it often goes unnoticed, alcohol and substance abuse is an increasing issue for seniors that can have serious consequences. Seeking out help is crucial to recovering and avoiding major health risks. All treatment options require considerable effort and motivation.

But don't think that you won't be able to conquer a substance problem or that it won't be worth it: Research shows that older people can be as successfully treated as younger adults. What's more, you can go on to lead a healthier and happier life. ■

of patients—a response rate similar to that of antidepressant drugs—and in 80–90% of people using it as first-line therapy. According to a recent report of 24 ECT patients, most said they were glad they had received the treatment, felt safe having it, and would choose ECT again in the future if recommended by a psychiatrist.

A major limitation of ECT treatment is that the benefits may be short-lived. Within a year, 50–60% of people experience a relapse, and they may have to take antidepressant medication or continue receiving ECT periodically to prevent relapse.

The immediate side effects of the procedure include headaches, nausea, muscle aches and soreness, disorientation, and confusion lasting about an hour. A person may also temporarily experience difficulty recalling newly acquired information. It is possible to lose memories formed up to six months before the procedure as well. But these learning and memory problems usually disappear within a few weeks or months following the last treatment. Memories of events immediately surrounding an ECT session may be permanently lost, however.

Problems with learning and memory can be moderated with unilateral ECT (electrodes placed on one side of the head) rather than bilateral ECT (electrodes placed on both sides of the head; see the "New Research" column on page 47). However, unilateral ECT may not be as effective and requires a higher current. New evidence shows that placing the electrodes near the front of the head lowers the risk of cognitive problems. Also, memory problems are less frequent when people undergo the procedure two rather than three times a week.

No one is sure how ECT helps certain mental disorders. It may flood the brain with neurotransmitters such as serotonin and dopamine, which are known to play a role in conditions such as depression and schizophrenia. ECT may also help regulate hormones that play a role in these disorders.

Light Therapy

Some people with seasonal affective disorder (SAD) can be successfully treated with exposure to bright light. In one study, 57% of 191 people with SAD responded to light therapy. In another study, light therapy was comparable in effectiveness to antidepressant therapy but worked faster and caused fewer side effects. And in a major review of 173 published studies, bright-light therapy yielded substantial relief for both SAD and mild to moderate depression that was not linked to seasonal changes.

Light therapy involves sitting in front of a bank of full-spectrum fluorescent lights for 30–60 minutes each day. Improvement can often be seen within a few days, with symptoms disappearing after two to three weeks. Continued light therapy is needed to prevent a relapse. Although commercially available light boxes are advertised for depressed people, these devices are not approved by the FDA. Light therapy should be used only with your doctor's guidance, as it can cause side effects when

ASK THE DOCTOR

Q. ***What can I do, in addition to medication and therapy, to alleviate depression and anxiety?***

A. Many lifestyle changes can help lessen depression and anxiety symptoms. To start, a healthy diet can contribute to good mental health. A low level of omega-3 fatty acids, found in fatty fish such as tuna and salmon, has been associated with depression, so eating more of these fish may help improve your mood.

Studies have also shown that low levels of the B vitamin folate are linked to depression and may prevent people from responding optimally to antidepressants. Supplements at doses of 400–800 mcg can be of benefit—although you should ask your doctor before trying any supplements to be sure they won't interact with medications you're taking.

Getting adequate sleep is also important: People who don't get enough rest tend to be irritable and moody, which can trigger major depressive episodes.

Finally, exercise is a key ingredient of a comprehensive program for depression and anxiety. Even though it can be difficult to motivate yourself to be physically active when you're feeling sad and lethargic, studies show that even taking a short, 10-minute walk may improve your mood. Mind-body exercises such as yoga may be particularly beneficial because they force you to breathe deeply, circulating oxygen to all parts of your body and potentially releasing endorphins that may help you feel better and more invigorated.

used improperly. For instance, light therapy may trigger manic symptoms in people who have bipolar disorder.

Supplemental Treatments

Other healthy behaviors that can improve recovery success rates include regular exercise, improved sleep, and good nutrition.

Exercise

Numerous studies have shown that exercise can alleviate depression and improve mood. One review of 14 studies, for example, found that aerobic exercise (walking or running three times a week for at least five weeks) was more effective than a placebo pill at relieving symptoms of mild to moderate depression and was just as effective as psychotherapy. The benefits of exercise in these studies lasted up to a year, especially among those who continued exercising. Exercise was also shown to be more cost effective than other treatments.

No one is sure exactly how exercise relieves depression. An increase in aerobic fitness may play a role, but it cannot be entirely responsible because nonaerobic exercise, such as weight training, can have similar effects. Some researchers have theorized that exercise, like most antidepressant medications, increases the activity of serotonin and/or norepinephrine. Exercise also stimulates the release of endorphins, which are hormones that reduce pain and can induce euphoria. Exercise may provide an outlet for pent-up anger and frustration as well. In addition, it may improve disturbed sleep, which can be a symptom of, and an aggravating factor in, depression. Finally, there are some reports that even brief exposure to natural daylight—as with a walk outside during the middle of the day or other outdoor exercise—helps people with SAD.

Some of the effects of exercise may have more to do with psychology than physiology. For instance, exercise may give people a sense of self-mastery or control over their depression or anxiety, which can lead to a reduction in symptoms.

To increase your level of physical activity, begin by making small changes in your daily life. Try parking your car further away from the store or mall to increase the amount of time you spend walking. When possible, take the stairs instead of an elevator. Also, try to decrease the amount of time you spend in sedentary activities, such as watching television. Your goal should be at least 30 minutes of moderately intense activity, such as swimming, bicycling, gardening, raking leaves, or brisk walking on most days of the week; however, any increase in activity can be beneficial.

NEW RESEARCH

Yoga May Ease Anxiety and Depression

Low levels of the neurotransmitter gamma-aminobutyric acid (GABA) have been associated with depression and particularly anxiety; antidepressants are shown to increase GABA levels. Now, preliminary research suggests that the regular practice of yoga may be an effective, nonpharmacologic way to raise GABA levels and potentially improve anxiety and depression symptoms.

Researchers recruited eight longtime yoga devotees who practiced twice a week for at least four months and 11 comparison participants. Both groups had a baseline brain scan done. Then the yoga participants performed a one-hour yoga session while the control group read books or magazines for the same time, and all participants were rescanned immediately after.

The yoga volunteers showed a 27% increase in GABA levels compared with baseline, but there was no change among the readers.

Several previous trials have demonstrated that yoga can reduce anxiety and depression symptoms, but this is the first study to identify a possible mechanism for the effects. The practice of yoga should be explored further and compared with other forms of exercise as a means of raising GABA levels and relieving anxiety and depression. Yoga may serve as a useful adjunct to standard treatment recommended by your doctor.

JOURNAL OF ALTERNATIVE AND COMPLEMENTARY MEDICINE
Volume 13, page 419
May 2007

Sleep

Most people experience mild irritability or mood changes when they have insomnia, but sleep deprivation can have an even greater impact on those with mood disorders. Chronic sleep deprivation and irregular sleep habits not only worsen depression but may also interfere with its treatment. Sleep disturbances can even trigger a manic episode in some people. Focusing on getting regular, adequate sleep is a crucial part of controlling symptoms and increasing the benefits of other mood disorder treatments. (In some depressed people, controlled sleep deprivation may result in very brief improvements in depressive symptoms, but these improvements do not last.)

Nutrition

If you suffer from depression, one of the most important things you can do to help yourself is to avoid alcohol. There is no question that alcohol exacerbates depression; it is, after all, a chemical depressant.

As for general nutrition, some people with mild depression or dysthymia report that they do better when they eat more foods containing omega-3 fatty acids (such as salmon and other fatty fish) or complex carbohydrates (such as beans and whole grains). However, the interplay between food and mood is not well understood.

Malnutrition, particularly folic acid and vitamin B_{12} deficiencies, has been associated with depression in older people. Eating a well-balanced diet will help provide the full range of nutrients your body needs to stay healthy in general.

Future Treatments

For individuals whose depression is not alleviated by standard therapies, new treatment options are under investigation. At the forefront of research are various brain-stimulating techniques, such as deep brain stimulation (DBS), which involves the implantation of a device that delivers electric current to the brain to normalize its activity. Like the heart, the brain is an electrical organ, so stimulating it with a small electrical current is an efficient way to precisely target areas that are malfunctioning—more efficient than drug therapy, in fact, which tends to affect the whole brain and often causes side effects. Although results of small trials have been encouraging, the finer points of the procedure are still being debated: the precise areas of the brain to stimulate, the optimal number of electrodes to implant, and the voltages to use. DBS is

Anxiety and Your Physical Health

Worry tries more than just the heart and soul

The link between depression and physical illness has been well explored, and now researchers are turning their attention to the role of anxiety disorders in prompting medical problems.

The latest research shows a strong connection between anxiety disorders—generalized anxiety disorder, panic disorder, agoraphobia, social phobia, post-traumatic stress disorder, and obsessive-compulsive disorder—and physical conditions. In fact, a 2006 study found that those with anxiety were up to twice as likely to have a physical illness, too.

What the Studies Say

Investigators from Canada looked at the association between anxiety disorders and physical conditions in 4,181 German adults (1,913 men and 2,268 women) between ages 18 and 65. The participants completed a survey that asked about 44 mental and physical health issues. They also underwent a physician's exam that included blood pressure measurements and urine and blood sample analysis to identify physical problems and a psychiatric evaluation to detect anxiety disorders.

Of the subjects, 429 (8%) reported having an anxiety disorder in the past month, and 2,610 (61%) noted having a physical condition. Anxiety was most commonly linked with lung and gastrointestinal illnesses, arthritis, allergies, thyroid problems, and migraine headaches. Most people with both anxiety and a physical illness said that the anxiety came first. Their mental distress also appeared to make their physical ailments worse: They had a poorer quality of life than those who suffered from just anxiety or a physical ailment alone, and were more likely to have one or more days of inactivity than those with physical problems alone.

A U.S. study of the link between anxiety and physical disorders by the same researchers in 2005 produced similar results and found that post-traumatic stress disorder, panic attack, and agoraphobia were more likely than other anxiety disorders to be linked with physical ailments. Other investigators have shown that people with anxiety are at greater risk for high blood pressure, heart attacks, fertility problems, autoimmune conditions (such as lupus and multiple sclerosis), and skin disorders.

The Chicken or the Egg?

The Canadian researchers said that while it is not entirely clear why anxiety is linked to physical illness, they suggested that it could trigger one or more processes in the body—like hormonal changes—that contribute to an illness. People may also try to self-medicate their anxiety with alcohol, drugs, or food and may develop a substance abuse disorder or obesity, which then could exacerbate both the physical and the mental illness. The same genetic or environmental factors could also cause both anxiety and a physical disorder.

Conversely, although most people in the study said that anxiety preceded physical illness, some may develop a medical problem first, and worrying about it may become serious enough to be classified as an anxiety disorder. For instance, migraine and arthritis may bring on anxious feelings about the severity of pain, when it may abate, or, if it goes away, whether it may return. Likewise, someone with an implantable cardiac defibrillator may worry about the unexpected shock that occurs when it detects an abnormal heart rhythm, not to mention the fear of the device malfunctioning.

Whether the anxiety comes before the physical condition or after, however, a vicious cycle may ensue, each aggravating the other.

Seek Medical Attention

Since anxiety isn't often recognized as a cause of physical illness, you need to let your doctor know if you're suffering from symptoms (see page 55), or if you think you have a physical condition that may be linked to anxiety.

You should also report symptoms such as numbness, tingling, or feeling hot, which could be signs of anxiety. This is especially important among older adults since anxiety is very common—in fact, it's more prevalent than depression, affecting 10–24% of the elderly—and tends to be characterized more by physical symptoms than by worry.

The bottom line: Getting help for anxiety and a physical illness may mean the difference between effective treatment of psychological symptoms or prolonged mental and physical suffering. It can bring tremendous relief from disquieting feelings, while also improving your overall health and quality of life. ■

also not without risks. It is, after all, brain surgery, which carries with it the chance of hemorrhage in the brain, infection, and even death. The DBS device can malfunction and the batteries typically need to be replaced after four to five years. In addition, doctors need to carefully monitor the multiple medications patients are typically taking to ensure drug side effects and interactions are minimized.

Besides DBS, recent studies have shown that vagus nerve stimulation (VNS) may help people with treatment-resistant depression. A vagus nerve stimulator is a small, surgically implanted device designed to stimulate the brain periodically through the vagus nerve—a major nerve that passes from the brain through the neck and chest into the abdomen. One VNS device was approved by the FDA in July 2005 for treatment-resistant depression.

Another treatment method under investigation is rapid transcranial magnetic stimulation (rTMS). In this technique, an electromagnetic coil is placed on the scalp (but not implanted). A high-intensity current passes through the coil and produces a powerful magnetic field that affects the function of the underlying brain cells. Some studies have shown that rTMS performed in the frontal areas of the brain can have antidepressant effects, although this research is still in its infancy.

Additional drugs are also being tested for treating depression. These include drugs that stimulate the production of gamma-aminobutyric acid (GABA, a neurotransmitter that suppresses the action of nerve cells); medications that block the action of glutamate (a neurotransmitter that stimulates nerve cells); drugs that block substance P (a protein originally investigated for its role in pain); and blockers of corticotropin-releasing factor receptors, which play a role in the body's reaction to stress.

Even the wrinkle fighter botulinum toxin (Botox) is under investigation. In one small preliminary trial of 10 women, it was injected into facial muscles to discourage frowning, resulting in a reduction in depressive symptoms.

ANXIETY DISORDERS

Anxiety is a common, normal, and often useful response to life's challenges and dangers. But in people who suffer from an anxiety disorder, anxiety levels spin out of control, causing psychological and physical symptoms that interfere with normal functioning, appear even in the absence of obvious external stressors, or are clearly excessive in the face of the stressors.

Researchers believe that anxiety disorders result from hyperactivity in certain areas of the brain, perhaps related to low levels of the chemical messenger (neurotransmitter) GABA, which is responsible for keeping activity levels of nerve cells in check. Anxiety disorders also run in families.

Despite how common it is, anxiety may be undertreated: In one study, almost 20% of patients visiting a primary care clinic were diagnosed with at least one anxiety disorder—but 41% were receiving no treatment.

Symptoms of Anxiety

Common psychological symptoms of anxiety include irritability, intense fear, worry, difficulty concentrating, and a general "keyed up" feeling. Physical symptoms include sweating, dry mouth, hot flashes or chills, dizziness, heart palpitations, muscle tension, trembling, nausea, and restlessness.

Some medical conditions and drugs can either cause anxiety or produce its symptoms. Alcohol withdrawal, asthma, a heart attack, an overactive thyroid, and a deficiency in folate or vitamin B_{12} are examples. Drugs that might cause or mimic anxiety symptoms include bronchodilators such as ephedrine and epinephrine, psychostimulants such as methylphenidate (Ritalin), and thyroid hormone.

Effects of Anxiety on Physical Health

Some evidence suggests that chronic anxiety may lead to long-term health problems such as high blood pressure (hypertension). An 18- to 20-year follow-up of people who participated in the Framingham Heart Study found such a connection in men ages 45–59. None of the men had high blood pressure at the start of the study. To evaluate psychological traits that might lead to high blood pressure, participants were asked about levels of anxiety, feelings of anger, and expression of anger. Men who had a high score for anxiety at the start of the study were twice as likely to develop high blood pressure than those with a low score for anxiety symptoms. Not all studies have found such an association, however.

Heart attack risk may also be increased by anxiety. A study of 30,000 men, ages 42–77, found that those who scored highest on a questionnaire measuring common phobias had triple the risk of a

NEW RESEARCH

Anxiety Worsens Heart Attack Risk

The first study to repeatedly measure anxiety levels in people with coronary artery disease (CAD) over several years has found that excessive worry nearly doubles the chances of having a fatal or nonfatal heart attack (myocardial infarction).

The 516 study participants with CAD (82% male, mean age 68) underwent cardiac tests and responded to a questionnaire to measure anxiety levels at the start of the study and at annual intervals.

During an average follow-up of three years, 12 participants suffered cardiac-related deaths and 44 had nonfatal heart attacks. Those with anxiety levels in the highest third had double the risk of heart attack or death of those with anxiety levels in the lowest third. More important in predicting a heart attack than high anxiety at the study's outset was a pattern of escalating anxiety after a CAD diagnosis, which increased the risk of heart attack or death by 10%. Likewise, participants who started out with the highest anxiety levels that then dropped to the lowest third in cumulative average levels were among the least likely to suffer a heart attack or die.

Regular anxiety assessments should be performed in individuals with heart disease to identify and treat anxiety and potentially prevent life-threatening events.

JOURNAL OF THE AMERICAN COLLEGE OF CARDIOLOGY
Volume 49, page 2021
May 2007

subsequent fatal heart attack than men with the lowest scores. Similar results were found in a smaller study of 1,408 men in the United Kingdom. It is possible that the fatal heart attacks resulted from some physical consequence of phobic anxiety, such as a disturbance in the heart's rhythm or hyperventilation, which led to spasm of a coronary artery. (For more, see "Anxiety and Your Physical Health" on page 53.)

Panic Disorder

The main features of panic disorder include sudden but short-lived attacks of terror and fear of losing control. Attacks begin without warning during non-threatening activities. Affected individuals often go to the emergency room or consult a cardiologist because the physical symptoms are similar to those of a heart attack. (If you ever suspect that you're having a heart attack, see a doctor or go to the nearest emergency room immediately.) Panic attacks generally peak within 10 minutes and dissipate within 20–30 minutes. They are characterized by some combination of the following symptoms:

- Shortness of breath or hyperventilation
- Heart palpitations or a racing pulse
- Discomfort in the chest
- Dizziness, lightheadedness, or feeling faint
- Choking, nausea, or stomach pain
- Sweating
- Hot or cold flashes
- Trembling or shaking
- A feeling of detachment from one's surroundings or a sense of unreality
- Tingling or numbness
- Fear of dying or losing one's mind.

Symptoms of depression and anxiety are common in people with panic disorder. Although both panic attacks and symptoms of depression and anxiety may improve with antidepressant medications, some people require separate medications.

According to the National Institute of Mental Health, six million adults (2.7% of adult Americans) suffer from panic disorder each year. It is twice as common in women as in men. Attacks commonly begin in the late teens or early 20s and often go undiagnosed and untreated. One study estimated that only one in four people with panic attacks receives appropriate care.

The most common complication of panic disorder is agoraphobia—fear of being in public places, especially when alone—

which develops as a result of trying to avoid situations that have triggered panic attacks in the past. Left untreated, panic attacks and agoraphobia can severely restrict a person's lifestyle. Panic disorder is also associated with an increased frequency of major depression, alcohol and drug dependency, and suicide.

Generalized Anxiety Disorder

Generalized anxiety disorder (GAD) is characterized by excessive, recurrent, and prolonged anxiety and worrying. People with GAD typically agonize over everyday concerns, such as job responsibilities, finances, health, or family well-being or even such minor matters as household chores, car repairs, being late for appointments, or personal appearance. The focus of anxiety may shift frequently from one concern to another, and sensations may vary from mild tension and nervousness to feelings of dread.

GAD affects 6.8 million adults (3.1% of adult Americans) each year. Although people with GAD know that the intensity, duration, and frequency of their anxiety and worry are out of proportion to the actual likelihood or impact of the feared event, they still have difficulty controlling their emotions. Perpetual anxiety may impair concentration, memory, and decision-making ability, decrease attention span, and lead to a loss of confidence. Normal activities, such as working, socializing with friends, and maintaining intimate relationships, may become difficult or even impossible.

GAD may also produce a range of physical symptoms, including heart palpitations, restlessness, sweating, headaches, and nausea. Some GAD sufferers, not realizing that GAD is a treatable illness, become accustomed to their condition and assume that it is normal to feel on edge all the time. But the constant anxiety can lead to alcohol or drug abuse. The physical symptoms of GAD, along with alcohol or drug abuse, are often what finally compel a person to seek treatment.

Obsessive-Compulsive Disorder

Obsessive-compulsive disorder (OCD) is marked by recurrent, repetitive thoughts (obsessions), behaviors (compulsions), or both. People with OCD recognize that their obsessions and compulsions are unreasonable, unnecessary, intrusive, and sometimes even foolish, yet they cannot resist them. Regardless of whether a person suffers from obsessions, compulsions, or both, the condition interferes with day-to-day activities and relationships with others.

Obsessions are defined as recurring and persistent thoughts,

The Power of Positive Thinking

How cognitive-behavioral therapy (CBT) can help conquer anxiety

When many people think of "therapy," they envision endless hours on the proverbial couch dredging up memories from childhood and reflecting on old wounds. But an increasingly popular alternative to psychodynamic therapy, cognitive-behavioral therapy (CBT) focuses on thought patterns in the present rather than feelings about the past as the root of anxiety or depression.

In short, advocates of CBT believe that chronic negative thinking leads to feeling unwell, both physically and emotionally, so CBT aims to help people change those thoughts to relieve troubling psychological symptoms. Recent research confirms earlier findings that CBT can be an effective treatment for an array of anxiety disorders.

CBT for GAD and PD

A review of 25 studies published last year examined the effectiveness of CBT for generalized anxiety disorder (GAD), a condition where excessive and uncontrollable worry about everyday life interferes with normal functioning. Researchers found that people undergoing CBT were significantly more likely to have reduced anxiety at the end of treatment than those receiving no treatment. The study also found that most people preferred individual instead of group CBT sessions.

CBT has also been shown to help people with panic disorder (PD), in which overwhelming bouts of fear or "panic attacks" are accompanied by physical symptoms like heart palpitations, dizziness, and sweating. A study published in the *Journal of the American Medical Association* revealed that PD subjects treated with CBT maintained their improvement significantly better six months after treatment ended than those taking imipramine (Tofranil): Only 4% saw their symptoms worsen compared to a 25% incidence of relapse among those on the medication. Perhaps this is because those in the CBT group learned coping mechanisms that they can use for the rest of their lives.

Beyond GAD and PD, numerous small studies have found CBT to be beneficial for a wide variety of anxiety disorders, including phobias, obsessive-compulsive disorder, and post-traumatic stress syndrome. Additional research conducted over the past 30 years has shown that CBT can relieve depression, bulimia, hypochondria, and insomnia, and more than 150 studies are currently underway to explore its effectiveness for other mental and physical conditions.

How CBT Works

A more concrete, goal-oriented type of therapy, CBT doesn't require a long term, open-ended commitment to a therapist the way psychoanalysis does. Typically, 10–25 weekly visits can help relieve symptoms (a fact health insurers appreciate). CBT therapists use a combination of "cognitive" methods, such as a guided discovery style of questioning to uncover a person's way of reasoning and thinking, and "behavioral" approaches, like helping the individual to feel safe enough to change his or her actions or face feared situations.

Many people with GAD, for instance, are prone to catastrophizing and imagining the worst-case scenario, as their minds are flooded with irrational thoughts. They tend to perceive themselves as powerless victims or failures and view the world as a dangerous place. Something as trivial as getting stuck on line at the post office can create anxiety. They may fear being late for their next

ideas, images, or impulses, sometimes of an aggressive nature, that seem to invade a person's consciousness. The sufferer will try to suppress or ignore these uncomfortable thoughts, often recognizing that they are unrealistic. Common obsessions are fear of contamination from germs, thoughts of violent behavior (such as killing a family member), fear of making a mistake or of harming oneself or others, and a constant need for reassurance.

appointment or that they won't be helped before the post office closes. They may overreact and feel like they never get a break in life. Or they may worry they'll have a panic attack and embarrass themselves. The stress makes them grumpy with the postal clerk—who responds in kind, creating a self-fulfilling prophecy that perpetuates their anxiety.

Many of these thought processes happen in a flash and are extremely subtle and habitual, making it seem to GAD sufferers like the external event is the problem when really it's the thoughts about the situation that are to blame. By learning to retrain their brains to refute negative self-talk, individuals with GAD can start to approach life with a more positive outlook—and be on the receiving end of more pleasant behavior from others.

Using CBT

More interactive than traditional therapy sessions, CBT utilizes homework assignments to encourage personal growth. Between sessions, individuals attempt to test out the new approaches they've learned in daily interactions.

The following techniques suggested by Edmund J. Bourne, Ph.D., author of *The Anxiety & Phobia Workbook*, are basic CBT practices you can use to help relieve anxiety:

- **Stop and ask yourself** whenever you start to feel anxious what thoughts you're having. By identifying your negative self-talk, you can begin to counter it with positive statements. For instance, if you find yourself worrying that the plane you are about to board is going to crash, remind yourself that the vast majority of planes arrive safely at their destinations. Tell yourself that even though you're worried, you know you can handle the situation. Don't put yourself down for feeling anxious and attempt to refrain from using statements like, "I'm not going to get anxious today," because the stress of trying to make something *not* happen can often create anxiety.
- **Create a list** of some of the negative things you most commonly tell yourself. Look at it objectively and rationally, and come up with positive counter statements. Then read the list every day at a set time and whenever you're feeling anxious.
- **Distract yourself** with relaxation techniques or physical exercise to break free of pessimistic self-talk.
- **Think about what would happen** if the worst-case scenario did come true. How would you cope with it? Many people with anxiety disorders overestimate the odds of a bad situation occurring and underestimate their ability to manage hardships, when in truth the worst that could happen isn't so horrible after all. So what if you have a panic attack at your friend's house? Yes, you might be embarrassed, but your friend would likely understand and try to help you.
- **Praise yourself** and reinforce positive thoughts and behaviors. Every time you do something without letting your worry get the best of you, congratulate yourself. Say something like, "I'm really proud of myself for handling this situation without getting anxious."
- **Gradually expose yourself** to things that make you fearful—then build on your successes. When you can control your anxiety in a given scenario, you become more confident that you can handle it the next time and in other circumstances, too. But when you avoid stressful situations, you reinforce your negative beliefs and self-talk, making the situation seem more dangerous than it actually is. ■

Compulsions are ritualistic, repetitive, and purposeful behaviors that are performed according to certain rules or stereotypical patterns. The behavior, although clearly excessive, temporarily relieves the tension and discomfort brought on by the obsessive thoughts. Common compulsions are rechecking to be sure doors are locked, windows are closed, or an appliance is turned off; excessive neatness and organization; and repetitive hand washing that accompanies an obsession with dirt and germs.

OCD occurs in about 2.2 million adult Americans (1% of the adult population) each year and affects men and women equally. It most often starts in the teens or early 20s. Embarrassed and upset by their behavior, most sufferers try to keep it a secret. Those with mild OCD often manage to function with only minimal interference in their daily lives. But in people with more pronounced OCD, obsessive thoughts or compulsive behaviors may be frequent or distressing enough to become incapacitating.

Probably the most common complication of the disorder is depression; another is marked interference with social and work behaviors. Although some people with OCD experience spontaneous remission, in most the illness has an episodic course with periods of partial remission. In about 10% of sufferers, the course of OCD is chronic and unchanged.

Post-Traumatic Stress Disorder

Post-traumatic stress disorder (PTSD) is a form of chronic psychological stress that follows exposure to a traumatic event, such as a natural disaster, a violent crime, an accident, terrorism, or warfare. The symptoms include the following:

- Recurrent, intrusive, distressing dreams and memories of the trauma
- A sudden sense that the event is recurring; experiencing flashbacks
- Extreme distress when confronted with events that symbolize or resemble the trauma
- Attempting to avoid thoughts, feelings, and activities associated with the event
- Inability to remember aspects of the trauma
- Markedly diminished interest in important activities
- Feelings of detachment and estrangement from loved ones
- Low expectations for the future
- Insomnia or excessive fatigue
- Extreme irritability
- Inability to concentrate
- Hypervigilance or an exaggerated startle response.

Symptoms must last at least one month for a diagnosis of post-traumatic stress disorder. In the acute version of the syndrome, symptoms begin within six months of the trauma. The chronic syndrome may be delayed in its onset until more than six months after the event or may persist for more than six months afterward. As many as

15% of the people involved in a major natural disaster suffer enough distress to need treatment. Complications include anxiety, alcohol or drug abuse, depression, and family or work problems.

Overall, 7.7 million adults (3.5% of adult Americans) develop PTSD each year. It can develop at any age and tends to affect women more than men.

Phobic Disorders

The hallmarks of phobic disorders are persistent, irrational fears and avoidance of the specific things or activities (for example, air travel, closed spaces, certain animals or insects) that induce these fears. The diagnosis of a phobic disorder is made only when the phobia significantly impairs the individual's social functioning or work performance.

A common type of phobia is social phobia (also called social anxiety disorder), which affects 15 million adults (6.8% of the population). Social phobia is an undue fear of embarrassment in social situations. Although many people feel some anxiety when placed in a situation that forces them to meet and talk to new people, social phobia causes such an extreme reaction to this everyday aspect of life that it interferes with daily functioning.

Treatment of Anxiety

Treatment of anxiety does not always require medication. The use of antianxiety drugs depends in part on whether the person can tolerate his or her symptoms while learning to manage them. Coping measures include psychotherapy and stress-reducing therapies such as progressive muscle relaxation, biofeedback, or, less commonly, yoga, self-hypnosis, or meditation. In general, these approaches are designed to give people with anxiety a feeling of control over their symptoms.

If you suffer from anxiety, you can help yourself by getting adequate sleep, exercising (which aids sleep and improves self-esteem), and avoiding caffeine and alcohol. Often a person has more than one anxiety disorder; determining exactly which disorders are present can lead to better treatment. As with mood disorders, a careful evaluation by a health professional is the first step in treatment. Depending on the severity of anxiety symptoms, treatment can be managed by your primary care physician or a specialist.

NEW RESEARCH

Smokers' Mental Health Fares Worse After Stress

While post-traumatic stress disorder (PTSD) is associated with increased smoking, a Dutch study suggests the reverse: that smokers are more likely than nonsmokers to develop severe anxiety, hostility, and PTSD after experiencing a major disaster or stressful event.

Researchers conducted surveys 1.5 and four years after a fireworks disaster in the Netherlands that killed 23 people and injured 900 others. They compared 662 adult victims of the disaster to 526 residents of another Dutch city. The surveys measured smoking habits; anxiety, depression, and hostility symptoms; and signs of PTSD.

Victims who smoked at the 18-month postdisaster mark were twice as likely to have severe anxiety and hostility symptoms and almost three times as likely to have PTSD as nonsmokers four years after the disaster. Smoking was also associated with severe anxiety symptoms among members of the control group: Those who smoked at 18 months were likely to have severe anxiety at four years when confronted with stressful life events.

More studies are needed to confirm these findings, but quitting smoking after a disaster or stressful time may help to prevent PTSD, anxiety, and hostility.

JOURNAL OF CLINICAL PSYCHIATRY
Volume 68, page 87
January 2007

General Medication Treatment

Although benzodiazepines are still commonly used to treat anxiety, two classes of antidepressant drugs—SSRIs and tricyclics—have become the first line of treatment. The serotonin and norepinephrine reuptake inhibitors and tetracyclics are also used to treat these conditions. These drugs are not habit forming and can be effective in low doses. Clearly, antidepressants are indicated when a person with anxiety is also depressed.

Tricyclics and SSRIs take several weeks to work, making them slower acting than benzodiazepines, but they do bring a fast-acting benefit to people with anxiety by promoting better sleep, which quickly improves daily functioning.

Benzodiazepines

It is thought that benzodiazepines relieve anxiety by enhancing the effects of the neurotransmitter GABA. The mechanism of action is not fully understood, however. The side effects of benzodiazepines are generally minor. They include mild disturbances of thinking and, in rare instances, slowed breathing. Two side effects of benzodiazepines, drowsiness and clumsiness, may lead to an increased risk of accidents while driving. A study from Quebec found that users of benzodiazepines had a 26% greater chance of having a car accident than non-users. The increased risk for those using benzodiazepines was highest (45%) during the first week of therapy.

The most troublesome issues with benzodiazepine treatment are the development of tolerance (decreased effectiveness of a given dose with continued use) and both physical and psychological dependence, especially with long-term use of a drug at high doses. Physical dependence is defined by the development of a specific set of physical symptoms upon withdrawal of a drug. Psychological dependence refers to a persistent desire for the drug after it has been discontinued.

Tolerance may cause a person to request, and at times receive, increasingly larger doses to maintain benefits. In this instance, the person may be switched to an SSRI or a tricyclic drug instead of higher doses of a benzodiazepine. The risk of side effects, such as drowsiness and confused thinking, rises with increased doses of benzodiazepines.

When a person is physically or psychologically dependent on benzodiazepines, he or she can experience serious symptoms during withdrawal, including irritability, agitation, restlessness, insomnia, loss of appetite, tremor, muscle aches, and, in some people, confusion or seizures. The danger of severe withdrawal symptoms can be diminished by using the smallest effective dose of a benzodiazepine for the shortest possible time and by slowly tapering the drug dose as it is discontinued.

Buspirone

The antianxiety drug buspirone (BuSpar) has fewer adverse effects than benzodiazepines, but it may be less effective, particularly for panic disorder. Common side effects of BuSpar are dizziness, headache, nervousness, and nausea. However, BuSpar causes less drowsiness than other drugs, and abuse is unlikely because it does not lead to tolerance or dependence. In switching from benzodiazepines to BuSpar, a person may be able to minimize anxiety symptoms by starting immediately on BuSpar while tapering the dose of a benzodiazepine. For more on the drugs used to treat anxiety, see the chart on pages 64–65.

Herbal treatments

Kava, which is prepared from the crushed root of *Piper methysticum* (a shrub-like pepper plant), is marketed as a natural remedy for anxiety and stress. However, the FDA has issued a warning that the supplement can damage the liver. In addition, long-term use of kava may result in allergic reactions, visual disturbances, or difficulties maintaining balance. Kava should not be used if you are pregnant, breastfeeding, or taking antidepressants.

Valerian is also sold as a natural antianxiety remedy. Most research on the herb, which is prepared from the dried root of the plant *Valeriana officianalis*, has focused on people with insomnia. Less is known about its effectiveness in treating anxiety.

As with all herbal products, kava and valerian aren't regulated by the FDA, and there's no guarantee of the products' purity or effectiveness. Drug–herb interactions are also a concern. It is important to discuss all herbal remedies with your doctor before trying them.

Treatment of Specific Anxiety Disorders

Psychotherapy, medication, and coping behaviors are used to treat all anxiety disorders. However, the disorders respond differently to the various treatment approaches.

Panic disorder

Treatment of panic disorder often involves both psychotherapy and medication. A therapist who specializes in treating panic disorder is

ASK THE DOCTOR

Q. *Do medications change your personality or who you are?*

A. Antidepressant and antianxiety medications don't alter your personality, but they may change your interactions with others. For example, depending on your initial symptoms, they may make you feel less anxious, sad, moody, irritable, or lethargic. That can help you get along with others better and be more productive and engaged in life. The medications don't artificially make you go from sad to happy; rather, they correct the chemical imbalance that, in turn, has thrown your emotional reactions out of balance. You should still be able to experience mood changes.

Sometimes, individuals taking antidepressants experience a sense of numbness, apathy, or dulling of moods. This side effect is not a goal of the treatment. It may mean that your depression has been partially treated and the dull mood will lift with time, or that you need to adjust your dosage. It could also mean that this particular medication is not the right one for you, and switching to another one might produce better results.

You also may not have received the correct diagnosis: For instance, you may have been diagnosed with depression when you are actually suffering from bipolar disorder, which requires a different approach to treatment. That's why it's imperative to be aware of your moods. If you feel like you're just not yourself when you're taking a medication, be sure to discuss it with your doctor.

Commonly Used Antianxiety Drugs 2008*

Drug type: Brand (generic)	Typical daily dosage†	How they appear to work
Benzodiazepines		
Ativan (lorazepam‡)	2–6 mg	Balance brain chemicals by enhancing effects of the neurotransmitter gamma-aminobutyric acid (GABA).
Gen-Xene (clorazepate‡)	15–60 mg	
Klonopin (clonazepam‡)	0.5–4 mg	
Librium (chlordiazepoxide‡)	15–100 mg	
Niravam (alprazolam‡)	0.75–4 mg	
(oxazepam§)	30–120 mg	
Tranxene, Tranxene-SD (clorazepate‡)	15–60 mg	
Valium (diazepam‡)	4–40 mg	
Xanax (alprazolam‡)	0.75–4 mg	
Buspirone		
BuSpar (buspirone‡)	15-60 mg	Affects the actions of the neurotransmitters serotonin and dopamine in the brain.
Selective serotonin reuptake inhibitors (SSRIs)		
Celexa (citalopram‡)	20–60 mg	Block the reabsorption and inactivation of the neurotransmitter serotonin by neurons. This increases the availability of serotonin to carry messages between nerve cells.
(fluvoxamine§)	50–300 mg	
Lexapro (escitalopram‖)	10–20 mg	
Paxil (paroxetine‡)	10–60 mg	
Paxil CR (paroxetine, controlled-release‖)	12.5–75 mg	
Prozac (fluoxetine‡)	10–60 mg	
Zoloft (sertraline‡)	25–200 mg	
Serotonin and norepinephrine reuptake inhibitors (SNRIs)		
Cymbalta (duloxetene)	30–120 mg	Block the reabsorption of serotonin and norepinephrine, increasing the availability of these neurotransmitters in the brain.
(trazodone§)	150–400 mg	
Effexor (venlafaxine‡)	75–375 mg	
Effexor XR (venlafaxine, extended-release)	75–225 mg	
Tetracyclics		
Remeron (mirtazapine‡)	15–45 mg	Blocks the reabsorption of serotonin and/or norepinephrine, increasing the availability of these neurotransmitters in the brain.
Remeron SolTab (mirtazapine‡)	15–45 mg	
Tricyclics		
Anafranil (clomipramine‡)	25–250 mg	Block the reabsorption of serotonin, norepinephrine, and, to a lesser extent, dopamine, increasing the availability of these neurotransmitters in the brain.
Aventyl (nortriptyline‡)	75–150 mg	
Norpramin (desipramine‡)	100–300 mg	
Pamelor (nortriptyline‡)	75–150 mg	
Sinequan (doxepin‡)	25–300 mg	
Tofranil (imipramine‡)	75–200 mg	

* Many of these drugs are not approved by the U.S. Food and Drug Administration (FDA) for anxiety disorders but are commonly used to treat them.

† These dosages represent an average range for the treatment of anxiety and may differ from the dosage prescribed by your doctor. The precise effective dosage varies from person to person and depends on many factors. Do not make any change to your medication without consulting your doctor. *Starting dosages tend to be lower for older patients.*

‡ Generic version available at lower cost.

§ Generic only available.

‖ Generic version approved as of press time.

Precautions	Common side effects
Chronic use of these drugs may lead to tolerance and dependence. Antacids may decrease effectiveness. Do not drink alcohol while using.	Sedation (often purposely prescribed for their ability to induce relaxation and sleep), dizziness, weakness, unsteadiness/clumsiness, depression, headache, dry mouth, decreased sex drive, dependence.
Do not take with MAO inhibitors.	Dizziness, nausea, headache, nervousness, lightheadedness, excitement. Nonaddictive, less sedating than other antianxiety drugs.
Do not take with MAO inhibitors, triptans, or St. John's wort. The development of a skin rash can be a sign of a serious medical problem; see a doctor immediately. If discontinuing use, reduce dosage gradually to prevent withdrawal symptoms.	Anxiety, nervousness, insomnia, drowsiness, weakness, headache, diarrhea, increased sweating, nausea, impaired sexual function, weight gain. Side effects appear to be lesser with escitalopram.
Do not take with MAO inhibitors or triptans. Effexor may increase blood pressure and/or cholesterol levels in some people; regular blood pressure and cholesterol monitoring is advised. If discontinuing use, reduce dosage gradually to prevent withdrawal symptoms.	Nausea, weakness, sweating, insomnia, drowsiness, dry mouth, dizziness, constipation, nervousness, impaired sexual function, appetite loss.
Do not take with MAO inhibitors. Caution advised with use of mirtazapine in the elderly because of delayed clearance of the drug, which may increase the risk of adverse effects.	Sleepiness, nausea, increased appetite, weight gain, dizziness, blurred vision, weakness, dry mouth, headache, constipation, shakiness, nervousness.
Do not take with MAO inhibitors. Do not stop treatment abruptly. It is not advisable to take tricyclic antidepressants if you have seizures, a heart disorder, glaucoma, or use alcohol excessively.	Dizziness on standing, drowsiness, weakness, headache, dry mouth, blurred vision, constipation, nausea, difficulty urinating, increased appetite (which may include a craving for sweets), impaired sexual function, increased heart rate. Skin is more sensitive to sunlight during use of these drugs, which may result in itching, redness, discoloration of skin.

optimal. According to a year-long study of 232 people with panic disorder treated at primary care clinics, sustained cognitive-behavioral therapy (gradual exposure to whatever brings on symptoms of anxiety) plus antianxiety medication is more effective than typical care (initial counseling and ongoing medication) for treating this type of anxiety.

Panic disorder may require more long-term drug therapy than other anxiety disorders (such as GAD). Tricyclic antidepressants and MAO inhibitors are sometimes used to treat panic disorder; both are 80–90% effective in blocking panic attacks but require six to 12 weeks to take effect. High doses of alprazolam (Xanax), a benzodiazepine, can be effective within a few days. While Xanax causes fewer side effects than antidepressants, it is usually addictive (like all benzodiazepines).

In addition to benzodiazepines, the SSRIs fluoxetine (Prozac), paroxetine (Paxil), and sertraline (Zoloft), as well as the SNRI venlafaxine (Effexor), are FDA approved for treating panic disorder. The tricyclics desipramine (Norpramin), imipramine (Tofranil), and nortriptyline (Aventyl, Pamelor) may also be used, although they do not have FDA approval for treating panic disorder. Beta-blockers, such as propranolol (Inderal) or atenolol (Tenormin), can halt the physical symptoms of panic attacks but do not prevent the fear or panic itself.

Regardless of the specific drug(s) used to treat panic disorder, about 30–60% of people with the disorder suffer a relapse of symptoms six to 12 months after they stop taking their medication.

Generalized anxiety disorder (GAD)

Despite its more chronic course, GAD responds better to treatment than does panic disorder. Psychotherapy helps many people, either by itself or in combination with medication. In addition, relaxation techniques, such as deep breathing exercises or meditation, may relieve symptoms of GAD.

The antidepressant medications duloxetine (Cymbalta), escitalopram (Lexapro), Paxil, and Effexor are FDA approved for the treatment of GAD, but other serotonin and norepinephrine reuptake inhibitors, SSRIs, tricyclics, benzodiazepines, and BuSpar are also commonly used to treat GAD.

Many people with GAD experience depression and self-medicate with alcohol, nicotine, or other drugs, particularly benzodiazepines. As a result, someone with GAD who is being treated with a benzodiazepine should be given limited prescriptions of the drug (five to seven days). BuSpar, though sometimes less effective, may be a better option, as it does not cause dependence or withdrawal symptoms.

In terms of self-care, cutting back on caffeine may help ease the symptoms of GAD. One study found that the effects of caffeine, such as raising blood pressure, pulse rate, and brain activity, were more pronounced in people with GAD. Moreover, people with GAD reported higher subjective levels of anxiety with greater caffeine intake.

Obsessive-compulsive disorder

As with panic disorder, OCD may improve with a combination of medication and cognitive-behavioral psychotherapy. SSRIs, such as citalopram (Celexa), Lexapro, Prozac, fluvoxamine, Paxil, and Zoloft, are now commonly used to treat this illness. The FDA has approved Paxil, Zoloft, Prozac, and fluvoxamine for the treatment of OCD (the first three are also approved for panic disorder). Improvements, which may take six to eight weeks of drug therapy, are more likely for compulsions than for obsessions. Higher doses of these medications (compared with those typically used to treat depression) may be necessary to treat OCD.

Post-traumatic stress disorder

Successful treatment requires a combination of psychotherapy—aimed at desensitizing the individual to the traumatic experience—and medication. A recent study in *Behavior Research and Therapy* found that eight to 12 sessions of cognitive-behavioral therapy (involving desensitization and progressive muscle relaxation) was better at reducing post-traumatic stress disorder symptoms than supportive therapy. Two SSRIs have been approved by the FDA for treating post-traumatic stress disorder: Zoloft and Paxil. The tricyclics amitriptyline and Norpramin are commonly used to treat the mood disturbances and anxiety that accompany the disorder.

Phobic disorders

When treatment is needed, cognitive and/or behavioral therapy may help desensitize the person to the thing or situation that causes the fear. Therapy involves gradually exposing the individual to the feared situation, while teaching the person how to use various relaxation techniques to confront the fear.

Social phobia

Recent studies have shown that people with social phobia respond to the SSRIs Paxil and fluvoxamine; other SSRIs, such as Zoloft,

NEW RESEARCH

Medication Response in OCD Determined By Genes

Although selective serotonin reuptake inhibitors (SSRIs) are the most effective medications for obsessive-compulsive disorder (OCD), up to 40–60% of people with OCD do not achieve relief, and more than a third do not respond when switched to another SSRI. According to a new study, their genetic makeup may be the reason why.

Dutch researchers enrolled 91 individuals with OCD in a double-blind study and randomly assigned them to receive the SSRI paroxetine (Paxil) or the serotonin and norepinephrine reuptake inhibitor (SNRI) venlafaxine, extended-release (Effexor XR) for 12 weeks. All participants underwent blood tests for genetic assessment of previously identified serotonin transporter genes, which have been associated with treatment responses to serotonin-related medications.

The investigators found that participants who responded favorably to Effexor XR carried the S/L genotype of the 5-HTTLPR polymorphism, or genetic variant, while those who benefited from Paxil carried the G/G genotype of the 5-HT2A polymorphism. Ten percent of participants had both genetic variations and responded to both medications.

In the future, if these results are replicated in other trials, genetic assessment might be used to help individualize the choice of medication for people with OCD, maximizing the chance that they respond well.

JOURNAL OF CLINICAL PSYCHIATRY
Volume 68, page 747
May 2007

and the extended-release serotonin and norepinephrine reuptake inhibitor Effexor XR, may provide benefits as well. Tricyclics and benzodiazepines may also be used.

Many people who suffer from stage fright (such as classical musicians) use beta-blockers, like Inderal, for performance anxiety. Although the drugs may reduce the physical symptoms of performance anxiety associated with a particular event, they are not recommended for ongoing treatment. ■

agoraphobia—Fear of being in public places.

Alzheimer's disease—A progressive neurological disease marked by deficits in cognition, especially in memory.

antidepressant—A drug used to treat depression.

atypical depression—A type of depression in which a person does not experience sadness or some of the other symptoms normally associated with the disorder.

behavioral therapy—A form of psychotherapy that involves training in social skills, problem solving, scheduling of activities, and self-control. The emphasis is on day-to-day improvements in behavior.

benzodiazepines—A class of drugs used to relieve anxiety.

beta-blockers—A class of drugs used to treat angina, high blood pressure, irregular heart rhythms, and migraine. Chronic use of these drugs may cause depression; they are sometimes used in combination with antidepressants or to treat performance anxiety.

bipolar disorder—A mood disorder with episodes of both depression and mania; it is also known as manic depression.

breakthrough depression—A depressive episode that occurs in someone with bipolar disorder or major depression who has been doing reasonably well with long-term treatment.

cognition—Mental abilities such as memory, attention, learning, awareness, and judgment.

cognitive therapy—A form of psychotherapy designed to reverse a person's belief that exaggerated weaknesses and inadequacies doom him or her to failure.

compulsion—Ritualistic, repetitive, and purposeful behavior that is performed according to certain rules or stereotypical patterns.

crisis intervention—See **interpersonal therapy**.

Cushing's disease—A medical condition caused by an overproduction of the steroid hormone cortisol by the adrenal gland.

deep brain stimulation (DBS)—A procedure in which an electrical stimulator (a pacemaker-like device) is implanted in the chest and programmed to send electrical impulses to a specific region of the brain. DBS is currently being tested for treating severe depression.

dementia—Deterioration of cognitive abilities resulting from a brain disorder or other disease.

depression—A mood disorder characterized by persistent low or sad mood, decreased or absent interest in almost all activities, loss of self-confidence, and a sense of worthlessness.

dopamine—A neurotransmitter; low levels are linked to depression and Parkinson's disease.

dopamine reuptake inhibitors—Antidepressant drugs that decrease the reabsorption of the neurotransmitter dopamine by the cell that released the dopamine.

double depression—Dysthymia with recurrent episodes of major depression.

dysthymia—A chronic disorder lasting two years or more, characterized by the presence of depressed mood for most of the day for more days than not. It may be intermittent, with periods of feeling normal, but relief lasts no more than two months. Symptoms are not severe enough to meet the criteria for major depression.

electroconvulsive therapy (ECT)—A series of sessions in which a controlled seizure is produced by attaching electrodes to the head and then sending brief electrical impulses through the skull into the brain. Used to treat depression and other psychiatric conditions when other treatments have failed or when immediate relief of symptoms is needed.

gamma-aminobutyric acid (GABA)—A neurotransmitter that suppresses the action of nerve cells. Decreased activity of GABA may contribute to anxiety disorders.

generalized anxiety disorder (GAD)—A condition characterized by persistent, excessive anxiety and worry.

glutamate—A neurotransmitter that stimulates nerve cells. High glutamate levels in the brain may contribute to depression.

group therapy—A form of psychotherapy in which people meet under the guidance of a therapist to share feelings, experiences, and solutions in a supportive environment.

Huntington's disease—A disease of the central nervous system characterized by jerky movements, personality changes, and dementia.

hypomania—Episodes of mild manic symptoms.

hypothalamus—A part of the brain located within the limbic system that regulates the pituitary gland and may be involved in hormonal imbalances sometimes associated with depression.

hypothyroidism—The condition of having an underactive thyroid gland. When untreated, it can trigger symptoms of a mood disorder.

interpersonal therapy—A form of psychotherapy that aims to help a person cope with immediate problems and difficult transitions (such as divorce). Also known as crisis intervention.

kava—An herb marketed as a remedy for anxiety; it is not approved by the FDA.

light therapy—A treatment for seasonal affective disorder (SAD) that involves exposure to sources of bright light.

limbic system—A group of structures deep in the brain that play a major role in processing memories and emotion. These structures include the hippocampus, amygdala, hypothalamus, and entorhinal cortex.

mania—A mood disorder characterized by elated or elevated mood, increased activity, overblown self-image, and exaggerated self-confidence.

manic depression—See **bipolar disorder**.

melatonin—A hormone that appears to play a role in the body's daily rhythms. In supplement form, it is marketed as a remedy for seasonal affective disorder. It is not approved by the FDA.

mixed state—A condition in bipolar disorder when simultaneous symptoms of mania and depression are manifest.

monoamine oxidase (MAO) inhibitors—Antidepressant drugs that increase brain levels of the neurotransmitters norepinephrine, serotonin, and dopamine by blocking the action of the enzyme monoamine oxidase, which normally inactivates these neurotransmitters.

neuroleptics—Antipsychotic drugs sometimes used to control the psychotic symptoms of bipolar disorder until other mood-stabilizing drugs begin to take effect.

neurons—Nerve cells in the brain.

neurotransmitters—Chemicals used for communication between neurons.

nonsteroidal anti-inflammatory drugs (NSAIDs)—A class of drugs (including ibuprofen and aspirin) that reduce pain and inflammation. NSAIDs can increase the risk of toxicity when taken with lithium.

norepinephrine—A neurotransmitter, low levels of which are linked to depression.

obsession—Recurring and persistent thoughts, ideas, images, or impulses, sometimes of an aggressive or violent nature, that invade a person's consciousness.

obsessive-compulsive disorder (OCD)—A condition characterized by recurrent, repetitive thoughts (obsessions), behaviors (compulsions), or a combination of both. A person with OCD recognizes that his or her obsessions and compulsions are unreasonable, intrusive, unnecessary, or foolish but cannot resist them.

omega-3 fatty acids—Polyunsaturated fatty acids that are found in certain foods, notably fish and flaxseed. Researchers are currently studying omega-3s as a potential treatment for depression and bipolar disorder.

panic disorder—A condition characterized by short-lived, sudden attacks of terror and fear of losing control; attacks begin without warning during non-threatening activities.

Parkinson's disease—A progressive neurological disease characterized by tremors, stooped posture, and slow movement.

phobic disorder—A condition characterized by persistent, irrational fears that significantly impair an individual's social or work performance.

pituitary gland—A small gland located at the base of the brain that releases hormones regulating growth and metabolism.

post-traumatic stress disorder (PTSD)—A form of chronic psychological stress that follows exposure to a traumatic event such as an earthquake, a violent crime (rape, child abuse, murder), torture, an accident, or warfare.

psychiatric nurse specialist—A registered nurse, usually with a master's degree in psychiatric nursing, who specializes in treating mental disorders.

psychiatric social worker—A social worker with specialized training in counseling.

psychiatrist—A medical doctor trained in the diagnosis and treatment of mental disorders; psychiatrists are authorized to prescribe medications and hospitalize patients.

psychoanalytic therapy—A form of psychotherapy in which a person meets with an analyst three to five times a week in a stream-of-consciousness, free-association atmosphere that involves minimal feedback from the therapist.

psychodynamic therapy—A form of psychotherapy that focuses on the patient's previous experiences in an attempt to understand current conflicts or feelings about recent changes, such as retirement or grief.

psychologist—A person with a doctorate degree in psychology who is trained in counseling, psychotherapy, and psychological testing; psychologists are not authorized to prescribe medication or hospitalize patients.

psychotherapist—A person who practices psychotherapy. Licensing and certification of psychotherapists vary from state to state.

psychotherapy—The treatment of an emotional, behavioral, personality, or psychiatric disorder by means of verbal and nonverbal communication, as opposed to the use of medication or physical interventions. Psychotherapy has many forms (see separate entries): interpersonal therapy; psychodynamic therapy; supportive therapy; behavioral therapy; cognitive therapy; psychoanalytic therapy; and group therapy.

rapid cycling—A condition that occurs in bipolar disorder and involves multiple episodes of depression and mania within a given year.

rapid transcranial magnetic stimulation (rTMS)—A procedure in which an electromagnetic coil is placed on the scalp and sends pulsed magnetic stimulation to the brain. TMS is currently being tested for treating depression.

reuptake—The reabsorption of a neurotransmitter by

the nerve cell that released it. Drugs that block reuptake allow the neurotransmitter in the synaptic cleft to continue stimulation of other nerve cells.

S-adenosylmethionine (SAM-e)—A supplement that is marketed as a treatment for depression; it is not approved by the FDA.

seasonal affective disorder (SAD)—Episodes of depression that occur during certain times of the year when there is less sunlight, usually beginning in November and lasting through the winter months.

selective serotonin reuptake inhibitors (SSRIs)—Antidepressant drugs that inhibit the reuptake of serotonin and thereby raise its concentration in the brain.

selective serotonin reuptake inhibitor (SSRI) withdrawal—Withdrawal symptoms experienced by about 25% of people who abruptly stop taking an SSRI. Most common symptoms are dizziness, nausea, lethargy, and headache.

serotonin—A neurotransmitter; low levels are linked to depression.

serotonin and norepinephrine reuptake inhibitors—Antidepressant drugs that inhibit the reuptake of serotonin and norepinephrine.

serotonin syndrome—A disorder that develops in some people who take a combination of drugs that raise the level of serotonin in the body. Symptoms include altered mental status and neuromuscular and nervous system problems.

social phobia—An undue fear of embarrassment in social situations. People with social phobia are so consumed by the fear of embarrassing themselves or being judged negatively that they avoid most social contact.

St. John's wort—An herbal remedy used for mild to moderate depression; it is not approved by the FDA.

supportive therapy—A form of therapy that teaches people about their illness, with the idea that a better understanding of the illness will enable them to set more realistic and tangible goals. The person's family members or close friends may be included in some counseling or education sessions.

synaptic cleft—The small gap between nerve cells; sometimes referred to as a synapse.

testosterone—The principal male sex hormone; it is currently being studied for its ability to treat depression in men.

tetracyclics—Antidepressant drugs with actions, effectiveness, and side effects similar to those of tricyclics.

tolerance—Decreased effectiveness of a given dose of a drug resulting from its continued use.

tricyclics—Antidepressant drugs that raise concentrations of the neurotransmitters norepinephrine and serotonin in the synaptic cleft by blocking their reuptake.

vagus nerve stimulator—A small, surgically implanted device that periodically stimulates the brain through the vagus nerve. It is used in the treatment of epilepsy and is being studied for treating depression.

valerian—An herb used to alleviate anxiety; it is not approved by the FDA.

HEALTH INFORMATION ORGANIZATIONS AND SUPPORT GROUPS

American Association of Suicidology
5221 Wisconsin Ave., NW
Washington, DC 20015
☎ 202-237-2280
☎ 800-273-8255 (crisis hotline)
www.suicidology.org
Nonprofit organization with both individual and organizational members. Publishes newsletters and journals on suicide prevention. Offers various services to suicide survivors.

American Psychiatric Association
1000 Wilson Blvd., Ste. 1825
Arlington, VA 22209-3901
☎ 703-907-7300/888-35-PSYCH
www.healthyminds.org
Medical specialty society that provides clinical patient information about mental illnesses, medication, and psychiatric treatment.

American Psychological Association
750 First St., NE
Washington, DC 20002-4242
☎ 800-374-2721/202-336-5500
www.apa.org
Professional organization that publishes books, pamphlets, and brochures on psychological issues.

Anxiety Disorders Association of America
8730 Georgia Ave. Ste. 600
Silver Spring, MD 20910
☎ 240-485-1001
www.adaa.org
Nonprofit organization that promotes the early diagnosis, treatment, and cure of anxiety disorders. Offers information on a variety of anxiety disorders and medications. Provides therapist referrals.

Depression and Bipolar Support Alliance
730 N. Franklin, Ste. 501
Chicago, IL 60610-7224
☎ 800-826-3632/312-642-0049
www.dbsalliance.org
Provides educational materials, support groups, and a hotline staffed by people with depressive or manic-depressive illness.

Depression and Related Affective Disorders Association
2330 W. Joppa Rd., Ste. 100
Lutherville, MD 21093
☎ 410-583-2919
Educates, informs, and offers support services to individuals, families, and professionals about depression and bipolar disorder. Works in cooperation with the Department of Psychiatry at Johns Hopkins School of Medicine.

National Alliance on Mental Illness
Colonial Place Three
2107 Wilson Blvd., Ste. 300
Arlington, VA 22201-3042
☎ 703-524-7600/800-950-6264
www.nami.org
Grassroots self-help support and advocacy organization dedicated to improving the lives of people with severe mental illness and their families.

National Institute of Mental Health
Science Writing, Press, and Dissemination Branch
6001 Executive Blvd.
Rm. 8184, MSC 9663
Bethesda, MD 20892-9663
☎ 866-615-6464/301-443-4513
www.nimh.nih.gov
Supports and conducts research on depression and other mental health disorders. Also distributes information on various mental health issues and mental disorders.

National Mental Health Association
2001 N. Beauregard St., 6th Fl.
Alexandria, VA 22311
☎ 800-969-NMHA/703-684-7722
www.nmha.org
Provides referrals to treatment services and support groups and offers literature on various mental health topics. Has branches in communities throughout the country.

LEADING HOSPITALS
for Psychiatry as Ranked by *U.S. News & World Report*

1. **Massachusetts General Hospital**
   Boston, MA
   ☎ 617-726-2000
   www.massgeneral.org

2. **Johns Hopkins Hospital**
   Baltimore, MD
   ☎ 410-502-4003/410-955-5464
   www.hopkinsmedicine.org

3. **McLean Hospital**
   (a Harvard Medical School affiliate)
   Belmont, MA
   ☎ 800-333-0338/617-855-2000
   www.mclean.harvard.edu

4. **New York-Presbyterian University Hospital of Columbia and Cornell**
   New York, NY
   ☎ 877-NYP-WELL
   www.nyp.org

5. **University of California, Los Angeles Neuropsychiatric Hospital**
   Los Angeles, CA
   ☎ 800-825-9989
   www.npi.ucla.edu

6. **Sheppard and Enoch Pratt Hospital**
   Baltimore, MD
   ☎ 410-938-3000
   www.sheppardpratt.org

7. **Menninger Clinic**
   Houston, TX
   ☎ 800-351-9058/713-275-5000
   www.menningerclinic.com

8. **Mayo Clinic**
   Rochester, MN
   ☎ 507-284-2511/507-538-3270
   www.mayoclinic.org

9. **Yale-New Haven Hospital**
   New Haven, CT
   ☎ 888-700-6543/203-688-4242
   www.ynhh.org

10. **Stanford Hospital and Clinics**
    Stanford, CA
    ☎ 650-723-4000
    www.stanfordhospital.com

INDEX

INDEX

NOTES

NOTES

ISBN 978-1-933087-61-0
1-933087-61-7

Printed in the United States of America

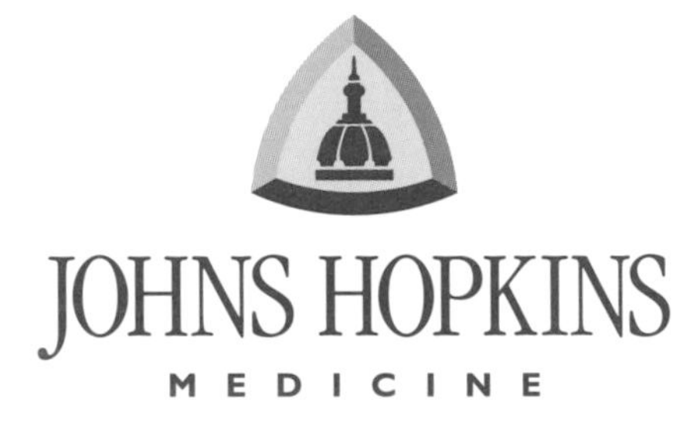

The Johns Hopkins White Papers are published yearly by Medletter Associates, LLC.

Visit our website for information on Johns Hopkins Health Publications, which include White Papers on specific disorders, home medical encyclopedias, consumer reference guides to drugs and medical tests, and our monthly newsletter *The Johns Hopkins Medical Letter: Health After 50*.
www.JohnsHopkinsHealthAlerts.com

DIABETES

Christopher D. Saudek, M.D.,

and

Simeon Margolis, M.D., Ph.D.

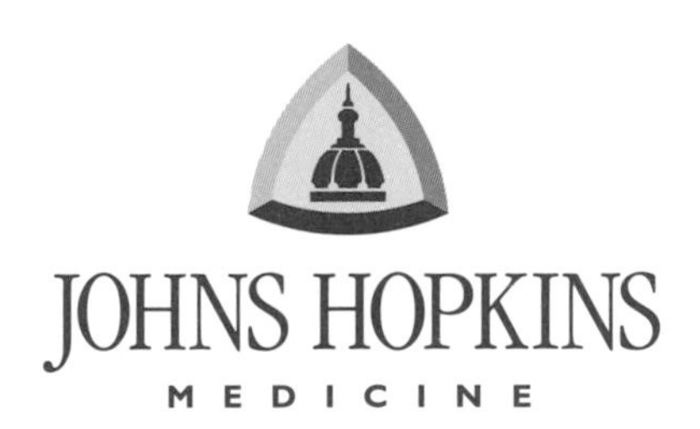

Dear Reader:

Welcome to the 2008 *Diabetes White Paper*—your Johns Hopkins guide to the prevention, diagnosis, and proper care of one of today's most widespread diseases, diabetes.

This year's highlights include:

- **Lab tests** and **exams**: When to go and what numbers to shoot for. (page 11)
- A plan for avoiding problems by getting your blood **glucose** under **tight control**. (page 16)
- How to know if a **continuous glucose monitor** is right for you. (page 22)
- How to feel full on fewer calories: **Weight loss strategies** that work. (page 28)
- The **antidepressant** that may help keep your blood glucose normal. (page 39)
- Making sense of the maze of diabetes **medications** available today. (page 42)
- Knowing when it's **time to start insulin** for type 2 diabetes. (page 46)
- Controlling your blood glucose levels when you have a **cold** or **flu**. (page 58)
- Exercises to **reduce** your **risk of falls**, an under-recognized diabetes complication. (page 66)
- **Foot care tips** to keep your feet happy and healthy. (page 73)
- Research on whether **Reiki** can provide relief from **nerve pain**. (page 75)

You'll also find a new "Ask the Doctor" column on pages 25, 27, 49, 63, and 71. This year's questions came from my patients, but next year we'd like to answer some of yours. If you have any diabetes-related queries you want answered in the White Papers, or comments about the White Papers in general, please e-mail the editors at whitepapers@johnshopkinshealthalerts.com.

Wishing you the best of health in 2008,

Christopher D. Saudek, M.D.
Director, Johns Hopkins Diabetes Center
Professor of Endocrinology and Metabolism, Johns Hopkins University School of Medicine

P. S. Please visit www.HopkinsDiabetes.com for the latest news on diabetes and other information that will complement your Johns Hopkins White Paper.

THE AUTHORS

Christopher D. Saudek, M.D., received his B.A. from Harvard University and his M.D. from Cornell University Medical College. He trained in internal medicine at Chicago's Presbyterian-St. Luke's Hospital and in metabolism at Boston City Hospital and Harvard Medical School. After serving on the faculty at Cornell and winning a Robert Wood Johnson Health Policy Fellowship, Dr. Saudek joined the faculty of the Johns Hopkins University School of Medicine, where he is currently the Hugh P. McCormick Family Professor of Endocrinology and Metabolism, Director of the Johns Hopkins Diabetes Center, and Program Director of the General Clinical Research Center.

A past president of the American Diabetes Association, Dr. Saudek is active in diabetes education and public health policy. His research focuses on the development of an implantable insulin pump, a topic on which he has published widely. He is author of *The Johns Hopkins Guide to Diabetes: For Today and Tomorrow.* In 1991, he was named Outstanding Clinician in Diabetes by the American Diabetes Association.

▪ ▪ ▪

Simeon Margolis, M.D., Ph.D., received his M.D. and Ph.D. from the Johns Hopkins University School of Medicine and performed his internship and residency at Johns Hopkins Hospital. He is currently Professor of Medicine and Biological Chemistry at the Johns Hopkins University School of Medicine and Medical Editor of *The Johns Hopkins Medical Letter: Health After 50.* He has served on various committees for the Department of Health, Education, and Welfare, including the National Diabetes Advisory Board and the Arteriosclerosis Specialized Centers of Research Review Committees. In addition, he has acted as a member of the Endocrinology and Metabolism Panel of the U.S. Food and Drug Administration.

A former weekly columnist for *The Baltimore Sun,* Dr. Margolis lectures to medical students, physicians, and the general public on a wide variety of topics, such as the prevention of coronary heart disease, the control of cholesterol levels, the treatment of diabetes, and the use of alternative medicine.

CONTENTS

DIABETES

Has your doctor told you that you are at risk for diabetes? Americans of all ages, even children, are generally more overweight and less active than previous generations—and this puts them at greater risk for diabetes. Fortunately, several preventive measures can significantly reduce the risk of developing diabetes. In addition, similar measures help people with diabetes keep their disease under control.

The goal of this White Paper is to show you how to prevent diabetes or, if you already have diabetes, how to manage your disease and improve your quality of life. In the following pages, you'll find information on the two main types of diabetes, common risk factors, and the best tests for detecting and monitoring the disease. You'll also read about the latest medications, diet, and exercise regimens that can help prevent diabetes complications.

What Is Diabetes?

Many people think of diabetes as the "sugar disease." But that's only part of the story. Diabetes mellitus, more commonly referred to simply as diabetes, is a chronic disease in which high levels of glucose (sugar) build up in the bloodstream. The term "diabetes" is derived from the Greek word for siphon (a tube bent in two through which liquid flows) and the Latin word "mellitus," which means sweet as honey.

The disease is aptly named: Persistent thirst and frequent passing of urine containing glucose are characteristic symptoms of diabetes. These symptoms result from insufficient production of insulin by the pancreas or resistance of the body's tissues to insulin action—or a combination of both. To understand what this means, you have to know where your body's glucose comes from, what it's used for, and how it is regulated by insulin.

What Is Glucose?

Glucose is a sugar serving as the fuel that provides energy for the body's cells. Your liver produces some glucose and your body gets the rest by digesting sugars, starches, and other foods you eat.

What Is Insulin?

Insulin is a hormone produced by beta cells in a part of the pancreas known as the islets of Langerhans. Insulin controls how much glucose the liver produces and also helps to move glucose from the bloodstream into your cells, where it is needed as a source of energy.

The uptake of glucose into your cells occurs through a complex series of events. It begins when insulin attaches ("binds") to receptor sites on the surface of cells in muscles and other tissues and causes carrier proteins (called glucose transporters) to move from inside the cell to the cell's surface. Like little dump trucks, these transport proteins deliver glucose from outside the cell to the inside. Without the initial binding of insulin to the receptor sites, glucose enters the cells too slowly.

In a healthy person

Normally, the pancreas makes enough insulin to keep the supply and use of glucose in balance. When the blood contains enough insulin, the liver temporarily shuts down its production of glucose, and glucose is transported from the blood into your cells. Cells use some of the glucose immediately. Most of the remainder is converted to a substance called glycogen in the liver and muscles, where it is stored for future use. The body's ability to store glycogen is limited, and any excess glucose that does not get stored as glycogen is converted to triglycerides and stored in adipose (fat) tissue.

Pancreatic cells in the islets of Langerhans continuously monitor blood glucose levels. After a meal, the carbohydrates you eat are digested and broken down into glucose and other sugars, which pass into the bloodstream. As your blood glucose levels rise, beta cells in the pancreas respond by secreting insulin into the blood. Glucose then passes into your cells and the liver shuts down glucose production. Between meals, insulin also prevents excessive release of glucose from the liver into the bloodstream. If blood glucose levels drop too low between meals, alpha cells in the pancreas release a hormone called glucagon. This hormone signals the liver to convert amino acids and glycogen into glucose that is sent into the blood.

When someone has diabetes

In diabetes, this glucose balancing system is disrupted, either because too little insulin is produced or because the body's cells do not respond to insulin normally (a condition called insulin resistance). The result is an unhealthy rise in blood glucose levels. If diabetes is left untreated, the two principal dangers are the immediate results of

How the Pancreas Regulates Blood Glucose

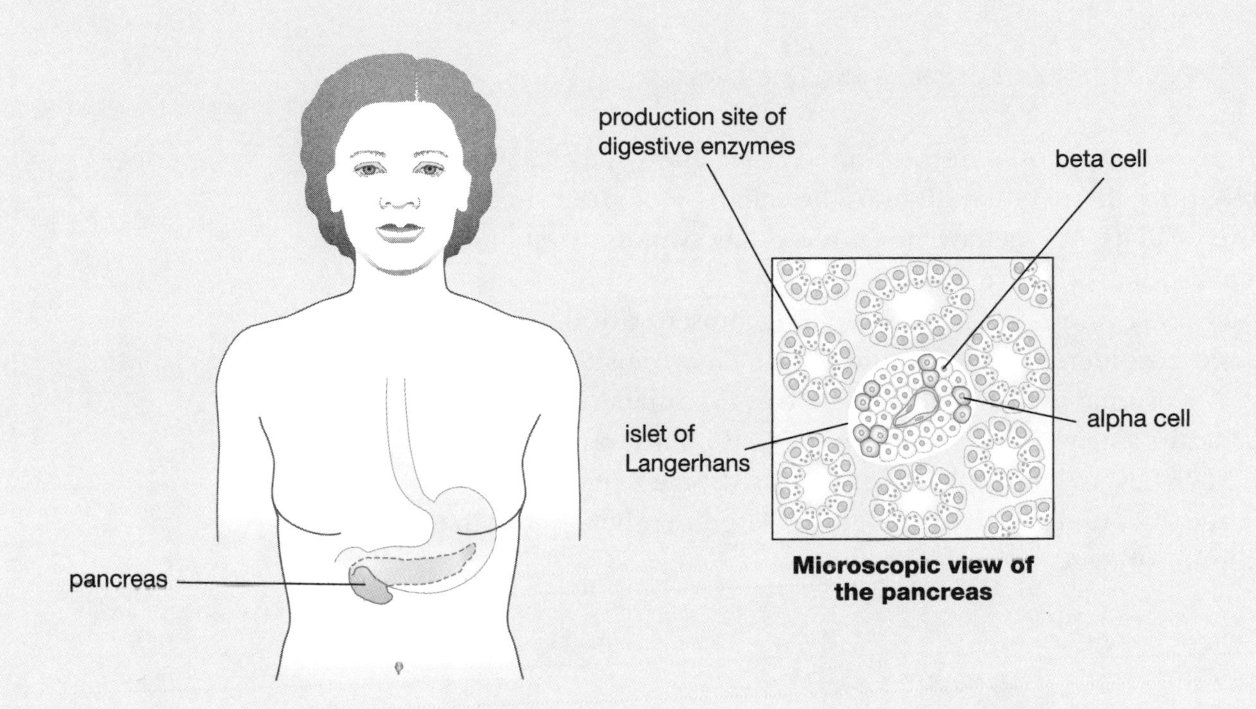

Microscopic view of the pancreas

The pancreas is an organ that stretches partway across the abdomen, just below the stomach. Because its main functions are to aid digestion and produce hormones that control blood glucose levels, the pancreas is a focal point for understanding diabetes.

In addition to secreting certain enzymes that help you properly digest food, the pancreas manufactures hormones that regulate blood glucose—the fuel that provides the body's cells with energy. Scattered throughout the pancreas are tiny nests of cells known as islets of Langerhans; the majority of the cells are beta cells that produce and store the hormone insulin until needed. Also located in the islets are alpha cells, which make and store glucagon, a hormone that counteracts the effects of insulin.

After a meal, carbohydrates in foods are converted into glucose in the intestine and liver and enter the bloodstream. Beta cells sense the rising blood glucose levels and secrete insulin into the blood. Once in the bloodstream, insulin helps glucose enter the body's cells, where it can be "burned" by the liver and muscles for energy. Liver and muscles can also convert glucose to glycogen, a type of reserve form of energy that is stored there for future needs. When the body is working as it should, blood glucose levels quickly return to normal, and insulin secretion decreases.

A drop in blood glucose levels—for example, when one hasn't eaten for several hours—stimulates an opposite effect: alpha cells secrete glucagon into the blood, which converts stored glycogen back into energy-producing glucose.

Normally, the secretion of these hormones by the pancreas is perfectly balanced: Beta and alpha cells continuously monitor blood glucose levels and release insulin or glucagon as needed. In diabetes, this balance is thrown off because beta cells produce little or no insulin or the body's cells are resistant to insulin action—or often both. Glucose then fails to enter cells effectively and the fuel for energy remains stuck in the bloodstream. The result is persistently high blood glucose levels (hyperglycemia). Without treatment, hyperglycemia can lead to serious long-term complications, such as eye, kidney, and heart disease and damage to nerves. ■

high blood glucose levels (which include excessive urination, dehydration, intense thirst, and fatigue) and long-term complications that can affect your eyes, nerves, kidneys, and large blood vessels.

Prevalence of Diabetes

About 21 million people in the United States have diabetes. Unfortunately, only about 14.6 million of them have been diagnosed with the disease. The others have not noticed any symptoms yet and do not realize that they have diabetes.

Since 1997, the number of people diagnosed with diabetes has increased considerably, rising from 5% of Americans to almost 7% today. An estimated 1.5 million new cases of diabetes in people age 20 and older were diagnosed in 2005, the most recent year for which statistics are available. In the United States, nearly 10% of adults age 20 and older have diabetes. A large number—more than 10 million—are age 60 or older.

Types of Diabetes

There are several kinds of diabetes, but the two most common are:

- **Type 1** diabetes, which usually develops before age 30 and tends to come on suddenly
- **Type 2** diabetes, which accounts for 90–95% of diabetes cases and usually starts later in life.

Type 1 Diabetes

In this type (formerly called insulin-dependent diabetes), the body's immune system attacks and destroys beta cells in the pancreas so it can no longer produce sufficient amounts of insulin. Type 1 diabetes is sometimes called juvenile-onset diabetes because it most often starts in childhood. It can develop in adults, but this is far less common.

Type 1 diabetes is a serious condition that cannot be treated simply by losing weight or watching what you eat. People with type 1 disease must take insulin injections several times a day to prevent blood glucose from rising to life-threatening levels.

Type 2 Diabetes

In this type (formerly called adult-onset diabetes), beta cells still produce insulin, but the quantity may be reduced or the body's cells may be insulin resistant. Most people with type 2 diabetes are obese. This type of diabetes develops gradually and is usually diagnosed in adulthood. However, more and more children are being diagnosed with the disease as the frequency of childhood obesity rises.

Type 2 diabetes can often be controlled without insulin treatment through exercise, a proper diet, weight loss, and oral medications. That's why type 2 diabetes has also been called non-insulin-dependent diabetes.

Causes of Diabetes

When our bodies are humming along smoothly, we rarely think about all the complex processes that are going on. But when we don't feel well and we're unable to perform our usual activities, we want to know what's causing the problem and how it can be fixed.

Type 1 Diabetes

Type 1 diabetes is an autoimmune disease. Something triggers the body to mount an immune system attack against itself, in the same way the immune system normally attacks harmful bacteria and viruses. In type 1 diabetes, the immune system produces antibodies that attack and destroy the insulin-secreting beta cells in the pancreas. As the number of beta cells decreases, the amount of insulin that is produced decreases as well. Since the pancreas can't make new beta cells, eventually only a small number of beta cells remain and little or no insulin is produced.

Fortunately, the immune system attack doesn't affect the body's ability to respond to insulin. That's why people with type 1 diabetes can compensate for the lack of insulin production by taking insulin injections.

Type 2 Diabetes

Type 2 diabetes is caused by a combination of insulin resistance (reduced sensitivity of the body's tissues, primarily the liver and muscles, to the action of insulin) and inadequate amounts of insulin. If you have insulin resistance, your pancreas must increase its production of insulin, because your body needs more insulin to accomplish the job of moving glucose into your cells. For example, the pancreas of a healthy person might produce 30 units of insulin a day. If that person develops insulin resistance, more insulin is required, because those same 30 units will no longer be sufficient to clear glucose from the bloodstream. Eventually, the pancreas can no longer keep up with the increasing demand for extra insulin, and glucose accumulates in the bloodstream. At that point, the person has type 2 diabetes.

Obesity is the major contributing factor to insulin resistance and type 2 diabetes. That's why obese people who have early signs of type 2 diabetes are told by their doctors to make dietary changes, lose weight, and exercise. If these lifestyle measures are not sufficient to control their blood glucose, the next step is oral diabetes medications. About 40% of people with type 2 diabetes eventually need insulin injections to keep their blood glucose at a safe level.

Risk Factors for Diabetes

Now that you know the causes of type 1 and type 2 diabetes, it is even more important to understand what makes them occur.

Type 1 Diabetes

Research scientists are still trying to identify the risk factors that lead to type 1 diabetes. Here are two possibilities.

Viral infection

Several studies suggest that type 1 diabetes may be triggered by a particular kind of viral infection that occurs during childhood or early adulthood or during a mother's pregnancy. Scientists think the virus may trigger changes in the child's immune system, perhaps by creating antibodies that are capable of attacking beta cells. When a similar viral infection occurs later in the child's life, it may reactivate these antibodies so they begin to destroy beta cells.

Heredity

Your family history plays a small role. If one of your parents or grandparents has type 1 diabetes—especially your father or grandfather—your risk of developing the disease is increased but only slightly. Most people with type 1 diabetes, however, have no family history of the disease. Yet research suggests that some genetic susceptibility to type 1 diabetes must be present for the disease to occur.

Type 2 Diabetes

Unlike the situation for type 1 diabetes, researchers have identified many risk factors for type 2 diabetes.

Heredity

Family history plays an important role in type 2 diabetes. In a study of more than 200 adults with type 2 diabetes, about two thirds reported at least one close relative with diabetes and nearly 50% had at least two relatives with the disease. In particular, people whose mother had diabetes were twice as likely to get the disease as those whose father had diabetes—33% vs. 17%. Eleven percent of the women with type 2 diabetes had at least one child with diabetes, whereas only 4% of the men with type 2 diabetes had a child with the disorder.

Genes

In a very fast-moving field of research, investigators have discovered changes in at least 10 genes that can raise the risk of diabetes. All told, these known genetic variations may account for a roughly 2–20% greater overall chance for developing the disease. Researchers hope that by knowing who is at risk for diabetes, they can target ways to prevent or delay it. So far, however, there is no reliable test to tell if these genetic variations will substantially up your chances of suffering from diabetes down the road.

Race and ethnicity

Race and ethnic background affect diabetes risk. For example, blacks, Hispanics, Asians, and Native Americans have a greater risk than whites of developing type 2 diabetes, although scientists aren't sure why this is so.

Obesity

Being overweight is the major contributing factor for type 2 diabetes. About 80% of individuals with type 2 diabetes are overweight or obese, and the risk of type 2 diabetes rises as a person's weight increases. Research suggests that having more fat cells somehow makes cells throughout the body more resistant to insulin.

Location of excess fat

Where your fat is located also makes a difference. People with abdominal obesity (excess fat within the abdomen) are more likely to develop type 2 diabetes than are those with extra weight in the hips and thighs. In fact, recent studies suggest that your waistline measurement is a better predictor of diabetes risk than your body weight.

NEW RESEARCH

Diabetes Risk Tied to Midlife Weight

For women, being overweight or obese in your late 40s is a greater risk factor for diabetes than quick weight changes later in life, suggests a new study.

The findings are based on data from the Australian Longitudinal Study on Women's Health, in which 7,239 women ages 45–50 at the study's outset filled out four separate questionnaires on their health and weight over a period of eight years.

The researchers found that a woman's body mass index (BMI) at the beginning of the study was strongly linked to developing diabetes within five to eight years. Indeed, very obese women with a BMI of 35 or above had a 12 times greater risk for developing diabetes than normal-weight participants. Weight gained during the course of the study, however, was not associated with the diagnosis of the disease.

Of course, any weight gain should be taken seriously and could potentially increase your chances of developing diabetes. But the importance of countering obesity at the earliest possible age should inspire people to make the small, necessary lifestyle changes.

DIABETES CARE
Volume 30, page 1418
June 2007

The metabolic syndrome

Scientists have found that abdominal obesity is often accompanied by insulin resistance, increased blood glucose levels, high blood pressure (hypertension), low levels of high-density lipoprotein (HDL) cholesterol (the "good" cholesterol), and elevated triglycerides (another fat found in the bloodstream). This cluster of abnormalities, known as the metabolic syndrome, is an important risk factor not only for diabetes but also for heart disease and stroke.

Doctors are starting to pay more attention to the metabolic syndrome because its presence often suggests that diabetes is starting to develop. If you have a large waist circumference and unhealthy HDL and triglyceride levels, your doctor may order a test of your blood glucose levels after you have fasted for at least eight hours.

Prediabetes

Anyone with a fasting blood glucose reading of 100–125 mg/dL has prediabetes—blood glucose levels higher than normal but not high enough for a diagnosis of diabetes. About 54 million Americans have prediabetes. Without lifestyle changes or medication, many of them will develop type 2 diabetes within 10 years.

Physical inactivity

A sedentary lifestyle also is a risk factor for type 2 diabetes. Physical activity uses glucose, and thus less glucose accumulates in the bloodstream. Exercise also builds muscles, and muscle cells take up and use large amounts of glucose. If you get little exercise, however, you will have less muscle tissue, you will use less glucose, and blood levels of glucose will increase.

Aging

Getting older is another diabetes risk factor. Age alone does not seem to be the problem. Instead, it is what you're doing and what you're eating, particularly after age 45, that makes the difference. As people get older, they often exercise less, eat more foods that are high in fats and carbohydrates, and gain weight (especially around the middle).

Pregnancy

Some women develop type 2 diabetes during pregnancy (a condition called gestational diabetes). Although the diabetes goes away after childbirth, studies show that these women have an increased risk of developing diabetes later in life.

Other health problems

A small number of people are at risk for diabetes because they have diseases that destroy the pancreas, such as hemochromatosis (excessive absorption and storage of iron), chronic pancreatitis (inflammation of the pancreas), or pancreatic cancer. Certain tumors increase the risk of diabetes because they result in the overproduction of hormones that interfere with insulin action. For example, growth hormone produced by tumors of the pituitary gland, cortisol or epinephrine from adrenal tumors, and glucagon from pancreatic tumors can all raise blood glucose levels.

Medications

Certain medications increase the risk of type 2 diabetes in people who are predisposed to the disease. Examples are corticosteroids (commonly used to treat asthma and arthritis) and thiazide diuretics (typically used in the treatment of high blood pressure and heart failure).

Prevention of Diabetes

If one or more people in your family have type 1 or type 2 diabetes, you're probably concerned about developing the disease yourself and are likely interested in taking measures to reduce your risk. Although there is no way to prevent type 1 diabetes, there are several proven steps you can take to reduce your risk of type 2 disease.

Type 1 Diabetes

The fact that researchers have not found a way to prevent type 1 diabetes is not for lack of trying. They've tested everything from low-dose insulin injections and drugs that suppress the immune system to vitamin supplements and lifestyle measures. In general, these approaches have not been found helpful, but a few lifestyle measures have shown a glimmer of promise.

For example, studies suggest that vitamin D deficiency may be a risk factor for type 1 diabetes. If you have a family history of type 1 and you don't get enough vitamin D in your diet, you may want to take vitamin D supplements. Sensible sun exposure (five to 10 minutes of exposure on the arms and legs, or the hands, arms, and face, two to three times per week) is also recommended as a safe way to increase vitamin D levels without increasing your risk of skin cancer.

NEW RESEARCH

Excess Weight a Bigger Risk Factor Than Lack of Exercise

Being overweight and not getting enough exercise can both raise your risk for type 2 diabetes, but a new study suggests that shedding pounds may be more important for preventing the disease.

Researchers followed close to 69,000 participants in the ongoing Harvard Nurses' Health Study. None of the women had a history of diabetes, cardiovascular disease, or cancer when the study began. Sixteen years later, 4,030 women had been diagnosed with diabetes.

After adjusting for age, smoking, and other diabetes risk factors, increased waist size and body mass index (BMI) had a substantial impact on developing the disease. Women who were considered very obese—with a body mass index (BMI) of 40, for example—had a 28 times higher risk of diabetes than normal or underweight women whose BMI was below 21. A lack of physical activity was not as big a factor. Even in those who exercised at least 20 hours a week, the risk of diabetes was 11 times greater in obese participants than in lean ones.

These findings don't mean you should scale back on physical activity, which often goes hand and hand with losing weight. But since exercise may not always be enough to help you drop the pounds, watching what you eat should be an equally important goal.

DIABETES CARE
Volume 30, page 53
January 2007

As you'll read below, eating less and exercising more can help keep weight under control and thus prevent type 2 diabetes. This same lifestyle approach may help delay the onset of type 1 diabetes. Research shows that type 1 diabetes occurs an average of one to two years earlier in overweight children than normal-weight children, suggesting that the insulin resistance that leads to type 2 diabetes may also accelerate the onset of type 1 disease.

Researchers are also working on ways to halt the loss of insulin-producing beta cells after the onset of type 1 diabetes. One approach under investigation is "blocking antibodies," which are being given intravenously in the hopes of heading off the autoimmune response to save any remaining beta cells.

Type 2 Diabetes

Diet and exercise are the cornerstones for preventing type 2 diabetes. These measures are especially important for people with risk factors for the disease, such as prediabetes, obesity, a family history of diabetes, diabetes during pregnancy (gestational diabetes), or an ethnic background (black, Hispanic, Asian, or Native American) that puts them at higher risk. Quitting smoking may be helpful, too.

Diet and exercise

Research studies from around the globe all show that modest weight loss and regular physical activity can help to prevent type 2 diabetes. The largest and best known of these studies is the Diabetes Prevention Program, which was done in the United States. Study participants who followed a low-calorie, low-fat diet, exercised 30 minutes a day, and lost an average of 15 lbs were almost 60% less likely to develop type 2 diabetes over a three-year period than people who did not make these lifestyle changes.

A high-fiber diet also may decrease the risk of developing type 2 diabetes. In a study of nearly 36,000 women, those who consumed the most fiber from cereal had a 36% lower risk of developing type 2 diabetes than those consuming the least fiber from cereal. A more recent study from Finland reported similar results in men. Fiber, commonly found in whole grains such as brown rice or wheat bread, may improve the body's sensitivity to insulin.

A Harvard study, involving 84,000 female nurses, found that women who supplemented their diets with at least 1,200 mg of calcium and 800 IU of vitamin D lowered their risk of type 2 diabetes by a third.

Lab Tests and Physical Exams for Diabetes Control

When to go and what your goals should be

To prevent or delay the development of complications from type 1 or type 2 diabetes, you need to take a proactive role in the management of your health care. This includes making regular visits to your primary care physician and other professionals on your healthcare team. How frequently you see each member of your team varies, but, in general, individuals with diabetes should have a comprehensive physical once a year and have their diabetes assessed at least every six months.

During these visits, you may undergo tests and exams that indicate how well you are maintaining your health and if any complications of diabetes are emerging or progressing. Individuals with diabetes should know about the tests and exams their doctors perform, the goal for each test and exam, and how often each is typically done.

Physical Exams	Desirable Result	Frequency
Blood pressure	≤130/80 mm Hg	Every visit
Foot inspection	No ulcers, skin abnormalities, joint problems, or loss of sensation	Every visit: Visual inspection Yearly: Assessment of pulses and sensation
Eye exam	—	Yearly
Dental exam	—	Yearly

Laboratory Tests	Desirable Result	Frequency
HbA1c	<7%	Every three to six months
Fasting blood glucose	90–130 mg/dL	Every visit
Fasting blood lipids:		Yearly, or more often if goals are not met
Low-density lipoprotein (LDL) cholesterol	<100 mg/dL	
High-density lipoprotein (HDL) cholesterol	Men: >45 mg/dL Women: >55 mg/dL	
Triglycerides	<150 mg/dL	
Urine microalbumin test (random, spot collection)	<30 mcg albumin/mg creatinine	Yearly

Quit smoking

Quitting smoking may reduce the risk of type 2 diabetes, too. A study of more than 21,000 U.S. male physicians found that those who smoked 20 or more cigarettes a day were 70% more likely to develop diabetes than those who had never smoked or were former smokers.

Medication

Several studies show that oral medications used to treat type 2 diabetes can also help prevent the disease. For example, participants in the Diabetes Prevention Program who took the diabetes drug metformin (Glucophage) reduced their risk of type 2 diabetes by about 30% over a three-year period, compared with people who received a placebo. Metformin was as effective as lifestyle measures for only a small percentage of people: those ages 24–44 and those who were obese (50–80 lbs overweight). The drug was just slightly effective in people age 60 and older and in those who were less overweight. Based on these findings, the American Diabetes Association does not recommend the use of oral diabetes drugs as a substitute for, or in addition to, lifestyle modifications like diet and exercise to prevent diabetes.

In another study, the Heart Outcomes Prevention Evaluation (HOPE), people taking the ACE inhibitor ramipril (Altace) were 30% less likely to develop diabetes than those taking a placebo. However, more research is needed before ACE inhibitors can be recommended for preventing diabetes.

Symptoms of Diabetes

The most common early symptoms of diabetes are increased thirst and frequent urination. These initial symptoms are usually related to hyperglycemia, the medical term for high blood glucose levels.

Type 1 Diabetes

The initial symptoms of type 1 diabetes often occur suddenly and are very serious. As insulin production decreases, glucose accumulates in the bloodstream instead of being transported into the body's cells, which need it for energy. To generate this missing energy, the body breaks down fat tissue and releases fatty acids. These fatty acids are then metabolized into toxic chemicals called ketones, which increase the blood's acidity to dangerous levels (a state called ketoacidosis).

The initial symptoms of diabetic ketoacidosis include excessive thirst and urination, dehydration, weight loss, nausea, vomiting, fatigue, dry or flushed skin, rapid breathing, abdominal pain, and mental confusion. One sure sign is breath that smells like fruit or nail polish remover. Diabetic ketoacidosis is a medical emergency that requires immediate hospitalization. If you or a loved one develops any of the symptoms of ketoacidosis, call your doctor or an ambulance immediately. Death can occur, but the vast majority of people recover with aggressive administration of insulin and fluids.

Type 2 Diabetes

Type 2 diabetes develops gradually over many years and the initial symptoms may be almost unnoticeable. In fact, many people find out that they have type 2 diabetes when a routine laboratory test shows high blood glucose levels.

As glucose levels continue to increase, most people develop the classic initial symptoms of increased frequency of urination, increased thirst and fluid intake, and, in later stages, weight loss despite increased hunger and food intake. Fortunately, these symptoms go away once blood glucose levels are brought under control. Other common symptoms of type 2 diabetes include blurred vision (due to changing levels of glucose in the eye), weakness and fatigue, recurrent vaginal yeast infections, and infections of the skin and gums. These symptoms are temporary, do not indicate any permanent damage, and can be eliminated by controlling blood glucose levels.

In some people, complications of diabetes such as peripheral neuropathy (nerve damage in the hands or feet) or coronary heart disease are the first indication of diabetes. These complications can be controlled but cannot be cured once they develop.

Another possible initial symptom of diabetes is hyperosmolar nonketotic syndrome. It occurs when the stress of an injury or major illness, such as a stroke, heart attack, or severe infection, causes extremely high blood glucose levels (above 1,000 mg/dL). Although insulin levels are adequate to avert excessive ketone production (as occurs in ketoacidosis), the insulin levels are not high enough to prevent high blood glucose and hyperosmolarity, a condition in which the blood has high concentrations of sodium, glucose, and other molecules that draw water from cells into the bloodstream.

Symptoms of hyperosmolar nonketotic syndrome include a dry, parched mouth; increased hunger; nausea or vomiting; and warm, dry skin. Severe dehydration worsens the problem, causing lethargy, confusion, and even loss of consciousness. In extreme cases, the result is a coma. Immediate treatment with insulin and large amounts of fluids is vital to prevent death. If you or a loved one develops any of these symptoms, call your doctor or an ambulance immediately.

Diagnosis and Office Follow-Up of Diabetes

If you have any of the common symptoms that suggest the presence of diabetes, your doctor will order laboratory tests to confirm the diagnosis. Regular screening tests to measure blood glucose levels are recommended for certain people who have no symptoms of diabetes.

To promote the early detection of diabetes and reduce the risk of long-term diabetes complications, the American Diabetes Association recommends that individuals age 45 and older be screened for the disease every three years. Screening is also recommended for individuals under age 45 who have an increased risk of diabetes because of obesity, high blood pressure (140/90 mm Hg or higher), or ethnicity (black, Hispanic, Asian, or Native American). Other examples of risk factors that merit early or more frequent screening (for example, every one to two years) include a history of diabetes in a first-degree relative (a parent or sibling), diagnosis of diabetes during pregnancy (called gestational diabetes), delivery of a baby weighing more than 9 lbs, low levels of HDL cholesterol (less than 40 mg/dL), high triglyceride levels (150 mg/dL or higher), or prediabetes. If screening tests show that you have diabetes, your physician will perform regular laboratory tests and physical examinations to monitor the progression of the disease.

Laboratory Tests

Three blood tests are available to diagnose prediabetes and diabetes:

- Casual plasma (blood) glucose
- Fasting plasma glucose (FPG)
- Oral glucose tolerance test.

To make a diagnosis, the results of each test must be confirmed by repeat testing on a different day, unless you have obvious symptoms of elevated blood glucose (hyperglycemia). If diabetes is diagnosed, you'll need periodic hemoglobin A1c (HbA1c) tests to monitor your blood glucose control.

Casual plasma (blood) glucose test

This test measures blood glucose levels at any time of day, no matter when you had your last meal. It is most often used in people who have classic diabetes symptoms such as excessive thirst, frequent urination, and unexplained weight loss. The criteria for a diagnosis of diabetes with this test is the presence of diabetes symptoms and a blood glucose level of 200 mg/dL or higher.

Fasting plasma glucose (FPG) test

The fasting plasma glucose test is the preferred method for diagnosing diabetes in children, men, and nonpregnant women. The test measures blood glucose levels after an overnight fast (no food intake for at least eight hours). A diagnosis of diabetes is made when the fasting blood glucose level is 126 mg/dL or higher on at least two tests. Values of 100–125 mg/dL indicate prediabetes. A normal fasting blood glucose level is less than 100 mg/dL.

Oral glucose tolerance test

This test is done when diabetes is suspected, but you have normal results on a fasting plasma glucose test. For the test, you'll have to fast overnight and then drink a very sweet solution containing 75 g of glucose. A sample of your blood will be drawn two hours later. Normal glucose levels are less than 140 mg/dL at two hours. The criterion for a diagnosis of diabetes with this test is a two-hour blood glucose level of 200 mg/dL or higher. Prediabetes is diagnosed if the two-hour blood glucose level is 140–199 mg/dL.

Hemoglobin A1c test

The HbA1c test measures the amount of glucose attached to hemoglobin—the oxygen-carrying protein in red blood cells that gives blood its color. The HbA1c test is used in people already diagnosed with diabetes and is not recommended for diagnosing diabetes. As blood glucose levels rise, so does the amount of glucose attached to hemoglobin. Since hemoglobin circulates in the blood until the red blood cells die (half of red blood cells are replaced every 120 days), the HbA1c test measures average blood glucose levels over the previous two to three months.

The American Diabetes Association recommends keeping your HbA1c levels at less than 7%, which is equivalent to an average blood glucose level of about 170 mg/dL or less. Your doctor may give you a different level to aim for, depending on your age, weight, and other factors. HbA1c tests are usually performed every three

NEW RESEARCH

Short-Term Stress Doesn't Affect Glucose Control

While chronic stress has been associated with high blood sugar levels and poor treatment adherence among those with diabetes, Swiss researchers have found that a short-lived stressful event such as a roller-coaster ride does not cause similar ups and downs in blood glucose in people with type 1 diabetes.

The team followed 20 thrill seekers with type 1 diabetes on intensified insulin treatment who took two separate roller-coaster rides within 15 minutes. In addition to strapping on seat belts, the volunteers wore continuous glucose monitors.

The researchers documented that the rides produced a typical stressful reaction, as the physiological markers of stress—blood pressure, heart rate, and levels of the stress hormone cortisol—all shot up afterwards. However, this stress barely affected glucose control.

The researchers caution that their study focused only on people with diabetes who already had good glucose control and cannot necessarily be applied to those with more elevated glucose levels who encounter short-term stress or for those with diabetes who endure more chronic forms of tension or anxiety. But this unique trial does suggest that individuals with type 1 diabetes who undergo a stressful experience can maintain good glycemic control without adjusting their insulin dose.

DIABETES CARE
Volume 30, page 1599
June 2007

Getting and Staying In Control

How to keep blood glucose at normal levels and avoid problems

Keeping a tight lid on your blood glucose level is a good way to remain healthy if you have diabetes. The evidence is clear: Those who maintain their glucose within a range of 90–130 mg/dL before meals—while allowing it to spike to no more than 180 mg/dL 90 minutes after eating—can protect against a wide range of diabetes complications, including damage to the eyes, nerves, and kidneys, and cut the risk of heart attacks and strokes.

The Challenge

Still, the task is not easy for many people. Keeping your blood glucose under tight control requires monitoring glucose, following a healthy lifestyle, and often, taking medication. Those with type 1 diabetes may need as many as four separate insulin injections a day. Most people with type 2 diabetes take daily pills, and four in 10 require at least one insulin shot a day. Over time, plenty of trips to the doctor are needed to control your glucose as well as two major risks for cardiovascular disease: low-density lipoprotein (LDL) cholesterol and blood pressure.

Moreover, keeping blood glucose in check has its own risks: Tight control can cause a dangerous drop in your glucose levels known as hypoglycemia, which needs to be recognized and treated quickly. However, the benefits of controlling your blood glucose and averting possible diabetes-related complications far outweigh the danger of hypoglycemia.

The bottom line: Better blood glucose control with the right management strategy can significantly cut your risk of diabetes complications.

The Benefits

The most important motivation for sticking with a strategy for tight control is to realize how much it can help. The Diabetes Control and Complications Trial (DCCT) randomly assigned 1,400 people with type 1 diabetes to either intensive or conventional therapy for 6.5 years. Intensive therapy consisted of three or more daily injections of insulin or treatment with an insulin pump, along with adjusting doses based on at least four self-monitored glucose readings each day; the target glucose range was 70–120 mg/dL before meals and 180 mg/dL after meals. In comparison, conventional therapy consisted of only one or two daily insulin injections, with no glucose goals beyond those needed to prevent symptoms of high or low blood glucose.

Compared with conventional treatment, intensive therapy significantly reduced the progression of retinopathy by 76%, clinical neuropathy by 60%, and kidney disease by 50%. After taking part in the study, the volunteers were allowed to choose whatever care they wished. The vast majority in the intensive therapy group decided to stick with it, while 94% of the conventional-treatment group also attempted tighter blood glucose control.

The Diabetes Control and Complications Trial/Epidemiology of Diabetes Interventions and Complications (DCCT/EDIC) Study Research Group then followed 93% of these subjects for an additional 11 years. Those who had been on intensive therapy during the original 6.5 years of the study reduced the risk of any cardiovascular disease event by 42% and the risk of nonfatal heart attacks, stroke, and deaths from cardiovascular disease by 57%.

Researchers have found that people with type 2 diabetes also benefit from tight glycemic control; in the United Kingdom Prospective Diabetes Study (UKPDS), intensive therapy with insulin, a sulfonylurea, or metformin reduced the risk of complications like retinopathy and neuropathy by 25%.

The Plan

The most effective strategy for glucose control involves the following basic steps.

- **Take medicine if needed.** For a few people with type 2 diabetes, diet and exercise may be enough to control blood glucose levels. However, most also need oral medications (which also work better with improved diet and exercise). Although taking insulin has usually been considered as a last resort, new studies indicate that starting such therapy early provides better glucose control in type 2 disease. Daily insulin shots are required by everyone with type 1 diabetes. People with both types of diabetes may need more or less insulin during the day, depending on what they eat and how much they exercise.

• **Test, test again.** If you have type 1 diabetes, you should test blood glucose levels often and at key points during the day, such as before meals, right before going to sleep, and immediately before and after you exercise. Many people with type 2 diabetes may only need to test glucose once a day or even less often. Testing around bedtime is particularly important if you take insulin because you might not recognize the symptoms of hypoglycemia, which may occur when the medication lowers blood glucose too much and can become severe if left untreated overnight. If your glucose is too low at night, eat a small snack before going to bed.

Your doctor should periodically test your hemoglobin A1c (HbA1c), which measures your average blood glucose levels over two to three months. Using both the HbA1c test and home monitoring is the best way to keep tabs on how well you are controlling your glucose.

• **Ensure accurate readings.** With a prescription, dozens of different types of self-monitoring glucose devices can be bought at your local pharmacy. These require a drop of blood from a simple prick to get a reading, which is either displayed on a meter or read aloud by a computer. Regardless of the device you choose, make sure you know how to use it properly. At-home tests are not as precise as the ones your doctor uses, so keep these tips in mind to avoid errors:

- Regularly calibrate your meter based on the instructions provided in the manual, and perform quality-control checks every couple of months.
- Clean your hands. Having food on your fingers can affect the results.
- Clean your meter even if it doesn't look dirty, and check the time and date functions. Sometimes changing the time can alter the readings.
- Keep the test strips in a cool, dark place. Light and humidity can affect their accuracy.

• **Eat a healthy diet.** People with diabetes should follow a diet that not only helps to control blood glucose, but also reduces blood pressure and cholesterol levels. To help achieve this goal, limit your total dietary fat to 25–35% of your caloric intake and saturated fat to less than 7% of calories. Also keep sodium consumption to no more than 2,300 mg a day (equivalent to slightly more than 1 tsp), and try to eat at least 3 oz of whole grains, 2 cups of fruit, and 3 cups of vegetables each day.

You can eat sweets in moderation, but not at the expense of other carbohydrates. The American Diabetes Association recommends getting nearly half to two thirds of your calories from carbohydrates because they are a valuable source of vitamins, minerals, and fiber. Clearly some carbohydrate-dense foods are healthier than others. Choose whole-grain breads over white bread, and snack on fruits, vegetables, whole-grain crackers, or low-fat popcorn. And, as always, make sure that you watch the amount of calories you eat. Being overweight makes it harder to control your blood glucose levels.

• **Exercise regularly.** Exercise improves both your glucose levels and the amount of high-density lipoprotein (HDL, or "good") cholesterol, while also helping you to maintain a healthy weight. Strive to exercise 30–60 minutes a day. The physical activity doesn't have to be strenuous or completed all at once. Working in the yard or around the home is good exercise, as long as such activities are performed at a level of intensity similar to a brisk walk. You may reduce your insulin dose or consume extra carbohydrates before your workout, depending on the intensity and duration of activities. Both insulin and certain oral drugs can lower your blood glucose, which might possibly affect your balance when exercising. ■

months to see if you are maintaining your blood glucose within the target range. If you have stable blood glucose levels and are meeting your treatment goals, you may need less frequent HbA1c testing.

Other laboratory tests

In addition to measures of blood glucose and HbA1c, initial and subsequent doctor visits may include tests to check for kidney damage, a common complication of diabetes. These tests include blood urea nitrogen (BUN), blood creatinine, and protein (albumin) in the urine. The risk of coronary heart disease is increased in people with diabetes, so you'll also need blood tests to measure levels of triglycerides, total cholesterol, low-density lipoprotein (LDL) cholesterol, and high-density lipoprotein (HDL) cholesterol.

Medical History and Physical Examination

If you are diagnosed with prediabetes or diabetes, your doctor will pay extra attention to factors in your medical history and physical examination that could affect your diabetes care.

In taking your medical history, the doctor will ask about the date and circumstances of your diabetes diagnosis, your dietary and exercise habits, your weight history, any medications you are taking, your alcohol and tobacco use, and your family history of diabetes, heart disease, and stroke. If you use oral diabetes drugs or insulin, the doctor will record when you take these medications and how much, the effectiveness of blood glucose control (based on symptoms of high blood glucose and blood glucose values), the frequency and timing of symptoms of hypoglycemia (low blood glucose) or ketoacidosis, and any symptoms of long-term diabetes complications.

Your physical examination should include measurements of your weight and blood pressure and a foot inspection to look for common diabetes-related problems such as ulcers and other skin abnormalities, joint problems, and loss of sensation. Because diabetes can affect your vision, you should have a dilated eye examination performed by an ophthalmologist (a medical doctor who specializes in diseases of the eye).

Treatment of Diabetes

Learning that you have an incurable, chronic disease like diabetes is understandably upsetting. On the positive side, diabetes is very treatable. What's more, as soon as you start telling people you have diabetes, you'll be surprised to discover how many people you know have it, too, and they are leading normal, productive lives. There's also a tremendous amount of new research on diabetes, and this means you'll continue to see new treatments in the years ahead.

The Goals of Treatment

The goals of treating diabetes are keeping your blood glucose under control and preventing the development of long-term complications. How you'll try to achieve these goals depends on your age, weight, current diet and exercise habits, work schedule, prior health problems, and whether you have type 1 or type 2 diabetes. You'll need a personalized treatment plan that takes all of these factors into consideration, and you'll need the patience and determination to follow through with that plan every day. For most people with diabetes, this means carefully monitoring blood glucose levels, limiting certain foods, losing weight, exercising, and taking oral or injected medication.

The Diabetes Health Care Team

Your primary care physician can probably handle the varied aspects of your diabetes treatment plan—but that doesn't mean he or she should assume that responsibility. Because even basic health care is more complicated in people with diabetes, it's better to be treated by a team of professionals who have specialized knowledge about various aspects of the disease.

Your ideal team captain is a board-certified endocrinologist—a physician with special training and expertise in managing conditions caused by abnormal hormone secretions (remember that insulin is a hormone). Some endocrinologists specialize in treating diabetes—they're called diabetologists. Your primary care physician or your local hospital can provide names of board-certified endocrinologists and diabetologists in your area.

Other people on your diabetes health care team may include:

- Your primary care physician
- A pharmacist
- A diabetes nurse educator, a registered nurse who specializes in providing instruction and advice on the day-to-day management of diabetes
- A registered dietitian to help you plan meals
- An exercise physiologist to give advice on an exercise program
- Mental health professionals to help you deal with the emotional stress of living with diabetes

- An ophthalmologist to monitor eye changes that could signal retinopathy (eye damage)
- A podiatrist to check your feet and lower legs for cuts and sores, which often fail to heal and can lead to amputations in people with diabetes.

Some of these health professionals will have the initials C.D.E. after their names, which means they have passed special examinations to become Certified Diabetes Educators. The American Diabetes Association can provide the names of C.D.E.s in your area. (See page 79 for contact information.)

Tight Glucose Control

The most important goal of diabetes treatment is tight glucose control. The American Diabetes Association recommends that most adults with diabetes keep their blood glucose levels between 90 and 130 mg/dL before meals (preprandial) and less than 180 mg/dL after meals (postprandial). Your doctor may recommend a higher or lower range, depending on your individual circumstances. The only way to tell if your blood glucose levels are under control is to test your blood sugar levels one or more times a day with a home blood glucose monitor and have your doctor test your HbA1c level at his or her office every few months.

If you've had diabetes for many years, you know that in the past doctors weren't this strict about glucose control. They knew that people with diabetes needed to check their blood levels to prevent sudden symptoms of high blood glucose (hyperglycemia) and low blood glucose (hypoglycemia). But they weren't sure whether preventing everyday highs and lows had any effect on preventing long-term diabetes complications, such as kidney disease (nephropathy), nerve damage (neuropathy), and eye damage (retinopathy), all of which are caused by injury to very small blood vessels (microvascular complications). The proof came in 1993, with the publication of the Diabetes Control and Complications Trial (DCCT), a 10-year study involving 1,441 men and women with type 1 diabetes, and in 1998, with the 10-year United Kingdom Prospective Diabetes Study (UKPDS) of 3,867 people with type 2 diabetes.

The DCCT

Participants with type 1 diabetes in the DCCT followed one of two treatment regimens: intensive or standard. Individuals in the intensive-treatment group monitored their blood glucose levels three or four times a day, injected insulin three or four times a day (or used an insulin pump), adjusted their insulin doses according to blood glucose levels, and followed daily dietary and exercise recommendations. Individuals in the standard-treatment group checked their blood glucose once a day, injected insulin once or twice a day, and followed the diet and exercise regimen.

Compared with the standard-treatment group, people who received intensive treatment had significantly lower fasting blood glucose and HbA1c levels during the study. In addition, they significantly reduced their long-term risks of retinopathy by 76%, nephropathy by 50%, and neuropathy by 60%. In a follow-up study, people who lowered their HbA1c from an average of 9.1% to 7.4% with intensive treatment over a 6.5-year period reduced their risk of heart attack, stroke, or dying of cardiovascular disease by 57%.

The UKPDS

Similar results were seen in the UKPDS, in which half of the participants with type 2 diabetes followed a conventional diet and exercise regimen, and the other half were treated with diabetes medication (a sulfonylurea drug, metformin, and/or insulin) in addition to the usual lifestyle regimen. Drug treatment plus the usual lifestyle regimen resulted in better blood glucose control and a 25% reduction in retinopathy and kidney disease, compared with lifestyle measures alone. In addition, every 1% reduction in HbA1c was associated with a 14% decrease in the risk of heart attacks.

The potential risks

It's important to realize that tight blood glucose control can increase your risk of hypoglycemia (low blood sugar). For example, participants in the intensive-treatment group of the DCCT had a threefold higher incidence of hypoglycemia than people in the standard-treatment group. This risk of hypoglycemia may outweigh the benefits of tight blood glucose control in elderly people, whose chance of living long enough to develop long-term complications may not be as great as hypoglycemia-related risks such as dizziness, fainting, and injuries due to falls.

Less aggressive blood glucose control may also be advised for individuals who do not recognize hypoglycemic reactions (a condition called hypoglycemic unawareness). As a result of nerve damage from diabetes or the use of beta-blockers, your body may stop providing the usual warning symptoms of low blood glucose such as anxiety, nervousness, sweating, and rapid heartbeat. Without these warnings, the risk of severe hypoglycemia increases. Fortunately, studies

NEW RESEARCH

Tight Control Doesn't Pose a Risk for Mental Decline

Treatment to keep blood glucose under tight control does not seem to harm mental abilities years later, according to new findings from the Diabetes Control and Complications Trial (DCCT) and Epidemiology of Diabetes Interventions and Complications (EDIC) study.

Although doctors recommend strict glycemic management as the best way to prevent diabetes complications, concerns arose that tight control might impair memory and cognitive function, especially if someone had repeated bouts of hypoglycemia, which limits the glucose supply to the brain.

Researchers used an array of cognitive tests to examine 1,144 people with type 1 diabetes at the study's outset and again an average of 18 years later. They reported that hypoglycemic comas or seizures occurred in 40% of the participants and were more common in those receiving intensive therapy. Nevertheless, the results showed that neither tight control nor repeated bouts of hypoglycemia had any effect on mental capacity. In fact, it was the higher glycemic levels that could lead to a modest decline in motor skills and mental efficiency.

These findings do not mean that hypoglycemia should be taken lightly. Dangerous drops in glucose can impair memory and increase the risk of accidents. But individuals can expect to be just as sharp after years of tight glucose control.

THE NEW ENGLAND JOURNAL OF MEDICINE
Volume 356, page 1842
May 2007

Keeping Tabs on Your Glucose 24–7

New continuous monitors can lead to better control

Several high-tech devices can monitor glucose levels 24 hours a day rather than at just one point in time, giving you unprecedented information on how well you are managing your diabetes. Most useful to avoid hypoglycemic episodes in those whose diabetes requires insulin, continuous monitoring can benefit all individuals with either type 1 or type 2 diabetes. The devices provide information on how diet, exercise, medication, and other factors affect blood glucose.

Continuous glucose monitors can enable you to spot general trends in how well you are controlling your blood glucose, recognize whether it is on its way up or down, and help determine adjustments in your treatment. Better yet, the new sensors even include alarms that can warn you if your blood glucose is too low or too high.

Such continuous monitoring has been compared to having your own security camera rather than just occasional snapshots of your home. Whereas traditional needlestick tests give a snapshot of your blood sugar levels, continuous monitors track fluctuations continuously over several days.

But is a continuous glucose monitor really right for you? Here's a guide to what you need to know before taking the next step in diabetes management.

Monitoring 101

Five continuous monitors are approved by the U.S. Food and Drug Administration (FDA): CGMS System Gold, Guardian REAL-time System, Guardian RT, MiniMed Paradigm REAL-Time System (all from Medtronic), and DexCom STS. One more with pending approval will be marketed soon: The Abbott FreeStyle Navigator.

All of the devices use a tiny, flexible sensor that is inserted via a needle under the skin of your abdomen to measure blood glucose levels in the fluid outside of cells (extracellular fluid). The sensor connects to a transmitter that is attached to the skin by an adhesive patch; the transmitter sends real-time data every one to five minutes to a pager-sized receiver with a visible display that attaches to your belt or the waistline of your pants. The amount of glucose in the extracellular fluid reflects the level in your bloodstream, although there is a lag time of 20–30 minutes before changes in blood glucose are reflected in the extracellular fluid—especially if the shifts are rapid, when the lag time is even longer.

The readings can be downloaded later to a computer to produce charts that show the average trends of a person's glucose levels over three days.

How long do the sensors last? The DexCom monitor is approved for seven days before the sensor has to be changed; the Medtronic monitors last about three days. Some users, though, find that the sensors remain accurate for longer periods, sometimes up to 10–12 days.

As with other home glucose tests, all continuous monitors must be calibrated with a fingerprick blood test and checked to make sure they are working properly. You also need to sort out several technical issues before using the device, including what to do with all of the blood glucose information you receive.

Unfortunately, continuous monitors are costly and health insurance coverage is presently a real problem. The few successes in obtaining coverage have required strong advocacy by the prescribing physician. You will definitely need a doctor's prescription and a strong letter of medical necessity before you can expect coverage. So carefully consider the cost not only of the device, which can run in the thousands, but also of the disposable supplies. The sensors may cost about $35 a day, which is a big expense over the course of a year.

Pros and Cons

Almost all of the controlled studies that examined the different devices showed better HbA1c levels with continuous monitoring than with conventional intermittent testing of three to four blood glucose measurements throughout the day, although investigator enthusiasm could play a role. One study, which followed 91 people with diabetes, also found that people who used the new devices were

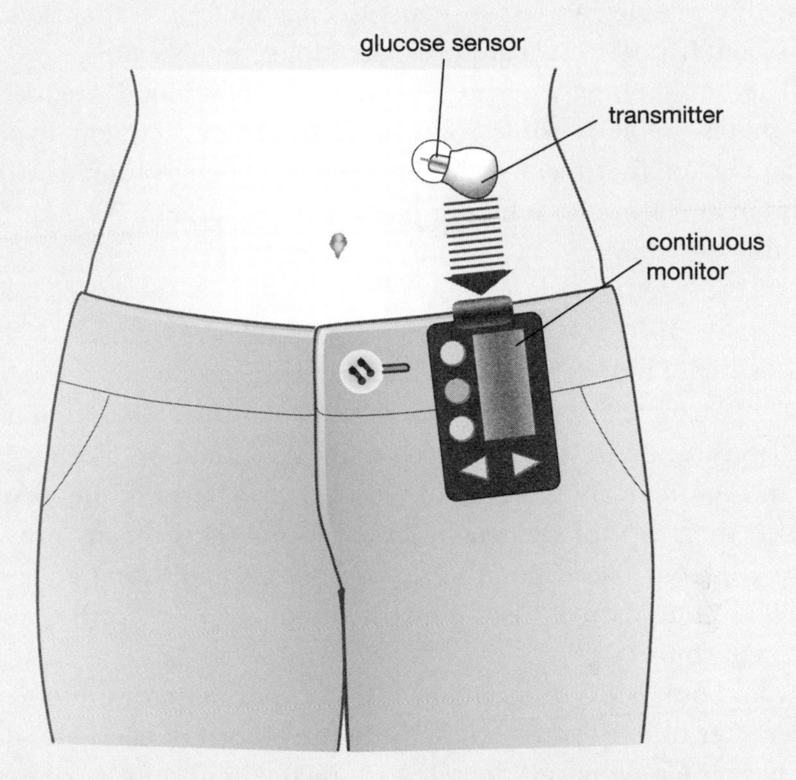

23% less likely to have high blood glucose levels and 21% less likely to suffer from low blood glucose than those who relied on standard tests.

Continuous monitoring is particularly helpful when your blood glucose patterns are poorly understood. Looking at the fluctuations over time, you can pinpoint what you ate or did that might have affected the readings—and then make changes accordingly.

But continuous monitoring devices are not without their issues. In addition to the cost, another main concern is that they can create information overload that causes people to overreact. Seeing a general drop or rise of blood glucose, some may feel the need to up their medication or grab a meal when it is not necessary because these tests only estimate blood glucose levels. They are not as accurate as traditional home glucose tests, so you will still need to use a needlestick in addition to the monitor before making a treatment decision in order to determine if any abnormal reading is accurate.

You must also understand how long your insulin dose should last to avoid repeated and excessive injections for high blood glucose that doesn't respond to the first dose; there is a slight delay between an insulin injection and a fall in your blood sugar, as well as between blood glucose changes registering in the extracellular fluid and on the meters.

Though the devices are increasingly popular, people may find them uncomfortable and more of a hassle than a help. Studies on children with type 1 diabetes found that the majority reduced their monitor usage from twice a week to once a week after a couple of months, and several stopped using them altogether. Many complained that the information gained was not worth the discomfort.

However, the sensors that transmit the glucose levels are becoming increasingly smaller, and the monitors that receive the information are also less bulky. As the technology is relatively new, the accuracy of the monitors should improve with time. Each device has its own unique advantages and disadvantages. So if you're planning on purchasing one, be sure to research the different models and get your doctor's input first.

Our Recommendation

Remember that using a continuous monitor doesn't mean the end of finger-prick testing. You will still need to do traditional finger glucose readings to calibrate the device and before making any treatment adjustments. Continuous monitoring also definitely does not cause automatic insulin delivery from a pump: You still have to choose what insulin dose to give.

At the moment, we consider continuous monitoring most useful for people who have had severe swings in their blood glucose despite good self-care patterns and, especially, for those who have been troubled by severe hypoglycemia. We are aware that insurance coverage is still spotty but hope that it will improve. ■

show that people can regain hypoglycemia awareness if episodes of significant hypoglycemia are prevented for several months.

The bottom line: You should aim for the best blood glucose control that is safely possible for you. If severe or frequent hypoglycemia occurs, that means you may need to change your treatment regimen and settle for a higher blood glucose target. (For more, see "Getting and Staying In Control" on pages 16–17.)

Self-Monitoring of Blood Glucose Control

Self-testing of blood glucose with a blood glucose meter is the backbone of diabetes management. Results from the DCCT and the UKPDS indicate that people with diabetes should be more aggressive in their daily monitoring of blood glucose levels if they want to reduce their risk of diabetes complications. This means not only more frequent blood glucose testing but also adjusting your diet, exercise, and doses of insulin or oral medications according to the results of your tests.

A logbook is often included with the purchase of a blood glucose meter to help you keep an accurate record of each blood test result. Some meters can download your readings onto a computer, and this is an excellent way to evaluate your results and share them with your doctor. Some meters can record, chart, and graph the results for you. When you display the downloaded information on a printout, it may be easier for you to notice patterns that affect control of your diabetes. For example, you may find that unexpected fluctuations in your blood glucose readings are caused by simple changes in your usual routine such as unusually large or small meals, variations in exercise, or mental stress.

Blood glucose testing

Using a glucose meter may seem complicated, but with practice you'll soon be doing it quickly and easily. Most glucose meters require only a single drop of blood, which is typically obtained by pricking your finger with a sharp-pointed lancet. After the finger stick, you place a drop of blood on a small test strip that has been treated with an enzyme called glucose oxidase. You then insert the strip into your meter, and within seconds a digital readout of the result appears on the screen.

A variety of devices make drawing blood as painless and simple as possible. For example, some lancets are spring-loaded and adjustable to give a shallow stick. Other lancets allow blood to be withdrawn from the forearm, which is less sensitive to pain than the fingertips.

Your doctor, however, may want you to use the finger-stick method, since blood from the fingertips shows decreases in blood glucose levels more quickly (30–60 minutes) than blood from other sites.

Choosing a blood glucose meter. Ask your doctor or diabetes educator to recommend a meter that suits your needs. Many new meters offer multistrip cartridges, large display screens, ultrashort test times (as little as five seconds), and other convenience features. Most meters display the results digitally, although audio meters (which read the results aloud) are available for people with vision problems. Before buying a meter, test it to make sure you feel comfortable using it. Also, find out how easy it is to maintain, clean, and calibrate the meter. Once you've purchased a meter, ask your doctor or diabetes educator to observe you testing yourself to make sure that you're doing it properly.

How often to self-test. People with diabetes are encouraged to check their blood glucose levels frequently. Recommendations for home monitoring vary from once a day or less in people with well-controlled type 2 diabetes to multiple times daily in people with type 1 disease. Most health insurance companies understand this and offer programs that provide reimbursement for certain meters plus sufficient free testing supplies. (Be sure to check with your own insurance company for details.) Prices for meters range from about $20–300, but many manufacturers offer rebates and special offers. Because the biggest expense over time is the test strips, manufacturers often offer a free meter and free replacement meters so that you will keep purchasing their brand of test strips.

Urine glucose testing

Testing urine for the presence of glucose is far less accurate than blood glucose monitoring and is not recommended.

Ketone testing

This testing is necessary only for people with type 1 diabetes and is done to detect early signs of ketoacidosis when a glucose meter indicates that blood glucose levels are higher than 250 mg/dL. You can easily measure your ketone levels by placing a ketone test strip or tablet in a urine sample and examining it for a color change. Home monitors that test blood for ketones are also available but may not be covered by health insurance. Although ketones show up in the blood more quickly than they appear in urine, the American Diabetes Association recommends either testing technique. Call your doctor immediately if a ketone test is strongly positive or

ASK THE DOCTOR

Q. *Why do my blood glucose levels sometimes go up for seemingly no reason?*

A. Blood glucose levels naturally fluctuate, so don't get exceptionally worried if they go up for no apparent reason—we can never explain every rise and fall. But when looking for the culprit, food and drink are an obvious starting point. "Harmless" energy drinks, for instance, often have more sugar or caffeine than you realize and can cause a spike in blood glucose. Bagels, which contain 60 g or even 90 g of carbohydrate, are a well-known offender. Stress or an illness can also provoke a temporary jump, and a cortisone injection (into a knee or shoulder, for instance) will predictably raise blood glucose a lot.

Your average blood glucose level (HbA1c) is the best indication of how well you are managing your diabetes over time. That doesn't mean you shouldn't monitor your blood glucose levels at various points in the day. Finger-stick tests can give an early indication that your glucose is rising faster than it should.

But keep in mind that blood glucose naturally goes up and down, and sometimes the fluctuations are unpredictable. No matter how hard you try, your levels will not be normal every time you test. As long as they don't stay too high, you should be in good shape.

if you have symptoms that suggest ketoacidosis—fruity breath, nausea, vomiting, or difficulty concentrating.

Dietary Measures

The right diet can help keep your blood glucose levels in check and help prevent obesity, high blood pressure, and elevation of blood lipids (total cholesterol, LDL cholesterol, and triglycerides), all of which increase your risk of developing diabetes complications. To find the best diet for your individual needs, consult a registered dietitian who is knowledgeable about diabetes.

Weight loss

Whatever dietary regimen you follow, it's important to control your intake of calories, saturated fat, and cholesterol. If you are overweight, controlling your calories is particularly important. Losing weight will improve your blood glucose control and blood pressure and reduce your triglycerides. It may also lower your total cholesterol and raise your HDL ("good") cholesterol.

Strict diets work temporarily for many people, but are extremely difficult to follow over the long term. Ultimately, the best approach to weight loss is to develop a balanced, healthy diet (again, consult with a dietitian) that you can follow for the rest of your life. The American Diabetes Association recommends a combination of reducing your intake of calories and increasing exercise. This combination not only produces faster and more permanent weight loss than dieting alone but also strengthens your cardiovascular system and prevents excessive loss of muscle mass. (Muscle cells burn more calories than fat cells, even at rest.) Approximately 1 lb of body weight is lost for every 3,500 calories of reduced food intake or increased energy expenditure. (See page 33 for exercise advice.)

Carbohydrates

Some people with diabetes think they can't eat foods containing sugars and starches (carbohydrates). But most experts now believe that people with diabetes should eat a diet high in carbohydrates and low in saturated fat.

The American Diabetes Association recommends that 45–65% of your total calories should come from carbohydrates. This may sound counterproductive, since people with diabetes need to control their blood glucose levels. However, carbohydrates are an important source of energy, water-soluble vitamins and minerals, and fiber, so restricting total carbohydrate intake to less than 130 g per day is not recommended. In addition, some experts have relaxed the allowance for ordinary sugar (sucrose) intake to as high as 10% of total calorie intake. That means people with diabetes can have a limited amount of sweets, chocolates, and desserts as part of a healthy meal plan.

Low-carb diets. Despite the more relaxed attitude toward carbohydrate intake, researchers continue to investigate low-carbohydrate, high-protein diets (that limit saturated fat) in people with diabetes. In one recent report, scientists asked a group of 16 people with type 2 diabetes to follow a diet that included just 20% of calories from carbohydrates. After 22 months, the participants had lost more than 17 lbs on average and cut their HbA1c levels from 8% to 6.9%.

However, the long-term effects of low-carbohydrate diets are not known. What's more, many doctors are concerned that low carbohydrate intake may cause ketosis and that high protein intake can damage the heart and the kidneys—all of which are already risks for people with diabetes. Studies have shown that people who have diabetes and chronic kidney disease may help prevent further damage to their kidneys by reducing the amount of protein in their diet. The American Diabetes Association does not recommend low-carbohydrate diets in the management of diabetes.

Glycemic index. A number of books and diet doctors advocate low-glycemic-index diets. Proponents of these diets claim that foods with a low glycemic index (such as whole grains and most fruits and vegetables) are more healthful than foods with a high index (such as white bread, candy, and soda) because they do not produce as rapid an increase in blood glucose levels when eaten. Based on this reasoning, proponents say that low-glycemic-index foods should comprise the greatest proportion of your carbohydrate intake.

The glycemic index can encourage better carbohydrate choices, such as consuming more fiber and fewer high-sugar foods, but it may also lead to worse choices, such as avoiding carbohydrates altogether and eating fattier foods. (For more, see the "Ask the Doctor" column at right.)

Sugars. Both the amount of carbohydrates (number of grams) and the type of carbohydrates you eat affect your blood glucose levels, although the total amount of carbohydrates you consume is more important than the type of carbohydrate.

If sugar is used as a replacement for other carbohydrates—gram for gram (calorie for calorie)—and is not simply added to the diet,

ASK THE DOCTOR

Q. ***What is the glycemic index, and should it be used?***

A. The glycemic index (GI) measures how much a given amount of a carbohydrate-containing food raises glucose levels within two hours in comparison to eating white bread, which is a reference point with a GI of 100. Foods with a GI higher than 100, such as instant rice, cause a faster and greater surge in blood glucose. Kidney beans score low at 38, as glucose jumps much less after eating them.

The GI can be complicated to use regularly since it is not listed on most food labels and the wide variability of numbers across websites makes it impossible to know what is correct. Foods are also rated as consumed individually, which is not how people usually eat—it does not take into account, for instance, the fat in a meal. Finally, carrots, corn, and raisins score at the high end of the GI, but these are clearly nutritious foods that don't need to be eliminated. A useful, related concept is "glycemic load," which multiplies the glycemic index by the *amount* of carbohydrate in a typical serving, thus more accurately reflecting its effect on blood glucose.

The most recent nutrition guidelines from the American Diabetes Association recommend monitoring carbohydrate intake as the key strategy for glycemic control, and that using the glycemic index and load may provide a modest, additional benefit. We agree.

Feel Full on Fewer Calories

Six strategies to help you eat less and lose weight

Cutting back on calories is the only way for you to shed pounds, which is crucial for keeping your blood glucose under control and preventing diabetes complications. But reducing calories can also mean hunger pangs—psychological more than physical—and we all know how hard it can be to keep from eating too much when available food beckons.

Fortunately, researchers are finding that you can fool your body into feeling full with fewer calories—and it may be easier than you think.

Think Smaller

First, start by looking at how much is on your plate. Overeating often has less to do with appetite than with the amount of food we have in front of us. That's because big meals can override the cues that tell us we are full and should stop eating. Research shows that when people reduce their portion sizes by about 20% or leave four to five bites on their plate, they feel just as satisfied as when they consume larger servings.

You can take advantage of this observation by using smaller plates that accommodate less food, ordering the small- or medium-sized meal instead of the large, and buying single-serving snacks.

Also, a major marketing trick is to offer a super size at little more cost than the regular size. Even though you appear to save money with the super-size, small portions do less damage to your body.

The 80% Rule

Along the same lines, residents of the Japanese island of Okinawa have perfected an eating habit known as *hara hachi bu*, which literally means "eat until you're 80% full." The Okinawans are famous for being among the oldest and healthiest people on the planet. Research suggests that part of the reason may be their diet.

In general, Okinawans eat 10–40% fewer calories than Americans. To follow their example, try eating until you feel mostly full, then wait 20 minutes to judge how satiated you feel. Studies show that many people are satisfied after following the 80% rule, even though they eat less. In contrast, overweight people report that they eat until they feel overstuffed far more often than lean people.

Super Size Right

Healthy foods like fruits and vegetables contain lots of water and fiber, which can quickly fill you up without the extra calories. For example, 1 cup of fruit contains only 45 calories, and 2 cups of lettuce with a sprinkling of tomatoes, skinless chicken, almonds, and a tablespoon of vinaigrette dressing has roughly 60 calories. So increase your intake of the right foods—fruits and vegetables—rather than fast food.

This recommendation does not come unfounded. A recent study found that people who stuck to a low-calorie meal plan involving plenty of fruits and vegetables lost more weight, despite eating a larger weight of food, than those on a high-calorie diet.

Try a variety of fresh produce to keep your diet interesting. Don't give up on all fruits and vegetables if you don't care for a few.

people with diabetes can safely eat foods that contain sugar. The downside is that sugary foods often contain "empty calories," whereas starchy foods are more nutritious because they also supply vitamins, minerals, and fiber.

Sugar is available in many forms—white, brown, granulated, and confectioners'. The chemical name for these sugars is sucrose. Many food products contain other types of sugar, all having chemical names that end in –ose, such as glucose (also called dextrose), fructose (in fruits and honey), lactose (in milk products),

Choose Lean Protein

A high-protein, low-carb diet is unhealthy in the long run and not necessary for controlling diabetes, despite what certain diet gurus may claim, often because what is billed as high-protein—such as a hamburger—is also high in fat. Yet eating a reasonable amount of lean protein—such as skinless chicken and turkey, fish, low-fat dairy and soy products, and lentils or other beans—may fill you up and help you cut back on fatty foods, according to some small studies.

For example, researchers at the University of Washington School of Medicine followed 19 people who kept to a 2,000-calorie diet for several months. At first, they got 15% of calories from protein. Then they upped their protein to 30%. Throughout the study, the men and women ate the same percentage of carbohydrates, while cutting back on fats. The volunteers reported feeling more full when they ate more calories from protein and also lost more weight.

Limit Sweets

Sweet treats like cookies and cake are a dieter's nightmare, and regular-calorie soft drinks may be the worst threat of all. Almost all sweets pack a lot of calories and do little to fill you up. But liquids are also much less filling than food to begin with, and research shows that people do not compensate for high-calorie beverages by cutting back on food calories.

A recent study in the *American Journal of Clinical Nutrition* showed that diners ate the same amount of food at lunch when they were given a sugary soda that added an extra 128–158 calories to the meal as they did when they drank a zero-calorie beverage like water or diet soda.

Moreover, people with a "sweet tooth" may have trouble stopping at one piece of candy. Researchers at the University of North Carolina asked 163 men and women to rate their tastes toward sweet foods. Those who had the highest preference for sweets reported the greatest mood-altering effects after eating sugary foods and had less control over their cravings than the rest of the group.

You can offset your sweet tooth by becoming a fruit lover—the two foods are a lot closer in taste than commonly believed, studies show. And the next time you grab a can of soda, think twice and reach for a glass of water or club soda instead.

Snack Smart

Snacking between meals can lead to weight gain, especially if you indulge in traditional snack foods like cookies or chips. But sensible snacking may keep your hunger in check between meals and leave you less tempted to overeat at mealtime.

To investigate the dietary habits of the French, generally noted for their thinness, researchers in France asked 54 of their countrymen to keep a diary of everything they ate for a month. On average, the participants ate nearly three meals and a little over one snack a day. The regular meals were about twice as high in calories than the snacks, but the participants said they felt more satisfied after snacking and gave the highest satiety ratings after having a little bite to eat in the afternoon.

To make sure that several small meals don't add up to just another big meal, try picking out a range of foods that are low in calories—carrots and celery—or potentially more filling to you, such as a handful of nuts or a slice of cheese. ■

and maltose (in starchy foods). During digestion, sucrose, lactose, and maltose are broken down into glucose and other simpler types of sugars. Some of these sugars have a lower glycemic index and reach the bloodstream more slowly than other sugars, but they still raise blood glucose levels. Unfortunately, some foods that are labeled "safe for diabetics" just replace sucrose with fructose, maltose, or other forms of sugar. That's why it's important to check food labels for hidden sugars such as honey, corn syrup, molasses, and ingredients ending in the telltale –ose.

Sugar alcohols. Also watch for sugar alcohols with names that end in –ol, such as sorbitol, mannitol, xylitol, and maltitol. These sweeteners are chemically related to alcohol, but they have no alcoholic effects. They are carbohydrates that are converted to ordinary sugar during digestion.

Sugar alcohols are used in many products labeled as "low carb," "low sugar," or "sugar free." Although they have a lower glycemic index than ordinary sugar, don't be fooled. Sugar alcohols have calories and will raise your blood glucose level. They are not "free foods" (a free food is any food or drink that contains less than 20 calories or less than 5 g of carbohydrate per serving). In addition, many low-carb foods that are sweetened with sugar alcohols are high in fat, and large quantities of sugar alcohols often cause diarrhea.

Noncaloric sugar substitutes. Some "sugar-free" beverages and packaged foods really are what they say. That's because they contain one of the products the U.S. Food and Drug Administration (FDA) has approved as non-nutritive sweeteners: saccharin (Sweet-'N Low, Sweet Twin, Necta Sweet), aspartame (Equal, NutraSweet, NatraTaste), acesulfame-K (Sunett, Sweet One), sucralose (Splenda) and neotame. According to the American Diabetes Association, all of these noncaloric sugar substitutes have undergone rigorous testing and are safe for consumption by people with diabetes.

Dietary fiber

Everyone, including people with diabetes, should eat a wide variety of foods that contain fiber—with a goal to consume at least 20–35 g of dietary fiber each day.

Fiber is a type of carbohydrate that is not broken down during the digestion process. Some studies show that a diet high in soluble fiber—found in oats, oat bran, legumes, barley, citrus fruits, and apples—can lower blood glucose and blood cholesterol levels. Insoluble fiber—found in whole wheat, wheat bran, vegetables, and fruit—can help prevent constipation. Both types of fiber are needed in a healthy diet.

Experts aren't sure exactly how fiber lowers blood glucose levels. It's possible that fiber slows the digestion of food and delays the breakdown of carbohydrates, which means that glucose enters the bloodstream more gradually. The resulting slower rise in blood glucose after a meal gives insulin a greater opportunity to convert the glucose into energy.

Fats

Everyone needs some fat in their diet, but saturated fats, cholesterol, and trans fats are unhealthy and increase your risk of a heart attack or stroke. A type of polyunsaturated fat called omega-3 protects the heart, however.

Saturated fats and cholesterol. Eating saturated fats and cholesterol increases blood levels of LDL cholesterol and insulin, which contribute to coronary heart disease (CHD). Because people with diabetes are at especially high risk for heart disease, the American Diabetes Association recommends a diet that includes less than 10% of calories from saturated fats and less than 300 mg a day of cholesterol. If your LDL cholesterol is above 100 mg/dL, your doctor may suggest that you lower your saturated fat intake to less than 7% and your dietary cholesterol to less than 200 mg a day. The American Heart Association recommends that you keep your saturated fat intake below 7% of total calories regardless of your LDL cholesterol level.

Rather than calculating the percentage of calories from saturated fat and counting milligrams of cholesterol, it may be easier to simply cut back on foods containing these fats. Foods high in saturated fat include red meats, dark-meat poultry, poultry skin, whole-milk dairy products, and products made with hydrogenated oils or coconut, palm, or palm kernel oils. Cholesterol is found only in animal foods and is particularly plentiful in egg yolks, organ meats, shrimp, crab, and lobster.

Another way to reduce saturated fats and cholesterol in your diet is to replace them with more healthful fats. Consuming monounsaturated fat—which is plentiful in olive and canola oils and in avocados and some nuts—lowers total blood cholesterol levels without reducing HDL cholesterol. It may also help prevent the accumulation of LDL in the walls of large arteries (one of the first steps in the development of atherosclerosis, or hardening of the arteries). Polyunsaturated fats, found in vegetable oils like safflower, corn, sunflower, and soybean oils, also help to lower total cholesterol levels but may reduce HDL cholesterol. Even though monounsaturated and polyunsaturated fats have beneficial effects, they're still high in calories, so intake must be limited.

Trans fats. Another unhealthy fat is trans fat. It is found in hydrogenated and partially hydrogenated oils and in margarines. Trans fats raise blood levels of LDL cholesterol and lower levels of HDL cholesterol. The American Heart Association recommends that trans fat intake make up no more than 1% of the calories you eat. So if you typically eat 1,500 calories a day, you should consume no more than 1.5 g of trans fat a day. All food labels now include the amount of trans fat (in grams) per serving.

Omega-3 fat. This polyunsaturated fat has heart-protective benefits, reducing blood levels of triglycerides and preventing life-threatening abnormal heart rhythms. Fatty fish such as salmon, mackerel, trout, and herring are the best sources of omega-3 fat. The American Diabetes Association recommends that people with diabetes eat two to three servings of fish each week to reap the heart benefits of omega-3 fat. If you're concerned about mercury contamination, eat a variety of fish and limit your consumption of tuna, swordfish, king mackerel, shark, and tilefish.

Antioxidants

Antioxidants are chemical compounds that can prevent cell damage. They inactivate harmful molecules called free radicals that are formed during the normal course of metabolism. Common antioxidants include vitamin C, vitamin E, selenium, and beta-carotene. Early research suggested that antioxidants might help prevent CHD. However, in three large studies, neither vitamin E nor beta-carotene supplements prevented heart attacks and strokes in people with CHD or in people with diabetes or others at high risk for CHD. The American Diabetes Association does not recommend antioxidant supplements or any other vitamin and mineral supplements for people with diabetes unless they have vitamin deficiencies.

Sodium

If you have high blood pressure, restricting your sodium intake to less than 2,400 mg per day may lower your blood pressure. You can do this by using less salt at the table and in cooking and by avoiding foods that are high in sodium (for example, processed meats such as sausages, cured ham, and hot dogs; canned or dried soups; ketchup; and most cheeses).

Protein

According to the American Diabetes Association, people with diabetes and normal kidney function can safely consume 15–20% of total calories from protein—the same amount recommended for people without diabetes. For people with kidney damage (nephropathy), however, reducing dietary protein to lower levels may help slow kidney damage.

Alcohol

People with well-controlled diabetes can drink alcoholic beverages as long as they do so in moderation and with food. However, you shouldn't drink alcohol if you are pregnant, have a history of alcohol abuse, or have additional medical problems such as pancreatitis (inflammation of the pancreas), advanced neuropathy (nerve damage), or elevated triglyceride levels. These same precautions apply to people who do not have diabetes.

Studies in adults with and without diabetes show that regular consumption of light to moderate amounts of alcohol (5–15 g a day) increases HDL cholesterol and decreases the risk of CHD. Although excessive consumption of alcohol on a regular basis increases blood pressure and triglyceride levels, moderate use of alcohol does not pose such risks. Based on these findings, the American Diabetes Association recommends that alcohol intake be limited to no more than two alcoholic drinks per day for adult men and no more than one drink per day for adult women. (One drink is defined as 12 oz of beer, 5 oz of wine, or 1.5 oz of distilled spirits.)

Alcohol is considered an addition to the diet for individuals with diabetes, so do not omit other foods in order to drink. Since alcoholic beverages are high in sugar, drink them along with food so that blood glucose levels won't rise as quickly. If you use insulin, you may also need to adjust your dosage.

For people with diabetes, drinks that contain smaller amounts of sugar, such as light beers and dry wines, are preferable to sweet mixed drinks. Remember, however, that all alcoholic beverages contain calories and can contribute to weight gain. When taking the oral diabetes drug chlorpropamide (Diabinese), alcohol can cause flushing of the face, arms, and neck.

Exercise

Exercise is beneficial for people with diabetes. One recent study found that people with type 2 diabetes who walked three miles a day or performed an equivalent amount of physical activity lost weight and lowered their heart rate, blood pressure, cholesterol and triglyceride levels, and HbA1c. Exercise is also good for your mental health.

How much is enough?

With a doctor's approval, most adults with type 1 or type 2 diabetes can follow the American Heart Association and American College

NEW RESEARCH

Exercise—and Focus—To Control Blood Glucose

More proof that regular exercise really does work: A recent meta-analysis showed that individuals with type 2 diabetes who increased their physical activity levels experienced improved blood glucose levels. Interestingly, individuals who focused only on boosting exercise achieved better results than those who tried to change their diet, exercise, and medication adherence at the same time.

The evaluation of 103 studies, encompassing 10,455 participants, compared exercise-only interventions with lifestyle measures that also targeted multiple health behaviors. This was the first meta-analysis to explore the effect of various methods of inspiring people to exercise, from sessions with a personal trainer to watching others exercise as a motivation method.

The researchers found that HbA1c levels dropped by 0.45% in those who exercised more compared with inactive participants. The type of approach used to get participants moving did not affect glucose readings. Blood glucose improved twice as much among individuals who focused on exercise only, compared with those who tried to improve other lifestyle factors as well.

Perhaps it may be more effective for people with type 2 diabetes to try to change one behavior at a time and avoid becoming overwhelmed by making multiple modifications all at once.

DIABETOLOGIA
Volume 50, page 913
March 2007

Oral Blood Glucose–Lowering Medications 2008

Drug type: Brand (generic)	Typical daily dosages*	How to take†	Monthly cost‡: Brand (generic)
Sulfonylureas			
First-generation sulfonylurea			
Diabinese (chlorpropamide)	250–375 mg	One or 1.5 250-mg tablets 1x/day with breakfast.	$35–53 ($10–15)
Second-generation sulfonylureas			
Amaryl (glimepiride)	1–4 mg	One 1-, 2-, or 4-mg tablet 1x/day with breakfast.	$18–35 ($10–15)
Glucotrol (glipizide)	10–20 mg	One 10-mg tablet 1–2x/day, 30 minutes before a meal.	$31–62 ($8–11)
Glucotrol XL (glipizide, extended-release)	5–20 mg	One or two 5- or 10-mg tablets 1x/day with breakfast. Swallow whole.	$18–64 ($17–63)
DiaBeta, Micronase (glyburide)	5–20 mg	One to four 5-mg tablets 1x/day with breakfast or 2x/day with meals.	$30–156 ($8–32)
Glynase (glyburide, micronized)	3–12 mg	One or two 3- or 6-mg tablets 1x/day with breakfast or 2x/day with meals.	$32–99 ($11–38)
Biguanides			
Glucophage (metformin)	1,500–2,550 mg	One 500-, 850-, or 1,000-mg tablet 2–3x/day with meals.	$49–176 ($34–45)
Glucophage XR (metformin, extended-release)	1,500–2,000 mg	Three or four 500-mg tablets or two 750-mg tablets 1x/day with evening meal. Swallow whole.	$70–96 ($60–80)
Glumetza (metformin, extended-release)	1,500–2,000 mg	Three 500-mg tablets or two 1,000-mg tablets 1x/day with evening meal. Swallow whole.	$107
Thiazolidinediones			
Actos (pioglitazone)	15–45 mg	One 15-, 30-, or 45-mg tablet 1x/day with or without meals.	$113–180
Avandia (rosiglitazone)	4–8 mg	One 4- or 8-mg tablet 1x/day or 2x/day in the morning and evening, with or without meals.	$111-413
Meglitinide			
Prandin (repaglinide)	3–12 mg	One 1-mg tablet or one or two 2-mg tablets 3x/day 1–30 minutes before each meal. Do not take if a meal is missed. If you plan to eat a fourth meal, take another dose up to 30 minutes beforehand.	$122–244

See chart legend on page 36.

Precautions	Most common side effects	Call your doctor if...
Can cause hypoglycemia (low blood glucose), which can recur for up to 24 hours, even after treatment. To prevent hypoglycemia, eat meals on a regular schedule, do not skip meals, and avoid alcohol. Symptoms of hypoglycemia include chills, cold sweat, blurred vision, dizziness, drowsiness, shaking, rapid heart rate, weakness, headache, fainting, tingling of the hands or feet, or hunger. Always carry a piece of hard candy or glucose tablets with you to treat an episode of hypoglycemia. Also wear sunblock and avoid prolonged sun exposure, because sulfonylureas can make your skin more sensitive to the sun.	Hypoglycemia. *Chlorpropamide only*: facial flushing with alcohol use.	You experience a fever, have an infection or injury, need to undergo surgery. These conditions can make your blood glucose more difficult to control, and a change in your medication may be necessary.
To minimize gastrointestinal side effects, ask your doctor to increase the dose slowly and take the medication with food. Before undergoing surgery or imaging tests, tell your doctor that you are on metformin. You may need to temporarily stop the medication before the procedure. People with kidney damage should not use metformin. Limit alcohol intake to prevent lactic acidosis (a potentially fatal buildup of lactic acid in the blood).	Diarrhea, nausea, bloating, gas, abdominal pain, metallic taste. These side effects usually go away in the first few weeks of treatment.	You experience signs of lactic acidosis: unusual tiredness or severe drowsiness, cold skin, muscle pain, breathing trouble or rapid breathing, unusually slow or irregular heartbeat, unusual or unexplained stomach upset.
Because another drug in this class now off the market was associated with potentially fatal liver disease, you should have a blood test to evaluate liver function before starting a thiazolidinedione and periodically thereafter. These drugs aren't recommended for people with heart failure. Avandia is also linked to increased heart attack risk.	Weight gain, fluid retention, sore throat, muscle pain, tooth problems.	You experience signs of liver problems: unusual tiredness, persistent nausea or vomiting, severe stomach or abdominal pain, yellowing of eyes or skin, dark urine. Signs of heart failure: unusually rapid increase in weight, extreme fluid retention, shortness of breath. *Avandia only:* changes in vision such as blurriness, decreased color sensitivity, decreased night vision.
To prevent hypoglycemia (low blood glucose), which this medication can cause, eat meals on a regular schedule (do not skip any) and avoid alcohol. Hypoglycemia symptoms are: chills, cold sweat, blurred vision, dizziness, drowsiness, shaking, rapid heart rate, weakness, headache, fainting, tingling of hands or feet, and hunger. Always carry hard candy or glucose tablets with you to treat an episode.	Hypoglycemia, headache, nausea, vomiting, diarrhea, upset stomach, joint pain.	You experience a fever, have an infection or injury, need to undergo surgery. These conditions can make your blood glucose more difficult to control, and a change in your medication may be necessary.

continued on the next page

Oral Blood Glucose–Lowering Medications 2008 (continued)

Drug type: Brand (generic)	Typical daily dosages*	How to take†	Monthly cost‡: Brand (generic)
D-phenylalanine derivative			
Starlix (nateglinide)	180–360 mg	One 60- or 120-mg tablet 3x/day 1–30 minutes before each meal. Do not take if a meal is missed. If you plan to eat a fourth meal, take another dose up to 30 minutes beforehand.	$120–123
Alpha-glucosidase inhibitors			
Glyset (miglitol)	150–300 mg	One 50- or 100-mg tablet 3x/day with the first bite of a meal.	$73–85
Precose (acarbose)	150–300 mg	One 50- or 100-mg tablet 3x/day with the first bite of a meal.	$82–94
Dipeptidyl peptidase-4 inhibitor			
Januvia (sitagliptin)	25–100 mg	One 25-, 50-, or 100-mg tablet 1x/day, with or without food.	$164
Combination products			
Actoplus Met (pioglitazone/metformin)	15–30 mg pioglitazone/ 500–1,000 mg metformin	One 15-mg/500-mg tablet 1–2x/day with meals.	$87–174
Avandamet (rosiglitazone/metformin)	4 mg rosiglitazone/ 1,000 mg metformin	One 2-mg/500-mg tablet 2x/day with morning and evening meal.	$132
Avandaryl (rosiglitazone/glimepiride)	4–8 mg rosiglitazone/ 1–4 mg glimepiride	One or two tablets (4 mg rosiglitazone/1–4 mg glimepiride) 1x/day with first meal of the day.	$121–242
Glucovance (glyburide/metformin)	10 mg glyburide/ 1,000 mg metformin	One 5-mg/500-mg tablet 2x/day with morning and evening meal.	$63 ($48)
Janumet (sitagliptin/metformin)	50–100 mg sitagliptin/ 500–2,000 mg metformin	One 50-mg/500-mg tablet 1–2x/day with meals, or one 50-mg/1,000-mg tablet 1–2x/day with meals.	$83–167
Metaglip (glipizide/metformin)	5 mg glipizide/ 1,000 mg metformin	One 2.5-mg/500-mg tablet 2x/day with morning and evening meal.	$60

* These dosages represent the usual daily dosages for the treatment of diabetes. The precise effective dosage varies from person to person and depends on many factors. Do not make any changes to your medication without consulting your doctor.

† These instructions represent the typical way to take the medication. Your doctor's instructions may differ. Always follow your doctor's recommendations.

‡ Prices per drugstore.com.

Precautions	Most common side effects	Call your doctor if...
To prevent hypoglycemia, eat meals on a regular schedule (do not skip any) and avoid alcohol. Symptoms are: chills, cold sweat, blurred vision, dizziness, drowsiness, shaking, rapid heart rate, weakness, headache, fainting, tingling of hands or feet, and hunger. Always carry hard candy or glucose tablets with you to treat an episode.	Hypoglycemia, nausea, vomiting, diarrhea, upset stomach.	You have a fever, infection, or injury or need to undergo surgery. These conditions can make your blood glucose more difficult to control, and a change in your medication may be necessary.
Glyset and Precose interfere with the breakdown of sucrose. If you experience an episode of hypoglycemia while taking one of these medications with another diabetes drug, sucrose-containing foods like table sugar or nondiet soda will not raise blood glucose quickly enough. Instead, use glucose tablets, honey, or orange juice.	Diarrhea, gas, upset stomach, stomach pain. These side effects disappear after a few weeks.	See Starlix (above). *Precose only*: You have signs of liver problems including unusual tiredness, persistent nausea or vomiting, severe stomach or abdominal pain, yellowing of eyes or skin, dark urine.
If you have kidney problems, you may need a dose of 25 mg or 50 mg. You should also have blood tests done from time to time to measure how well your kidneys are working.	Upper respiratory infection, headache, stuffy or runny nose, sore throat.	See Starlix (above).
See separate entries for pioglitazone and metformin.		
See separate entries for rosiglitazone and metformin.		
See separate entries for rosiglitazone and glimepiride.		
See separate entries for glyburide and metformin.		
See separate entries for sitagliptin and metformin.		
See separate entries for glipizide and metformin.		

of Sports Medicine recommendation to get at least 30 minutes of moderate physical activity on most, and preferably all, days of the week or at least 20 minutes of vigorous intensity aerobic activity three days a week. These guidelines define "moderate" as equivalent to walking at a pace of three to four miles per hour.

It does not matter whether the 30 minutes is continuous or divided into short bursts of 10 minutes each, three times a day. Brisk walking, jogging, biking, and calisthenics are good aerobic activities, but so are walking short distances instead of driving, walking up stairs instead of taking the elevator, and pedaling on a stationary bicycle while watching television or reading. Gardening, housework, raking leaves, dancing, and playing with children also count as part of the 30-minute total—if they are performed at a level of intensity similar to brisk walking and for at least 10 minutes each.

If you need to lose weight, the Institute of Medicine recommends getting even more exercise—an hour a day—but you should work up to that amount gradually.

Precautions

Before starting any exercise program, you should check with your doctor. If you have arthritis or damage to nerves and blood vessels in your feet and legs, you may need to avoid foot trauma. That might mean replacing brisk walking or jogging with swimming or bicycling. People with heart disease or blockages in major blood vessels may need a similar, low-stress exercise program. Your doctor can refer you to an exercise physiologist to help you plan an exercise regimen that will minimize any risks.

During exercise your cells take in glucose and use it for energy, which causes a drop in your blood glucose level. Therefore, if you use insulin or oral diabetes medications, you must test your blood before and after exercise. You'll probably need to adjust your medication dosages and your food intake to prevent blood glucose highs and lows. For example, many people with diabetes find that after vigorous exercise, their blood glucose drops dramatically and then shoots up because the body compensates for running out of energy. This can often be avoided by having a small snack before you exercise to boost your blood glucose level.

Oral Medications

Diet and exercise may be enough to control blood glucose levels in some people with type 2 diabetes. But if you're still not meeting your HbA1c goal or if you're having diabetes symptoms, your doctor will start you on oral medications, either alone or in combination with insulin injections.

There are seven classes of oral drugs for diabetes—sulfonylureas, meglitinides, D-phenylalanine derivatives, biguanides, thiazolidinediones, alpha-glucosidase inhibitors, and dipeptidyl peptidase-4 (DPP-4) inhibitors, as well as combination products. You probably know these drugs better by their brand names, which you can find in the chart on pages 34–37.

The classes of oral diabetes drugs work in different ways, so it's often helpful to take drugs from more than one class. For example, if a sulfonylurea stops working, you may be switched to metformin (Glucophage) or continued on the sulfonylurea in combination with metformin, an alpha-glucosidase inhibitor, or a thiazolidinedione. (For a quick guide to how these drugs work, see "Making Sense of Diabetes Medications" on pages 42–43. More in-depth explanations follow below.)

Adding insulin is usually a last resort, but many new studies show that starting insulin early in the course of type 2 diabetes provides better glucose control, protects beta-cell function, and helps to prevent diabetes complications. That's why many experts now recommend early treatment with a combination of an oral drug plus insulin.

Sulfonylureas

These drugs stimulate beta cells in the pancreas to secrete more insulin. They are classified as either first-generation (drugs that were introduced long ago) or second-generation (newer drugs). If you've been taking oral medication for many years, you may have used chlorpropamide (Diabinese), a popular first-generation sulfonylurea. Today, most physicians prescribe second-generation drugs such as glimepiride (Amaryl), glipizide (Glucotrol, Glucotrol XL), and glyburide (DiaBeta, Glynase, Micronase), which are stronger than the first-generation sulfonylureas and require lower dosages.

About 85% of people with type 2 diabetes who take a sulfonylurea have an initial favorable response. However, the medication gradually loses its effectiveness in more than one quarter of people because beta cells in the pancreas continue to be destroyed. Sulfonylureas rarely work in people with fasting blood glucose levels above 300 mg/dL.

Sulfonylureas can cause weight gain, excessive water retention, and flushing after drinking alcohol. The most common and serious side effect is low blood glucose (hypoglycemia), which typically

NEW RESEARCH

Antidepressant Linked to Better Glycemic Control

Individuals with diabetes who are depressed may benefit from the antidepressant bupropion (Wellbutrin XL), which can lift their spirits and improve blood glucose control, new findings suggest.

While similar results have been reported before, lower glucose levels were thought to result from the weight loss and improved self-care that often accompany successful depression treatment. But researchers are now finding that a better mood alone may lead to improved glycemic control over the long haul.

In a two-phase, open-label trial, 93 participants with type 2 diabetes and major depression took Wellbutrin XL, an antidepressant associated with weight loss, for just over two months. Of the 75 volunteers who stayed on Wellbutrin XL for 10 weeks, 84% reported improved mood, weight loss, and better self-care with diet and exercise. At the same time, the participants experienced a 0.5% reduction in HbA1c levels.

Looking at whether these improvements would last if they took the medication longer, a positive mood was most important for keeping glucose under control for another six months, regardless of weight loss or self-care changes. While the exact mechanisms behind better glycemic control need further study, treating any accompanying depression is clearly important for managing diabetes.

DIABETES CARE
Volume 30, page 459
March 2007

occurs during the first few months of treatment. If hypoglycemia persists, reducing the dosage often helps. The risk of hypoglycemia is highest in frail, elderly people and in those who are malnourished or have reduced pituitary, adrenal, liver, or kidney function. Alcohol consumption, skipped meals, and exercise also can trigger hypoglycemia in people taking a sulfonylurea.

Meglitinides

Meglitinides work in the same way as sulfonylureas, by stimulating the pancreas to release more insulin into the bloodstream. Repaglinide (Prandin) is the only meglitinide approved by the FDA. It is taken before meals and increases insulin levels much faster than sulfonylureas.

Hypoglycemia, the most common side effect, occurs less often with Prandin than with sulfonylureas. Prandin takes effect quickly, so you must eat soon after taking it and consume carbohydrate-rich foods to prevent blood glucose levels from falling too low. If Prandin doesn't sufficiently control your blood glucose, your doctor may add another drug such as metformin, an alpha-glucosidase inhibitor, or a thiazolidinedione.

D-phenylalanine derivatives

Nateglinide (Starlix) is the only D-phenylalanine derivative approved by the FDA. Like sulfonylureas and Prandin, it stimulates secretion of insulin from the pancreas. Starlix is taken before eating. It is most effective in people who have very high postmeal blood glucose levels (more than 200 mg/dL). It can be taken by itself or in combination with metformin.

Because Starlix stimulates rapid release of insulin, its most common side effect is hypoglycemia. The drug should be used with caution in people with serious liver disease. In rare cases, it may cause upper respiratory infection, flu symptoms, dizziness, and joint pain.

Biguanides

Metformin (Glucophage), which is also available in an extended-release form (Glucophage XR, Glumetza), is the only biguanide sold in the United States. It acts primarily by decreasing the liver's production of glucose. It also increases the amount of glucose that is transported into cells. Metformin is often the first drug that doctors prescribe for type 2 diabetes because of the following advantages:

- Its effects do not involve beta cells, so it works even in people with little beta-cell function.

- It doesn't cause hypoglycemia when used alone.
- It doesn't cause weight gain and may even produce weight loss. (In one study, people taking metformin lost almost 6 lbs, on average.)

On the negative side, about 30% of people taking metformin develop gastrointestinal side effects such as diarrhea, nausea, bloating, and gas, which often disappear over time. Metformin should not be taken by people with alcoholism, kidney or liver disease, heart failure, or severe emphysema or other chronic lung diseases, because it increases the risk of life-threatening lactic acidosis (buildup of lactic acid in the blood).

Metformin is often prescribed for obese people who are insulin resistant—that is, people who develop high blood glucose levels because their body's cells have become less sensitive to the action of insulin. It can be used either as a first-line treatment (the first drug tried) or as a second-line choice for people who do not achieve adequate glucose control with a sulfonylurea. Studies have shown that metformin, taken alone, can reduce blood glucose levels by about 20% and can boost the glucose-lowering effects of a sulfonylurea by an additional 25%.

Metformin is also prescribed in combination with a meglitinide, an alpha-glucosidase inhibitor, a thiazolidinedione, or insulin. Several of these combinations are sold as a single pill: Actoplus Met (metformin and pioglitazone), Avandamet (metformin and rosiglitazone), Glucovance (metformin and glyburide), and Metaglip (metformin and glipizide).

Thiazolidinediones

Pioglitazone (Actos) and rosiglitazone (Avandia) are the two thiazolidinediones currently available. They work by decreasing the body's resistance to the actions of insulin. Since obese people with diabetes are insulin resistant, they are often treated with Actos or Avandia. One welcome outcome of treatment is redistribution of body fat from around the midsection. However, thiazolidinedione drugs often cause an overall weight gain due partly to fluid retention, which can lead to heart failure or worsen existing heart failure. As a result, thiazolidinediones aren't recommended for people with heart failure.

Further concerns were raised with a review of studies on Avandia, which found that the drug was associated with an increased chance of heart attacks compared with other diabetes treatments. (See the "New Research" column at right.) The FDA's review of Avandia and the risk of heart attack is ongoing.

NEW RESEARCH

Avandia May Boost Heart Attack Risk

A review of rosiglitazone (Avandia) found that the widely prescribed diabetes medication is associated with a greater risk of heart attacks.

Researchers from the Cleveland Clinic examined 42 controlled trials on Avandia, which was approved for use in 1999. In the trials, 15,565 people with type 2 diabetes received Avandia, while 12,282 used a different treatment.

There were 86 heart attacks with Avandia compared with 72 in the control group. Thirty-nine people died of cardiovascular events while taking Avandia, compared with 22 on another medication. The researchers say that the risk of cardiovascular death with Avandia is of "borderline significance." A second report found similar results for people with prediabetes, and another study found that the other drug in the same class, pioglitazone (Actos), was *not* associated with increased heart attack risk.

As of press time, the FDA had issued a black-box warning on the risk of heart attack and heart failure for Avandia while a safety assessment continued. Actos carries a warning for heart failure only. If you are concerned about your use of Avandia or Actos, do not stop taking it unless your doctor determines that, *for you*, the risks outweigh the benefits.

THE NEW ENGLAND JOURNAL OF MEDICINE
Volume 356, page 2457
June 2007

JOURNAL OF THE AMERICAN MEDICAL ASSOCIATION
Volume 298, pages 1180 and 1189
September 2007

Making Sense of Diabetes Medications

A quick guide to the different types, what they do, and their effectiveness

There has been a veritable explosion of new oral medications to help control blood glucose levels in people with type 2 diabetes. Since those with type 2, unlike people with type 1 diabetes, are still able to produce insulin, more options are available for lowering glucose levels. (People with type 1 disease must still rely only on insulin, almost always given by injection.)

But the number of treatment choices can cause confusion over which ones to take. At least 21 different diabetes medications are now on the market; in addition, weight loss medications can also help lower your blood glucose if you lose weight. And all the medications show better effects when combined with a healthy lifestyle, meaning that simply taking pills is not enough. Your doctor can help you choose the right medication, based on your own particular needs.

How They Work

Various types of oral diabetes drugs work to control blood glucose levels in different ways (see the chart on pages 34–37 for information on specific medications):

- **Sulfonylureas and short-acting sulfonylurea-like medications** all stimulate cells in the pancreas to release more insulin. Sulfonylureas (such as glimepiride [Amaryl], glipizide [Glucotrol, Glucotrol XL], and glyburide [DiaBeta, Micronase, Glynase]) are the oldest class of diabetes medication. Short-acting sulfonylurea-like medications (nateglinide [Starlix], repaglinide [Prandin]) are used immediately before meals. The main side effects of all these drugs, because they stimulate insulin secretion, are hypoglycemia and weight gain.
- **Metformin** (Glucophage, Glucophage XR, Glumetza) is a venerable diabetes drug used around the world since the 1960s and in the United States since the 1980s. The most widely prescribed pill to control blood glucose, it works primarily by decreasing the liver's production of glucose as well as increasing the amount of glucose that is transported into cells. The main side effects, which happen in about 15% of people, are bloating, loose stools, and diarrhea. Also, individuals with a number of conditions, such as kidney disease or heart failure, and even those facing elective surgery should not use metformin.
- **Alpha-glucosidase inhibitors** such as acarbose (Precose) and miglitol (Glyset) slow the breakdown of starches and certain sugars, which help keep glucose levels from spiking after a meal. They often cause unpleasant gas and gastrointestinal upset.
- **Thiazolidinediones,** one of the newer classes of pills, lower insulin resistance by helping

Liver failure was a rare but catastrophic effect of the first thiazolidinedione to be approved, troglitazone (Rezulin), prompting it to be withdrawn from the market. Cases of liver failure have not been reported with Actos or Avandia, but the FDA still requires blood testing to measure liver function during the first year of treatment.

Thiazolidinediones are used alone or in combination with a sulfonylurea, a meglitinide, metformin, an alpha-glucosidase inhibitor, or insulin. When a thiazolidinedione is added to insulin, it may take up to eight weeks before the full effects are seen. So it's important to check frequently for hypoglycemia, which signals the need to decrease the insulin dosage. People who take the cholesterol-lowering medications cholestyramine (Questran, Questran Light) or colestipol (Colestid) should be aware that these drugs inhibit the absorption of thiazolidinediones and should not be taken at the same time of day.

insulin work better in muscle and fat. The two available forms are rosiglitazone (Avandia) and pioglitazone (Actos). Side effects of both include fluid retention and weight gain. Recent evidence indicates that they also increase the risk of heart failure and, possibly, heart attacks.

• **Dipeptidyl peptidase-4 (DPP-4) inhibitors** are the newest class of treatments that boost insulin levels after blood glucose rises. The most recently approved drug, sitagliptin (Januvia), is a DPP-4 inhibitor that works by prolonging the action of hormones, called incretins, which help increase insulin production and release. The medications are new, but so far they seem to be free of major side effects.

• **Combination products** that contain medications from different classes in one pill include pioglitazone/metformin (Actoplus Met), rosiglitazone/glimepiride (Avandaryl), metformin/glyburide (Glucovance), and metformin/glipizide (Metaglip).

Effectiveness

All of the oral medications have been shown to improve blood glucose control and reduce the risk of diabetes complications, namely kidney disease and retinopathy. The glucose-lowering effects of these drugs are roughly similar; trials have shown an average reduction in HbA1c levels of 1–1.5 percentage points. The exceptions are the alpha-glucosidase inhibitors, which do not lower HbA1c levels quite as much. But since all oral diabetes drugs work in broadly different ways, some people might respond better to one type of treatment than to another.

Metformin is usually the first drug tried, because it does not promote weight gain or cause hypoglycemia. But a mix of lifestyle measures and metformin is often not enough to keep blood glucose under control. That's where drug combinations come into play.

Recent studies have found that combination pills are particularly beneficial. For example, while metformin can reduce blood glucose levels by about 20% when used alone, it can also boost the effectiveness of a sulfonylurea by 25%. If lifestyle changes and metformin are not effective in maintaining blood glucose, the next steps are to add another medication: either insulin, a sulfonylurea, or a thiazolidinedione.

Oral diabetes medications help to control blood glucose levels when diet and exercise fail to do so alone. But they should not be seen as replacing these measures. In a recent review of nearly 17 studies that followed more than 8,000 people with impaired glucose tolerance, lifestyle interventions were at least as effective in preventing or delaying type 2 diabetes as drug treatments. ■

Alpha-glucosidase inhibitors

The drugs acarbose (Precose) and miglitol (Glyset) block the action of the alpha-glucosidase enzymes that break down carbohydrates (starches and sucrose) in your digestive tract. As a result, digestion is delayed, glucose passes into the bloodstream more slowly, and blood glucose levels stay lower after a meal. On the negative side, the undigested carbohydrates often cause gas, diarrhea, and abdominal discomfort. Although these side effects tend to lessen over time, Precose and Glyset are not recommended for people with inflammatory bowel disease, liver or kidney disease, or other serious intestinal disorders.

When taken alone, Precose and Glyset do not cause hypoglycemia. However, hypoglycemia may occur when either drug is used in combination with a sulfonylurea, a meglitinide, or insulin. It is important to remember that alpha-glucosidase inhibitors block the digestion of sucrose, so don't reach for a candy bar if you develop hypoglycemia. You need to eat glucose (dextrose) or drink milk or fruit juice (fruit contains fructose and glucose).

Dipeptidyl peptidase-4 (DPP-4) inhibitors

The newest diabetes drug is sitagliptin (Januvia), which prolongs the activity of proteins that boost the release of insulin after blood sugar rises. By blocking an enzyme—dipeptidyl peptidase 4, or DPP-4—that breaks down these proteins, the drug leads to better blood sugar control. Januvia can be used alone or in combination with two other commonly prescribed oral diabetes medications, metformin or Starlix, when either of these treatments fails to provide adequate blood sugar control by itself.

The most common side effects from Januvia seem to be mild and include a possible increase in upper respiratory infections, headache, stuffy or runny nose, and sore throat. If you have kidney problems, you may need lower doses of the drug. You should also have periodic blood tests to measure how well your kidneys are working.

Byetta

When oral medication is not enough to control blood glucose levels, your doctor may prescribe an injected medication other than insulin. Called exenatide (Byetta), this medication belongs to a new class of type 2 diabetes drugs known as incretin mimetics. Drugs in this class mimic the action of glucagon-like peptide-1 (GLP-1), a hormone that triggers insulin production after a meal. Byetta acts only when blood glucose levels are high. This is an important difference from other diabetes drugs, which often cause hypoglycemia by triggering insulin secretion even when blood glucose levels are low.

Byetta is a synthetic version of a protein derived from the saliva of a venomous lizard known as the Gila monster. It is an injected medication that is taken in addition to metformin and/or a sulfonylurea. In one study, nearly half of individuals who had previously been unable to control their blood glucose with oral medication reduced their HbA1c levels to 7% or lower after taking Byetta for 30 weeks. Byetta users also lost 3–6 lbs on average.

Byetta is not recommended for people with type 1 diabetes, severe kidney disease, or severe gastrointestinal disease. Nausea is the most common side effect. Vomiting and diarrhea may also occur. Because Byetta slows the absorption of oral drugs, you may need to take certain medications at least one hour before an injection of Byetta.

Insulin

Everyone with type 1 diabetes needs insulin treatment to control his or her disease. In addition, about 40% of those with type 2 diabetes eventually require some type of insulin treatment to control their blood glucose, either because their diabetes gets worse or it no longer responds to oral drugs. Many people with type 2 diabetes take insulin in combination with a sulfonylurea, metformin, or a thiazolidinedione.

Types of insulin

Insulin cannot be taken by mouth because digestive enzymes would break it down before it reaches the bloodstream. Therefore, insulin must be taken via injections under the skin (subcutaneous) or via a pump that dispenses insulin under the skin.

There are four main types of insulin:

- Regular (short-acting)
- Rapid-acting
- Intermediate-acting
- Long-acting.

Insulin was once obtained exclusively from pig or cow pancreas. Today, regular and intermediate-acting insulins are referred to as human insulins, because they are manufactured to be identical to the insulin produced by the human pancreas. Rapid- and long-acting insulins are chemically modified forms of human insulin.

Most individuals need to use more than one type of insulin, so they either mix two types of insulin together or buy prepared (premixed) insulin mixtures.

The insulin types differ in three ways:

- Onset—the length of time it takes for the insulin to reach the bloodstream and begin lowering blood glucose.
- Peak activity—the period of time during which insulin has its maximum effect in lowering blood glucose.
- Duration—the amount of time the insulin continues to lower blood glucose.

Regular or short-acting insulin. This type of insulin is manufactured to be similar to the insulin produced in the human body. Popular brands have an "R" (for regular) in their names, for example, Humulin R and Novolin R.

Regular insulin is typically injected 30–60 minutes before meals and usually reaches the bloodstream within 30 minutes, in time to cover the rise in blood glucose that begins after food is eaten. Insulin action peaks one and a half to two hours after injection and

When To Start Insulin for Type 2 Diabetes

If the time comes for insulin, don't delay

Despite the importance of diet and nutrition in controlling blood glucose—and the growing number of easy-to-take drugs that are available when lifestyle changes are not enough—everyone with type 1 diabetes and many people with type 2 diabetes do need insulin.

Insulin treatment, which is a necessity for type 1 diabetes, has traditionally been thought of as a last resort for type 2 disease when lifestyle and oral medications no longer manage blood glucose levels effectively and complications threaten to develop. Individuals with diabetes, unfortunately, resist taking insulin all too often. They may view it as punishment for not controlling the condition through diet and exercise. They may (mistakenly) associate taking insulin with the bad outcome they heard about from a friend or relative. They may exaggerate the difficulty or pain of insulin injections. But for whatever reason, starting insulin too late in type 2 diabetes often causes unnecessary diabetes complications to develop.

As Diabetes Progresses

It's true that standard oral drugs like metformin (Glucophage, Glucophage XR, Glumetza) allow more people to keep their average blood glucose within the target range compared with diet alone, at least for a while. And combinations of pills may keep levels in a good range for even longer. But if you find that your diabetes medication isn't doing what it used to, you're not alone.

According to the landmark United Kingdom Prospective Diabetes Study (UKPDS) Group, which followed 4,075 patients newly diagnosed with type 2 diabetes, as many as half of them needed to add other medications to get the same blood glucose control after three years of taking a single drug. What's more, by nine years after diagnosis, even with the combination of medications, a significant number of individuals needed insulin to reach target HbA1c levels. Clearly this decline in glucose control is not a matter of personal defeat, but rather the natural progression of the disease.

Timing Is Everything

The key is not waiting too long to start. Adding insulin at the first signs that other medications are ineffective is your best shot at getting the disease back under control. Know your HbA1c level, and if it is persistently over about 7%, consider whether the next step is more pills or starting insulin.

Keeping insulin as a last resort strategy can be dangerous. If blood glucose levels have been too high for years, diabetes complications are more likely to appear. Compared with individuals who use oral drugs alone, studies have shown that people with diabetes who started insulin early achieved optimal blood glucose levels, potentially lowered the risk of some heart disease complications, and found it easier to attain glucose control later on.

The general guidelines for when you should consider adding insulin therapy are as follows:

- If your average glucose levels are above 7%, as measured by your doctor with an HbA1c test
- If your fasting glucose levels fail to stay between about 90 and 130 mg/dL
- If your glucose levels are more than 180 mg/dL after eating.

According to research, people

the effects last about eight to 10 hours.

Rapid-acting insulin. Insulin aspart (Novolog), insulin lispro (Humalog), and insulin glulisine (Apidra) are called insulin analogues, because their chemical structure is a modified form of human insulin that is designed to work more quickly and peak faster than regular insulin. These manufactured insulins are safer to use because they work more closely to how natural insulin functions in the body. Consequently, they are more effective in preventing high who are less likely to achieve these targets tend to be younger, more obese, or have higher blood sugar levels to begin with than others with diabetes.

Other deciding factors for starting insulin early in the disease include additional health problems such as heart or kidney disease, a new diagnosis of severe hyperglycemia and other diabetes symptoms, and allergies to or an inability to tolerate oral diabetes medications.

Treatment Steps

The American Diabetes Association recommends the following protocol to initiate insulin therapy.

• **If your control of the disease is very poor**, you may start insulin without first trying oral medications and lifestyle changes. This approach is considered when fasting blood glucose levels greater than 250 mg/dL, random glucose levels consistently higher than 300 mg/dL, or HbA1c levels greater than 10% are accompanied by symptoms like frequent urination, excessive thirst, weight loss, and the presence of ketones in the urine. All this means is that at least for the moment, you are less likely to respond to pills.

• **If after two to three months of lifestyle changes and treatment** with metformin or another oral medication your HbA1c levels are still above 8.5%, you should consider starting insulin therapy.

• **If you have added a second oral medication to metformin and lifestyle changes** but your HbA1c levels are still above 7%, consider insulin therapy as the next step.

• **If you start on insulin therapy, oral medication can be continued** and the insulin doses can be intensified gradually by adding injections of rapid-acting insulin before meals.

Before You Begin

Of course, cautions must be observed when starting insulin, just like with any other medicine. The most common side effects are hypoglycemia (a sharp drop in blood glucose) and weight gain, but both can be managed. Low blood sugar episodes are less frequent and less severe among people with type 2 diabetes than in those with type 1. Weight gain is less likely with the newer longer-acting insulins like insulin detemir (Levemir). Also, combining insulin with metformin helps minimize weight gain.

You should take the correct amount of insulin, eat meals at generally regular times, and have a snack before exercise to prevent hypoglycemia. You need to know the kind(s) of insulin you are taking and how quickly they act.

People with type 2 diabetes are often started on a long-acting insulin such as insulin glargine (Lantus) or Levemir, which act continuously over most or all of the day. NPH insulin (Humulin N, Novolin N) is an intermediate-acting insulin that is usually effective for about 12 hours. You can then add short-acting insulins such as regular insulin (Humulin R, Novolin R), insulin aspart (Novolog), or insulin lispro (Humalog), which are taken directly before meals to "cover" the rise in blood glucose provoked by eating.

In most cases, the benefits of insulin therapy far outweigh the risks. Taking insulin doesn't have to be a hindrance, and it can be tailored to fit your lifestyle. Very thin needles and insulin pens make it much more convenient to take insulin these days. (See the chart on pages 50–53 for complete information on different types of insulin.) ■

blood glucose (hyperglycemia) after meals and are less likely to produce hypoglycemia.

Rapid-acting insulin must be injected immediately before meals because it starts to work within five to 15 minutes. You must eat right away after injecting or your glucose will drop too low. Peak action occurs in 30–60 minutes, with a short duration of action of four to six hours. Novolog, Humalog, and Apidra are sold only by prescription, as their effects in children and pregnant women aren't known.

Intermediate-acting insulin. This type of human insulin called NPH insulin contains protamine, which makes the solution cloudy and slows the absorption of insulin. NPH insulins have an "N" in their names, for example, Humulin N and Novolin N.

After injection, intermediate-acting insulins reach the bloodstream within two to four hours and show peak action in four to eight hours. Duration of action is from 12–20 hours. Intermediate-acting insulin is often used in combination with regular or short-acting insulin.

Long-acting insulin. Both insulin glargine (Lantus) and insulin detemir (Levemir) are long-acting insulin analogues. They are often used alone in people with type 2 diabetes, or in combination with a more quick-acting insulin.

Lantus is a clear solution in the vial, but it precipitates in the skin after injection. This precipitation greatly slows the absorption of Lantus, making it very long acting, usually 18–24 hours. Levemir also is absorbed slowly, because it binds to the protein albumin in the skin. Its effects last 14–18 hours.

Insulin combinations. Most individuals with diabetes use a combination of insulin types. Regular or rapid-acting insulin is generally needed before meals to reduce the after-meal increase in blood glucose levels. Intermediate- or long-acting insulin is the usual choice at bedtime to control blood glucose levels overnight.

Regular or rapid-acting insulin can be combined in the same syringe with intermediate-acting NPH insulin but not with the long-acting insulins Lantus and Levemir. Because NPH insulin can modify regular and rapid-acting insulin, it's best to inject the combination within five minutes of mixing the two insulin types.

Combining regular or rapid-acting insulin with intermediate-acting insulin can be simplified with the use of premixed products. Your physician can prescribe a 70/30 mixture, which contains 70% NPH and 30% regular insulin, or a 50/50 mixture, which contains 50% NPH and 50% regular insulin. Premixed products containing insulin aspart or insulin lispro with an intermediate-acting insulin also are available. However, the fixed ratio of the two insulin types in premixed products is unsuitable for many people because the quantity of each insulin cannot be adjusted to match the specific foods eaten at each meal.

Insulin adjuncts. Symlin (pramlintide) is for people who inject insulin but have not achieved adequate glucose control. It is a synthetic version of a hormone produced by the pancreas called amylin, which blocks the release of glucose from the liver, slows the passage of food from the stomach to intestines, and suppresses appetite. Symlin must be injected before meals. A recent review found that Symlin users lowered their HbA1c levels by up to 0.7% and lost 4 lbs, on average.

Modes of insulin administration

The most common way to take insulin is as a subcutaneous (under the skin) injection at a site where there is fat tissue. The most common injection sites are the abdomen (except for a 2-inch area around the navel), the front and outer side of the thigh, the upper part of the buttocks, and the outer side of the upper arm. Many people find that insulin is absorbed fastest from the stomach area.

When you first begin insulin treatment, you'll probably use a needle and syringe for your injections. Your doctor or nurse educator will show you how to load the syringes, how to inject yourself, and how to rotate injection sites to prevent damage to any one area and to provide the absorption speed that meets your needs. When you become more experienced at the injections, you may explore other options, such as insulin pens, jet injectors, or an external insulin pump.

Insulin syringes. For years, injection of insulin with a needle and syringe was the only option. Syringes are still the best choice for most people who mix different types of insulin for a single injection. Fortunately, the syringes currently available—disposable, lightweight syringes with shorter, ultrafine needles—make daily injections more convenient and less painful. They come in a wide variety of sizes and styles, so you'll want to experiment to find the size that works best for you. For example, individuals who are overweight may not be able to use very short needles.

Insulin pens. Insulin pens combine an insulin container and syringe in one compact device. Two types are available: reusable and prefilled. With reusable pens, you load a cartridge of insulin into the pen, attach a needle, dial in your insulin dose, and press the plunger to administer the injection. Prefilled pens contain a built-in insulin cartridge and are even easier to use, although they can be expensive. After the insulin is used up, you throw the prefilled pen away.

Jet injectors. Jet injectors use a high-pressure jet of air to send a fine stream of insulin through the skin. Although jet injectors eliminate the need for needle sticks, they cause as much pain as insulin injections and often result in bruises. In addition, jet injectors are bulky and expensive, adding to the reasons they are not widely used.

External insulin pumps. Some people who require frequent insulin injections do better with an external insulin pump, which

ASK THE DOCTOR

Q. ***Am I a good candidate for an insulin pump?***

A. Insulin pumps have been used to treat type 1 diabetes for the past 20 years. The external pumps are small, computerized devices that deliver insulin through a thin tube inserted via a needle into the skin of the stomach or thigh. Their big draw is that they offer flexibility, convenience, and an insulin flow that is completely predictable since you program it yourself.

Most people with type 2 diabetes who require insulin have fairly stable blood glucose levels, often requiring just one or two injections per day, so an insulin pump isn't needed. But in hard-to-treat type 2 individuals, when glucose levels become very unstable and multiple doses of insulin are needed daily, the device may be beneficial. One study found that insulin pumps were comparable to multiple daily injections in keeping type 2 diabetes under tight control, and most of the participants preferred the devices to shots.

Individuals must be knowledgeable about their diabetes and committed to regular glucose monitoring when using an insulin pump. Unlike shots, you have to make sure to set the delivery rate correctly, check the tubing for blockages and change it regularly, and keep the insulin storage chamber full. Since pumps only use rapid-acting insulin, any malfunction can cause a rapid drop in insulin levels, so you need to monitor your blood glucose several times a day. If you think you would benefit from using an insulin pump, discuss it with your doctor.

Injected Medications for Diabetes 2008

Drug type: Brand (generic)	Peak activity*	How to take†	Cost‡
Rapid-acting injected insulin			
Apidra (insulin glulisine)	30–60 minutes	Inject just before starting a meal.	5 3-mL cartridges (100 mg/mL): $167
Novolog (insulin aspart)	30–60 minutes	Inject within 5–10 minutes of eating a meal.	10-mL vial (100 mg/mL): $89 5 3-mL syringes (100 mg/mL): $158
Humalog (insulin lispro)	30–60 minutes	Inject within 15 minutes before or immediately after eating a meal.	10-mL vial (100 mg/mL): $79 3-mL cartridge (100 mg/mL): $31
Regular or short-acting injected insulin			
Humulin R (regular insulin)	1.5–2 hours	Inject within 30–60 minutes of eating a meal or immediately after the meal.	10-mL vial (100 mg/mL): $35 20-mL vial (500 mg/mL): $185
Novolin R (regular insulin)	1.5–2 hours	Inject within 30–60 minutes of eating a meal or immediately after the meal.	10-mL vial (100 mg/mL): $39 3-mL cartridge (100 mg/mL): $16
Intermediate-acting injected insulin			
Humulin N (NPH insulin)	4–8 hours	Gently mix until milky. Then inject in the morning and before bedtime. Inject quickly over 2–4 seconds.	10-mL vial (100 mg/mL): $35 5 3-mL cartridges (100 mg/mL): $90
Novolin N (NPH insulin)	4–8 hours	Same as for Humulin N (see above).	10-mL vial (100 mg/mL): $39 5 3-mL cartridges (100 mg/mL): $81–107
Long-acting injected insulin			
Lantus (insulin glargine)	No peak	Gently mix and then inject 1x/day before breakfast, dinner, or bedtime.	10-mL vial (100 mg/mL): $80 5 3-mL cartridges (100 mg/mL): $157
Levemir (insulin detemir)	No peak	Inject 1x/day with dinner or at bedtime or 2x/day in the morning and with dinner, at bedtime, or 12 hours after the morning injection.	10-mL vial (100 mg/mL): $84 5 3-mL syringes (100 mg/mL): $159
Premixed insulin			
Humulin 50/50 (50% NPH/50% regular)	Varies	Gently mix until milky. Then inject 2x/day within 15 minutes before eating breakfast and dinner.	10-mL vial: $32
Humulin 70/30, Novolin 70/30 (70% NPH/30% regular)	Varies	Gently mix until milky. Then inject 2x/day within 15 minutes before eating breakfast and dinner.	10-mL vial: $37–40 5 3-mL cartridges: $81–108
Novolog 70/30 (70% aspart protamine/ 30% aspart)	Varies	Gently mix until milky. Then inject 2x/day within 5–10 minutes before eating breakfast and dinner.	5 3-mL syringes: $167
Humalog 75/25 (70% lispro protamine/25% lispro)	Varies	Gently mix until milky. Then inject 2x/day within 5–10 minutes before eating breakfast and dinner.	10-mL vial: $84 5 3-mL syringes: $148

Precautions	Most common side effects	Call your doctor if...
To prevent hypoglycemia, do not delay eating after the injection. Do not use if the solution is cloudy or colored. Do not mix rapid-acting insulin with insulin glargine (Lantus) or insulin detemir (Levemir). If you mix rapid-acting insulin with NPH insulin, draw the rapid-acting insulin into the syringe first; then, inject the mixture right away.	Hypoglycemia	You experience an injection site reaction (for example, pain, redness, irritation); have severe or recurrent hypoglycemia.
Do not use if the solution is cloudy or colored. To prevent hypoglycemia, do not delay eating after the injection. Do not mix short-acting insulin with other types of insulin besides NPH insulin. If you mix short-acting insulin with NPH insulin, draw the short-acting insulin into the syringe first; then, inject the mixture right away.	Hypoglycemia	You experience an injection site reaction (for example, pain, redness, irritation); have severe or recurrent hypoglycemia.
May be mixed only with short- or rapid-acting insulin. Draw the short- or rapid-acting insulin into the syringe first, followed by the intermediate-acting insulin, and inject right away.	Hypoglycemia	You experience an injection site reaction (for example, pain, redness, irritation); have severe or recurrent hypoglycemia.
Do not use if the solution is cloudy or colored. Do not mix with other types of insulin.	Hypoglycemia	You experience an injection site reaction (for example, pain, redness, irritation); have severe or recurrent hypoglycemia.
To prevent hypoglycemia, do not delay eating after the injection.	Hypoglycemia	You experience an injection site reaction (for example, pain, redness, irritation); have severe or recurrent hypoglycemia.

* The length of time the insulin has its maximum blood glucose–lowering effect.

† These instructions represent the typical way to take the medication. Your doctor's instructions may differ. Always follow your doctor's recommendations.

‡ Prices per drugstore.com.

continued on the next page

Injected Medications for Diabetes 2008 (continued)

Drug type: Brand (generic)	Peak activity*	How to take†	Cost‡
Other injected medications			
Byetta (exenatide)	Not applicable	Inject 5–10 micrograms (mcg) 2x/day within 1 hour before your morning and evening meals.	1.2 mL cartridge (250 mcg/mL): $200 2.4 mL cartridge (250 mcg/mL): $226
Symlin (pramlintide)	Not applicable	Inject 15, 30, 45, 60, or 120 mcg immediately before a major meal (containing more than 250 calories or more than 30 g of carbohydrate).	5 mL solution (600 mcg/mL): $115

* The length of time the insulin has its maximum blood glucose–lowering effect.

† These instructions represent the typical way to take the medication. Your doctor's instructions may differ. Always follow your doctor's recommendations.

‡ Prices per drugstore.com.

more closely mimics the work of the pancreas. The pump is a small, portable device (usually worn at the waist) that delivers insulin through a tube (a catheter) attached to a small needle inserted just below the skin of the abdomen or thigh. The pump is easy to use. It is programmed to automatically deliver a continuous amount of insulin throughout the day. Before meals, the user presses a button to deliver the extra insulin needed.

Insulin pumps are primarily used by people with type 1 diabetes, but more type 2 patients are starting to use the pump. The biggest advantage of the pump is improved blood glucose control. For example, in a four-month study of 79 people, pump users had an average HbA1c level that was 0.8 percentage points lower than that of people on injected insulin therapy.

There are drawbacks to insulin pumps, including the need for frequent blood glucose monitoring. However, some newer pumps are equipped with glucose meters; one, the Medtronic Minimed Paradigm, recommends bolus dosages based on current blood glucose levels, how much insulin remains in your body, and how many carbohydrates you expect to eat in your next meal. Users must also be vigilant for skin infections, pump malfunctions, leaks in the catheter, and inadvertent removal of the needle from its site beneath the skin. Any of these interruptions in the insulin infusion can cause a rapid fall in blood insulin levels that could result in ketoacidosis in people with type 1 diabetes. (See the "Ask the Doctor" column on page 49.)

Precautions	Most common side effects	Call your doctor if...
Do not inject after a meal. Do not use if cloudy or colored.	Nausea, vomiting, diarrhea. Can also produce mild to moderate hypoglycemia when used with a sulfonylurea.	Any of the side effects mentioned at left persist or worsen. You experience signs of pancreatitis: persistent, severe abdominal pain which may be accompanied by vomiting.
Do not mix with insulin. Do not use if cloudy or colored. Do not inject in your upper arm.	Hypoglycemia, nausea, vomiting, lack of appetite, headache.	You experience an injection site reaction (for example, pain, redness, irritation).

Now that long-acting insulins like Lantus and Levemir are available, they may be a more practical choice than the pump for some people. Studies have shown that once-a-day injections of Lantus plus Humalog or Novolog injections prior to meals is a close second to the efficacy of pump treatment.

Inhaled insulins. In 2006, the FDA approved Exubera, the first inhaled insulin. Exubera was a dry powder administered with a device similar to an asthma inhaler. It could take the place of premeal insulin injections but could not be used as a substitute for longer-acting insulin needed in the morning or before bed. Exubera was pulled from the market in late 2007 due to low sales, partly because of concerns from doctors whether it was safe for the lungs. Other inhaled insulins are currently in development and seeking FDA approval as early as 2009.

Techniques under development. Researchers are working on several new approaches to insulin delivery, including nasal sprays, pills, and skin patches.

Also in the works is an implantable insulin pump, which is placed under the skin on the left side of the abdomen. The pump delivers insulin in small, intermittent pulses at a constant rate via a catheter. The insulin pulses are supplemented by mealtime doses of insulin that are controlled with an external device that transmits commands to the pump. Needle injections are required only every few months to refill the pump.

About 1,500 people worldwide have been treated with implantable pumps. In fact, the device is approved for use in several European countries. Currently, the manufacturer is not pursuing FDA approval of the pump in the United States. Thus, for now, these implantable pumps are available only to people participating in clinical trials. Results so far suggest that implantable insulin pumps may be a good long-term option for people with poorly controlled blood glucose levels.

Adverse effects of insulin

People taking insulin are susceptible to hypoglycemia when they administer too much insulin, delay or miss a meal, exercise without first eating a snack, or drink alcohol on an empty stomach. That's why insulin treatment requires careful attention to the timing of meals, exercise, and alcohol intake. If you're taking insulin, you'll also need to test your blood glucose at home, perhaps several times a day. Your doctor will also perform periodic HbA1c tests to check your overall glucose control and to help you find the best doses of insulin that will keep your blood glucose low, but not so low that you have episodes of hypoglycemia.

Other adverse effects of insulin include loss or overgrowth of fat tissue at injection sites, allergic reactions, and insulin resistance. If you inject in the same area over and over again, you may develop fat deposits there, which reduce insulin absorption. This effect is less common with the types of insulin used today, and you can prevent it by rotating injection sites. Allergic reactions are also less common with the newer insulins. If you suffer reactions, you can be treated with a desensitization procedure that involves starting with injections of small doses of insulin and gradually increasing to higher doses. Insulin resistance, which may be caused by the formation of antibodies against insulin, is usually managed by increasing the insulin dose.

Dealing With Episodes of Hypoglycemia

Insulin treatment is not the only cause of hypoglycemia (low blood glucose). Hypoglycemia can also result from treatment with an oral sulfonylurea, a meglitinide, or a D-phenylalanine derivative. But unexplained "lows" frequently occur even in people who carefully control their medications and regularly monitor their blood glucose levels. That's why it's important to recognize the early signs of hypoglycemia and know what to do when they occur.

There are two types of hypoglycemic symptoms: adrenergic and neurologic.

Adrenergic symptoms

Sweating, heart palpitations, nervousness, hunger, faintness, and weakness are the earliest signs that your blood glucose has dropped below about 60 mg/dL. When your blood glucose is this low, a hormone called epinephrine is released into the bloodstream. Epinephrine triggers the liver to increase its glucose production and the pancreas to release glucagon, another hormone that increases blood glucose.

These unpleasant adrenergic symptoms warn you that you must immediately eat or drink something with sugar to raise your blood glucose level. The best choices are sugars that are rapidly absorbed into the bloodstream, such as 4 oz of orange juice, 6 oz of nondiet soda, five to seven hard candies, or two to five glucose tablets. You should always have one of these fast-acting carbohydrates on hand. But do not reach for chocolate or nuts to treat an episode of hypoglycemia. These high-carbohydrate foods contain fat that slows down their digestion.

Neurologic symptoms

If your blood glucose drops to below 40 mg/dL, you may develop severe neurologic symptoms such as headache, lack of coordination, double vision, slurred speech, confusion, and numbness in your fingers and around your mouth. This can happen if you are taking a beta-blocker (a heart medication) or have diabetes-related nerve damage. It can also happen if you have had diabetes for five to 10 years, because the body's response to low blood glucose, particularly the release of glucagon, may no longer occur.

Neurologic symptoms are a sign of a dangerous situation because you may be too sick or too confused to realize what is happening and know what to do about it. Without treatment, extreme hypoglycemia can cause seizures, coma, and, in rare cases, permanent brain damage and death. If you are taking insulin or an oral diabetes drug that can cause hypoglycemia, your doctor or diabetes educator will train you (and family members or friends who would be available to help you) on how to give a glucagon injection, which can rapidly raise blood glucose levels. It's easy to do, because you can inject glucagon almost anywhere (in the abdomen, thigh, buttocks, or upper arm), and it's nearly impossible to take an overdose.

You'll need a prescription to buy prefilled glucagon syringes, which you should keep on hand at all times. The glucagon syringe should be kept cool but need not be refrigerated and should be replaced on the expiration date. If glucagon is unavailable or its use does not revive the person with diabetes, an ambulance must be called immediately.

Pancreas and Islet Transplants

For some people with type 1 diabetes, even frequent insulin injections or use of an insulin pump can no longer prevent serious, life-threatening glucose highs (hyperglycemia) and lows (hypoglycemia). Since there is currently no way to get the beta cells in the pancreas to work again, researchers hypothesized that getting a new pancreas would solve the problem. Years ago, that was only a dream. But thanks to advances in transplantation surgery, it's now a possibility, although a complicated one.

Pancreas transplantation

First, you need to be fairly young (the best candidates are age 45 or younger) and in relatively good health. Second, you need a donor. Since each person has only one pancreas, a living person cannot donate a whole pancreas. But if a close relative is a good match for you, based on your human leukocyte antigen (HLA) type, he or she could provide a partial pancreas transplant. That's often done if a relative is also donating one of his or her kidneys to you, since many people with type 1 diabetes also have severe "end-stage" kidney disease that requires a kidney transplant. But if a living donor is not available, you'll have to wait for a nonliving (cadaver) donor whose pancreas is a good match for you.

Donor organs of all types are scarce and pancreas transplant surgery is technically difficult. However, more than 1,000 pancreas transplants a year are performed in the United States, and yours may be one of them. If so, be sure to choose an experienced surgical team that has performed a large number of pancreas and kidney transplants and has a high rate of successful outcomes. However, even if your pancreas transplant surgery is a success, you'll be trading your daily insulin injections for a lifelong regimen of powerful immune-suppressing drugs to help prevent your body from rejecting the new pancreas. These drugs can cause serious side effects, including an increased risk of infections and cancer, elevated blood pressure and cholesterol levels, and more rapid deterioration of kidney function. Even with the immunosuppressant treatment, as many as half of all pancreas transplants are rejected.

People who get a combined pancreas-kidney transplant have better survival rates than those who undergo a pancreas transplant alone. If you qualify for a pancreas transplant, it is best to undergo the combined procedure rather than having two separate transplant surgeries. Another advantage is that the same immunosuppressant drugs work for both kidney and pancreas transplants.

There is no evidence that a pancreas transplant (or a combined pancreas-kidney transplant) can halt or reverse any diabetes complications you already have, such as kidney damage (nephropathy), eye damage (retinopathy), or blood vessel damage (macrovascular disease). Indeed, about 5% of people who undergo pancreas or pancreas-kidney transplantation will die within a year, either because of complications of immunosuppressant treatment or of diabetes. A recent study showed that people still waiting for a pancreas transplant had a lower risk of dying within one to four years than people who had received a transplant. As all of these findings indicate, transplantation is not a perfect solution.

Islet transplantation

Researchers are now focusing on transplantation of pancreatic islets (clusters of insulin-secreting beta cells) rather than transplanting a whole or partial pancreas. With islet transplants, pancreases from two or three deceased donors are treated with an enzyme that breaks up connective tissue so that islet cells can be separated out for removal. Then the surgeon injects the islets through a blood vessel in the patient's abdomen and into the liver via a small plastic tube (a catheter). Direct injection into the pancreas is not possible because of the risk of inflammation. The procedure was developed at the University of Alberta in Edmonton, Canada.

Several hundred islet cell transplants have been done using the Edmonton protocol. One year after transplantation, a majority of patients no longer need insulin injections, although they do need powerful immunosuppressant drugs to prevent transplant rejection. However, within five years, most patients are again back on insulin, because the transplanted islets stop working or are damaged by the immunosuppressant drugs.

One possible way to overcome these problems is to obtain a large number of islet cells from just one nonliving donor, which would decrease the risk of rejection. In a 2005 study, researchers treated people who had type 1 diabetes with inflammation-preventing drugs, then performed transplants using islet cells from single donors. In the study, five of the eight patients maintained good blood glucose control one year later, without the need for insulin injections. In another recent study, Japanese doctors successfully

How To Control Blood Glucose During an Illness

Getting sick can trigger rises in blood glucose levels

People with diabetes must be especially careful when suffering from an illness like a cold or the flu. Illness not only affects your eating, sleeping, and exercise habits—which are closely linked to blood glucose control—but it may also cause the liver to make and release glucose into the bloodstream. This increase in glucose released from the liver provides extra energy to combat the stress of an illness, but in people with diabetes it can cause blood glucose to rise too high, whether or not you are eating.

At the same time, an illness decreases the sensitivity of cells to insulin and makes it more difficult for these cells to remove glucose from the bloodstream. A person without diabetes can produce extra insulin to help the additional glucose enter cells. But people with diabetes are less able to produce extra insulin or respond to it effectively. The resulting rise in blood glucose increases the risk of diabetic ketoacidosis in people with type 1 diabetes and hyperosmolar nonketotic state in those with type 2 diabetes. To prevent these serious complications as well as to minimize fluctuations in blood glucose levels, follow these sick-day precautions.

- **Inform your healthcare professional when you become sick.** This precaution is particularly important if you are unable to eat regular foods, have diarrhea or vomiting for more than six hours, or have had a fever for a couple of days that is not improving.
- **Follow the treatment plan for the sickness.** For example, take any necessary medications, such as antibiotics for an infection, according to schedule. If you are treated by a doctor you have never seen before, make sure he or she is aware of your diabetes.
- **Test blood glucose levels more often than usual.** If you have type 1 diabetes, test levels of blood glucose and urine ketones every four hours, even during the night. (Set an alarm clock or have someone wake you up.) If you have type 2 diabetes, testing blood glucose levels four times during the day is probably enough; if blood glucose levels exceed 250 mg/dL, test urine for ketones. Call your health care professional if blood glucose levels are consistently above 250 mg/dL and are accompanied by ketones in the urine.

transplanted islet cells taken from a *living* donor into a woman with type 1 diabetes.

Stem-cell transplants

The shortage of organs from living and nonliving pancreas donors is also spurring research into other means of producing beta cells, either by using donor cells to grow new cells in the lab (culturing human islet cell lines) or by growing beta cells from stem cells. This research is in its infancy, and many more laboratory and animal studies are needed before these techniques can be attempted in humans.

Alternative and Complementary Treatments

The use of alternative therapies for many diseases, including diabetes, is increasingly popular. People often turn to therapies that are outside the medical mainstream, especially when conventional medications cause troubling side effects or aren't sufficiently effective.

The problem, however, is that few nontraditional treatments have

Preventing Illness in the First Place

To prevent flu and pneumonia, the American Diabetes Association strongly recommends that people over six months of age who have diabetes receive a flu vaccine once a year. The vaccine is available at doctors' offices, clinics, and pharmacies, among other places. The best time to get vaccinated is at the beginning of the flu season—between September and November. The pneumonia vaccine is also recommended for people with diabetes. If you are over age 65 and have not had a pneumonia vaccination in the past five years, you need a second one.

• **Take your diabetes medication as usual,** unless, of course, your health professional advises otherwise. Being sick causes blood glucose levels to rise, even if you are not eating.

• **If you use insulin, keep a bottle of rapid- or very rapid–acting insulin handy.** You should take this precaution even if you do not take these types of insulin regularly. Use the rapid- or very rapid– acting insulin if your health professional tells you to take an extra sick-day dose or if you need to lower your blood glucose levels quickly.

• **Watch for any symptoms of dehydration, ketoacidosis, or hyperosmolar nonketotic state.** The symptoms of dehydration include dry mouth, cracked lips, and dry or flushed skin. Ketoacidosis symptoms include nausea, vomiting, and lack of appetite, while hyperosmolar nonketotic state is characterized by increased hunger, nausea, or stomach pain. Contact your health professional if any of these symptoms occur.

• **Prevent dehydration by drinking plenty of liquids.** You should consume at least one large (8 oz) glass of clear fluid each hour while awake. If your usual diet is not disrupted by the illness, drink water, tea, broth, or other sugar-free beverages. If you are unable to eat meals, alternate sugar-containing fluids with those that are sugar free.

• **Try to consume a normal amount of carbohydrates.** Eating many small portions throughout the day may help. Eat easy-to-digest foods such as gelatin, crackers, soup, and applesauce.

• **Rest as much as possible.** If necessary, get someone—such as a family member or friend—to help care for you. ■

been evaluated in well-designed research studies. So if you want to try any alternative or complementary treatments, talk to your doctor beforehand and do not discontinue your regular therapies. These alternative therapies should be used in addition to—not instead of—your prescribed treatment regimen, and your doctor needs to check for potential interactions with your diabetes drugs that could cause hypoglycemia or hyperglycemia.

Supplements

Dietary supplements being marketed for blood glucose control include *Gymnema sylvestre*, psyllium, garlic, cinnamon, cherry extract, and Chinese ginseng. Alpha-lipoic acid, evening primrose oil, ginkgo biloba, and chelation therapy also are purported to treat or prevent the major complications of diabetes. But be aware that there is little or no research showing that any of these treatments is beneficial for people with diabetes.

What's more, because the FDA does not regulate supplements,

there's no guarantee these products are free of toxic contaminants or that they contain the amount of active ingredients listed on the label. You can avoid these problems by buying supplements that meet U.S. Pharmacopeia standards (look for the USP symbol) or by checking results from ConsumerLab, an independent testing laboratory, at www.consumerlab.com. Keep an eye on your pocketbook, too. Many unproven remedies are sold at high prices to make them appear more valuable.

Vitamins and minerals

Some vitamins and minerals such as vanadium and chromium are advertised as beneficial for people with diabetes. But as you read in the section on dietary measures, the American Diabetes Association does not recommend vitamin and mineral supplements for people with diabetes unless they have vitamin or mineral deficiencies. If you do decide to take vitamins and minerals, be sure you purchase brands that meet U.S. Pharmacopeia standards.

Prevention and Treatment of Long-Term Diabetes Complications

After the initial shock of discovering that you have diabetes, you may settle into a less careful routine of watching your diet, exercising, taking prescribed medications, and seeing your doctor for regular checkups. Although you may feel fine, do not be fooled. Whenever your blood glucose levels go above normal, many organs in your body are affected. Each episode of hyperglycemia may cause minor damage, which over time can lead to major long-term complications, including macrovascular disease (abnormalities of large arteries supplying blood to the heart, brain, and legs), microvascular disease (abnormalities of small blood vessels in the kidneys and eyes), neuropathy (nerve damage), and changes in the skin, gums, teeth, and feet.

These complications of both type 1 and type 2 diabetes typically appear only after someone has had diabetes for years or even decades. Fortunately, their development is not inevitable. Strong evidence suggests that good control of blood glucose and other risk factors, such as high blood pressure and high LDL cholesterol, can prevent or delay the onset of long-term complications and may reduce the severity of complications that do occur. However, improved glucose control may not reverse complications once they appear.

The following section discusses all of the long-term complications of diabetes and the best ways to prevent and treat them.

Macrovascular Disease: Coronary Heart Disease, Stroke, and Peripheral Arterial Disease

People with diabetes are highly susceptible to atherosclerosis—the buildup of deposits called plaques, which form in large arteries. Plaques narrow arteries and can reduce blood flow to the heart, a condition called coronary heart disease (CHD). Partial blockage of the coronary arteries produces angina (chest pain); complete blockage results in a heart attack. Atherosclerosis can also lead to strokes (blockage of blood flow to the brain) and peripheral arterial disease (poor blood flow to the legs). These complications are the cause of death in three quarters of people with diabetes. That's why experts say controlling cardiovascular disease risk factors is just as important as controlling your blood glucose levels.

People with diabetes have a two to four times greater likelihood of CHD than people without diabetes. CHD also tends to appear at an earlier age in people with diabetes. Studies show that diabetes adds significantly to other CHD risk factors such as smoking, high blood pressure, elevated LDL cholesterol levels, and low HDL cholesterol levels. In fact, a Finnish study found that people with type 2 diabetes who have no history of CHD have the same risk of a heart attack as those without diabetes who have already had a heart attack. When elevated blood glucose levels occur together with high blood pressure, abdominal obesity, high blood triglyceride levels, and low HDL cholesterol levels, this is called the metabolic syndrome. This cluster of risk factors puts people at an especially high risk for CHD (and diabetes).

People with diabetes are also two to four times more likely to have a stroke than those without diabetes. High blood glucose likely increases the risk of stroke by promoting atherosclerosis. Also, high blood pressure—one of the most important stroke risk factors—is twice as common in people with diabetes.

Prevention

To reduce the risk of CHD, stroke, and peripheral arterial disease, people with diabetes need to control their ABCs:

- Maintain HbA1c below 7%
- Keep **b**lood pressure lower than 130/80 mm Hg
- Aim for an LDL ("bad") **c**holesterol level below 100 mg/dL (and ideally below 70 mg/dL).

NEW RESEARCH

Don't Count on Chromium To Treat Diabetes

The question of whether a chromium supplement can help people with diabetes in Western cultures was met with a resounding no, according to a new study from the Netherlands.

Previous research from China, where the treatment is popular, had suggested some success in lowering blood glucose levels. However, two other large-scale reviews found chromium to be ineffective.

In this trial, researchers randomly assigned 57 participants with type 2 diabetes who had moderate glycemic control while taking oral medication to take either 400 mcg of chromium yeast or a placebo daily for six months. The volunteers were overweight and had about 34% body fat on average.

At the end of the study, there were no significant differences between the chromium and placebo groups in fasting blood glucose, HbA1c, cholesterol levels, blood pressure, body fat, or insulin resistance.

This research confirms that there is no evidence that taking chromium supplements will improve glycemic control—so avoid these products and stick to your doctor's recommended treatment.

DIABETES CARE
Volume 30, page 1092
May 2007

You may be able to achieve these goals through diet and exercise alone, but most people require medication. Other steps you can take to reduce your risk include quitting smoking, taking an aspirin every day (only with a doctor's advice), keeping triglyceride levels below 150 mg/dL, and increasing HDL ("good") cholesterol levels to higher than 40 mg/dL (for men) or 50 mg/dL (for women).

Treatment

With few exceptions, the treatment of CHD and stroke is the same for people with diabetes as for the general population. High blood pressure and high cholesterol levels are initially treated with diet and other lifestyle measures in an effort to get these conditions under control without medication. Many of these lifestyle measures—for example, diet, weight loss, and exercise—are the same as the ones recommended by the American Diabetes Association for everyone with diabetes. Medication is needed when elevated blood pressure or blood cholesterol persists despite making the necessary lifestyle changes.

Blood pressure control. The latest American Diabetes Association guidelines recommend that people with diabetes have their blood pressure checked at every doctor's visit. If your blood pressure is higher than 130/80 mm Hg, you need drug treatment in addition to lifestyle measures. People with diabetes often need two or more blood pressure–lowering drugs to achieve blood pressure control. The guidelines recommend using drugs such as ACE inhibitors, angiotensin II receptor blockers, beta-blockers, diuretics, and calcium channel blockers.

An ACE inhibitor is one of the best drugs for lowering high blood pressure in people with diabetes. These drugs decrease production of angiotensin II, a hormone that increases blood pressure. ACE inhibitors also help to prevent or delay progression of kidney damage (nephropathy). If an ACE inhibitor cannot be used, the best substitute is an angiotensin II receptor blocker. Diuretics can raise blood glucose levels and reduce serum potassium levels, and beta-blockers can reduce the warning symptoms of hypoglycemia, so extra caution is needed with these medications. If you haven't been taking an ACE inhibitor or a beta-blocker and you have a heart attack, studies show that immediately starting treatment with these drugs can significantly reduce your risk of dying.

Cholesterol control. If your LDL cholesterol is not at the target of less than 100 mg/dL (or less than 70 mg/dL if you have had a heart attack), the American Diabetes Association recommends treatment with a statin drug. (Also, see the "Ask the Doctor" column at right.) Several large studies have shown a significant reduction in heart attacks and strokes in people with diabetes who took statin drugs to lower their LDL cholesterol. Six statins are available: atorvastatin (Lipitor); fluvastatin (Lescol); lovastatin (Mevacor); pravastatin (Pravachol); rosuvastatin (Crestor); and simvastatin (Zocor).

The American Diabetes Association recommends niacin (nicotinic acid) for people with diabetes who have low levels of HDL cholesterol (less than 40 mg/dL in men or 50 mg/dL in women) and fibrate drugs (Lopid, Lofibra, Tricor) for elevated levels of triglycerides (more than 200 mg/dL). Since niacin can increase blood glucose levels, your doctor will monitor you while you are using the drug.

Other cholesterol-lowering drugs are available, including bile acid sequestrants (Colestid, Questran, Welchol), ezetimibe (Zetia), and a combination of ezetimibe and simvastatin (Vytorin).

Blood clot prevention. Diabetes produces changes in your blood that make it more prone to clotting, which increases your risk of a heart attack and stroke. Taking a daily aspirin tablet can reduce the risk. The American Diabetes Association recommends preventive treatment with aspirin for people with type 1 and type 2 diabetes who have a high risk of cardiovascular disease or who have had a heart attack, stroke, or bypass surgery. The recommended dosage is 75–162 mg a day.

Always talk to your doctor before starting treatment with aspirin. You should not take aspirin if you are allergic to it, are taking anticoagulant drugs like warfarin (Coumadin), or have a bleeding disorder.

Angina treatment. Chest pain due to reduced blood flow to the heart is called angina. Most often, angina results from the buildup of plaque in the coronary arteries that carry blood to the heart. Nitrate drugs (such as nitroglycerin) can alleviate angina when it occurs. Nitrates can also be used preventively before you engage in activities that are likely to cause chest pain, such as rapid walking or playing tennis. Many people with diabetes take a beta-blocker to treat high blood pressure; these drugs help to prevent angina as well.

If angina cannot be controlled with drug treatment, it's often a sign that you have severe blockages in one or more of your coronary arteries. When this happens, you may need angioplasty or bypass surgery to maintain adequate blood flow and prevent a heart attack.

Angioplasty involves inserting a catheter with a balloon at its tip into a femoral artery in your groin and guiding it to the narrowed portion of the coronary artery. The surgeon then inflates

ASK THE DOCTOR

Q. ***I've read that because I have type 2 diabetes, I should take a statin medication even though my cholesterol levels are normal. Is this true?***

A. That depends on what you mean by "normal" and on your own individual risk. Type 2 diabetes is itself a major risk factor for coronary heart disease (CHD). In fact, recent research has shown that people with type 2 diabetes *without* a history of CHD have as much risk for heart attack as people without diabetes but *with* CHD. Reducing this risk is perhaps the most important thing you can do to improve your longevity.

Target LDL ("bad") cholesterol levels are lower for people with diabetes than for the general public: below 100 mg/dL and under 70 mg/dL if risk is especially high. Many people take statins to achieve these goals. If you have one risk factor for CHD—hypertension, physical inactivity, obesity, or being over age 55 or a smoker—you should take a statin in a modest dose, according to the American College of Physicians.

Any drug has potential downsides and for statins, the most common side effects are muscle aches, diarrhea, and upset stomach. Be sure to discuss with your doctor whether statin therapy is the best treatment decision for you.

the balloon several times to squeeze the plaque against the wall of the artery, thus widening the artery opening and increasing blood flow to the heart. In most angioplasty procedures, a metal tube called a stent is placed in the artery to keep it propped open.

In bypass surgery, the surgeon connects a healthy artery in your chest to an area beyond the blocked portion of the coronary artery. Alternatively, the surgeon may remove a portion of one of your large leg veins and attach the vein on each side of the blocked area. Blood flow is then rerouted through this new blood vessel, "bypassing" the blockage.

The choice between angioplasty and bypass surgery depends on many factors, including how many blockages you have, the location of the blockages, and your overall health. Studies show an advantage for bypass surgery in people with diabetes who can withstand this major invasive procedure. One ongoing study of more than 1,800 people found that survival at seven years was significantly better with bypass surgery (74%) than with angioplasty (56%) for people with diabetes. However, recent developments in angioplasty, including the use of stents coated with drugs that prevent arteries from reclogging, may make this alternative to bypass surgery an option for more people with diabetes.

Peripheral arterial disease. Just as plaques can build up in the coronary arteries, similar fatty deposits can develop in the arteries of the legs. This reduces blood flow to your feet and legs.

Narrowing of the leg arteries is called peripheral arterial disease. The characteristic symptom is intermittent claudication—cramping pain in the thighs, calves, and, sometimes, the buttocks that is brought on by exercise and subsides promptly with rest. It's called intermittent because it comes and goes. You may also feel numbness, tingling, burning, or cold in your feet and lower legs.

Smoking is the major risk factor for peripheral arterial disease, but diabetes doubles the risk. Peripheral arterial disease is most common in people with high blood pressure and high blood cholesterol levels (especially in cigarette smokers), so it's not surprising that people with peripheral arterial disease have a higher risk of CHD and heart attack, as well as strokes.

An estimated one of every three people with diabetes over age 50 will develop peripheral arterial disease. That's why the American Diabetes Association recommends that people with diabetes who are older than age 50 have an ankle brachial index (ABI) test. The test compares systolic blood pressure in your arm to that in your lower legs. If blood pressure in your ankle is lower than that in your arm, you may have peripheral arterial disease.

Symptoms of peripheral arterial disease usually progress slowly, but eventually the pain can interfere with normal activities and may even occur at rest. Reduced blood flow in the legs can also result in slow healing of foot blisters and other skin injuries and can lead to open sores (ulcers) and tissue death (gangrene) in the feet and legs. In severe cases, amputation may be necessary.

Treatment is identical to the "ABCs" mentioned earlier for preventing peripheral arterial disease: HbA1c less than 7%, blood pressure below 130/80 mm Hg, and "bad" LDL cholesterol levels lower than 100 mg/dL (ideally, less than 70 mg/dL), with medication given if these goals aren't achieved. Quitting smoking is absolutely essential. In addition, antiplatelet drugs such as aspirin or clopidogrel (Plavix) may be prescribed to reduce the risk of blood clots.

Although it may seem surprising, walking a prescribed distance several times a week gradually increases the pain-free distance you can walk. Your doctor may also prescribe medications such as pentoxifylline (Trental) and cilostazol (Pletal) to relieve walking-related leg pains. But if exercise and drug treatments fail to prevent severe blockages, you may need leg surgery using angioplasty or bypass procedures to treat the plaque buildup.

Microvascular Disease: Nephropathy and Retinopathy

Tiny blood vessels throughout the body also become blocked and damaged in people with diabetes. This is known as microvascular disease (micro means small) and often causes severe damage to the kidneys and the eyes.

Kidney damage (nephropathy)

About 30–40% of people with type 1 diabetes and 20% of those with type 2 diabetes eventually develop kidney damage that can lead to kidney failure. The damage occurs in tiny blood vessels (called capillaries) throughout the kidneys, which act as filters to remove waste products from the bloodstream. The risk of heart attack and stroke is also increased in people with kidney damage.

The first detectable sign of kidney damage is the appearance of small amounts of a protein called albumin in the urine (microalbuminuria), which usually develops after you have had diabetes for five to 10 years. Over the next eight to 10 years, worsening of kidney damage may cause leakage of larger quantities of protein into the urine (proteinuria), accumulation of waste products in the blood (azotemia), and finally kidney failure, which requires

NEW RESEARCH

Diabetes-Specific Statin Drug Advice Improves Adherence

Although using statin drugs to reduce cardiovascular risk is currently recommended for all individuals with type 2 diabetes, many have issues with starting and sticking to a medication regimen. That's why researchers at the Mayo Clinic developed and tested a decision-aid brochure to help people with diabetes make informed decisions about cholesterol-lowering medications.

Statin Choice predicts the chances of having a heart attack over the next 10 years, then explains the benefits of taking statins. It also details the potential downsides of the drug, which include muscle aches and other minor side effects as well as the rare chance of more serious muscle inflammation that can cause life-threatening kidney damage.

The Mayo Clinic team randomly assigned 98 participants with diabetes to use either Statin Choice or a standard medical pamphlet about cholesterol management. After three months, 63% of both groups reported taking statins. Only two of the 33 participants who went on to take statins in the Statin Choice group forgot to take them at one point during the week. In comparison, six of 29 patients who read the standard pamphlet failed to take the drug every day.

Those who used the diabetes-specific decision aid also had a better understanding of the dangers of high cholesterol and the risk reduction with statins.

ARCHIVES OF INTERNAL MEDICINE
Volume 167, page 1076
May 2007

Keeping Your Balance and Reducing Your Risk of Falls

Ten tips and four exercises to try

Diabetes can raise your risk of various complications, but you should also pay attention to a less recognized issue: your risk of falls. That's because diabetic neuropathy or severe hypoglycemia can affect your balance and lead to falls that can result in broken bones.

The Diabetes-Falls Link

The link between diabetes and falls is usually related to peripheral neuropathy, a common diabetes complication that damages nerves in the legs and feet. As nerve injury worsens, the legs and feet may begin to feel numb. The nerve damage also reduces messages to the brain about exactly where the legs and feet are positioned. As a result, many people with peripheral neuropathy feel unsteady on their feet and have an increased risk of falls.

Although middle-aged people with diabetes may suffer from balance problems, the elderly with diabetes are at especially high risk. For example, in a recent study, researchers at Columbia University discovered that nursing home residents were four times more likely to fall if they had diabetes. A separate study from England found a surprisingly high incidence of falls in seniors who lived at home and had poorly controlled diabetes.

The many other factors that can raise the risk of falls include hypoglycemia, obesity, loss of flexibility, poor strength, and the use of multiple medications. Still, studies show that neuropathy is one of the top reasons why seniors with diabetes are more likely to stumble.

Maintaining Your Balance

Keeping diabetes under control is one important way to prevent nerve damage that can affect your balance. Specific exercises also are thought to lower your risk of falls by boosting your strength and balance.

The following is a simple exercise routine recommended by Jennifer Millar, a Johns Hopkins physical therapist who specializes in balance problems. Practicing this routine three to five times per week will help improve your strength, range of motion, and stability. Be sure to talk to your doctor or physical therapist before attempting any of these exercises. Also, you should take extra precautions so that you do not fall while exercising.

When you begin doing the first two exercises, hold on with both hands to a table, kitchen countertop, or back of a chair. As your balance improves, you can try holding on with just one hand. ■

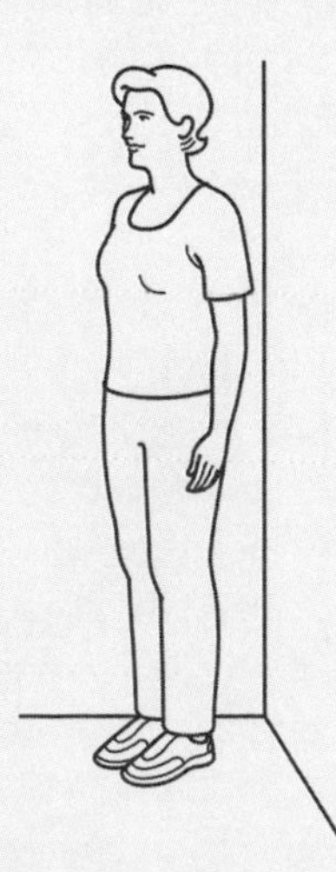

Static standing balance. Stand with your back in a corner, but not touching it, away from any furniture or other objects. Place your feet as close together as you can without falling or touching the wall, and keep your arms at your side. Gradually build up to holding this position for one minute.

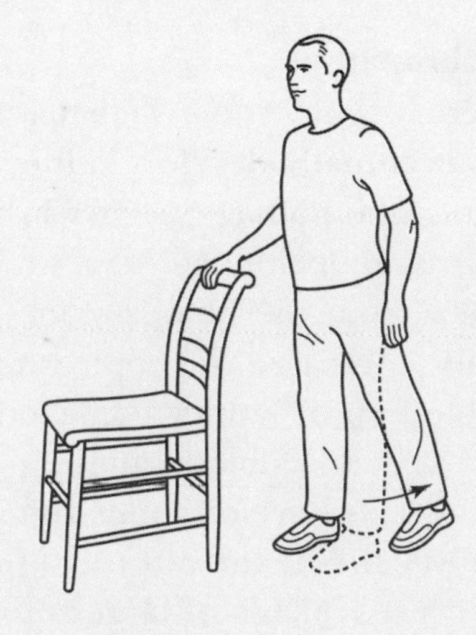

Side leg lift. Stand with your legs shoulder-width apart. Slowly lift one leg to the side, aiming to hold your leg at a 45-degree angle for five seconds. Then slowly lower your leg to the starting position. Gradually build up to eight to 15 repetitions on each leg.

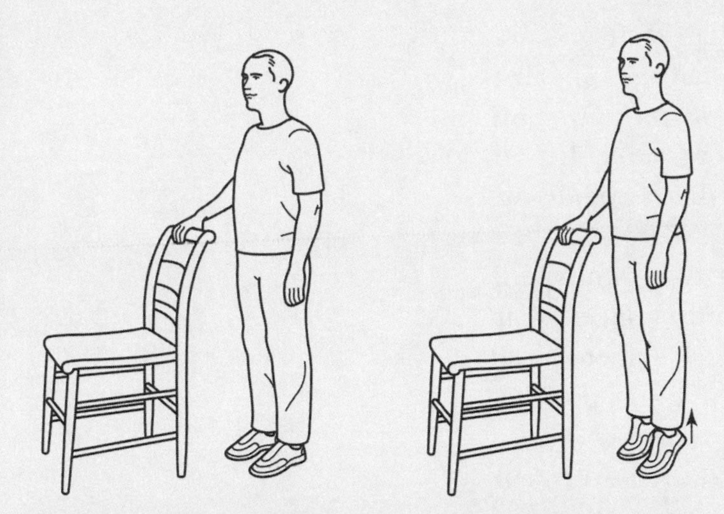

Heel raises. Stand with your legs shoulder-width apart. Slowly lift your heels until you are standing on your tiptoes. Hold for five seconds, and then slowly lower your heels to the starting position. Gradually build up to eight to 15 repetitions.

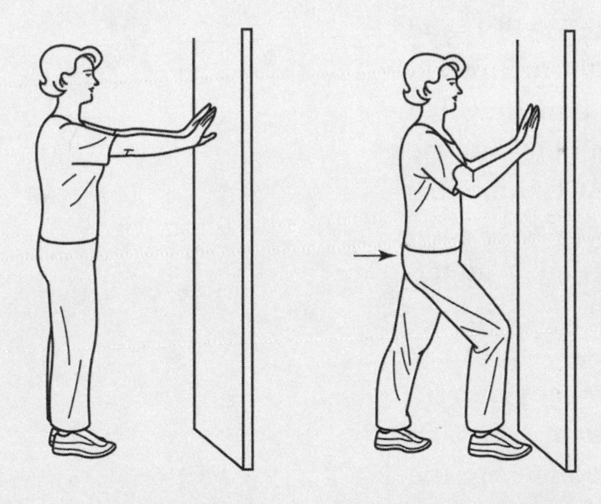

Heel cord stretch. Stand facing the wall, hands on the wall. Step forward with one foot, leaning hips towards the wall, keeping your back straight. Keep rear leg straight with heel on floor. Hold this position for 20 seconds. Repeat three times on each leg.

10 Steps To Prevent Falls

Here is some helpful advice on preventing falls from the U.S. Safety Council.

1. Wear supportive, low-heeled, soft-soled shoes that fit properly and have good traction. Avoid walking in stocking feet.
2. Be cautious of spills. Clean up spills as soon as they occur.
3. Make sure all carpet edges in your home are tacked down.
4. Use a rubber mat or nonslip decals in the tub or shower. Use a nonskid rug on the bathroom floor.
5. Make sure there is an obstacle-free traffic lane in the hallways leading from your bedroom to the bathroom.
6. Keep telephone and appliance cords away from areas where people walk.
7. Make sure you have adequate lighting in your house. Have a light switch or lamp within easy reach of your bed. Use night-lights in your bathroom and in the hallway leading from the bedroom to the bathroom. Make sure you have light switches near every doorway and at both the top and bottom of each stairway.
8. Make sure that securely fastened handrails extend the full length of the stairs on each side of the stairway. Use them whenever going up or down stairs.
9. When young grandchildren visit, be alert for children playing on the floor as well as toys left in your path.
10. If you wear eyeglasses, make sure your prescription is up to date.

Illustrations: Susan Blubaugh

treatment with dialysis or a kidney transplant.

Prevention and treatment of kidney damage. Four strategies are used to prevent and slow the progression of kidney damage. The first three are: tight glucose control, treating high blood pressure, and restricting protein in the diet. The fourth is treatment with either an ACE inhibitor or angiotensin II receptor blocker, drugs commonly prescribed for high blood pressure.

To detect kidney damage in its early stages, people with type 2 diabetes should have a urine test for microalbuminuria once a year as soon as diabetes is diagnosed. In people with type 1 diabetes, testing should start within five years of diagnosis. If the test is positive, your doctor will tell you to lower your blood glucose and blood pressure and may recommend a low-protein diet to decrease protein loss in the urine and decrease the kidneys' workload. All adults with diabetes should also undergo a serum creatinine test at least once a year to measure the filtering capacity of the kidneys.

If you have type 1 diabetes with hypertension or protein in the urine, you should take an ACE inhibitor or angiotensin II receptor blocker. Studies have shown that two ACE inhibitors, captopril (Capoten) and enalapril (Vasotec), can slow kidney damage in its early stages. ACE inhibitors decrease pressure in the small blood vessels that filter blood in the kidneys. This effect can prevent destruction of these blood vessels. Some experts recommend that people with diabetes start treatment with an ACE inhibitor at the first sign of microalbuminuria. Others believe that ACE inhibitors will delay the onset of kidney disease if they are prescribed as soon as diabetes is diagnosed. Additional studies are needed to determine which approach is more effective.

If an ACE inhibitor causes intolerable side effects—the most common is a dry cough—your doctor may prescribe an angiotensin II receptor blocker, such as irbesartan (Avapro), losartan (Cozaar), or valsartan (Diovan). Angiotensin II receptor blockers prevent the actions of angiotensin by inhibiting it from binding to receptors. These drugs are effective in protecting the kidneys from further damage and in controlling blood pressure.

Many medications you take are excreted from the body via the kidneys. So if your kidneys are failing, the drug dosage you take must be decreased to avoid buildup to toxic levels. Many people with chronic kidney failure develop weakness and fatigue from anemia. If this happens, your doctor may prescribe erythropoietin, a hormone that stimulates the production of red blood cells.

If your kidney function deteriorates to less than 10% of normal—

a condition called end-stage kidney (renal) disease—you'll need kidney dialysis or a kidney transplant. One type of dialysis, hemodialysis, does the work your kidneys can no longer do by passing your blood through a machine that filters out waste products and then returns the cleaned blood to your bloodstream. Hemodialysis is performed in special treatment centers and usually requires three weekly sessions of three to five hours each.

Another procedure called peritoneal dialysis requires surgical implantation of a catheter in your abdomen through which dialysis solution (called dialysate) is delivered. The solution passes through the lining of your abdomen (the peritoneal membrane), which filters out wastes and excess fluid from the blood. The fluid is then drained out through the catheter and discarded. The process requires about half an hour every day, but you can do it yourself at home or almost anywhere. Peritoneal dialysis can also be performed with a machine called a cycler, which you can use at night while you are sleeping.

Dialysis can cause side effects, and it is time consuming and tiring. The best remedy for end-stage kidney disease is a kidney transplant. Unfortunately, many people with kidney failure must wait years until a donated kidney becomes available.

Retinopathy (eye damage)

Diabetic retinopathy, which affects more than four million Americans age 40 and older, is the most common eye complication of diabetes. Almost everyone with type 1 diabetes and more than 70% of people with type 2 disease will eventually develop retinopathy—in most cases without experiencing any vision loss. However, diabetic retinopathy can cause blindness and is the most frequent cause of new cases of blindness in adults ages 20–74.

The word "retinopathy" refers to damage in the retina, the light-sensitive nerve tissue at the back of the eye that transmits visual images to the brain. The damage is caused by changes in the tiny blood vessels that carry blood to the retina.

In the early stages—called nonproliferative retinopathy—these blood vessels weaken and develop bulges that may leak blood or fluid into the surrounding tissue. Vision is rarely affected during this stage. But if your diabetes isn't tightly controlled, eye damage is likely to get worse. Fragile new blood vessels may begin to grow on the retina and into the vitreous humor (the gel-like substance inside the back of the eye). This condition is called proliferative retinopathy. The abnormal blood vessels often rupture and bleed into the

NEW RESEARCH

Diabetes Decreases Life Expectancy

In a study that re-emphasizes the importance of cardiovascular prevention, people over age 50 with diabetes were found to have a shorter lifespan than those without the disease, mostly because of an increased incidence of cardiovascular disease.

Researchers concluded that men with diabetes lived about 7.5 years less—and women with diabetes lived 8.2 years less—than those without diabetes. Individuals with diabetes had nearly twice the risk of developing heart problems and dying prematurely than those who were diabetes free.

The conclusions are based on data from the Framingham Heart Study, a massive trial that began in the 1950s and followed some 5,200 Massachusetts residents for more than 46 years. Participants were analyzed at three follow-up periods of 12 years each until they developed cardiovascular disease or died; their diabetes status was measured again at the beginning of each interval.

Women with diabetes were more likely to have heart problems and pass away earlier than men. The researchers attributed the poorer outcome in women to a number of factors, including the traditionally better care men receive. This study shows that with the increasing prevalence of diabetes, preventing the disease is fundamental for healthy aging.

ARCHIVES OF INTERNAL MEDICINE
Volume 167, page 1145
June 2007

vitreous humor, causing blurred vision or temporary blindness. Scar tissue resulting from the bleeding can pull the retina away from the back of the eye (a condition called retinal detachment), which may cause permanent vision loss.

At any stage of retinopathy, fluid may accumulate around the macula, the most sensitive portion of the retina and crucial for seeing fine detail. This condition, called macular edema, causes severe blurring of vision.

Prevention of retinopathy. If you have diabetes, you should see an ophthalmologist (eye doctor) every year for an eye examination, during which special eyedrops are used to open (dilate) your pupils. This allows the doctor to get a better look at the retina to detect any damage when the disease is in its early, treatable stages and to monitor progression of the disease. People with type 1 diabetes should have an initial eye exam within three to five years of the onset of diabetes. People with type 2 diabetes should start annual eye examinations when their diabetes is first diagnosed.

Keeping your blood pressure below 130/80 mm Hg can help prevent the onset and progression of damage to the retina. Some—but not all—studies indicate that lowering blood cholesterol levels and quitting smoking may be helpful as well. However, the most important way to prevent diabetic retinopathy or keep it from getting worse is to maintain tight blood glucose control. For example, in the Diabetes Control and Complications Trial (DCCT), people with type 1 diabetes who injected insulin multiple times each day or used an insulin pump had a 76% lower risk of developing diabetic retinopathy and a 54% lower risk that existing retinopathy would worsen than people who followed a less rigorous treatment program. In addition, the United Kingdom Prospective Diabetes Study (UKPDS) showed that people with type 2 diabetes who controlled their blood glucose levels with medication were 30% less likely to have retinopathy that required laser treatment than people who relied on diet and exercise alone.

Treatment of retinopathy. One of the major reasons why annual vision exams are so important is that proliferative retinopathy can be effectively treated with laser photocoagulation procedures, but only if it is detected early. Prompt treatment can also preserve vision following a retinal detachment. However, laser photocoagulation surgery won't help if vision is already impaired.

Laser photocoagulation is an outpatient procedure in which an ophthalmologist dilates the pupils of your eyes. The doctor then aims bursts of laser light at a series of points on the retina, causing tiny scars to form. The procedure prevents small vessels from rupturing and bleeding into the vitreous humor. Although extensive photocoagulation usually diminishes peripheral vision and may decrease night vision, its success in preserving visual acuity makes it worthwhile.

If the extent or location of the retinopathy makes photocoagulation ineffective or if the vitreous humor of the eye is too clouded with blood, vision may be improved with vitrectomy, a surgical procedure that removes the vitreous humor and replaces it with a saline solution. Roughly 70% of people who undergo vitrectomy notice an improvement in or stabilization of their eyesight, and some recover enough vision to resume reading and driving.

Cataracts and Glaucoma

Cataracts and glaucoma also are more common in people with diabetes. A cataract is a clouding of the lens of the eye that impairs vision. Cataract formation associated with diabetes often occurs because of excess levels of sorbitol (a sugar formed from glucose), which form deposits within the lens. If a cataract begins to interfere with your vision, you may need surgery to remove the affected lens and replace it with a lens implant.

In glaucoma, abnormally high pressure within the eyeball damages the optic nerve, which carries visual information from the retina to the brain. Your ophthalmologist can easily measure the pressure in your eye (called intraocular pressure) during a routine eye exam. It's important to have your eye pressure tested regularly, since irreversible eye damage from glaucoma may occur before any symptoms appear. Treatment with medicated eyedrops often helps to reduce the intraocular pressure, but some people also need laser treatment to prevent severe loss of vision.

Nerve Damage (Neuropathy)

Neuropathy is a serious consequence of diabetes. The best way to prevent it is to maintain control of your blood glucose levels. Research shows that tight blood glucose control decreases the risk of diabetic nerve damage by as much as 60%. Once you have neuropathy, however, tight glucose control will do little to cure your symptoms.

About 60–70% of people with diabetes develop neuropathy, although they may not notice any symptoms at first. Diabetes can cause three types of nerve damage: peripheral neuropathy, focal neuropathy, and autonomic neuropathy.

ASK THE DOCTOR

Q. ***I have had diabetes for 20+ years and have had some bloating, heartburn, and nausea after I eat. Could this be related to my diabetes?***

A. Possibly. You could be suffering from gastroparesis—essentially a "paralyzed stomach." This problem can occur in long-term diabetes as a kind of nerve damage called autonomic neuropathy. Food remains in your stomach longer than normal, and it is often unpredictable how quickly it will be absorbed. No easy cure exists for gastroparesis, but various approaches such as eating a low-fat, high-fiber diet can help. Also, try eating six smaller meals a day versus the traditional breakfast, lunch, and dinner.

Specific treatments also can speed stomach emptying. Medications like metoclopramide (Reglan) and erythromycin (Erythrocin) help you digest food faster. Another option, Enterra Therapy, uses electrodes to stimulate the stomach muscles to contract. Other treatments are under investigation. If you suffer from nausea, your doctor can prescribe promethazine (Phenergan) and prochlorperazine (Compazine).

Keep in mind that delayed and unpredictable stomach emptying can make it more difficult to control blood glucose levels, while conversely, high glucose can worsen gastroparesis symptoms. To maintain your target glucose levels, you may need more frequent insulin injections. Also, using insulin after meals, rather than before, might be more effective.

Peripheral neuropathy

This is damage to the peripheral nerves, the nerves that connect your spinal cord to the rest of your body. It is the most common type, and it is a serious disorder that causes a slow, progressive loss of function in the sensory nerves in the arms and legs due to a lack of oxygen or nutrients, compression, and inflammation. Symptoms include numbness, tingling, and pain—most commonly in the legs, hands, and feet—but it can affect any part of the body. Symptoms range from mild to severe, depending on what nerves are affected, and may be worse at night.

Further nerve damage can lead to total loss of feeling in the affected areas. It can also lead to loss of reflexes and muscle control, loss of muscle tone and strength, foot ulcers and injuries to the feet that can become infected, loss of coordination and balance, and hair loss in the affected area.

Focal neuropathy

This refers to a disruption of blood supply to a single nerve or nerve group. It leads to sudden pain or weakness in the area of the body served by the affected nerve. Focal neuropathy often improves gradually over two to six months without any treatment.

Autonomic neuropathy

This type of neuropathy develops when diabetes damages the autonomic nervous system, which regulates body functions that are not under your voluntary control—for example, digestion, heart rate, and blood pressure. Symptoms of autonomic neuropathy include slow emptying of your stomach, poor bladder control, erectile dysfunction, rapid or irregular heartbeat, and abnormal sweating. Most individuals with autonomic neuropathy also have peripheral neuropathy.

Treatment of nerve damage

Improved control of blood glucose is the first step in treating neuropathy, but unfortunately it is rarely helpful. Thus, medication is usually needed.

Peripheral neuropathy. Amitriptyline, a medication also used to treat depression, is the most effective drug for relieving symptoms of peripheral neuropathy. The medication works by making more norepinephrine available to nerve cells. (Norepinephrine is a neurotransmitter, which is a chemical that carries messages between nerve cells.) Amitriptyline can cause drowsiness, urinary retention

Happy Feet

Foot care tips for people with diabetes

Individuals with diabetes need to pay special attention to their feet for a number of reasons. Diabetes can damage nerves in the feet, leading to a reduction in feeling that makes it difficult to know if you have a foot injury. Diabetes can also impair circulation and wound healing by narrowing the arteries supplying blood to the legs. A wound on the foot that does not heal can turn into an ulcer (deep sore) that may become infected and possibly even require an amputation if untreated.

You can reduce your risk of these complications by keeping your diabetes well controlled, having your feet inspected by a family doctor or podiatrist at least twice a year, and taking care of your feet as described below.

Inspect your feet each day. Contact your doctor or podiatrist if you notice any infected toenails, swelling, sores, cuts, bruises, blisters, or red spots that do not heal after a day. Also, notify your doctor if you experience tingling, numbness, or pain in your feet. If you cannot see your feet well, use a mirror or ask for help from a family member or friend.

Wear shoes and socks. Always wear well-fitting footwear, even indoors. If you walk barefoot, it is easy to injure your feet without realizing it. Before putting on your shoes, check for pebbles, gravel, or anything that could potentially cause a cut or sore. Break in new shoes slowly and carefully. To prevent blisters, you should always have on socks or stockings when wearing shoes. Avoid tight socks, garters, or elastic bands to hold up socks because they can cut off circulation to your feet.

Wash your feet daily. Use a gentle soap and warm water. If you have nerve damage, hot water can scald your skin without your even noticing it, so always be sure to test the temperature of the water using your elbow or a thermometer. Avoid soaking your feet, which can cause your skin to become dry and crack.

Treat calluses and corns gently. If recommended by your doctor, gently file calluses and corns after bathing, using an emery board or pumice stone. To avoid irritating your skin, rub in one direction only. Do not use chemlcals, razor blades, or other harsh methods to remove corns or calluses. If calluses or corns are particularly troublesome, you can have them removed by a healthcare professional.

Dry your feet thoroughly after bathing. Use a nonabrasive towel to gently blot dry your skin. Avoid rubbing, which can damage the skin. Don't forget to dry the spaces in between your toes.

Moisturize your feet. Apply a thin layer of skin cream, lanolin lotion, or petroleum jelly to the top and bottom of each foot after drying your feet. Avoid putting lotion between your toes, where excess moisture can contribute to infection. Cornstarch may help to minimize moisture in between your toes.

Cut your toenails once a week. Toenails should be cut after washing and drying your feet, when the nails are soft. Cut the nails straight across without curving in at the edges. Cutting into the corners of the nails can lead to ingrown toenails. Also, avoid cutting your nails too short. If you have trouble trimming your toenails, ask a family member or friend for assistance or have a health care professional trim them for you.

Carefully wash any cuts or blisters using soap and water. For cuts, use a mild antiseptic like Bactine and cover the cut with a dry, sterile dressing and paper tape. Do not pop a blister. Instead, rub an antibiotic cream on the blister a few times daily until it heals.

Avoid heat and cold. Never place a hot-water bottle or heating pad on your feet or place your feet near a radiator or fire because you may not be able to feel any damage that occurs. Instead, wear warm socks. Also, avoid sunburns by keeping your feet out of direct sunlight or by applying sunscreen. Feet can be damaged easily by cold surfaces or frostbite during the winter. Be sure to protect your feet from the cold during winter by wearing extra-warm socks and shoes. ■

(an inability to empty the bladder completely), and a severe drop in blood pressure upon standing (orthostatic hypotension). Starting with a small dose and then gradually increasing the dose can minimize these effects. Taking amitriptyline at bedtime also helps.

Desipramine (Norpramin) is another antidepression drug used to treat peripheral neuropathy. It has fewer side effects and is almost as effective as amitriptyline. When antidepressants are ineffective or cause too many side effects, your doctor may prescribe gabapentin (Neurontin). Neurontin, an anticonvulsant drug used for epilepsy, can be taken alone or in combination with amitriptyline. If side effects occur (typically, drowsiness and confusion), they usually can be minimized by lowering the dosage. A gabapentin-like drug called pregabalin (Lyrica) was recently approved for treating pain in people with diabetic neuropathy.

Autonomic neuropathy. When autonomic neuropathy affects nerves in the digestive system, eating frequent, small, low-fat meals instead of three large meals a day can help prevent the nausea and vomiting caused by slowed emptying of the stomach. Treatment with metoclopramide (Reglan) or the antibiotic erythromycin can also improve stomach emptying. (See the “Ask the Doctor” column on page 71.) Diarrhea sometimes responds to antibiotics such as tetracycline (which counteract the overgrowth of intestinal bacteria that may contribute to diarrhea) or conventional antidiarrhea drugs.

Men with autonomic neuropathy may have damage to nerves that control erections. Poor blood glucose control appears to worsen the problem. In a recent study, men who had HbA1c levels over 8% had the greatest risk of severe erectile dysfunction.

Skin Changes

As many as one out of every three people with diabetes develop skin disorders, even if they maintain tight glucose control. Diabetic dermopathy, which is caused by changes in small blood vessels, is the most common diabetes-related skin problem. Also called shin spots, diabetic dermopathy appears as reddish-brown, scaly lesions about half an inch in diameter that typically occur on the front of both legs. They don’t hurt, open up, or itch, and they don’t need to be treated.

People with diabetes are also more susceptible to bacterial skin infections, such as styes on the eyelids and boils in hair follicles, which can be treated with antibiotics. They also have more fungal and yeast infections, including vaginal yeast infections in women, jock itch in men, athlete's foot, and ringworm. Most fungal infections require drug treatment.

Dental Changes

Just as diabetes increases your risk of skin infections, it also increases infections in your mouth and gums. Normally, saliva protects against bacterial growth in the mouth, but if you have insufficient saliva (dry mouth), food particles will collect around your teeth, causing cavities and gum infections as well as dental plaques that can damage your gums. Individuals with diabetes are highly susceptible to cavities and to gum infection or inflammation (known as gingivitis), which can spread to the ligaments and bones that support the teeth (periodontitis). Dry mouth and diabetic nerve damage can also cause burning sensations in the mouth or on the tongue.

Once again, controlling glucose levels is the best way to prevent these complications. Of course, preventing cavities and gum infections also means avoiding candy, soda, and other sugary foods as well as brushing and flossing your teeth every day.

Foot Problems

Foot infections are another important concern for people with diabetes. Diabetes-related nerve damage can reduce feeling in the feet, making it difficult to detect a foot injury. Diabetes can also impair blood circulation and wound healing by narrowing the arteries that carry blood to the legs. This combination is extremely serious, because a wound on your foot or leg that doesn't heal can turn into an ulcer (deep sore) that quickly becomes infected. Amputation is often necessary. In fact, one fifth of all hospitalizations in people with diabetes are for foot infections, resulting in over 80,000 lower-limb amputations each year.

Blood glucose control, quitting smoking, and proper foot care can greatly reduce these risks. That's why everyone with diabetes, and especially those with neuropathy or poor circulation, should follow a routine of inspecting each foot and lower leg every day and carefully treating and monitoring even the most trivial blister, cut, or abrasion. Any injured areas should be washed with warm water and soap, cleaned with a mild antiseptic (such as Bactine), and covered with a dry, sterile dressing and paper tape. (See "Happy Feet" on page 73 for more foot care tips.)

If you do develop a foot or leg ulcer, call your doctor immediately. Because people with diabetes often have poor blood circulation, ulcers can become infected rapidly. Although treatment with

NEW RESEARCH

Reiki Found Ineffective for Diabetic Neuropathy

An alternative approach to treating diabetic neuropathy—a hands-on, Eastern technique of transmitting healing energy known as Reiki—is no more effective than a placebo in relieving pain, researchers from Great Britain report.

A total of 207 people with type 2 diabetes suffering from nerve pain were randomized into one of three treatment groups: Reiki, mimic Reiki, or usual care. For Reiki, participants laid on a comfortable bed while trained practitioners moved their hands over various points on the body. In the mock-Reiki group, actors trained to copy the technique performed it. Participants in the Reiki and mock-Reiki groups received two 25-minute sessions the first week and then a weekly session during the following 11 weeks.

Pain initially improved for the two treatment groups, but not for the usual-care group. But at the end of the study, there were no differences in the pain scores among the three groups. However, those who received Reiki and mock-Reiki were able to walk 12% further after treatment was completed.

Although Reiki produced no measurable results over placebo, the researchers note that the overall pain relief found in both Reiki groups suggests that therapeutic benefits can come from a sustained partnership between doctor and patient.

DIABETES CARE
Volume 30, page 999
March 2007

antibiotics is needed, it's not enough to cure these serious infections. Incision and drainage procedures are the best treatment. Severe ulcers usually require wearing a boot to protect the foot. These wound-care treatments are so complex that most doctors now send people with infected ulcers to specialized wound care centers. Treatment can take many months because wound dressings must be applied and changed frequently, and dead tissue may have to be removed from the wound (a process called debridement). Considering that the alternative to treatment is amputation, this expensive and time-consuming process is definitely worthwhile. ■

GLOSSARY

ACE inhibitors—Medications commonly prescribed to treat high blood pressure; this class of drugs also slows the progression of kidney disease in people with diabetes.

adrenergic symptoms—Symptoms, including sweating and heart palpitations, that occur when low blood glucose levels trigger the release of the hormone epinephrine into the blood.

alpha-glucosidase inhibitors—Oral diabetes drugs that inhibit intestinal enzymes that digest complex carbohydrates and sucrose, delaying the absorption of carbohydrates into the blood. Examples are acarbose (Precose) and miglitol (Glyset).

antioxidants—Substances that help the body neutralize free radicals, which can cause cell damage. Naturally occurring antioxidants include beta-carotene, vitamin C, vitamin E, and selenium.

atherosclerosis—An accumulation of deposits of fat and fibrous tissue, called plaques, within the walls of arteries that can narrow these blood vessels and reduce blood flow.

autonomic neuropathy—Damage to nerves that control involuntary actions in the body, such as digestion, heart rate, and blood pressure.

biguanides—Oral diabetes drugs that decrease glucose production by the liver and increase glucose uptake by cells. Metformin (Glucophage, Glucophage XR, Glumetza) is the only available biguanide.

cardiovascular disease—Disease affecting the arteries that supply blood to the heart and other organs. Coronary heart disease, stroke, and peripheral arterial disease are the most common types of cardiovascular disease.

cataract—A cloudiness (opacification) of the lens of the eye that can lead to visual impairment.

coronary heart disease (CHD)—A narrowing of the arteries that supply blood to the heart. Caused by atherosclerosis, CHD can reduce or completely block blood flow to the heart.

diabetic foot ulcer—An open sore on the foot that occurs in people with diabetes who have damage to nerves and/or have poor blood flow to the feet.

diabetic ketoacidosis—An acute complication of diabetes (usually type 1) that results from a nearly complete lack of insulin. The body is forced to use fatty acids instead of glucose as a major source of energy. The resulting breakdown of fatty acids to ketone bodies raises the acidity of the blood to dangerous levels. Symptoms include nausea, vomiting, heavy breathing, dry or flushed skin, and fruity breath.

diuretics—Drugs that increase urine production by enhancing loss of sodium through the kidneys. Diuretics are used to eliminate excess fluid from the body and to treat high blood pressure.

D-phenylalanine derivatives—Oral diabetes drugs that stimulate rapid insulin secretion to reduce the rise in blood glucose that occurs soon after eating. The only such drug available is nateglinide (Starlix).

external insulin pump—A pump, usually worn on a belt, that delivers a continuous flow of insulin (plus additional amounts before meals) through a needle inserted under the skin of the abdomen or thigh.

fasting plasma glucose (FPG) test—Measures blood glucose levels after an overnight fast. Diabetes is diagnosed if blood glucose is above 125 mg/dL on at least two tests.

free radicals—Chemical compounds that can damage cells and oxidize low-density lipoproteins, making them more likely to be deposited in the walls of arteries.

gestational diabetes—A type of diabetes that occurs during pregnancy. About 2–5% of pregnant women develop the condition, which goes away after childbirth. It signals a high risk of type 2 diabetes later in life.

glaucoma—An eye disease characterized by damage to the optic nerve. Increased pressure within the eyeball is a risk factor for developing glaucoma.

glucagon—A hormone that raises blood glucose levels by signaling the liver to convert amino acids and glycogen to glucose, which is then released into the bloodstream. Glucagon may be given by injection to raise blood glucose levels when severe hypoglycemia occurs.

glucose—A simple sugar that circulates in the blood and provides energy to the body. Excess glucose is converted to glycogen or triglycerides.

glucose transporters—Proteins that carry glucose from the outside of a cell to the inside.

glycogen—A complex carbohydrate that is stored in the liver and muscles until it is needed for energy.

hemoglobin A1c (HbA1c) test—A test that measures the amount of glucose attached to hemoglobin. The test is routinely used to assess blood glucose control over the previous two to three months.

high-density lipoprotein (HDL)—A lipid-carrying protein that protects against atherosclerosis by removing cholesterol deposited in artery walls.

hyperglycemia—High blood glucose levels.

hyperosmolar nonketotic state—A medical emergency characterized by extremely high blood glucose levels in people with type 2 diabetes. It is usually caused by the physical stress of an injury or major illness. Symptoms include dry or parched mouth, nausea, vomiting, rapid and shallow breathing, and warm, dry skin.

hypoglycemia—Low blood glucose levels that can cause symptoms such as shaking and sweating and may progress to confusion, sleepiness, or even coma. Can be reversed by eating a fast-acting carbohydrate or, if necessary, by injecting glucagon.

implantable insulin pump—A pump placed under the skin of the abdomen that delivers insulin at a constant rate (with added amounts for meals) through a catheter into the abdominal cavity. Not approved for use in the United States.

insulin—A hormone produced by the pancreas that regulates the production of glucose by the liver and the utilization of glucose by cells. Insulin is also a medication used by people with diabetes when the pancreas does not make enough insulin.

insulin pen—A combined insulin container and needle that makes injection of insulin more convenient.

insulin syringe—A syringe with a needle used to inject insulin; the most common way to administer insulin.

intermediate-acting insulin—Insulin medication that begins working in two to four hours, peaks at four to eight hours, and lasts for about 12–20 hours. NPH insulin is an example.

islets of Langerhans—Cellular masses in the pancreas that contain insulin- and glucagon-secreting cells; also called pancreatic islets.

jet injector—A needle-free way of injecting insulin that uses a high-pressure jet of air to send a fine stream of insulin through the skin.

ketoacidosis—Dangerously increased acidity of the blood, which occurs when extremely low insulin levels cause the breakdown of triglycerides in fat cells, releasing fatty acids into the bloodstream.

ketones—Toxic substances formed from the breakdown of fatty acids.

laser photocoagulation—A treatment for proliferative retinopathy or macular edema that slows or halts vision loss by destroying diseased blood vessels in the retina.

long-acting insulin—Insulin medication that has no peak activity and lasts for up to 18–24 hours. Examples are insulin glargine (Lantus) and insulin detemir (Levemir).

low-density lipoprotein (LDL)—A protein that transports cholesterol in the blood; excessive amounts are a major contributor to atherosclerosis.

macular edema—Swelling around the macula, a small area at the center of the retina of the eye that is responsible for central and fine-detail vision.

meglitinides—Oral diabetes drugs that promote the secretion of insulin by the pancreas when blood glucose is elevated after a meal. The only approved drug in this class is repaglinide (Prandin).

metabolic syndrome—A condition characterized by a group of findings, including elevated blood glucose levels, high triglycerides, low HDL cholesterol, high blood pressure, and obesity. Associated with an increased risk of diabetes, heart attack, and stroke.

microalbuminuria—Small amounts of a protein called albumin in the urine that are a first sign of kidney dysfunction.

nephropathy—Kidney disease.

neuropathy—Nerve damage.

oral glucose tolerance test—A test in which a person fasts overnight and then drinks a solution containing 75 g of glucose. Diabetes is diagnosed if two hours later blood glucose is 200 mg/dL or higher.

pancreas—An organ located behind and beneath the lower part of the stomach that produces and secretes insulin and glucagon.

pancreatic islets—see islets of Langerhans.

peripheral arterial disease—Atherosclerosis in the arteries leading to the legs and feet.

peripheral neuropathy—A slow, progressive loss of function of the sensory nerves in the limbs that causes numbness, tingling, and pain in the legs and hands.

prediabetes—A condition in which blood glucose levels are higher than normal (100–125 mg/dL) but not high enough for a diagnosis of diabetes (126 mg/dL or more).

rapid-acting insulin—Insulin medication that begins working in five to 15 minutes, peaks at 30–60 minutes, and lasts for about four to six hours.

regular insulin—Insulin medication that begins working in 30 minutes, peaks at 1.5–2 hours, and lasts for about eight to 10 hours.

retinopathy—Damage to the retina caused by changes in the tiny blood vessels that supply the retina.

statins—Drugs that reduce blood levels of cholesterol by blocking its formation.

sulfonylureas—Oral diabetes drugs that stimulate the pancreas to secrete more insulin. Examples are chlorpropamide (Diabinese) and glyburide (DiaBeta, Glynase, Micronase).

thiazolidinediones—Oral diabetes drugs that increase the sensitivity of cells to insulin. Examples are pioglitazone (Actos) and rosiglitazone (Avandia).

tight glucose control—Achieving near-normal levels of blood glucose by monitoring blood glucose several times a day and adjusting doses of insulin or oral diabetes drugs accordingly.

type 1 diabetes—An autoimmune disease that destroys the ability of beta cells in the pancreas to make insulin and occurs most commonly in children and young adults. Daily insulin injections are necessary to stay alive.

type 2 diabetes—The most common type of diabetes. Develops when the pancreas cannot make enough insulin to overcome the body's resistance to insulin action.

vitreous humor—A thick, gel-like substance that fills the back of the eyeball behind the lens.

HEALTH INFORMATION ORGANIZATIONS AND SUPPORT GROUPS

American Association of Diabetes Educators
200 West Madison St., Ste. 800
Chicago, IL 60606
☎ 800-338-3633
www.diabeteseducator.org
Organization of health professionals educating people on diabetes management. Provides referrals to local diabetes educators.

American Diabetes Association
1701 North Beauregard St.
Alexandria, VA 22311
☎ 800-342-2383
www.diabetes.org
National organization that funds research, provides information and publications, and offers referrals to support groups and education classes. Look in the white pages for your local chapter.

American Dietetic Association
120 S. Riverside Plaza, Ste. 2000
Chicago, IL 60606-6995
☎ 800-877-1600
www.eatright.org
Provides nutrition and weight control information, direct access to a registered dietitian, recorded nutrition messages, and referrals to local dietitians.

Joslin Diabetes Center
One Joslin Place
Boston, MA 02215
☎ 617-732-2400
www.joslin.org
Diabetes treatment, research, and education center affiliated with Harvard Medical School that has treatment centers nationwide. Also produces publications.

National Diabetes Information Clearinghouse
1 Information Way
Bethesda, MD 20892-3560
☎ 800-860-8747
www.diabetes.niddk.nih.gov
Collects and disseminates information on diabetes, responds to requests for information, and provides publications.

National Institute of Diabetes & Digestive & Kidney Diseases
Office of Communications
& Public Liaison
Building 31, Rm. 9A06
31 Center Dr., MSC 2560
Bethesda, MD 20892-2560
www.niddk.nih.gov
Conducts and supports research on diabetes as well as kidney, metabolic, and endocrine diseases.

National Kidney Foundation
30 East 33rd St.
New York, NY 10016
☎ 800-622-9010/212-889-2210
www.kidney.org
Health organization working for the prevention, treatment, and cure of kidney disease. Provides information and education on diabetes and kidney disease as well as on organ donation.

LEADING HOSPITALS
for Endocrinology as Ranked by *U.S. News & World Report*

1. **Mayo Clinic**
Rochester, MN
☎ 507-284-2511/507-538-3270
www.mayoclinic.org

2. **Massachusetts General Hospital**
Boston, MA
☎ 617-726-2000
www.massgeneral.org

3. **Johns Hopkins Hospital**
Baltimore, MD
☎ 410-502-4003/410-955-5464
www.hopkinsmedicine.org

4. **University of California, San Francisco Medical Center**
San Francisco, CA
☎ 888-689-UCSF
www.ucsfhealth.org

5. **New York-Presbyterian University Hospital of Columbia and Cornell**
New York, NY
☎ 877-NYP-WELL
www.nyp.org

6. **Cleveland Clinic**
Cleveland, OH
☎ 800-223-2273/216-444-2200
www.clevelandclinic.org

7. **Barnes-Jewish Hospital/ Washington University**
St. Louis, MO
☎ 314-747-3000/314-TOP-DOCS
www.barnesjewish.org

8. **University of Virginia Medical Center**
Charlottesville, VA
☎ 434-924-0211
www.med.virginia.edu

9. **Brigham and Women's Hospital**
Boston, MA
☎ 617-732-5500
www.brighamandwomens.org

10. **Hospital of the University of Pennsylvania**
Philadelphia, PA
☎ 215-662-4000
www.med.upenn.edu

INDEX

P

Q

R

S

T

U

V

W

X

Z

NOTES

NOTES

NOTES

NOTES

NOTES

NOTES

NOTES

Please address inquiries on bulk subscriptions and permission to reproduce selections from this White Paper to Medletter Associates, LLC, 6 Trowbridge Drive, Bethel, CT 06801.
The editors are interested in receiving your comments at whitepapers@johnshopkinshealthalerts.com or the above address but regret that they cannot answer letters of any sort personally.

ISBN 978-1-933087-62-7
1-933087-62-5

Printed in the United States of America

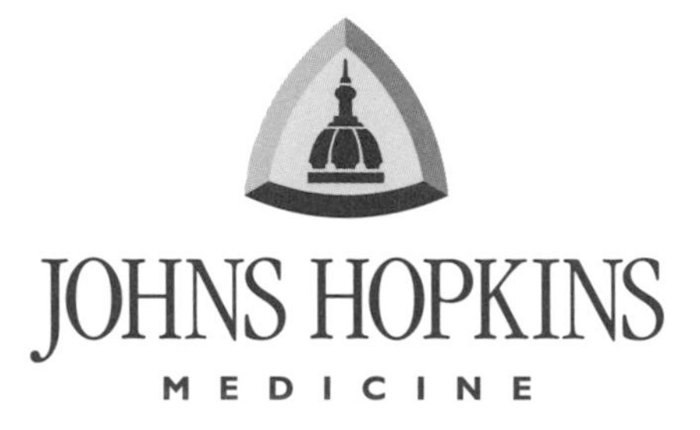

The Johns Hopkins White Papers are published yearly by Medletter Associates, LLC.

Visit our website for information on Johns Hopkins Health Publications, which include White Papers on specific disorders, home medical encyclopedias, consumer reference guides to drugs and medical tests, and our monthly newsletter *The Johns Hopkins Medical Letter: Health After 50*.
www.JohnsHopkinsHealthAlerts.com

DIGESTIVE DISORDERS

Sergey V. Kantsevoy, M.D.

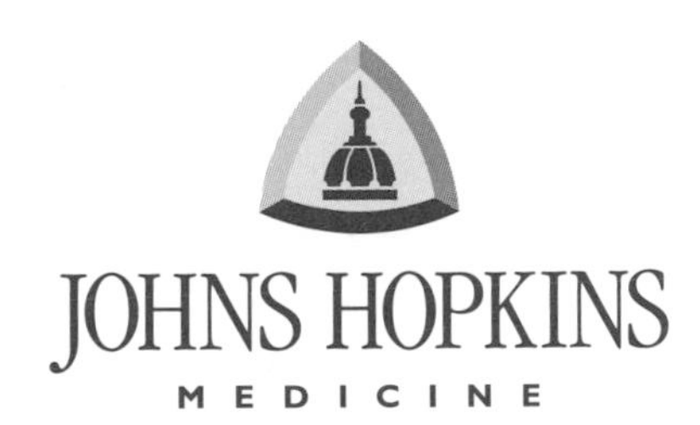

Dear Reader:

Welcome to the 2008 *Digestive Disorders White Paper*—your Johns Hopkins guide to the prevention, diagnosis, and management of conditions that affect your upper and lower digestive tract, liver, gallbladder, and pancreas.

This year's highlights include:

- What to expect before, during, and after an **upper endoscopy**. (page 6)
- How **excess pounds** can lead to **acid reflux**. (page 12)
- Special **precautions** to avoid digestive problems if you take **NSAIDs**. (page 23)
- How to fight **ulcers** with **friendly bacteria**. (page 26)
- What you need to know about **acetaminophen** and your **liver**. (page 36)
- Specific steps that can thwart **turista**, the dreaded **traveler's diarrhea**. (page 42)
- Why your **bones** need **extra care** if you have digestive problems. (page 48)
- Necessary **immunizations** for those with **inflammatory bowel disease**. (page 54)
- **Relaxation techniques** to keep stress from triggering digestive woes. (page 68)
- Not just for wrinkles: **Botox** can relieve **digestive symptoms**, too. (page 76)
- Protecting yourself with the **anti-colorectal cancer diet**. (page 79)

You'll also find a new "Ask the Doctor" column on pages 14, 27, 29, 47, and 80. This year's questions came from my patients, but next year we'd like to answer some of yours. If you have any digestive-related queries you want answered in the White Papers, or comments about the White Papers in general, please e-mail the editors at whitepapers@johnshopkinshealthalerts.com.

Wishing you the best of health in 2008,

Sergey V. Kantsevoy, M.D.
Assistant Professor of Medicine
Johns Hopkins University School of Medicine

P. S. Please visit www.HopkinsDigestion.com for the latest news on digestive disorders and other information that will complement your Johns Hopkins White Paper.

THE AUTHOR

Sergey V. Kantsevoy, M.D., Ph.D., received his M.D. and Ph.D. from the Gorky State Medical Institute in the former Soviet Union. He completed extensive training in the former Soviet Union and the United States, including an internship and residency in internal medicine at Washington Hospital Center in Washington, D.C., and a fellowship in gastroenterology at the Johns Hopkins University School of Medicine, where he is now Assistant Professor of Medicine and Director of Endoscopy Training and Certification. He specializes in advanced diagnostic and therapeutic endoscopy, including endoscopic ultrasound, endoscopic retrograde cholangiopancreatography, and biliary and pancreatic manometry.

His areas of research include pancreatic and biliary diseases, intestinal ischemia, and innovative endoscopic techniques such as cryotherapy and natural orifice transluminal endoscopic surgery (NOTES). He has published multiple scientific papers and presented research at numerous medical conventions around the world, including the Unites States, Canada, and the former Soviet Union.

CONTENTS

DIGESTIVE DISORDERS

A wide array of disorders can affect your digestive tract, a long tube of organs that begins at your mouth and ends at your anus. Some of these disorders, such as an occasional bout of heartburn or constipation, are minor annoyances. But many digestive disorders, such as Crohn's disease or irritable bowel syndrome, can severely affect your ability to go about your daily activities, and some, like colorectal cancer or a perforated ulcer, can be life threatening. This White Paper covers many conditions that affect the digestive tract, including diseases of the esophagus, stomach, liver, gallbladder, bile ducts, pancreas, small intestine, large intestine, rectum, and anus. You will learn how to prevent these diseases and, when symptoms arise, the best ways for you and your doctor to diagnose and treat them.

Approximately 70 million Americans have digestive disorders, which prompt nearly 60 million visits to doctors' offices and hospitals each year. Doctors who treat digestive disorders are called gastroenterologists. Although digestive disorders can affect people of any age, many of these problems occur more frequently as we get older.

There are many possible causes of digestive disorders. The most common are infections and a low-fiber, high-fat diet. Some people have a genetic predisposition that makes them more susceptible to these and other environmental triggers. But the causes of some digestive disorders are still unknown.

Although many of the symptoms of digestive disorders—gas, diarrhea, constipation, and blood in the stool—can be embarrassing to discuss, it's important to contact your doctor if you develop any of them. These symptoms can be a sign of something wrong with your digestive tract, and detecting the problem early will improve the success of treatment. Fortunately, there are many treatment options, ranging from lifestyle measures to medications and surgery that can alleviate (in many cases completely) the symptoms.

The Digestive Tract

The digestive tract consists of a series of hollow and solid organs that spans the length of the body from your mouth to your anus (see the illustration on page 3). The major organs along the tract are the esophagus, stomach, small intestine, large intestine (colon), and rectum. The role of the digestive tract is to break down food and fluids to provide your body with the energy it needs to function properly as well as the substances required to build and nourish cells. In a process called peristalsis, rhythmic muscle contractions push the food through the length of the digestive tract. Nutrients from food are absorbed in the small intestine, and what remains undigested passes into the colon and ends up in the stool.

Anatomy of the Upper Digestive Tract

Your upper digestive tract consists of your mouth, pharynx (throat), esophagus, stomach, and duodenum (first part of the small intestine).

Mouth and Pharynx

Your mouth is the first part of your digestive tract. It is where food is chewed and mixed with saliva until it becomes a soft mass that can be swallowed. Saliva is released into the mouth even before food enters it—the odor (or even the thought) of food can make you salivate. An enzyme in saliva called amylase starts breaking down the carbohydrates from food in your mouth. When you swallow, food moves into your pharynx, a passageway that is 5 inches long and carries both food and air.

Esophagus

From the throat, food enters the esophagus—a hollow, muscular tube about 10 inches long. At the upper end of the esophagus is a circular area of muscle tissue called the upper esophageal sphincter. When you swallow, this sphincter relaxes to allow food to enter the esophagus. After you swallow, the sphincter contracts to prevent air in the throat from entering the esophagus. Peristalsis pushes food through your esophagus.

The esophagus descends into the stomach through an opening in the diaphragm (a thin muscle that separates your chest cavity from your abdominal cavity). At the lower end of the esophagus is a ring of muscle tissue called the lower esophageal sphincter. When food reaches the lower esophageal sphincter, it relaxes to allow food to pass through to the stomach. It then contracts to prevent reflux (the backflow of stomach contents into the esophagus).

The esophagus contains a protective inner lining called the mucosa. In a healthy esophagus, the mucosa is smooth and pink. The

The Digestive System

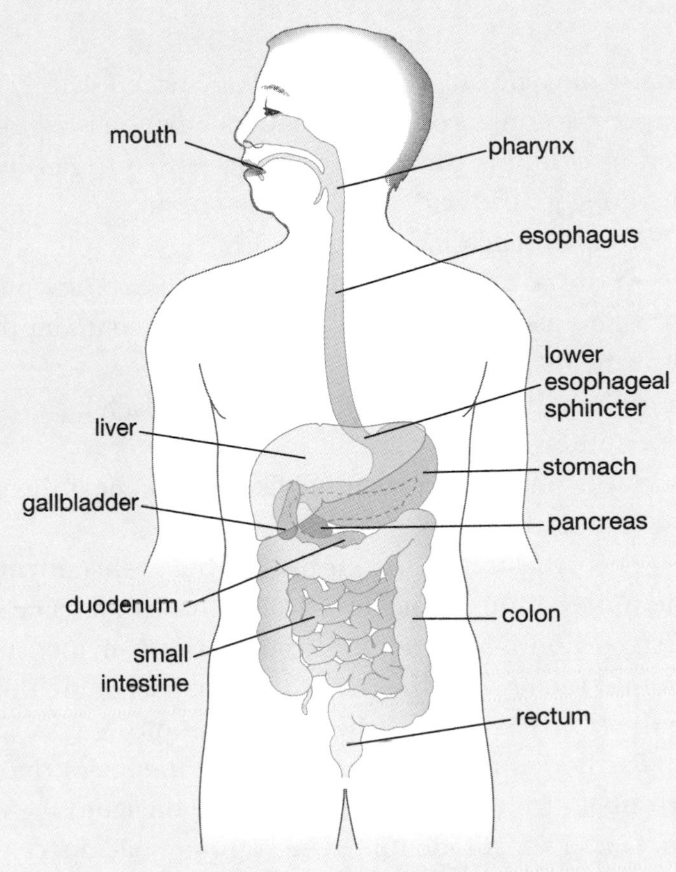

The process of digestion starts with saliva production, which occurs before food even enters the mouth. Saliva helps moisten food and contains an enzyme that breaks down starches. The teeth grind and chop the food, and the tongue mixes it with saliva until the food becomes a soft mass that can be swallowed into the pharynx (throat) and then into the esophagus.

Muscles in the wall of the esophagus then relax in front of the food and contract behind it to propel the mass of food toward the stomach. (These rhythmic muscle contractions, called peristalsis, occur throughout the digestive system.) Within a few seconds, the swallowed food reaches the juncture between the esophagus and stomach, a muscular ring called the lower esophageal sphincter. As food approaches, the sphincter's muscles relax to allow the contents to enter the stomach. In between meals, however, the lower esophageal sphincter generally remains contracted to prevent digestive juices produced in the stomach from entering the esophagus.

Once in the stomach, the food is broken down both chemically (by hydrochloric acid and the enzyme pepsin) and physically (by contraction of muscles in the lower stomach). When the food becomes a thick liquid, it passes from the stomach into the first part of the small intestine, known as the duodenum.

In the small intestine, the food is exposed to digestive juices from the liver, the pancreas, and the cells of the small intestine itself. Bile, a type of digestive juice manufactured in the liver, is stored in the gallbladder and released into the small intestine through the common bile duct.

The partially digested food components then move through the duodenum to the lower two sections of the small intestine (the jejunum and the ileum) over a period of about three to six hours. During this time, enzymes from the pancreas and intestinal cells break down the protein, carbohydrate, and fat components of food into smaller, more easily absorbed substances. Specialized cells then absorb these substances (nutrients) through the intestinal wall and deliver them into the bloodstream and lymphatic system. The nutrients are then transported to cells throughout the body.

The remaining mass of undigested matter (such as fiber), water, and electrolytes then passes from the ileum into the large intestine, also called the colon. Over the next one to two days, this residue moves through the length of the large intestine, where most of the water and salts from the residue are absorbed into the bloodstream.

The remaining solid waste accumulates in the rectum, the last portion of the large intestine. As waste material gathers, the walls of the rectum stretch, signaling the need to pass the stool. To have a bowel movement, the sphincter muscles in the anus—the last component of the digestive system—must relax as the muscles in the walls of the rectum contract to push out the stool.

The entire digestive process, beginning with chewing and ending with a bowel movement, can take anywhere from 18 hours to a number of days. ■

place where the esophagus makes contact with the stomach is called the gastroesophageal junction; it forms an irregular white line called the Z-line that can be seen by your doctor with an endoscope.

Stomach and Duodenum

Your stomach is a large, stretchy bag located slightly to the left in the upper portion of your abdomen. Its function is to hold ingested food and to continue the digestive process that began in your mouth by secreting gastric acid and digestive enzymes.

Your stomach has four sections:

- Cardia, a short segment next to the gastroesophageal junction
- Fundus, the top of the stomach located under the left dome of the diaphragm
- Body, the largest portion of the stomach located between the fundus and antrum
- Antrum, a short, channel-like portion near the bottom of the stomach.

The pylorus is a circular muscle below the antrum that connects the outlet of the stomach with the duodenum. The duodenum, the first portion of the small intestine, is a C-shaped tube that curves around the head of the pancreas. The part of the duodenum closest to the stomach is called the duodenal bulb.

Farther along in the duodenum is the major duodenal papilla, a protuberance where the common bile duct and the main pancreatic duct enter the duodenum. The common bile duct carries bile secreted from the liver via the gallbladder into the duodenum; the main pancreatic duct carries enzymes formed in the pancreas. The bile and pancreatic enzymes help digest food in the duodenum.

Tests for Examining the Upper Digestive Tract

Your doctor cannot determine the health of your upper digestive tract by examining you externally. He or she needs an internal view of your digestive tract. Ways to do this include an upper endoscopy, an upper gastrointestinal (GI) series, esophageal manometry, and pH monitoring.

Upper Endoscopy

An upper endoscopy examines the inside lining of the esophagus, stomach, and duodenum. It uses an endoscope—a long, thin, flexible tube with a tiny light and video camera at its tip—to look for abnormalities such as inflammation, ulcers, and tumors. If you're experiencing difficulty swallowing, nausea, vomiting with or without blood or coffee grounds-like material, heartburn, indigestion, upper abdominal pain, or chest pain, your doctor may perform an upper endoscopy. (See "Upper Endoscopy: What to Expect" on pages 6–7.)

Capsule Endoscopy

An upper endoscopy does not provide information about the small intestine beyond the duodenum. For this, the U.S. Food and Drug Administration (FDA) approved the use of a tiny ingestible camera in a capsule that takes close-up pictures of the small intestine as the capsule moves through the digestive tract. For more, see page 41.

Upper Gastrointestinal (GI) Series

An upper GI series (also called a barium x-ray) is usually used to evaluate areas of the small intestine that an endoscope cannot reach. In addition, if you cannot undergo an upper endoscopy—perhaps because you tend to bleed excessively or the number of platelets in your blood is low—an upper GI series may be performed to examine the esophagus, stomach, and duodenum.

An upper GI series is performed by a radiologist. First, you drink a solution containing barium (a heavy metal). The radiologist follows the passage of the barium through the upper digestive tract using a machine called a fluoroscope. X-rays also are taken. The barium coats the inner layer of the digestive tract, making it visible on the x-rays. The x-rays can reveal ulcers, tumors, strictures (abnormal narrowings due to scar tissue), areas of swelling and inflammation, and fistulas (abnormal connections between two organs).

Esophageal Manometry

This test measures pressure and evaluates contractions within the esophagus. It is typically performed to diagnose gastroesophageal reflux disease (GERD; see pages 10–15) and swallowing problems. During the test, a physician or specially trained nurse inserts a thin, pressure-sensitive probe through the nose and into the esophagus. The probe measures pressure within the esophagus while it contracts; it also measures pressure of the lower esophageal sphincter. Abnormal muscle contractions in the esophagus and decreased lower esophageal sphincter pressure indicate weakening of the antireflux barrier. The test takes about an hour.

Upper Endoscopy: What To Expect

If you are having problems with your upper digestive tract, you may need to undergo an upper endoscopy which examines the inside of the esophagus, stomach, and duodenum (the first part of the small intestine). Problems that might require an upper endoscopy include difficulty swallowing, nausea, vomiting, acid reflux, gastrointestinal bleeding, indigestion, upper abdominal pain, and chest pain.

Most people are nervous about having an upper endoscopy because it involves inserting a tube, about the thickness of your finger, down the throat and into the digestive tract. But the procedure usually produces little or no discomfort.

What Is An Upper Endoscopy?
An upper endoscopy, also known as esophagogastroduodenoscopy, is a way to examine the inside lining of the upper digestive tract. The procedure uses an endoscope—a long, thin, flexible tube with a light and tiny video camera at one end. The doctor guides the endoscope into the upper digestive tract and looks for abnormalities such as inflammation, ulcers, and tumors. In some cases, the doctor uses the endoscope to treat the abnormality.

What Happens Before?
Before you are scheduled for the endoscopy, your doctor will ask if you have any health problems or allergies and whether you are taking any medications. This information lets the doctor know what precautions to take before, during, and after the procedure.

The most important step is to make sure that you do not eat or drink anything for at least six to eight hours before the procedure. Food in the stomach or duodenum can block the view of the upper digestive tract and could cause you to vomit. You must also make arrangements for someone to drive you home afterwards because the sedative used during the procedure can affect your judgment and reflexes for the rest of the day.

What Happens During?
An upper endoscopy is performed in a hospital or a doctor's office and takes about 30 minutes. A numbing agent will be sprayed into your throat to prevent gagging when the endoscope is inserted. You'll also receive a pain medication and a sedative to keep you relaxed. Then, while you are lying on your left side, the doctor will slowly and gently insert the endoscope into the upper digestive tract. Air will be blown into the stomach through the endoscope to make it easier for the doctor to see the lining of the digestive tract.

The images from the endoscope are viewed on a television monitor. If the doctor notices anything abnormal in the lining of the upper digestive tract, a sample of the tissue (a biopsy sample) may be taken for

Esophageal Impedance Testing

This test also involves having a tiny tube inserted into your esophagus and measures whether gas or liquid is backing up into the esophagus. It is a helpful diagnostic tool for those with non-acidic reflux, since these substances wouldn't be detected by pH monitoring.

pH Monitoring

A pH monitoring test is often given to diagnose the severity of heartburn and GERD. A tiny tube or wireless capsule is placed in your esophagus for 24 hours, while you go about your daily activities, to record fluctuations in acid backing up into your esophagus from your stomach. Two-day pH monitoring is another option to detect GERD more accurately than standard 24-hour pH monitoring.

examination under a microscope. Instruments can be inserted into the endoscope to stop bleeding from an ulcer, to remove a non-cancerous growth, or to stretch a narrowed area of the esophagus. When the procedure is done, the endoscope is removed.

During the procedure the doctor and a nurse will administer pain medicine and sedatives while closely monitoring your vital signs (rate of your heart contractions, blood pressure, oxygen content in your blood, and so on) to ensure safety.

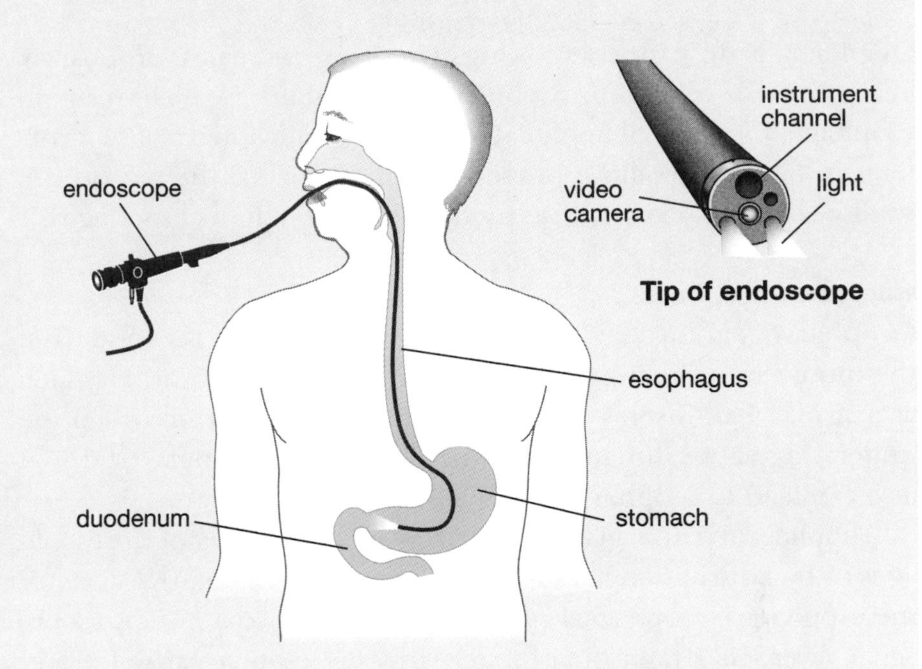

What Happens Afterward?
After the procedure, you will be taken to a recovery room to rest until the sedative wears off. This usually takes about one to two hours. Before you go home, your doctor will tell you the results. If a tissue sample was taken, your doctor will call you with results in a couple of days. You should rest for the remainder of the day and avoid driving.

An upper endoscopy is safe when performed by a doctor trained and experienced in the procedure. Serious complications, such as excessive bleeding, aspiration of stomach contents or saliva into the lungs, and puncture of the intestinal wall, are extremely rare. Some people have mild complications, such as a sore throat or bloating (due to the air introduced during the procedure), which usually disappear within 24 hours. Contact your doctor immediately if you experience signs of a serious complication (such as fever, difficulty swallowing, or increasing throat, chest, or abdominal pain). ■

Duodenal Gastroesophageal Reflux Testing

Duodenal gastroesophageal reflux (or bile reflux) can be a complicating factor in GERD. This test detects whether contents of the duodenum, such as bile or pancreatic enzymes, are backing up into the esophagus. You go about your daily activities while wearing a tiny tube in your esophagus. The fiberoptic tool attached detects the yellow color of bilirubin, the major component of bile.

Disorders of the Upper Digestive Tract

A number of disorders can arise in the upper digestive tract. They include dysphagia (difficulty swallowing), a hiatal hernia, GERD and other esophageal problems, gastritis, and peptic ulcers.

Dysphagia

Dysphagia is difficulty swallowing. There are two types: oropharyngeal (which is related to problems in the mouth or pharynx) and esophageal. In oropharyngeal dysphagia, individuals have problems initiating a swallow; in esophageal dysphagia, the person can swallow but problems arise as food passes through the esophagus.

Causes of dysphagia

Oropharyngeal dysphagia is caused by problems getting food from the mouth into the upper esophagus. Neurological disorders, such as a stroke, Parkinson's disease, or multiple sclerosis, are often the underlying cause. Inflammation or cancer of the mouth or throat also can lead to oropharyngeal dysphagia.

Esophageal dysphagia can be caused by a narrowing of the esophagus or by a disruption in esophageal motility (movement). Cancer of the esophagus, esophageal strictures (caused by scar tissue), esophageal diverticula (abnormal pouches in the esophageal wall), and esophageal rings or webs (thin, fragile mucosal folds that partially or completely block the esophagus) all can narrow the esophagus, making the passage of food more difficult. Esophageal motility can be disrupted by scleroderma (an autoimmune disease that affects the skin and internal organs), diffuse esophageal spasm (prolonged and excessive contractions of the esophagus), and achalasia (the inability of the lower esophageal sphincter to relax).

Symptoms of dysphagia

Typically, the first symptom of both oropharyngeal and esophageal dysphagia is a problem in swallowing solid food. Difficulty in beginning a swallow, coughing or inhaling food into the lungs while attempting to swallow, and food coming up through the nose are common symptoms of oropharyngeal dysphagia. If you have esophageal dysphagia, it may feel as if food is stuck in the esophagus, and you may have to strain or eat with your head turned to one side to propel food through the esophagus into your stomach.

Diagnosis of dysphagia

Your doctor will ask you some questions about your swallowing difficulties. For example: Is swallowing a problem with both liquids and solids? Difficulty swallowing both liquids and solids usually results from a motility problem. Difficulty swallowing only solids suggests a structural problem. The doctor will also perform an upper endoscopy or an upper GI series to determine the cause of dysphagia.

Treatment of dysphagia

The treatment of dysphagia depends on what is causing the problem. If the cause is esophageal strictures, rings, or webs or if you have achalasia, a procedure called endoscopic dilation may be performed to expand the esophagus. In this procedure, the esophagus is gradually stretched using special dilators or a balloon inserted through an endoscope and then inflated. Surgery may be necessary to treat esophageal tumors that have narrowed the esophagus.

You also may be referred to a speech-language pathologist who diagnoses and treats dysphagia in addition to dealing with language, voice, and speech problems. Therapy may involve learning exercises, body positions, and other techniques to improve your ability to swallow. The speech-language pathologist may also recommend foods and liquids with textures that are safer and easier to swallow.

Hiatal Hernia

The esophagus passes through a small opening in the diaphragm, which separates the chest cavity from the abdominal cavity. Normally, the lower esophageal sphincter at the bottom of the esophagus is aligned with this opening in the diaphragm (the hiatus). The rest of the esophagus is located above the diaphragm in the chest cavity,and the stomach is located below the diaphragm in the abdominal cavity.

If you are one of the 25% of people over age 50 who have a hiatal hernia, your lower esophageal sphincter and a small portion of your stomach have slipped through the opening in the diaphragm and are now protruding into your chest cavity. This creates a separation between the lower esophageal sphincter and the diaphragm, which weakens the barrier against reflux of acid from the stomach into the esophagus, increasing the risk of GERD and erosive esophagitis (damage to the lining of the esophagus).

Causes of hiatal hernia

A hiatal hernia can be congenital, meaning that you are born with it, or it can develop later in life. When it occurs later in life, a hiatal hernia is the result of either a weakening of the muscle that surrounds the opening of the diaphragm or a rise in pressure in the abdominal cavity. Risk factors for a hiatal hernia include being overweight and lifting heavy objects.

Symptoms of hiatal hernia

Most hiatal hernias produce no symptoms and are found by chance during tests for other health problems. However, when the lower esophageal sphincter is significantly displaced from its normal position in the hiatus, reflux symptoms (such as heartburn) can occur.

Diagnosis and treatment of hiatal hernia

Hiatal hernias are diagnosed by an upper GI series or an upper endoscopy. If a hiatal hernia is not causing any symptoms, treatment is not needed. When symptoms such as recurrent heartburn arise, they can often be relieved with lifestyle measures and medication (see the section on GERD below). If the hiatal hernia is causing severe reflux, it can be repaired surgically by pulling the stomach back into the abdominal cavity and repairing the defect in the diaphragm that allowed the stomach to slip into the chest cavity. To prevent future slippage and to strengthen the lower esophageal sphincter to reduce reflux, the surgeon may also perform a Nissen fundoplication, in which the top portion of the stomach is wrapped around the bottom of the lower esophageal sphincter.

Gastroesophageal Reflux Disease (GERD)

The contents of your stomach are emptied into the small intestine, but sometimes they flow backwards into your esophagus. This phenomenon, known as gastroesophageal reflux, happens to everyone from time to time. It usually produces no symptoms other than occasional heartburn—a burning sensation behind the breastbone.

When gastroesophageal reflux occurs frequently, however, you may begin to experience significant discomfort related to the acid reflux—then, it is considered gastroesophageal reflux disease (GERD). Many people in the United States have GERD: Heartburn affects about 7–10% of U.S. adults every day and up to 44% at least once a month. Symptoms of reflux are more common in individuals who are obese, smoke, or drink alcohol.

GERD is a serious condition because the acid and digestive enzymes from the stomach can damage tissues in the esophagus as well as in adjacent organs such as the mouth, pharynx (throat), larynx (voice box), trachea (windpipe), and lungs.

Causes of GERD

Coordinated contractions of the lower esophageal sphincter and the diaphragm produce an area of high pressure in the lower segment of the esophagus that prevents stomach contents from entering the esophagus.

This "antireflux barrier" does not always work properly. When it fails occasionally, the esophagus has several defenses to help it deal with the harsh stomach contents. First, the esophageal secretions and your saliva are alkaline, which helps to neutralize the acid and inactivate the enzymes from the stomach. Second, peristalsis and gravity work together to rapidly clear the esophagus of the acid and enzymes, minimizing the length of time the lining of the esophagus is exposed to the stomach contents. Third, the esophageal mucosa is able to regenerate quickly following injury from acid or enzymes. However, frequent reflux of the acidic stomach contents can overwhelm these protective measures, resulting in damage to the tissues of the esophagus and adjacent organs.

A recent survey of 43,000 people found that smoking and excessive use of table salt can increase the risk of GERD by 70%. A 2005 study found that a diet high in calories and fat (especially saturated fat) is linked to GERD. Medications that relax the lower esophageal sphincter, such as the bronchodilator theophylline (Theo-24, Theo-Dur, Uniphyl) used to treat asthma, emphysema, and chronic bronchitis), calcium channel blockers (for angina or high blood pressure), nonsteroidal anti-inflammatory drugs (for arthritis and pain), bisphosphonate drugs (for osteoporosis), some medications to treat menopausal symptoms, and a class of antidepressant drugs called tricyclics also can trigger GERD. If you are at risk for GERD or develop it while taking any of these medications, discuss with your doctor the possibility of discontinuing, switching from, or reducing the dosage of the medication. (Excess weight also can cause GERD; see "Obesity and Gastroesophageal Reflux Disease" on pages 12–13.)

Symptoms of GERD

GERD most often produces heartburn, indigestion (discomfort in the upper abdomen, nausea, and sometimes vomiting), and regurgitation of food from the stomach into the esophagus and mouth. Acid from the stomach can even regurgitate into organs connected to the esophagus, such as the larynx, trachea, and lungs. This can cause voice changes such as hoarseness, a chronic cough, episodes of asthma, or pain behind the sternum bone that resembles a heart attack. In fact, 10–15% of people with GERD experience these symptoms instead of heartburn and regurgitation, making diagnosis and treatment more difficult.

The chest pain associated with an intense episode of heartburn can feel like a heart attack. If you think you are having a heart attack, seek medical assistance immediately. Much of the damage done by a heart attack occurs in the first hour. Therefore, waiting

NEW RESEARCH

Nonacid Reflux May Increase on Proton Pump Inhibitors

Some people with GERD may find that their symptoms persist even while taking proton pump inhibitors, which are usually very effective. A new study suggests that the symptoms may be caused by a relative increase in nonacid reflux events—bile salts and pancreatic enzymes that back up into the esophagus—primarily during sleep.

Researchers randomly assigned 15 people with GERD to take esomeprazole (Nexium) or a placebo. After one week of treatment, the participants were given a reflux-causing dinner of pizza, brownies, and grape juice, then were monitored in their sleep for the frequency and type of all reflux events. The participants then switched treatments and took part in a repeat sleep study one week later.

As expected, acid reflux was significantly less common in the Nexium group compared with the placebo group (12 vs. 67)—but nonacid reflux events were more frequent among the Nexium users (27 vs. 6).

However, all participants were equally likely to wake up following either acid or nonacid incidents and produce saliva and swallow, which protects the esophagus. So nonacid reflux poses no increased risk of damage to the esophagus.

CHEST
Volume 131, page 460
February 2007

Obesity and Gastroesophageal Reflux Disease

How excess pounds may lead to acid reflux

Eating too much food once in a while might give you occasional heartburn, but eating too much on a regular basis may give you gastroesophageal reflux disease (GERD). With both obesity and GERD on the rise in the United States, medical researchers have wondered if a link exists between the two. The answer to this question appears to be "yes."

A December 2006 review article in *The American Journal of Gastroenterology* examined the results of 20 studies involving more than 18,000 people with GERD. Overall, people who were overweight were 50% more likely to have GERD than normal-weight people; obese individuals were more than twice as likely. An August 2005 review of nine studies in the journal *Annals of Internal Medicine* found almost identical results.

Excess Weight and Reflux

Several possible theories may explain the link between GERD and obesity.

For example, extra fat in the abdomen may increase pressure on the stomach and cause the lower esophageal sphincter to relax, allowing stomach contents to flow back up into the esophagus. In addition, body fat may release chemicals that decrease pressure in the lower esophageal sphincter or slow the clearance of acid from the esophagus.

Another possibility: Estrogen levels may play a role in the connection between obesity and GERD. One study found that obese women were more likely than obese men to have GERD; the risk was highest in premenopausal women and in postmenopausal women taking estrogen.

Will Weight Loss Help?

Whatever may be causing the increased risk of GERD in obese people, losing weight seems to help. A 2006 review article in the *Archives of Internal Medicine* found that losing weight and elevating the head of the bed were the only lifestyle measures that helped relieve GERD symptoms.

How much weight loss is enough? According to a 2006 study in *The New England Journal of Medicine,* decreasing BMI by 3.5 points (the equivalent of losing about 20 lbs) may significantly improve your GERD symptoms.

Starting a Program

The best way to lose weight and to keep it off is to make changes in both your diet and level of physical activity. To lose about 1 lb per week—a gradual and safe rate of

to see if chest pain is due to heartburn could prove fatal.

How can you distinguish between a heart attack and GERD? Your chest pain is more likely to be heartburn if it is accompanied by a bitter or acid taste in your mouth or other symptoms such as belching and difficulty swallowing, and if the pain worsens when you lie down or bend over and improves when you take an antacid. But if the pain is accompanied by a cold sweat, a fast heartbeat, shortness of breath, or lightheadedness and the pain radiates down one or both arms, there's a good chance you're having a heart attack. Again, if you have any doubt about the cause of your chest pain, you should err on the side of caution and call 911 immediately, chew an aspirin, and lie down until an ambulance arrives.

Diagnosis of GERD

To diagnose GERD, your doctor will perform an upper endoscopy as well as other tests to measure the motility and pH (acid concentration) of your esophagus.

weight loss—you must cut out about 500 calories per day.

You could just eat 500 fewer calories, but combining exercise with diet results in greater losses of body weight and fat than dieting alone. By adding a half hour or more of moderate exercise each day (enough to burn 250 calories), you can reduce your calorie restriction to a more manageable 250 calories daily.

Cutting calories. Instead of embarking on a fad diet, simply make sensible food choices: Replace dietary fat with complex carbohydrates (for example, fruits, vegetables, and whole grains), which automatically lowers your calorie intake but allows you to eat a satisfying volume of food.

In addition, eat lean instead of fatty cuts of meat, choose reduced-fat or reduced-calorie products when possible, opt for non-calorie beverages such as water, diet soda, or seltzer, and fill up on less energy-dense foods like fruits, vegetables, salads, and soups. Also, learn to read nutrition labels and stick to the portion sizes on the label.

Adding exercise. When planning an exercise routine, choose activities that are convenient and enjoyable. The following are some popular exercises and the calories burned after 30 minutes of activity:

- Swimming: 301 calories
- Walking (brisk): 149 calories
- Tennis (singles): 275 calories
- Yoga: 180 calories
- Golf: 120 calories
- Dancing: 185 calories

Gradually build up to 60–90 minutes of exercise daily. Don't be discouraged, though; you don't need to get all your exercise at one time. Breaking it up over the course of the day is just as effective. ■

Are You Overweight or Obese?

The easiest way to find out is to calculate your body mass index (BMI), a measure of your weight in relation to your height.

1. Multiply your weight in pounds by 703.
2. Multiply your height in inches by itself.
3. Divide the result in step 1 by the result in step 2.

If your BMI is between 25 and 29.9, you are overweight. You're considered obese if your BMI is 30 or more.

Treatment of GERD

There are four types of treatments for GERD: lifestyle measures, medication, surgery, and endoscopic procedures. Treating GERD is important. Untreated GERD can lead to serious complications, such as esophageal ulcers (nonhealing mucosal defects), esophageal strictures, Barrett's esophagus (a disorder of the cells lining the esophageal mucosa, which may lead to cancer), and esophageal cancer.

Lifestyle measures. The treatment of GERD starts with lifestyle measures, which may eliminate symptoms in some people with mild reflux. Traditionally, doctors recommended avoiding large meals as well as acidic foods (such as tomato-based products and citrus fruits), fatty or spicy foods, table salt, garlic, onions, peppermint, spearmint, chocolate, cinnamon, coffee, tea, carbonated beverages, alcohol, and smoking. But a recent study found little evidence for these and other lifestyle measures. The only ones that worked for relieving GERD symptoms were sleeping with the head of the bed elevated and losing weight. Nonetheless, lifestyle measures are worth a try before resorting to medication and other treatments for GERD.

Medication. If lifestyle modifications do not eliminate all of your symptoms, your doctor will recommend that you take medication to neutralize or decrease acid production in the stomach. These medications include antacids, histamine H_2-receptor antagonists (also known as H_2-blockers), mucosal protectants, proton pump inhibitors, and promotility agents. Sometimes a single medication will work, but if it doesn't control your symptoms, you may need to take a second medication. Although there have been concerns over long-term suppression of gastric acid, a recent study suggests that use of H_2-blockers and proton pump inhibitors does not increase the risk of esophageal or stomach cancer. (Also, see the "Ask the Doctor" column at right.)

Antacids. Over-the-counter antacids containing aluminum oxide, magnesium carbonate, and sodium bicarbonate (for example, Gaviscon, Gelusil, Maalox, Mylanta) rapidly neutralize stomach acid and are taken after meals when you experience heartburn. These medications provide fast relief, but their effect is short lived.

H_2-blockers. Over-the-counter or prescription H_2-blockers, which include cimetidine (Tagamet), famotidine (Pepcid), nizatidine (Axid), and ranitidine (Zantac), have a longer-acting effect on gastric acid than antacids. They usually need to be taken twice a day. A combination antacid/H_2-blocker, Pepcid Complete, also is available that appears to be more effective at relieving symptoms than H_2-blockers or antacids alone.

Mucosal protectants. A prescription mucosal protectant called sucralfate (Carafate), which is taken one hour before a meal, coats the esophagus, increasing its resistance to reflux from the stomach.

Proton pump inhibitors. These prescription drugs, which include esomeprazole (Nexium), lansoprazole (Prevacid), omeprazole (Prilosec), pantoprazole (Protonix), rabeprazole (AcipHex), and an omeprazole/sodium bicarbonate combination (Zegerid), are the most potent suppressors of gastric acid. They have a long-lasting effect and need to be taken only once a day. Prilosec is now available without a prescription in a 20-mg formulation.

Promotility agents. The effects of H_2-blockers and proton pump inhibitors can be enhanced by taking a promotility agent, such as metoclopramide (Reglan). This medication increases the clearance of acid from the esophagus, raises the pressure of the lower esophageal sphincter, and speeds emptying of the stomach. (For more on medications to treat GERD, see the drug chart on pages 18–22.)

ASK THE DOCTOR

Q. ***What are the risks of taking reflux medication over the long term?***

A. Medications like proton pump inhibitors and H_2-blockers are generally very safe. But as with any drugs, their beneficial effects are often offset by some negative consequences.

The most serious potential complications of reflux medication result from the reduction of stomach acid that actually protects your body from bacteria and viruses that may be present in food. Without sufficient acid levels, stomach bacteria are allowed to grow—and travel up or down the digestive tract.

For example, there's a small chance that stomach bacteria may enter your trachea and upper airways, resulting in pneumonia. Or you may not have enough acid to fight off a serious intestinal infection from a bacterium like *Clostridium difficile (C. difficile)*, which causes colitis, diarrhea, and cramps.

Your body also needs stomach acid to help digest vitamin B_{12}. Without sufficient levels of stomach acid, you could develop low vitamin B_{12} levels and, subsequently, anemia.

All of these potential complications are rare and treatable, so for most people, taking reflux medication does more good than harm—especially if you have esophagitis or Barrett's esophagus. If your reflux isn't severe, talk with your doctor about taking your medication as needed, rather than continuously.

Surgery. Lifestyle measures and medications are so effective at controlling reflux symptoms that only a small number of people need to undergo surgery. When surgery is required, the most common procedure is Nissen fundoplication. It involves lifting a portion of the stomach and tightening it around the gastroesophageal junction to increase pressure in the lower esophageal sphincter. The procedure is typically performed using laparoscopy. Five small incisions are made in the abdomen, and the surgeon inserts a tiny camera and specialized instruments through the incisions to perform the procedure.

Nissen fundoplication is performed in a hospital. You will receive general anesthesia and need to stay in the hospital for one to three days. Serious complications are rare but can include a negative reaction to the anesthesia, blood loss, infection, and injury to the esophagus, stomach, or spleen. More common complications are stomach bloating, difficulty swallowing, belching, and vomiting. These complications usually improve within one to three months.

Surgery reduces reflux symptoms in most people, but it does not always eliminate the symptoms. About a third of people who undergo Nissen fundoplication still require medication on a regular basis to control their symptoms.

Endoscopic procedures. These procedures are performed during an upper endoscopy on an outpatient basis and do not require incisions, general anesthesia, or a hospital stay like surgery does. However, these procedures are relatively new and their long-term effectiveness is not yet fully known.

One of these procedures is called endoscopic gastroplication. In the procedure, a gastroenterologist places a pair of stitches in the upper stomach about a centimeter below the lower esophageal sphincter and pulls the stitches together to form a "pleat." Usually, two to four pleats are created. By reducing the size of the opening between the stomach and esophagus, the pleats help prevent reflux of stomach contents into the esophagus.

A second procedure, full-thickness plication, also places a stitch in the gastroesophageal junction to prevent the reflux of acid into the esophagus. (See the "New Research" column at right.)

A third treatment, known as the Stretta procedure, delivers radiofrequency energy to the far end of the esophagus as well as to the upper stomach, creating multiple burns in the tissue there. As the tissue heals, it contracts and narrows the esophagus, helping to reduce reflux. The procedure works moderately well, but serious side effects, including death, have been reported.

NEW RESEARCH

Benefits of New GERD Surgery Extend to Three Years

When lifestyle changes and medication aren't enough to control GERD, endoscopic therapy may be a good option. One newer procedure, full-thickness plication, has been shown to reduce GERD symptoms and medication use one year later; now a new study shows that the benefits may extend to three years.

The study involved 29 people with GERD who took medication—either a proton pump inhibitor or an H_2-blocker—every day. All of the participants underwent the full-thickness plication procedure, which endoscopically places a stitch in the gastroesophageal junction to prevent acid reflux into the esophagus. They were evaluated for symptoms and medication use 12 and 36 months later.

Three years after endoscopic correction of GERD, 57% of the participants no longer needed daily medication, and 50% did not require any medication at all. These results are similar to those one year after surgery. There were no long-term adverse effects from the procedure, and any side effects (such as sore throat, abdominal pain, and chest pain) resolved within several days.

Full-thickness plication may be a viable option for people with mild GERD, and more research is needed to investigate the procedure in people with advanced reflux.

SURGICAL ENDOSCOPY
Volume 21, page 439
March 2007

Esophageal Motility Disorders

In a healthy esophagus, peristalsis propels food and fluid down the esophagus. Sometimes, however, these contractions become ineffective, and you have an esophageal motility disorder.

The two most common esophageal motility disorders are diffuse esophageal spasm and achalasia. In diffuse esophageal spasm, several segments of the esophagus contract strongly and simultaneously, preventing the normal, wave-like contractions from moving food and fluid down the esophagus. In achalasia, there is an absence of normal, wave-like contractions in the lower half of the esophagus, and the lower esophageal sphincter fails to relax and allow food to enter the stomach.

Causes of esophageal motility disorders

The causes of esophageal spasm and achalasia are unknown, and there are no known risk factors.

Symptoms of esophageal motility disorders

People with diffuse esophageal spasm experience intermittent episodes of dysphagia (difficulty swallowing), usually with both liquids and solids, as well as pain behind the breastbone. People with achalasia have gradually worsening swallowing problems with both solids and liquids, regurgitation of ingested food, and weight loss.

Diagnosis of esophageal motility disorders

The best test for diagnosing achalasia is esophageal manometry. In people with achalasia, manometry reveals very weak esophageal peristalsis as well as persistent elevated pressure in the lower esophageal sphincter (which indicates that the sphincter muscle cannot relax). Esophageal manometry is also helpful in diagnosing diffuse esophageal spasm. In this case, the test will show intense contractions of the esophageal wall.

An upper GI series also can be used to diagnose these disorders. In people with diffuse esophageal spasm, the radiologist will see strong contractions of the esophagus, which interfere with the movement of barium through the esophagus. Barium x-rays in people with achalasia often reveal widening of the upper portion of the esophagus with a gradual narrowing at the lower end.

In older people with suspected achalasia, an upper endoscopy to obtain a tissue sample from the gastroesophageal junction is necessary to rule out cancer.

NEW RESEARCH

Theophylline: A New Treatment for Esophageal Chest Pain?

Noncardiac chest pain—caused not by a heart attack but hypersensitivity of the esophagus—sends millions to the emergency room each year. A study now suggests that theophylline (Theo-24, Theo-Dur, Uniphyl), used to treat asthma, chronic bronchitis, emphysema, and other lung diseases, may help relieve esophageal chest pain.

In the first of two double-blind studies, 16 participants with esophageal hypersensitivity were randomly given intravenous theophylline or a placebo. A balloon was placed into the esophagus and inflated to reproduce typical chest pain. Those taking theophylline found that their threshold for pain greatly increased—63% had no pain—while the placebo group saw no improvement.

In the second study, 24 participants with esophageal hypersensitivity were randomly treated for four weeks with oral theophylline or a placebo. Overall, 58% of the participants had less chest pain while taking theophylline, while only 6% improved on the placebo.

Theophylline may help by increasing pain thresholds in the esophagus, decreasing hypersensitivity, and relaxing the esophageal wall. However, side effects may be common with theophylline—26% of the participants reported them—and experts question whether it will become a standard treatment owing to its potential for toxic reactions.

THE AMERICAN JOURNAL OF GASTROENTEROLOGY
Volume 102, page 930
May 2007

Treatment of esophageal motility disorders

Achalasia is initially treated with drugs like calcium channel blockers and nitroglycerin to relax the lower esophageal sphincter. Unfortunately, they are often ineffective, and most people require an endoscopic or surgical procedure to relax the lower esophageal sphincter.

The two endoscopic procedures for achalasia are dilation and injection of botulinum toxin A (Botox). Dilation involves insertion of a balloon device to expand the lower esophageal sphincter. Botox is injected into the lower esophageal sphincter to paralyze and relax it. Because the effects of Botox appear to be temporary, it is only recommended for people who are not good candidates for endoscopic dilation or surgery. (For more, see "Botox: Not Just a Wrinkle Eraser" on pages 76–77.)

Heller myotomy is the surgical procedure for achalasia. An incision is made through the muscle of the lower esophageal sphincter to weaken it. It can be done using a traditional surgical approach (making a large incision in the abdomen) or through small incisions in the abdomen (laparoscopy) or chest (thoracoscopy).

Unfortunately, there is no effective treatment for diffuse esophageal spasm. Medications such as calcium channel blockers and nitrates may be prescribed but are typically not helpful.

Esophageal Stricture

An esophageal stricture is a narrowing of the esophagus, typically in the lower third of the organ.

Causes and symptoms of esophageal stricture

Esophageal stricture is the result of chronic inflammation and scar tissue due to poorly controlled GERD. People with the disorder have ongoing difficulties in swallowing solid food, and the problem gradually worsens over time.

Diagnosis and treatment of esophageal stricture

An upper endoscopy must be performed to obtain a tissue sample from the stricture to rule out cancer. Treatment may require esophageal dilation followed by aggressive control of GERD with medications to prevent recurrence of the stricture. If dilation cannot widen the esophagus, surgery is recommended.

Barrett's Esophagus

Barrett's esophagus occurs when cells in the lining of the esophagus, also known as the esophageal mucosa, are replaced by cells

NEW RESEARCH

Celebrex Does Not Help Lower Barrett's Esophagus Cancer Risk

Nonsteroidal anti-inflammatory drugs (NSAIDs) such as aspirin and ibuprofen are thought to decrease the risk of developing esophageal cancer. But a study suggests that people with Barrett's esophagus—which is known to increase the risk of esophageal cancer—won't get any protection from taking the popular COX-2 inhibitor NSAID celecoxib (Celebrex).

Researchers at Johns Hopkins took biopsy samples from 100 people with Barrett's esophagus, then randomly assigned them to take either 200 mg of Celebrex or a placebo twice daily. Participants received upper endoscopies every three or six months throughout the study, depending on the severity of their condition.

Nearly a year later, repeat biopsy samples showed that people in the Celebrex group were no less likely to have dysplasia (precancerous cell changes) or cancer than people in the placebo group. Celebrex also did not appear to change the surface area affected by Barrett's esophagus.

The researchers theorize that the dosage of the drug used in the study may have been too low to be effective.

JOURNAL OF THE NATIONAL CANCER INSTITUTE
Volume 99, page 545
April 4, 2007

Prescription Drugs for the Treatment of Gastroesophageal Reflux Disease 2008

Drug type: Brand (generic)	Typical daily dosages*	How to take†	Monthly cost‡: Brand (generic)
Proton pump inhibitors			
AcipHex (rabeprazole)	20 mg	One 20-mg tablet 1x/day with or without food. Swallow whole (do not crush, chew, or split).	$140
Nexium (esomeprazole)	40 mg	One 40-mg capsule 1x/day at least 1 hour before a meal. Swallow whole.§	$137
Prevacid (lansoprazole)	15–30 mg	One 15- or 30-mg capsule 1x/day 1 hour before eating. Swallow whole.§	$142–148
Prilosec (omeprazole)‖	20 mg	One 20-mg capsule 1x/day 1 hour before a meal. Swallow whole.§	$131 ($21)
Protonix (pantoprazole)	40 mg	One 40-mg tablet 1x/day with or without food. Swallow whole.	$120
Zegerid (omeprazole/ sodium bicarbonate)	Capsule: 20 mg/1,100 mg Powder: 20 mg/1,680 mg	Capsule: One 20-mg/1,100-mg capsule on an empty stomach 1x/day at least 1 hour before a meal and with a full glass of water. Swallow whole. Powder: Empty one 20-mg/1,680-mg packet into 1–2 Tbsp of water 1x/day. Mix and take immediately with a full glass of water.	Capsule: Not available Powder: $145
Histamine H_2-antagonists (H_2-blockers)¶			
Axid (nizatidine)	300 mg	One 150-mg capsule 2x/day with or without food for up to 12 weeks.	$161 ($52)
Pepcid (famotidine)	40–80 mg	One 20- or 40-mg tablet 2x/day with or without food for 6–12 weeks.	$110–204 ($40–52)
Tagamet (cimetidine)	1,600 mg	Two 400-mg tablets 2x/day or one 400-mg tablet 4x/day with or without food for up to 12 weeks.	$230 ($34)
Zantac (ranitidine)	300 mg	One 150-mg tablet 2x/day with or without food.	$183 ($35)
Promotility agent			
Reglan (metoclopramide)	40–60 mg	One 10-mg tablet or one 10-mg and one 5-mg tablet 30 minutes before symptoms usually occur (e.g., before meals and sleep) not more than 3–4 times a day.	$143–230 ($21–41)

Precautions	Most common side effects	Call your doctor if...
If you are taking warfarin (Coumadin), your doctor may monitor your prothrombin time (a measure of how fast your blood clots) more closely. *Zegerid only:* This medication contains sodium and thus may not be appropriate for people on a low-salt diet.	Headache, diarrhea.	You experience a skin rash or signs of a B_{12} deficiency (unusual weakness, sore tongue, numbness or tingling of the hands or feet).
People with kidney disease need to take a lower dosage to prevent side effects such as confusion and dizziness.	Headache, dizziness, diarrhea.	You experience signs of liver problems: unusual tiredness, persistent nausea or vomiting, severe stomach or abdominal pain, dark urine, yellowing eyes or skin.
Avoid alcohol, because it can add to the drowsiness side effect.	Diarrhea, drowsiness, fatigue.	You experience involuntary movements of the eyes, face, or limbs; muscle spasms; trembling of the hands.

See next page for legend.

continued on the next page

Prescription Drugs for the Treatment of Gastroesophageal Reflux Disease 2008 (continued)

Drug type: Brand (generic)	Typical daily dosages*	How to take†	Monthly cost‡: Brand (generic)
Mucosal protectant			
Carafate (sucralfate)	4 g	One 1-g tablet 4x/day on an empty stomach (1 hour before each meal and at bedtime).	$144 ($44)

* These dosages represent the usual daily dosages for the treatment of gastroesophageal reflux disease. The precise effective dosage varies from person to person and depends on many factors. Do not make any changes to your medication without consulting your doctor.

† These instructions represent the typical way to take the medication. Your doctor's instructions may differ. Always follow your doctor's recommendations.

‡ Prices per drugstore.com.

§ If you have difficulty swallowing pills, empty the contents of the capsule onto 1 Tbsp of cold applesauce. Mix and take immediately.

|| Over-the-counter formulation available: Prilosec OTC. Do not take for more than 2 weeks straight or more often than every 4 months unless directed by your doctor.

¶ Over-the-counter formulations are available: Axid AR, Pepcid AC, Pepcid Complete, Tagamet HB, Zantac 75, Zantac 150. Do not take for more than 2 weeks straight unless directed by your doctor.

that are more resistant to acid, a process that is formally called metaplasia.

Causes of Barrett's esophagus

Normally, the esophageal mucosa is lined with multiple layers of flattened, scale-like cells. When these cells are damaged by gastric acid in individuals with GERD, they are replaced with a single layer of cells that are similar to those that line the stomach and small intestine.

Symptoms and diagnosis of Barrett's esophagus

Typically, Barrett's esophagus causes no symptoms, but it should be suspected in people with chronic GERD. An upper endoscopy is used to diagnose Barrett's esophagus. If the condition is present, the doctor will see tongue-like protrusions above the gastroesophageal junction. Samples of tissue (called biopsy samples) will be taken from these projections and examined under the microscope to look for precancerous changes called dysplasia.

Treatment of Barrett's esophagus

Barrett's esophagus increases your risk of esophageal cancer. In fact, about 0.5% of people with Barrett's esophagus develop cancer of the esophagus each year. To reduce the risk, it's important to control GERD and undergo an upper endoscopy and a biopsy

Precautions	Most common side effects	Call your doctor if...
Can interfere with the absorption of other medications; take other drugs 2 hours before or 2 hours after using Carafate. Can be taken with an antacid, but take the antacid 30 minutes before or after Carafate.	Constipation, dry mouth, upset stomach.	You experience an unusual or persistent feeling of fullness in the stomach, nausea or vomiting, stomach pain (especially after meals).

of the esophageal mucosa every three to five years.

When biopsies indicate that dysplasia is severe or that esophageal cancer is present, surgery is usually performed. It involves removing most of the esophagus and pulling the stomach up into the chest cavity to attach it to what remains of the esophagus.

A less invasive option is photodynamic therapy, a relatively new treatment that uses a light-sensitizing agent (for example, Photofrin) and then a laser to kill sensitized cancerous and precancerous cells. The light-sensitizing agent is injected into a vein. When the agent is exposed to the laser, it produces a chemical reaction that destroys the cancerous and precancerous cells. In a recent study, individuals who underwent photodynamic therapy were more likely to have a complete reversal of their dysplasia than people who did not receive the therapy. Two years after treatment with Photofrin, only 20% of these patients had cancer compared with 50% of those who did not receive the therapy. The risks of photodynamic therapy include esophageal strictures and temporary sensitivity to the sun.

Two new ablation therapies—which use heat or radiofrequency energy to destroy the abnormal cells on the esophageal walls—showed promise in a 2006 clinical trial. About 70% of participants who had radiofrequency ablation or argon plasma coagulation benefited, but these procedures are still considered experimental.

Gastritis

Gastritis occurs when the gastric mucosa, the inner lining of the stomach, becomes inflamed.

Causes of gastritis

Gastritis has many causes, including infections, medications, autoimmune reactions (in which the body begins to attack its own tissues), and food hypersensitivities or allergies.

The most common infection of the stomach is caused by a bacterium called *Helicobacter pylori* (*H. pylori*). This bacterium is found in feces, and ingesting food or water contaminated with *H. pylori* can result in a lifelong infection. Infection irritates and inflames the stomach lining and leads to overproduction of gastric acid, which increases the risk of developing peptic ulcers (ulcers in the stomach or duodenum; see pages 23–26) and gastric cancer.

The medications that most often cause gastritis are nonsteroidal anti-inflammatory drugs (NSAIDs) such as aspirin, ibuprofen (Advil, Motrin), and naproxen (Aleve, Naprosyn). NSAIDs interfere with the protective substances in the stomach that prevent damage to the mucosal lining; these drugs also inhibit the body's ability to stop bleeding. The combination of NSAIDs and *H. pylori* is especially damaging to the gastric mucosa and may lead not only to gastritis but also to the development of erosions (superficial defects) and ulcerations (deep defects) in the mucosal lining of the stomach and duodenum.

Newer types of NSAIDs called COX-2 inhibitors were developed to reduce the risk of gastritis and stomach ulcers associated with traditional NSAIDs. However, not all studies have shown COX-2 inhibitors to be safer for the stomach than other NSAIDs. In fact, the only COX-2 inhibitor currently available, celecoxib (Celebrex), carries a "black box" warning on its label informing consumers of the potential for gastrointestinal side effects. Two other COX-2 inhibitors—rofecoxib (Vioxx) and valdecoxib (Bextra)—were taken off the market, because they increase the risk of heart attacks and strokes.

Symptoms and diagnosis of gastritis

The symptoms of gastritis include indigestion (upset stomach) and a worsening of abdominal pain after meals.

The best way to diagnose gastritis is with an upper endoscopy. Your doctor will look for changes in the gastric mucosa, such as swelling, redness, brittleness, and erosions. A definitive diagnosis is made by microscopic examination of a sample of tissue removed during the endoscopy. The pathologist who examines the tissue will

NEW RESEARCH

Celebrex and Nexium May Be Best for Those With High Ulcer Risk

Current recommendations suggest that individuals at high risk for recurrent ulcer bleeding—i.e., those who have had ulcers before—take either a COX-2 inhibitor like celecoxib (Celebrex) alone or a traditional NSAID (such as ibuprofen) combined with a proton pump inhibitor to prevent ulcer bleeding. But a new study suggests that a combination of a COX-2 inhibitor and a proton pump inhibitor may be the most effective route.

Researchers recruited patients who had been admitted to the hospital for upper gastrointestinal tract bleeding and had been taking an NSAID for arthritis. They randomly gave 273 participants either Celebrex plus a placebo or Celebrex plus esomeprazole (Nexium) twice daily for one year.

During the treatment and a one-month follow-up period, 12 people (9%) in the control group had recurrent ulcer bleeding while no one in the combination group did. Side effects were similar in both groups.

While a COX-2 inhibitor plus a proton pump inhibitor may be the best treatment for people with a high risk of ulcers, the increased cardiovascular risk associated with COX-2 inhibitors may necessitate a different approach for those at high risk for heart disease.

THE LANCET
Volume 369, page 1621
May 12, 2007

look for signs of inflammation, the presence of *H. pylori* (using special stains), or evidence of autoimmune gastritis. *H. pylori* infection can also be diagnosed by a blood test that detects antibodies to the bacterium, a breath test, or a stool test.

Treatment of gastritis

Infection with *H. pylori* can be cured with medications that suppress gastric acid production and oral antibiotics to eradicate the infection. If a medication you are taking is causing gastritis, your doctor may lower the dosage of the medication or switch you to another one. Your doctor may also recommend that you start taking medication to decrease gastric acid production and protect the lining of the stomach. (See the chart on pages 18–21.)

Peptic Ulcer Disease

Peptic ulcers are deep, nonhealing defects or sores in the lining of the stomach and duodenum. When these defects occur in the stomach, they are called gastric ulcers. Ulcers that develop in the duodenum are known as duodenal ulcers. Duodenal ulcers tend to affect young people, especially males. Gastric ulcers are more common with age, because older people are more likely to be infected with *H. pylori* or to use NSAIDs. Both gastric and duodenal ulcers tend to recur even after they've been treated.

Causes of peptic ulcer disease

Peptic ulcers occur when the lining of the stomach or duodenum becomes damaged, usually by acid. Between 70% and 80% of gastric ulcers and nearly all duodenal ulcers result from *H. pylori* gastritis. NSAIDs and the osteoporosis drug alendronate (Fosamax) also can damage the lining of the stomach, increasing the risk of gastric ulcers. Smoking increases the risk of slow-healing duodenal ulcers.

Symptoms of peptic ulcer disease

The symptoms of a peptic ulcer depend on whether the ulcer is in your stomach or duodenum. A gastric ulcer results in pain in the upper abdomen 15–30 minutes after eating. Because of the pain, you may be afraid to eat and you may lose weight. With a gastric ulcer, pain rarely occurs at night or when you are fasting. A duodenal ulcer, on the other hand, results in pain in the upper abdomen two to three hours after meals, when the stomach is empty. The pain can awaken you at night and is relieved by eating.

If not treated, peptic ulcers can lead to complications such as

NEW RESEARCH

Preventing Ulcers Among NSAID, Aspirin, and Antiplatelet Users

Various medications such as aspirin, NSAIDs, and antiplatelet agents can promote peptic ulcer bleeding, but a new study suggests that several drugs—especially proton pump inhibitors—can help lower the risk.

In a case-controlled study, researchers in Spain gathered and analyzed data on 2,777 people with bleeding ulcers and 5,532 controls without ulcers. Participants taking aspirin or NSAIDs lowered their ulcer risk by 82% if they took a proton pump inhibitor, by 61% if they took an H_2-blocker, and by 49% if they took a nitrate.

The researchers also looked at the ulcer risk associated with heart medications: antiplatelet agents such as clopidogrel (Plavix) and anticoagulants such as warfarin (Coumadin). In people taking an antiplatelet agent, proton pump inhibitors lowered ulcer risk but H_2-blockers and nitrates did not. In those taking an anticoagulant, none of the three drug types offered any protection.

While the use of aspirin and traditional NSAIDs has increased following the removal of drugs like rofecoxib (Vioxx) and valdecoxib (Bextra) from the market, research suggests that too often prevention strategies are not employed to avoid gastrointestinal side effects. This study provides further evidence that proton pump inhibitors, H_2-blockers, and nitrates can protect against bleeding peptic ulcers.

THE AMERICAN JOURNAL OF GASTROENTEROLOGY
Volume 102, page 507
March 2007

bleeding, perforation, or penetration. Bleeding occurs when the ulcer causes a blood vessel to rupture in the lining of the stomach or duodenum. Perforation results when an ulcer erodes through the wall of the stomach or duodenum and into the abdominal cavity, leading to infection and inflammation of the abdominal cavity (peritonitis). Penetration happens when an ulcer erodes through the wall of the stomach or duodenum and into adjacent organs, such as the liver, pancreas, or colon (large intestine).

Less often, an ulcer can deform the stomach or duodenum and block the passage of food through the gastric outlet or duodenum, resulting in nausea and vomiting that do not improve with treatment.

Diagnosis of peptic ulcer disease

Peptic ulcers can be diagnosed using an upper endoscopy or an upper GI series. During endoscopy, a peptic ulcer appears as a round or elongated defect in the lining of the stomach or duodenum. On an upper GI series, barium accumulates inside the ulcer or shows changes in the normal appearance of the folds of the lining (such as convergence of the folds toward the ulcer).

Treatment of peptic ulcer disease

Peptic ulcers can be healed temporarily by suppressing gastric acid production. The medications most commonly used to do this are H_2-blockers and proton pump inhibitors (see the chart on pages 18–21). Ulcers usually return once these drugs are stopped.

Therefore, the more common way to treat ulcers is to eradicate *H. pylori* from the stomach. Once the infection is treated, gastric secretion returns to normal levels and peptic ulcers are usually cured. The treatment regimen to eradicate *H. pylori* includes antibiotics and acid-reducing medications (see the chart on the facing page). Usually doctors first prescribe triple therapy, which consists of a proton pump inhibitor and two antibiotics. This approach cures ulcers more than 90% of the time.

If triple therapy does not produce a cure, a second triple therapy containing different drugs may be tried. Another option is quadruple therapy: bismuth subsalicylate (Pepto-Bismol and other brands), two antibiotics, and a proton pump inhibitor or H_2-blocker. If the *H. pylori* infection is not eradicated, the likelihood is high that peptic ulcers will recur. Continued use of NSAIDs lowers the chances that gastric ulcers will heal.

Ulcers were once commonly treated with surgery: either partial gastrectomy or vagotomy. Partial gastrectomy involves removing the

NEW RESEARCH

Sequential Therapy May Be Best for Treating Ulcers

As antibacterial resistance continues to increase, the bacterium *Helicobacter pylori (H. pylori)*—often the main cause of peptic ulcers and gastritis—is becoming more difficult to combat. Now a study suggests that when the standard treatment of 10-day triple-drug therapy fails, sequential therapy might be more effective.

Researchers randomly assigned 300 people with peptic ulcers or gastritis to either the standard 10-day therapy with the proton pump inhibitor pantoprazole (Protonix) and the antibiotics clarithromycin (Biaxin) and amoxicillin or a sequential treatment of five days of Protonix, amoxicillin, and placebo followed by five days of Protonix, Biaxin, and the antibiotic tinidazole (Tindamax). Participants took breath tests to detect the presence of *H. pylori* four and eight weeks after the treatment ended.

People taking sequential therapy were more likely to have complete eradication of *H. pylori*—from 89–93% of the group—vs. 79% of those taking standard therapy.

The researchers aren't sure whether the improved success rate was a result of the order of the medications or the addition of a second antibiotic. But they assert that since sequential therapy is more successful and less expensive than standard therapy, it should be considered as a first-line treatment.

ANNALS OF INTERNAL MEDICINE
Volume 146, page 556
April 17, 2007

Drug Regimens for Treatment of Peptic Ulcers 2008

Regimen	Medications	Dosage	Cost*	Side effects/precautions
Triple therapy (two antibiotics and one proton pump inhibitor for 7–14 days. The duration of the regimen including AcipHex is 7 days; the duration of the other regimens is 10–14 days.)	1) Biaxin (clarithromycin)	One 500-mg tablet 2x/day.	$138 ($103)	*Biaxin, amoxicillin, metronidazole:* Side effects include diarrhea, nausea, vomiting, stomach upset, changes in taste, headache. Call your doctor immediately if you experience persistent diarrhea, abdominal pain or cramping, blood or mucus in your stool. *Biaxin only:* Take with milk if stomach upset occurs. *Amoxicillin only:* Drink plenty of liquids. *Metronidazole only:* Avoid alcohol while taking and for at least one day after finishing the medication.
	2) amoxicillin ***or***	Two 500-mg capsules 2x/day.	$15 ($15)	
	metronidazole	One 500-mg tablet 2x/day.	$121 ($9)	
	3) AcipHex (rabeprazole) ***or***	One 20-mg tablet 2x/day.	$65	
	Nexium (esomeprazole) ***or***	One 40-mg capsule 1x/day.	$64	
	Prevacid (lansoprazole) ***or***	One 30-mg capsule 2x/day.	$133	
	Prilosec OTC (omeprazole) ***or***	One 20-mg tablet 2x/day.	$20	
	Protonix (pantoprazole)	One 40-mg tablet 2x/day.	$112	*Proton pump inhibitors:* See the chart on pages 18–21.
Quadruple therapy (bismuth, two antibiotics, and one proton pump inhibitor or H_2-blocker for 14 days)	1) Pepto-Bismol (bismuth subsalicylate)	Two 262-mg tablets 3-4x/day or 30 mL liquid 3-4x/day.	*T:* $10–16 *L:* $18–23 ($10–14)	*Bismuth:* May cause stools to become gray-black.
	2) metronidazole	One 250-mg tablet 4x/day.	$138 ($31)	*Metronidazole:* See above.
	3) tetracycline	One 500-mg capsule 4x/day.	$38 ($15)	*Tetracycline:* Makes skin more sensitive to sunlight. Wear sunscreen.
	4) proton pump inhibitor (AcipHex, Nexium, Prevacid, Prilosec OTC, Protonix, Zegerid) ***or***	Same as for triple therapy (see above).	Same as for triple therapy (see above)	*Proton pump inhibitors:* See the chart on pages 18–21.
	Axid (nizatidine) ***or***	One 150-mg capsule 2x/day.	$75 ($24)	*H_2-blockers:* See the chart on pages 18–21.
	Pepcid AC (famotidine) ***or***	One 20-mg tablet 2x/day.	$10 ($12)	
	Tagamet (cimetidine) ***or***	One 400-mg tablet 2x/day.	$18 ($8)	
	Zantac 150 (ranitidine)	One 150-mg tablet 2x/day.	$21 ($15)	
Combination products	Helidac (bismuth/metronidazole/tetracycline) for 14 days	Chew two 262-mg bismuth tablets, then swallow one 250-mg metronidazole tablet and one 500-mg tetracycline capsule with a glass of water 4x/day (at breakfast, lunch, dinner, and bedtime).	$63	Side effects include nausea, diarrhea, abdominal pain. Do not take if you have kidney or liver problems. For other precautions, see separate entries for bismuth, metronidazole, and tetracycline.
	Prevpac (amoxicillin/Biaxin/Prevacid) for 14 days	Swallow two 500-mg amoxicillin capsules, one 500-mg Biaxin tablet, and one 30-mg Prevacid capsule 2x/day before eating.	$300	Side effects include diarrhea, headache, changes in taste. For precautions, see separate entries above for amoxicillin, Biaxin, and proton pump inhibitors.

*Prices per drugstore.com. Generic cost is in parentheses. Cost is for 14 days, except for AcipHex in triple therapy, which is used for only 7 days.

acid-producing portion of the stomach; vagotomy involves cutting the vagal nerve to decrease acid production. Now that ulcers can be effectively treated with medication, surgery is rarely needed. Surgery is still used, however, for people with ulcer complications—for example, to stop bleeding, close perforations, or open up the gastric outlet if an ulcer is blocking it. But these days, ulcers rarely progress to this stage.

Anatomy of the Liver, Gallbladder, and Pancreas

To digest food, your digestive tract needs some help from nearby organs. These organs, which include the liver, gallbladder, and pancreas, produce or store enzymes and other substances that help break down the food you eat.

Liver

The liver is a large organ located on the upper right side of your torso, opposite your stomach and behind your ribcage (see the illustration on page 31). One of its main functions is to make a substance called bile, which is composed mostly of bilirubin, bile salts, and cholesterol and is needed to digest food in the small intestine.

The liver is divided into two sections: a right lobe and a left lobe. Both lobes are made up of cells called hepatocytes. These cells produce bile and secrete it into the bile ducts, which carry bile to the gallbladder, where it is stored until used by the small intestine.

Gallbladder and Bile Ducts

The gallbladder is a pear-shaped sac located under the right lobe of the liver (see the illustration on page 31). Between meals, it stores and concentrates bile, which is produced at a constant rate by the liver. When it isn't full of bile, the gallbladder is about 3 inches long and 1 inch wide at its thickest part. After meals, the gallbladder releases bile into the duodenum to help with digestion.

The cystic duct carries bile from the gallbladder to the common bile duct, which empties into the duodenum. Entry of bile into the duodenum is regulated by layers of muscle called the sphincter of Oddi. Between meals, the sphincter of Oddi closes and prevents bile from entering the duodenum. During and after meals, this sphincter opens and allows bile to enter the duodenum.

NEW RESEARCH

Lactoferrin and Probiotics May Improve Ulcer Treatment

The standard therapy for peptic ulcers and gastritis caused by the bacterium *Helicobacter pylori (H. pylori)*—two antibiotics and a proton pump inhibitor—is sometimes unsuccessful. However, a new study suggests that simply adding two supplements to this treatment may improve results and reduce side effects.

Researchers randomly assigned 206 people with *H. pylori* infection to either treatment with esomeprazole (Nexium), clarithromycin (Biaxin), and amoxicillin for seven days or the same treatment plus bovine lactoferrin (a glycoprotein involved in immune defense) and probiotics (beneficial bacteria).

Eight weeks later, 89% of the supplement group tested negative for *H. pylori* compared with 73% of the control group. The supplement takers also reported significantly less side effects such as nausea, diarrhea, abdominal pain, tongue inflammation, and a metallic taste in the mouth. As diarrhea is a known side effect of antibiotic use, the probiotic may have helped reduce its occurrence by restoring balance in the gut flora.

The researchers suggest that probiotics and lactoferrin may help eradicate *H. pylori* synergistically by attacking the bacterium in different ways from the antibiotics and proton pump inhibitor, leading to a complete clearance of the infection.

THE AMERICAN JOURNAL OF GASTROENTEROLOGY
Volume 102, page 951
May 2007

Pancreas

The pancreas is a long, thin gland that lies horizontally behind the bottom part of your stomach (see the illustration on page 31). It makes digestive enzymes that flow through the pancreatic duct to the small intestine. These enzymes, along with bile from the gallbladder, break down food for use as energy by the body. The pancreas also makes insulin and glucagon, hormones that help regulate blood glucose (sugar) levels.

Disorders of the Liver, Gallbladder, and Pancreas

Disorders of the liver (such as cirrhosis and hepatitis), the gallbladder (gallstones, for example), and the pancreas (for instance, pancreatitis) can affect the proper function of your digestive tract.

Cirrhosis

Cirrhosis is a disease that causes the liver to slowly deteriorate and eventually malfunction. This happens when healthy tissue in the liver is replaced by scar tissue.

Causes of cirrhosis

Heavy alcohol use is the leading cause of cirrhosis, but the disease can also be caused by the hepatitis viruses (see pages 28–30), malnutrition, certain medications (such as isoniazid [Laniazid, Nydrazid] for tuberculosis, methyldopa for high blood pressure, and amiodarone [Cordarone, Pacerone] for irregular heart rhythms), parasites, exposure to toxic chemicals, and heart failure.

Symptoms of cirrhosis

Typically, people experience few symptoms in the early stages of cirrhosis. However, as more and more healthy cells are replaced by scar tissue, symptoms such as loss of appetite, weight loss, nausea, vomiting, weakness, fatigue, intense itching, indigestion, and stomach bloating may occur. Small, red lines may appear on your face, upper body, and arms, and you may bleed and bruise more easily than usual. Jaundice (yellowing of the eyes and skin because of an excess of bilirubin in the blood), memory problems, and hand tremors may develop as the disease worsens. Eventually, the liver may fail completely or you may develop life-threatening bleeding or liver cancer.

ASK THE DOCTOR

Q. ***Do the benefits of aspirin for your heart outweigh the risks to your gut?***

A. Low-dose aspirin can help reduce the risk of heart attack or stroke for many people. But aspirin, like other nonsteroidal anti-inflammatory drugs (NSAIDs), can also cause stomach upset, bleeding in the digestive tract, ulcers, or injury to the lining of the small intestine.

Aspirin has this potential because it disables the stomach's protective mechanisms that shield it from the acidic juices used to digest foods. NSAIDs also inhibit the blood's ability to clot properly, which can lead to excessive internal and external bleeding.

A recent study found that low-dose aspirin treatment was associated with one extra digestive complication (such as bleeding ulcers) in every 50 people in a given high-risk group—such as men, adults over age 60, individuals with a history of peptic ulcers, or those who take other NSAIDs. If you're in one of these groups, you and your doctor need to discuss whether aspirin is really right for you.

Aspirin-related complications often don't produce recognizable symptoms. If they do develop, they can include: stomach pain; dark black, tarry, or bloody stools; vomit that contains blood or material that looks like coffee grounds; weakness; dizziness; chest pain; or shortness of breath. If you experience any of these symptoms, see your doctor immediately.

Diagnosis of cirrhosis

Cirrhosis is typically detected by a physical exam, looking for outward signs of the disease such as jaundice. Your doctor may also perform blood tests to determine how well your liver is functioning. These blood tests measure the levels of certain enzymes that are released into the bloodstream when the liver is damaged. A liver biopsy—where a small sample of liver tissue is removed for laboratory analysis—also may be performed, to evaluate how badly the liver is damaged and whether cancer has developed.

Treatment of cirrhosis

Although scarring of the liver is irreversible, cirrhosis is a disease that progresses slowly and its early symptoms can be controlled. First, you must stop drinking alcohol, even if your cirrhosis is not caused by alcohol abuse. Always get your doctor's approval before taking any new prescription or nonprescription drugs, since many medications can affect liver function. In addition, eat a well-balanced, nutritious diet that is rich in fresh fruits and vegetables, whole grains, and beans, and low in fat and sodium. Also, avoid raw shellfish, as it can contain a bacterium, *Vibrio vulnificus,* that can be dangerous for people with cirrhosis.

If you are experiencing bloating, your doctor may prescribe a diuretic, which helps to reduce the fluid level in your body. Antacids may be recommended to relieve stomach discomfort. If hepatitis is the cause of cirrhosis, corticosteroids to reduce inflammation and immunosuppressive drugs such as interferon alpha may be prescribed to suppress the virus. Hospitalization may be necessary for severe cases of cirrhosis (for example, if you vomit blood or have bleeding in the digestive tract). People with severe cirrhosis also may need a liver transplant.

Hepatitis

Hepatitis is a virus that causes inflammation in the liver. Six types have been identified: hepatitis A, B, C, D, E, and G. About 42,000 new cases of hepatitis A, 56,000 new cases of hepatitis B, and 20,000 new cases of hepatitis C occur each year in the United States. The other three types rarely occur in the United States.

Causes of hepatitis

Hepatitis A is spread through contact with the saliva or feces of someone who has the virus or ingesting food or water contaminated with the virus. On rare occasions, hepatitis A can be transmitted through blood transfusions or blood products (although blood is now screened for the hepatitis viruses).

Hepatitis B is transmitted through tainted blood that enters the body via contaminated needles (illegal injection drug use or accidentally being stuck with a used needle), blood transfusions, transplants, hemodialysis, tattooing, body piercing, and acupuncture. You can also become infected when you have sex with someone who has the virus. Vaccines are available to prevent hepatitis A and B.

Hepatitis C is the leading cause of chronic liver disease. Like hepatitis B, it is transmitted through exposure to infected blood (most cases are linked to illegal injection drug use) and sexual contact with an infected person.

Symptoms of hepatitis

Hepatitis A may not cause any symptoms at all. If symptoms are present, they include fever, fatigue, appetite loss, nausea, stomach discomfort, dark urine, and jaundice (yellowing of the skin and whites of the eyes). The symptoms typically come on suddenly.

Hepatitis B tends to produce symptoms more slowly (and symptoms occur in only about half of people who have the virus). The symptoms are similar to those produced by the hepatitis A virus and include mild fever, loss of appetite, sluggishness, nausea and vomiting, stomach pains, muscle or joint aches, and dark urine. Up to a third of people with hepatitis B also develop jaundice.

Most people with hepatitis C don't have initial symptoms of infection or have just mild symptoms such as jaundice, fatigue, dark urine, stomach pain, loss of appetite, and nausea. But 75% of people with the infection develop symptoms of cirrhosis 20 or more years after they've been exposed to the virus. These people are at risk for chronic liver disease (which may require a liver transplant) and liver cancer.

Diagnosis of hepatitis

All three types of hepatitis can be detected with blood tests. A home test is available for detecting hepatitis C.

Treatment of hepatitis

There is no treatment for hepatitis A beyond getting rest and drinking plenty of fluids. Most people get over the virus within two to six months.

Most adults with hepatitis B recover within six months, but up to 10% can become chronically infected with the virus and are at risk for chronic liver disease.

ASK THE DOCTOR

Q. ***Should I be concerned about contracting hepatitis on my upcoming trip abroad, and what can I do to protect myself?***

A. Hepatitis B and C are spread by exposure to infected blood or sexual contact with an infected person, so the risk is low. The exception is in countries with intermediate or high rates of chronic hepatitis B and C, where travelers should be cautious about contaminated injections and healthcare equipment, blood transfusions, and unprotected sex.

Hepatitis A is the greater threat, since it is spread through the saliva and feces of an infected person—meaning that food and water can easily become contaminated. The risk is very low in North America (except Mexico), Japan, Australia, New Zealand, and Western Europe—the same as if you were traveling within the United States—but much higher in Africa, South and Central America, Eastern Europe, and Asia. (Look up your destination at wwwn.cdc.gov/travel/destination list.aspx.)

There is no vaccine for hepatitis C, but the hepatitis A and B vaccines are recommended for all unvaccinated people traveling to countries at intermediate or high risk. You should receive two or three shots starting as soon as travel is considered, but your doctor may also put you on an accelerated schedule. And while traveling to higher-risk countries, be sure to avoid beverages that aren't sealed or boiled, ice cubes, uncooked shellfish, and fruits or vegetables that you haven't peeled or prepared yourself.

For people with acute hepatitis B (of less than six months' duration), there are few treatments. Immediately after exposure to the virus (if you know you've been exposed), getting the vaccine for the virus can reduce the risk of infection by 75%. In some people, the antiviral drug interferon alpha (Infergen, Intron-A, Roferon-A) helps stop the virus from reproducing in the body. However, it also causes many side effects, including flu-like symptoms, depression, fatigue, and suppression of bone marrow function.

Chronic hepatitis B (lasting longer than six months) can be treated with interferon alpha and/or lamivudine (Epivir-HBV) or a new drug called telbivudine (Tyzeka). Both reduce levels of the virus in the body but don't cause as many side effects as interferon alpha.

Hepatitis C is treated with interferon alpha as early as possible after infection, in the hopes of preventing acute disease from becoming chronic. If chronic disease develops, interferon alpha may be given; however, only 15% of people respond. A new form of interferon alpha, peginterferon alpha (Pegasys, Peg-Intron), is more effective because it stays in the body longer; it appears to be beneficial in 30–40% of people. The most effective treatment, however, may be a combination of peginterferon alpha and the antiviral drug ribavirin (Copegus, Rebetol), which can suppress levels of the virus in the blood in about half of patients. Unfortunately, ribavirin, like interferon alpha, can lead to serious side effects, including hemolytic anemia (low blood count caused by rapid destruction of red blood cells), suppression of the bone marrow, kidney failure, and depression.

If medication is unsuccessful and the disease becomes chronic, liver cells may become so damaged that a liver transplant is needed.

Gallstones

Gallstones are small, pebble-like substances that develop in the gallbladder. An estimated 20.5 million Americans have gallstones. Women are two to three times more likely than men to have them. In fact, 10–30% of women develop gallstones in their lifetime.

There are two types of gallstones. Between 70% and 80% are cholesterol gallstones, which are made up mostly of cholesterol. The remaining 20–30% are black- or brown-pigment gallstones, which have a much lower cholesterol content and are primarily made of bilirubin (a component of bile made by the liver).

Causes of gallstones

Gallstones form when the liquid (bile) stored in the gallbladder hardens into stones. This occurs when there is too much cholesterol

The Gallbladder and the Bile Ducts

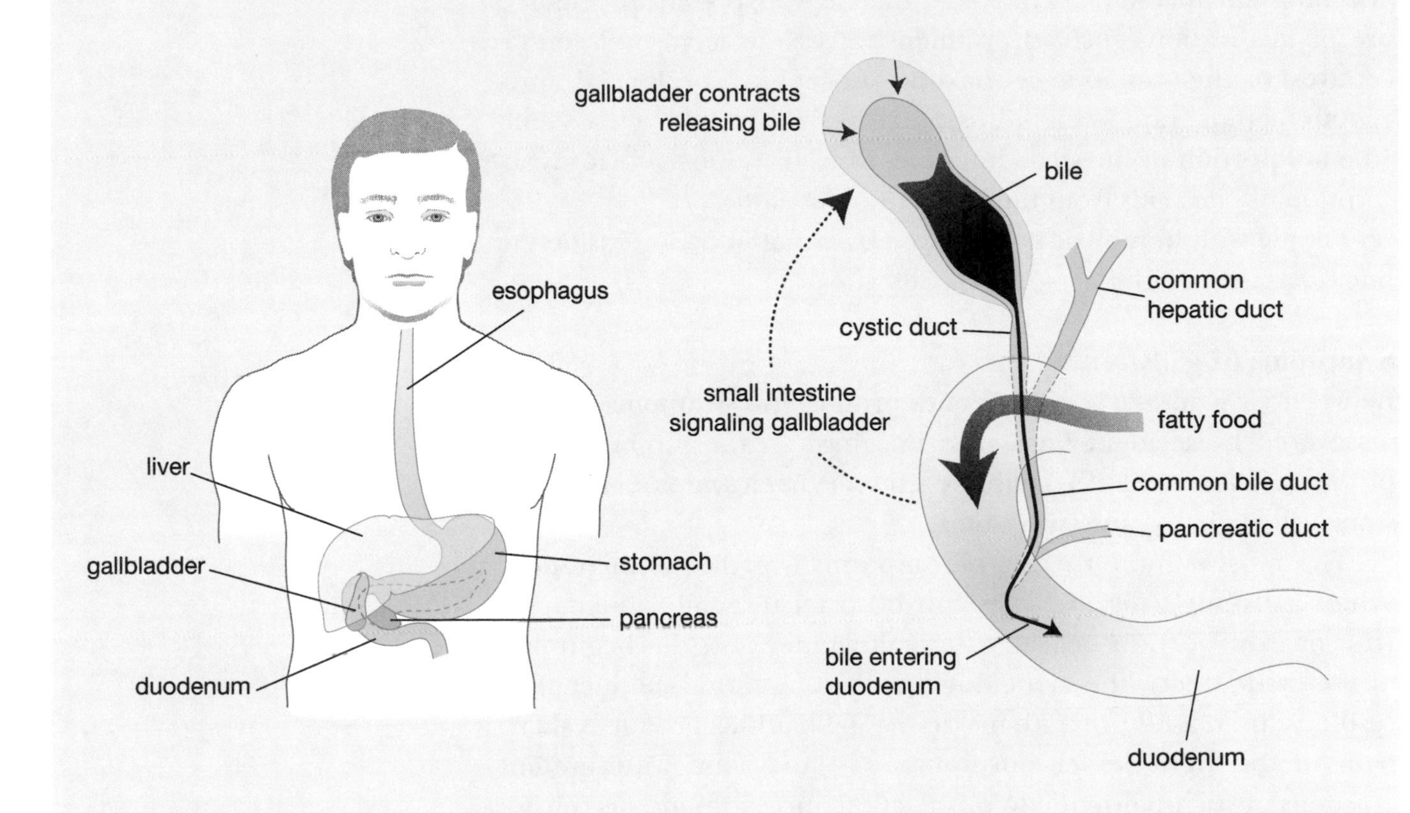

The gallbladder is a small, pear-shaped structure located underneath the liver. The main function of the gallbladder is to store bile, a fluid containing bile salts, cholesterol, lecithin, and bilirubin. Bile salts are needed to digest fat from your diet. In combination with lecithin, they also help keep cholesterol in solution to prevent gallstones.

The liver makes about 3 cups of bile each day and secretes it into the right and left hepatic ducts. Bile travels from these ducts to the gallbladder via the common hepatic duct and the cystic duct. In the gallbladder, bile is concentrated by the absorption of water and stored until it is needed for digestion.

After you eat a meal containing fat, the small intestine sends signals to the gallbladder that cause it to contract. The contractions push the bile back into the cystic duct, along the common bile duct, and into the duodenum (the first part of the small intestine). A layer of muscles called the sphincter of Oddi controls the entry of bile into the duodenum.

In the small intestine, bile salts help break down dietary fat into smaller particles that can be more easily digested and absorbed into the bloodstream. Once fat leaves the duodenum, the gallbladder stops contracting and begins to store bile again. About 95% of the bile salts in the intestine are absorbed into the bloodstream and returned to the liver to be reused. ■

or bilirubin in the bile or when the gallbladder doesn't empty as it should. It's not known why these imbalances occur. Diet may play a role: For instance, eating a diet high in cholesterol and fat and low in fiber may increase the risk of gallstones.

Risk factors for the development of cholesterol gallstones include a genetic predisposition (particularly in people of Pima Indian or Scandinavian ancestry); being older than age 50; obesity; pregnancy; use of medications such as postmenopausal estrogen, oral contraceptives, or the antibiotic ceftriaxone (Rocephin); prolonged intravenous feeding; rapid weight loss; and diseases of the terminal ileum (the last portion of the small intestine, which is responsible for reabsorption of bile acids from the bowel into the blood).

People with hemolytic anemia or a bacterial infection inside the bile ducts are at risk for pigment gallstones.

Symptoms of gallstones

Between 70% and 80% of gallstones produce no symptoms and are discovered by accident during an imaging test for another health problem. There's a 1–4% chance each year that a symptom-free gallstone will begin to cause symptoms.

The most common cause of symptoms is gallstone migration. When gallstones migrate, they can obstruct the gallbladder neck (the narrow portion between the gallbladder and the beginning of the cystic duct), the cystic duct, or the common bile duct. The resulting increased pressure inside the gallbladder produces sharp pain in the right upper portion of the abdomen. Intermittent episodes of such pain, due to obstruction and spontaneous release (when the stone dislodges itself), are called biliary colic.

When stones migrate from the gallbladder into the common bile duct, they can cause partial or complete obstruction of bile flow. Signs and symptoms of bile duct obstruction are intermittent abdominal pain, jaundice (yellow discoloration of the skin and eyes), and cholangitis (inflammation of the bile ducts). Gallstones that lodge in the major duodenal papilla (a small elevation in the second portion of the duodenum, where both the common bile duct and the pancreatic duct openings are located) can cause acute pancreatitis (inflammation of the pancreas; see pages 34–36), with abdominal pain, nausea, and vomiting.

If the obstruction persists, a condition called acute cholecystitis may develop. In this condition, rising pressure inside the gallbladder leads to decreased blood flow to the gallbladder wall, inflammation, bacterial infection, and, in some cases, a hole in the wall of the gallbladder (perforation). Symptoms of acute cholecystitis include severe pain, fever, nausea, and vomiting. The pain is located below the bottom edge of the right rib cage and often spreads to the back, right shoulder, or right side of the neck.

Diagnosis of gallstones

The best test to diagnose gallstones in the gallbladder is an abdominal ultrasound, which uses sound waves to create images of the inside of the gallbladder. It is a noninvasive, painless test that is performed by placing an ultrasound probe on the outside of your abdomen. No special preparation is required aside from fasting for six to eight hours. Abdominal ultrasound can detect gallstones as small as 2 mm.

If you have acute cholecystitis, ultrasound can detect thickening of the gallbladder wall as well as the presence of inflammatory fluid (pus that contains bacteria and inflammatory cells) in and around the gallbladder. Abdominal ultrasound cannot visualize stones in the bile ducts, but it can detect widening of the common bile duct due to obstruction by a stone.

If your doctor suspects that there is a gallstone in your common bile duct, an endoscopic ultrasound may be performed. This test uses a special endoscope with an ultrasound probe at its tip.

Computed tomography (CT) produces cross-sectional images of the human body using high-resolution x-rays that are processed by a computer. It involves lying on a special table while x-rays are passed through your body. Like abdominal ultrasound, CT is painless and noninvasive. It is better than ultrasound at detecting complications of acute cholecystitis, such as perforation of the gallbladder or bile ducts and the formation of an abscess (a localized accumulation of pus).

A hepatobiliary scintigram, also called a hepato-iminodiacetic acid (HIDA) scan, is used to evaluate the passage of bile through the bile ducts and gallbladder and to detect obstruction of the cystic duct. This test involves the intravenous injection of a small amount of a radioactive substance into a vein in your arm. The radioactive substance is removed from the blood by the liver and then secreted into the bile ducts. A special camera detects the presence of the radioactivity and creates a computer image of the bile ducts. The procedure is safe and exposes you to only small amounts of radioactivity.

Endoscopic retrograde cholangiopancreatography (ERCP) is the best way to diagnose stones in the bile ducts. It uses a special side-viewing endoscope to locate the opening to the duodenum and to place a thin catheter in the bile ducts. A contrast agent is then injected into the bile ducts and x-rays are taken, allowing your doctor to study the anatomy of the ducts and identify any defects or blockages caused by stones, strictures, or masses.

A noninvasive, painless alternative to ERCP is magnetic resonance cholangiopancreatography (MRCP). It uses radiofrequency waves to create pictures of the bile and pancreatic ducts. During the procedure, you will lie very still in the magnetic resonance imaging (MRI) scanner. The test takes about 20 minutes and may not require the injection of a contrast agent.

Treatment of gallstones

If you have gallstones but no symptoms, you do not need treatment. But if you're having frequent episodes of biliary colic, your physician will likely recommend that you have your gallbladder removed, an operation called a cholecystectomy, to prevent recurrences. Nearly all cholecystectomies are performed by laparoscopy, which decreases the amount of pain following the surgery and allows for a faster recovery than traditional open surgery. Other, less-preferred treatment options include dissolving the gallstones with chemicals or breaking them up with ultrasonic shock waves. These techniques are not that effective and frequently lead to recurrences of stones.

Pressure within the gallbladder, caused by stones that obstruct the bile ducts, can also be relieved by using ERCP to place a small tube (stent) into the gallbladder to keep it open. If stones are present in the bile ducts, they can also be removed during ERCP. (This is a supplemental procedure; if stones in the gallbladder are also causing pain, they still need to be taken out by removing the gallbladder.)

ERCP uses a special device called a sphincterotome to cut the bile duct sphincter and then extract the stones from the bile duct with a special basket or balloon. The procedure is normally done on an outpatient basis and causes few complications.

A study suggests that for those over age 60 who have had ERCP for common bile duct stones, watchful waiting may be a good alternative to gallbladder removal. Symptom recurrence after ERCP is relatively uncommon, and life expectancy was not improved by surgery.

Acute cholecystitis usually requires a hospital stay. Fluids and nutrients are given intravenously to let the digestive tract rest, and antibiotics are administered to eliminate the bacterial infection. If complications develop, the gallbladder is removed. If you are unable to undergo surgery, the gallbladder can be drained by passing a tube into the gallbladder through a small incision in the abdomen. Ultrasound or CT is used to guide placement of the draining tube.

Pancreatitis

Pancreatitis is an inflammation of the pancreas. When inflamed, the digestive enzymes produced by the pancreas become active within the pancreas instead of in the small intestine as they should. As a result, the pancreas starts to attack itself.

Pancreatitis can be acute or chronic. Acute pancreatitis causes attacks of pain within several hours of eating a large meal or drinking a large amount of alcohol. Chronic pancreatitis occurs in people with acute pancreatitis when the pancreas develops scar tissue and slowly starts to malfunction. Eventually, the pancreas may stop producing digestive enzymes. About 80,000 people in the United States suffer a bout of acute pancreatitis each year, and between three and 10 people per 100,000 suffer from chronic pancreatitis. Both types of pancreatitis are more common in men than in women.

Causes of pancreatitis

Gallstones blocking the bile duct and excessive alcohol consumption are the major causes of pancreatitis. Less frequently, certain medications (in particular, the aminosalicylate anti-inflammatory compounds used to treat Crohn's disease and ulcerative colitis; see the chart on pages 60–63), a duodenal ulcer, an overactive parathyroid gland, or a stomach injury can cause pancreatitis.

Symptoms of pancreatitis

Acute pancreatitis is hard to miss. It causes excruciating pain in the center of your upper abdomen extending through to your back, in addition to nausea and vomiting. You may develop a fever or bruising on your stomach from internal bleeding. You may also go into shock. If you experience severe abdominal pain that lasts more than 20 minutes, go to your doctor or a hospital emergency room for treatment.

With chronic pancreatitis, the abdominal pain can come on suddenly or gradually, usually after eating. It may develop into persistent abdominal pain. You can also develop jaundice, lose weight, and experience symptoms of diabetes (increased thirst and frequent urination) as the pancreas gradually deteriorates.

Diagnosis of pancreatitis

Pancreatitis is diagnosed with blood tests to assess levels of enzymes made by the pancreas as well as other chemicals in the body. X-rays, ultrasound, or CT scans of the pancreas are also done.

Treatment of pancreatitis

For acute pancreatitis, you will probably need a hospital stay of a few days to completely rest your bowels (that is, no food by mouth) and to receive intravenous fluids, antibiotics, and painkillers. If you have gallstones, they may need to be removed. Likewise, collections of fluid around the pancreas that develop from acute pancreatitis may be

NEW RESEARCH

Surgery Is a Must for All People With Early Pancreatic Cancer

Individuals who are treated with surgery for early pancreatic cancer have a 30% survival rate after five years, compared with less than 5% for people who don't undergo surgery. But nearly 40% of people with early-stage pancreatic cancer aren't even offered the surgery by their doctors, according to a recent study.

Researchers studied information from the National Cancer Data Base for 1995–2004. During that time, 9,559 people were diagnosed with pancreatic tumors that were potentially operable, but 3,644 of them (38%) were not presented with the option. Patients that were least likely to be offered surgery were over age 65, black, less educated, had lower incomes, were on Medicare or Medicaid, and were treated at small or community hospitals.

The authors say the underutilization of surgery may be due to lack of access to centers experienced in the procedure or to the long-held view that pancreatic cancer—and surgery to treat it—have poor long-term outcomes. However, mortality rates for the procedure have fallen from 25% in the 1960s to less than 3% at some high-volume centers today.

The importance of offering and encouraging surgery for all people with early pancreatic cancer must be emphasized, since it is the best hope for long-term survival.

ANNALS OF SURGERY
Volume 246, pages 173 and 181
August 2007

Avoiding Acetaminophen Dangers

Liver toxicity is more common than you think

Acetaminophen, the most frequently used pain reliever in the United States, has a well-deserved safety reputation. In any given week, 48 million adults use a medication containing acetaminophen, and the vast majority of them are fine. But if you take too much, you could do serious damage to your liver.

Apparently, that's not hard to do. Acetaminophen misuse is the number one cause of acute liver failure in this country. According to some estimates, roughly 56,000 Americans end up in the hospital each year as a result of acetaminophen overdoses, and about 100 die. And these numbers are on the rise: A recent study in *Hepatology* found that acetaminophen was the cause of 51% of acute liver failure cases in 2003, up from 28% in 1998.

Perhaps that's because acetaminophen can be found in more than Tylenol—it's in hundreds of medications, including cold and flu preparations (Theraflu) and headache remedies (Excedrin). There's also a fine line between a therapeutic dose and a harmful one: The maximum daily dosage is eight extra-strength or 12 regular-strength pills (4,000 mg of acetaminophen), but fatal liver damage can occur after taking just twice that amount.

In addition, many people think it's no big deal to mix alcohol with an over-the-counter drug, while in fact it can be a lethal combination, increasing the risk of liver problems. One study reports that almost a third of people have taken over-the-counter pain drugs on the same day they consumed alcohol.

Unfortunately, many more people aren't aware of the risks of acetaminophen. A January 2007 study in the *Journal of the American Pharmacists Association* found that out of 104 adults surveyed, 53% weren't aware that high doses of acetaminophen can harm the liver. Nearly 70% of the participants overestimated the maximum dose, and less than 15% knew that the drug is also found in prescription drugs like Vicodin and Percocet.

The Damage Done

Acetaminophen is rapidly absorbed from the stomach and small intestine and then metabolized in the liver by binding to nontoxic agents that are eliminated in urine. But excessive amounts of acetaminophen can overwhelm this normal binding process, forcing it to be processed and converted to a substance that is toxic to the liver. Most of the time, the liver can clear out this toxin before it does any harm. But if you take too much acetaminophen or if your liver is already busy metabolizing alcohol, more toxins form and accumulate in the liver. As a result, people who consume alcohol while taking acetaminophen can overdose on the drug even when taking the recommended doses.

Troublingly, a 2006 study in the *Journal of the American Medical Association* suggests that some healthy people may experience liver damage even if they don't exceed the recommended dosage. Researchers gave 106 adults either a prescription painkiller containing acetaminophen, Extra Strength Tylenol, or a placebo every six hours for 14 days. Both the prescription painkiller and the Tylenol contained 4 g of acetaminophen, the maximum daily dosage.

After two weeks, 39% of the participants who took one of the acetaminophen medications more than tripled their levels of alanine aminotransferase (ALT) liver enzymes—the point at which liver damage is a concern. Twenty-five percent of the

drained or surgically removed. You'll also need to stop drinking alcohol and follow a nutritious, low-fat diet.

If you are diagnosed with chronic pancreatitis, you will likely be prescribed medications that contain pancreatic enzymes to help your body absorb food. If the pain persists, surgery to remove damaged tissue in the pancreas or to cut the nerves that transmit pain may be needed. As with acute pancreatitis, stopping alcohol use and eating a nutritious, low-fat diet are important.

participants had enzyme levels five times the normal level, and 8% had eight times the normal level. Even after the participants stopped taking the acetaminophen, it took up to 11 days for their enzyme levels to return to normal.

These results are surprising, given that many people take recommended amounts of acetaminophen for long periods of time with no liver damage. The researchers stress the importance of not exceeding 4 g daily (and they recommend no more than 2 g per day for heavy drinkers).

The signs of liver damage resemble those of the flu: muscle aches, fatigue, tiredness, sweating, appetite loss, nausea, and vomiting. You may also have dark urine, light-colored stools, and yellow eyes and skin. Symptoms often come on quickly—you may feel fine, or perhaps a bit nauseous, the day before the situation becomes life threatening.

If you do experience any of these symptoms, call your doctor immediately. Acetaminophen overdoses are best treated in the first eight to 12 hours. After that, the medication used to treat it—N-acetylcysteine—loses its effectiveness. If treated quickly, the liver may repair itself. Otherwise, a liver transplant may be needed; more serious cases may lead to coma or death.

Staying Safe

It's not hard to take too much acetaminophen, particularly if you're on more than one medication. But these steps can help you benefit from acetaminophen without risking your liver:

Don't exceed the maximum dosage. It's easy enough to remember not to take more than 4 g (4,000 mg) daily, but it can be tricky to keep track of all sources of acetaminophen. Know what the active ingredient is in all of your drugs and the dose in each pill. For example, an Extra Strength Tylenol contains 500 mg of acetaminophen. But some drugs contain up to 750 mg, so you need to take fewer pills in 24 hours to stay under the maximum dosage.

Read the label. Before you take any medication, check to see if it contains acetaminophen. This may soon become simpler: In December 2006, the U.S. Food and Drug Administration (FDA) proposed stronger safety warnings for over-the-counter painkillers that require manufacturers to label more prominently that their products contain acetaminophen and use standard language for safety warnings that highlight the potential for liver problems.

Look at the package directions for information on how much to take, when to take it, and for how long. Some people experience liver and other side effects (like an allergic reaction) from taking too much, not waiting long enough between doses, or taking the medication for longer than they should. The label will also let you know what side effects to look for.

Avoid or limit alcohol. Those who have three or more drinks a day are especially at risk for toxicity. If you drink alcohol regularly, reduce your intake or talk to your doctor about using another type of pain reliever. And never take Tylenol or another acetaminophen product to ease a hangover.

Talk to your doctor. If you have a history of liver problems or feel the need to use an over-the-counter pain reliever for more than 10 days, consult with your doctor before taking acetaminophen. Your condition may need to be evaluated and your doctor may recommend a different treatment. Let your doctor know about any other medications you are taking, since there may be a risk of interactions between these drugs and acetaminophen. ■

Anatomy of the Lower Digestive Tract

Your lower digestive tract, also known as your bowel, is approximately 25 feet long and consists of the small and large intestines (see the illustration on page 3). Food from the stomach passes through the pyloric valve into the small intestine, a 20-foot tube with three sections: the duodenum, the jejunum, and the ileum. The walls of the small intestine are lined with muscles that contract and relax to carry food along its path. The walls are also covered in microvilli, hairlike projections that help to absorb nutrients into the bloodstream.

When food reaches the duodenum, it begins to get broken down by digestive enzymes and bile. This process turns proteins into amino acids, fats into fatty acids, and carbohydrates into simple sugars. The digested food then moves into the jejunum, where most of its nutrients are absorbed. Vitamins (such as A, D, K, and B_{12}) and other remaining nutrients are absorbed in the ileum.

The material left behind—mostly water, electrolytes (such as sodium and potassium), and waste (such as fiber and dead cells)—moves into the cecum, the first part of the colon (also called the large intestine). It then passes through the ascending, transverse, and descending colons; the sigmoid colon; and the rectum. No nutrients are absorbed by the colon. Its job is to remove excess water from the intestinal waste and return it to the bloodstream. Thus, as the material moves along the colon, it slowly dries out and forms a more solid substance called stool. Waste usually spends a day or two in the colon before it is expelled from the body.

When stool moves into the rectum, it stretches the walls of the rectum, which signals the need for a bowel movement. The stool then moves into the anal canal. At the end of the canal is the anal sphincter, a muscle that usually remains closed but opens to allow stool to pass out of the body.

Tests for Examining the Lower Digestive Tract

Various tests are available to obtain an inner view of the lower digestive tract: barium enema, sigmoidoscopy, colonoscopy, virtual colonoscopy, and capsule endoscopy. All of these procedures can be performed on an outpatient basis at your doctor's office or a hospital.

The colon must be emptied before all of these procedures so that your doctor can obtain a clear view of the inside of your lower digestive tract. Your doctor will give you specific instructions on how to do this, but the process typically involves consuming a liquid diet for up to three days before the procedure. Water, fat-free broth or bouillon, Jell-O, black coffee, plain tea, soda, and fruit juice are all usually allowed. In addition, you will be told not to eat or drink anything after midnight the night before the test and to use laxatives the day before the procedure to cleanse the colon. On the morning of the procedure, an enema (a liquid solution passed into the anus) will be needed to cleanse the colon completely.

Barium Enema

Your doctor may order a barium enema, also called a lower gastrointestinal (GI) series, to detect structural problems at the far end of your bowel. If a colonoscopy (see page 40) cannot be performed, a barium enema may also be used to diagnose inflammatory bowel disease (Crohn's disease and ulcerative colitis) and colon cancer.

Barium sulfate—a type of contrast dye—is administered through the anus and into the colon to help produce x-ray images of the lower digestive tract. During the exam, you lie on your side with your knees bent toward your chest. A lubricated tube is gently inserted through the anus and into the rectum. Barium is then passed through the tube into the rectum, allowing the colon to fill with contrast dye. No sedation or pain medication is needed, but you may feel some abdominal discomfort or an urge to pass stool during the test.

A radiologist will take continuous x-rays of your abdomen and view them on a screen. If any abnormalities are seen, the radiologist will take spot x-rays for later analysis. When the procedure is complete (it typically takes 30–45 minutes), you will be taken to the bathroom to expel some of the barium into the toilet. If a buildup of barium prevents you from having a bowel movement in the days after the test, your doctor may recommend a laxative or an enema. Also, your stool may be whitish in color for up to three days after the procedure because of the barium. Serious complications, such as perforation of the colon, are rare.

Sigmoidoscopy

During a sigmoidoscopy, a gastroenterologist examines the inside of the rectum and sigmoid colon (the last part of the large intestine) using a 2-foot, flexible viewing tube called a sigmoidoscope. You might have this test to screen for colorectal cancer (although a colonoscopy is the preferred method) or to investigate suspicious rectal bleeding, diarrhea, or pain.

Usually no sedation is required for a sigmoidoscopy, although you can request a sedative if you feel anxious or are in pain. While you lie on your left side, the doctor manually inspects the anus and rectum for any blockages and then gently inserts the sigmoidoscope into the anus and then into the rectum and lower colon to view the inner lining of these parts of the digestive tract. The physician may take biopsy samples and remove any polyps (abnormal growths).

The procedure takes up to 30 minutes, and, if no sedation was necessary, you usually can drive home afterward. If you do receive sedation, you won't be able to leave until it wears off, and you'll need someone to drive you home. Some people experience gas or a small amount of bleeding or abdominal cramping following a sigmoidoscopy. More serious complications, such as excessive bleeding and perforation of the colon or rectum, can occur but are rare.

Colonoscopy

A colonoscopy is similar to a sigmoidoscopy, but a longer flexible viewing tube called a colonoscope is used to examine the entire colon and (if necessary) the lower portion of the small intestine. It is typically performed to detect colorectal cancer and to determine the causes of rectal bleeding, chronic diarrhea, chronic constipation, or abdominal pain.

Pain medication and a mild sedative are usually given intravenously just before colonoscopy. While you lie on the examining table, the doctor manually checks for blockages in the anus and rectum. He or she then gently inserts the tube through the anus and rectum and into the colon. As the colonoscope is slowly withdrawn, the physician inspects the lining of the intestines and may take biopsy samples of any abnormal tissue and remove any polyps. You may experience abdominal cramping, bloating, and a need to pass stool or gas during the procedure. The whole process can take up to an hour.

The sedation will wear off about an hour after the procedure. You'll need to have someone drive you home because of the lingering effect of the sedative. It is common to have gas after the procedure and to have minor rectal bleeding if a biopsy was performed. Serious complications are rare (occurring in fewer than 0.1% of all colonoscopies) and can include excessive bleeding, labored breathing (from the sedative), and perforation of the colon or rectum.

Virtual Colonoscopy

A virtual colonoscopy requires the same preparation to empty the bowels as a standard colonoscopy, but instead of inserting a viewing tube into the colon and rectum, a CT scan of the abdomen is done to obtain two- and three-dimensional images of the intestines. Because the test will cause only minor discomfort, sedation is not needed.

You might be wondering why your doctor wants to perform a standard colonoscopy when a virtual colonoscopy sounds like an easier test to endure. Even though a 2003 study found that a three-dimensional CT virtual colonoscopy was as accurate as a standard colonoscopy for detecting abnormal growths in the colon and rectum, the test has a number of drawbacks. First, biopsy samples cannot be taken with a virtual colonoscopy. This means that if any abnormalities are detected, you will need to undergo a standard colonoscopy for confirmation of the diagnosis. Second, polyps cannot be removed during virtual colonoscopy as they can during a standard colonoscopy. Third, virtual colonoscopy may not be able to distinguish stool from polyps or cancers. Because of these drawbacks, your doctor won't perform a virtual colonoscopy unless you have a medical condition that makes a standard colonoscopy risky or physically difficult.

Capsule Endoscopy

When symptoms, such as gastrointestinal bleeding or chronic abdominal pain, cannot be explained using standard diagnostic procedures, capsule endoscopy may be a useful technique. It allows for a full view of the small intestine, particularly the areas that are usually unreachable with an upper endoscopy or colonoscopy. However, capsule endoscopy cannot be used to view the esophagus or the stomach, and biopsy samples cannot be taken.

Similar to the other imaging techniques described above, you will need to follow a liquid diet and take a laxative to empty your bowels before the procedure. On the day of the procedure, you will swallow a camera-containing capsule with a full glass of water. The capsule is then propelled through the digestive tract by peristalsis. You can go about your normal daily activities, although you must wait two hours before drinking clear liquids and four hours before eating a light meal.

The capsule is somewhat larger than a vitamin pill and contains a video camera, light, and radio transmitter. It takes pictures (two per second) of the digestive tract and transmits these images to a Walkman-like device that is worn at your waist. After about eight hours, you return the recording device to your doctor, who downloads the information from the device to a computer. The capsule is eliminated in your stool and does not need to be returned. Your doctor, however, may ask you to watch for the capsule in your stool; it gets stuck in the intestines of about 0.5% of people.

Thwarting Turista

How to prevent and treat the dreaded traveler's diarrhea

When you think of vacation, visions of fabulous meals and sumptuous buffets may dance in your head. But beware: Turista—also known as traveler's diarrhea or food poisoning—may be on the menu.

According to the Centers for Disease Control and Prevention (CDC), turista is the most common illness among vacationers. It affects about 10 million Americans a year, especially those venturing to exotic locales. Common culprits are:

- Bacteria, such as *Escherichia coli*, Shigella, Campylobacter, and Salmonella
- Viruses, such as the Norovirus, found on cruise ships.

Simply overindulging or eating foods and spices that your digestive tract is not accustomed to—whether you are on vacation or at home—also can lead to diarrhea. But these symptoms are mild and are not due to food poisoning.

Location, Location, Location!

Although you can develop traveler's diarrhea right here in the states, certain spots worldwide are notorious for causing food poisoning in travelers: Mexico tops the list, followed by other Latin American countries, Africa, the Middle East, and Asia. The risks in these countries are related to poor sanitation and hygiene, which can lead to contaminated food and water.

Cruise ships and resorts also are breeding grounds for outbreaks of turista, because infected and healthy individuals are in such close proximity to each other. In these environments, bacteria and viruses can spread quickly through exposure to foods and surfaces (for example, door handles and eating utensils) that have been touched by infected individuals.

The Symptoms

Once you've had turista, you'll never forget it. The symptoms may be severe and come on abruptly. Diarrhea, frequent and strong feelings of needing to defecate, nausea, vomiting, abdominal cramps, bloating, fever, and general malaise may all be part of the the illness.

The good news is that turista is rarely serious. It usually comes and goes in two to seven days, even without treatment. But it can interrupt your plans with days spent suffering in your hotel room.

Who's at Risk

Men and women are equally prone to turista, but certain people are more susceptible. For example, those taking proton pump inhibitors (esomeprazole [Nexium], rabeprazole [Aciphex], lansoprazole [Prevacid] or omeprazole [Prilosec]), H_2-blockers (famotidine [Pepcid] and cimetidine [Tagamet]) or antacids (Gaviscon, Maalox) for heartburn or ulcers are more likely to get turista because these products reduce the amount of stomach acid that normally would kill off bacteria in contaminated food. In addition, people who have illnesses or are taking medications that weaken the immune system are at increased risk.

When Turista Strikes

Staying hydrated and possibly taking medication (antibiotics or over-the-counter antidiarrhea products) are your options when traveler's diarrhea strikes.

Stay hydrated. The most important step is to make sure you're getting enough fluids (since diarrhea can lead to a rapid loss of body fluids and essential electrolytes, such as sodium and potassium). Contrary to popular belief, water and Gatorade will not do the trick. Water does not contain electrolytes, and Gatorade is designed to replace fluids and electrolytes lost through sweat—not diarrhea.

According to R. Bradley Sack, M.D., Sc.D., Director of the International Travel Medicine Service at Johns Hopkins, fruit juices and salty liquids such as clear vegetable or chicken broth are your best choices to replenish fluids.

When diarrhea is severe, he recommends an oral electrolyte solution, CeraLyte, available over the counter at your pharmacy. Before leaving on vacation, purchase it in a powdered form and bring a packet or two. If diarrhea strikes, mix the powder with water and then drink it to replace the fluids and electrolytes lost in your stool.

Take antibiotics. Most cases of traveler's diarrhea are due to bacteria, and taking antibiotics is the most effective treatment for this. Dr. Sack recommends asking your doctor for a prescription for an antibiotic and filling it before you leave. Then you'll be able to treat yourself without having to find a physician while away. (See the inset box at right for advice on finding a doctor abroad.)

Typically, doctors prescribe floroquinolone antibiotics. A typical prescription: One 500-mg tablet of ciprofloxacin (Cipro) at the onset of symptoms and another 500-mg tablet 12 hours later. Azithromycin (Zithromax) and rifaximin (Xifaxan) also are sometimes prescribed. All of them usually relieve diarrhea within 24 hours.

It's important to take the antibiotics exactly as prescribed by your doctor and for the full duration of the prescription—*even if you start feeling better*—to ensure the bacteria are fully eradicated.

Try an over-the-counter antidiarrhea product. Those containing bismuth subsalicylate (Pepto-Bismol) or loperamide (Imodium A-D) can be taken for *mild* traveler's diarrhea. They provide symptom relief but, unlike antibiotics, do not kill off the bacteria responsible, so they're not your best option.

These products shouldn't be used if you have a fever or bloody diarrhea because they can make you sicker by slowing the removal of the bacteria or virus that's causing your illness. But taking Imodium A-D along with an antibiotic can help you get better more quickly.

See your doctor. If you're still sick when you return home or after you've finished antibiotic therapy, you might have an infection with a parasite or bacteria resistant to antibiotics, so call your doctor. He or she will ask you to collect a stool sample; if it reveals a parasite or drug-resistant bacteria as the cause of the diarrhea, you will be prescribed appropriate medication.

Finding a Doctor in Another Country

You can easily find a qualified, English-speaking doctor on a cruise ship. But if you are traveling in less-developed countries, you can obtain lists of local clinics where English is spoken by:

- Contacting the local U.S. embassy
- Visiting the International Society of Travel Medicine website (www.istm.org) or the International Association for Medical Assistance to Travelers website (www.iamat.org).

You may want to check these sites before you travel and print out the contact information for clinics in the countries you're planning to visit.

You also may wish to purchase travel health insurance. Your usual health insurance won't cover airlifting to a medical facility if you become very ill or get injured while traveling outside of the United States. For information on policies, visit www.insuremytrip.com.

Prevention Is Key

To minimize the chances you'll get traveler's diarrhea in high-risk locales, follow advice from the CDC:

- Drink only bottled water or water that has been treated (boiled, chlorinated, or filtered). Do not drink tap water or even brush your teeth with tap water.
- Avoid ice cubes, unpasteurized milk, and dairy products made from unpasteurized milk.
- If you can't peel, boil, or cook it, don't eat it. That means forgoing any raw fruits or vegetables that you can't peel first.
- Don't buy food or drinks from street vendors, who may not follow proper hygiene practices.
- Don't eat raw or undercooked meat or seafood.
- Beware of buffets, especially if the food has been sitting out for a long time.
- Don't overeat—overindulgence and eating unfamiliar foods can upset your stomach, even if they don't lead to food poisoning.
- Wash your hands frequently to clean them of bacteria and viruses. Carry antibacterial wipes and gels with you to use if you can't find a washroom prior to eating. Some cruise lines now have antibacterial gel dispensers located throughout the ship, especially at entrances to the restaurants, so use them.

The CDC doesn't encourage taking antibiotics during your trip to prevent traveler's diarrhea, primarily because of the risk of allergic reactions when antibiotics are used for prolonged times.

Dr. Sack and the other doctors at the International Travel Medicine Service at Johns Hopkins sometimes recommend preventive antibiotic therapy to people who could become deathly ill from a bout of diarrhea (like those who are taking immunosuppressive medications) or have a crucial engagement they can't miss (such as an important meeting or family affair). For these individuals, taking an antibiotic such as Cipro daily at the start of the trip and for up to three weeks during the trip can prevent diarrhea up to 90% of the time. If you think you might benefit from preventive antibiotic therapy, ask your doctor what's best for you.

For More Information

Try visiting the CDC website, www.cdc. gov/travel, or the World Health Organization's website, www.who.int/ith/en/, for travel-related health advice and updates. ■

Disorders of the Lower Digestive Tract

A large number of disorders can afflict your lower digestive tract, including diverticulosis and diverticulitis, celiac disease, Crohn's disease, ulcerative colitis, irritable bowel syndrome, hemorrhoids, anal fissures, and colorectal cancer. Many of these disorders have constipation or diarrhea as a symptom.

Constipation

Nearly everyone has had a bout of constipation—infrequent bowel movements and difficulty passing stool—at some point in their life. This common problem is not a disease but rather a symptom that can stem from a number of medical conditions. It becomes more common with age and occurs in at least 25% of people over age 65. In most cases, constipation is not a serious condition and can be treated with lifestyle measures, such as increasing your intake of dietary fiber and level of physical activity or taking a laxative. In rare cases, surgery may be necessary to relieve symptoms.

Causes of constipation

Constipation typically occurs when fecal matter moves too slowly through the colon. This allows the body to absorb too much water from the stool, leaving it dry and hard. Many experts no longer believe that a low-fiber diet is a *major* contributor to constipation. However, ignoring the urge to have a bowel movement and changing one's daily routine, such as during travel, are contributing factors.

Constipation can also be a side effect of medication, including pain medications (mainly narcotics), antidepressants, diuretics, iron supplements, and aluminum-containing antacids. Some experts believe that excessive use of laxatives also may lead to constipation, because the colon becomes dependent on the laxative to initiate defecation. Overuse of enemas can have the same result.

Various medical conditions also can cause constipation. These include Parkinson's disease, diabetes, multiple sclerosis, stroke, lupus, decreased thyroid function, and spinal cord injuries. Constipation can also be a symptom of irritable bowel syndrome. Tumors in the colon and diverticulosis can cause constipation by blocking the passage of fecal matter. Last, constipation can result from mental health problems such as depression and eating disorders.

Symptoms of constipation

What is considered normal when it comes to the frequency of bowel movements varies from person to person. In fact, having only three bowel movements a week is just as normal as having three bowel movements a day. Therefore, a sudden decrease in your typical number of bowel movements is a better indicator of constipation than your actual number of movements.

If untreated, constipation can lead to complications. Straining during bowel movements can irritate or cause hemorrhoids or rectal prolapse (when part of the lining of the rectum pushes out of the anus). Hard stools may lead to anal fissures—tears in the skin near the anus. All of these conditions can cause pain, bleeding, or excessive secretion of mucus. Another potential complication is fecal impaction, an inability to have a bowel movement because the stool has formed a large, dense mass in the colon or rectum.

You should call your doctor if you experience sudden and unexplained constipation, especially if it is accompanied by blood in the stool or severe abdominal pain, or if you experience constipation that lasts longer than a week despite making changes in your diet and physical activity.

Diagnosis of constipation

You are considered to have chronic constipation if you consistently average one or fewer bowel movements per week for at least a year or have at least two of the following signs of constipation:

- Two or fewer bowel movements per week
- Straining during at least one quarter of bowel movements
- Passage of pellet-like or hard stools during at least one quarter of bowel movements
- Feeling like not all of the fecal material is eliminated during at least one quarter of bowel movements.

If you have a bowel movement fewer than three times a week but experience no discomfort or change in the pattern of your bowel movements, you likely aren't constipated.

Diagnostic tests like blood tests, abdominal x-rays, sigmoidoscopies, colonoscopies, and barium enemas are not helpful—or necessary—for the diagnosis of constipation.

Treatment of constipation

The first therapies your doctor will recommend if you have constipation are diet and lifestyle modifications. One of these is an increase in fiber consumption. The average American consumes

FDA APPROVAL

Laxative MiraLax Available Without a Prescription

The U.S. Food and Drug Administration (FDA) recently approved the switch of polyethylene glycol (MiraLax) from a prescription to an over-the-counter medication. MiraLax is a bulk-forming laxative that can be helpful for some people with occasional constipation. The OTC version is the same strength as the prescription medication, 17 g.

MiraLax is the first laxative to switch from prescription to OTC status in 30 years. The medication gently increases the frequency of bowel movements and softens the stool so it is easier to pass, without causing cramps and gas. To be taken once daily, it comes in a powder form that dissolves in any common beverage (coffee, tea, juice, etc.) without changing the color or taste of the drink.

MiraLax does not usually cause any serious side effects and is not habit forming. Like any other fiber supplement or laxative, it should only be used for a week at a time. If you are still experiencing constipation after a week, consult your doctor.

U.S. FOOD AND DRUG ADMINISTRATION
October 6, 2006

5–20 g of fiber a day; however, the Institute of Medicine recommends that men over age 50 get at least 30 g of fiber daily and that women over age 50 consume at least 21 g. (Younger men and women should aim for 38 g and 25 g of fiber daily, respectively.)

Although a 2006 review concluded that a lack of dietary fiber probably does not contribute to chronic constipation, fiber may help treat constipation by adding bulk (increased volume) and softening the texture of your stools. Fresh fruits and vegetables, whole grains, and beans are examples of fiber-rich foods that you should add to your diet. Avoiding foods with a high-fat and low-fiber content, including meat and full-fat dairy products, also may be helpful. Also, don't ignore the urge to have a bowel movement or delay a trip to the bathroom when the urge develops.

Fiber supplements that act as laxatives (such as Citrucel, Fiberall, Konsyl, or Metamucil) or a prescription-strength laxative such as polyethylene glycol (MiraLax, now available over the counter) are useful for some people with constipation. These laxatives add bulk to the stool and are generally safe to use for a week at a time. If you need to use them for longer than that, you should consult your doctor. You should also slowly increase the amount of fiber you take to avoid problems with gas, and be sure to drink plenty of water or other fluids every day.

If bulk-forming laxatives fail to help, your doctor may recommend an enema or a nonbulk-forming laxative, including stimulants, stool softeners, lubricants, and saline laxatives. Stimulants such as bisacodyl (Correctol, Dulcolax) cause rhythmic muscle contractions in the intestines, stool softeners such as docusate sodium (Colace, Dialose, Surfak) add water to the stool which makes it easier to pass, lubricants such as mineral oil (Fleet) allow stool to move more easily through the colon, and saline laxatives such as magnesium hydroxide (Milk of Magnesia) draw water into the colon which provides a flushing action. Even though these laxatives are available without a prescription, they should be used for only a week at a time. If you need them for longer than that, ask your doctor for guidance.

Fiber supplements and laxatives are the primary treatments for chronic constipation. For many people who weren't helped by these medications, a drug called tegaserod (Zelnorm) was the next step. But Zelnorm was withdrawn from the market in April 2007 because it was linked to a higher risk of heart attacks, strokes, and chest pain.

If constipation results in fecal impaction, your doctor may recommend a stool softener or enema. Then he or she will manually remove the hardened stool. If a drug you are taking for another health problem is the suspected cause of your constipation, your doctor may be able to lower the dosage of the medication or switch you to another drug that does not have constipation as a side effect. (Never stop taking a medication or change the dosage without first consulting your doctor.) When a medical condition is the source of the problem, treating that condition may relieve the symptoms.

Biofeedback—in which you learn to strain more effectively, coordinate your breathing, and properly relax and contract the muscles involved in a bowel movement—may help a small number of people with constipation, particularly the type caused by the inability to relax the pelvic floor muscles.

Diverticulosis and Diverticulitis

As we age, most of us develop small pouches (diverticula) that bulge outward through weak points in the wall of the large intestine—a condition called diverticulosis. The condition is present in about half of Americans ages 60–80 and in virtually everyone older than age 80. A disorder called diverticulitis, an infection or inflammation of diverticula, develops in about 10–25% of people with diverticulosis. Diverticulosis and diverticulitis are referred to as diverticular disease.

Although diverticulosis can occur anywhere along the length of the colon, the pouches typically develop in the sigmoid colon, the last portion of the colon before the rectum. The number of diverticula can range from one (called a diverticulum) to hundreds. Diverticula are usually 5–10 mm in diameter but can exceed 2 cm.

Causes of diverticulosis and diverticulitis

A low-fiber diet is the major culprit in diverticulosis because it leads to hard stools. When you strain to move hardened stool, pressure inside the colon increases, which can cause weak spots in the colon wall to bulge outward and become diverticula. Diverticulosis primarily affects people in affluent, industrialized areas like the United States, Europe, and Australia, where diets low in fiber are common.

Diverticulitis occurs when bacteria or hardened stool is trapped in a diverticulum, causing an infection or inflammation. This may ultimately lead to a small hole in the tip of a diverticulum, which allows bacteria to enter the abdomen and cause infection (peritonitis).

Symptoms of diverticulosis and diverticulitis

Although most people with diverticulosis have no discomfort or symptoms, some experience mild abdominal pain, bloating, and

ASK THE DOCTOR

Q. ***Should people with diverticulosis avoid certain foods?***

A. It was once thought that people with diverticulosis should avoid seeds and nuts because they can become lodged in diverticula, the pea-sized pouches in the intestinal wall that characterize this condition, and may often lead to more serious inflammation and infection known as diverticulitis. But it's now understood that some of the very foods that were once thought inappropriate for diverticulosis may actually be beneficial.

Diverticulosis is strongly associated with a low-fiber diet. Stool formed from refined grains and fatty foods moves slowly through the intestine and leads to constipation. The increased pressure required to keep stool moving can prompt the formation of diverticula. Fiber bulks up the stool, encourages it to move through the intestine, and helps prevent constipation. Therefore, adequate fiber intake of 20–30 g a day may prevent diverticula from developing as well as existing pouches from worsening or progressing to diverticulitis.

Fruits and vegetables, including ones with small seeds like tomatoes, strawberries, and raspberries, pose no problems for people with diverticulosis and are good sources of fiber, as are whole grains. Be sure to chew foods well.

If you need to increase your fiber intake, do so gradually—a quick increase can cause gas and bloating. You can also use a psyllium-containing bulk-forming laxative (such as Metamucil and others). And be sure to drink about 64 oz of fluid a day.

Osteoporosis and Digestive Disorders
How your gut can affect your bones

When you think of the ways a digestive disorder can affect your life, bone fractures probably don't come to mind. But some digestive problems—or their treatments—can increase your risk of osteoporosis and lead to broken bones.

The Biggest Culprits

Lactose intolerance is the most common example of a digestive disorder that can weaken bones, but it's not the only one. People with untreated celiac disease and those who take corticosteroids or proton pump inhibitors for their digestive ills are also at risk.

Lactose intolerance. Up to 50 million Americans have trouble digesting lactose, a sugar found in milk and foods made with milk. Unfortunately, these foods are the most plentiful sources of calcium, a mineral that helps keep bones strong. As a result, people with lactose intolerance who avoid dairy products may be more likely to develop osteoporosis.

Untreated celiac disease. People with celiac disease are unable to digest gluten (a protein in wheat, rye, barley, farina, and bulgur), causing the body to attack and damage the small intestine lining. The small intestine then cannot properly absorb nutrients, including calcium and vitamin D. A study in the *Archives of Internal Medicine* found that the prevalence of celiac disease was much higher in people with osteoporosis than in those without (3.4% vs. 0.2%).

Corticosteroids. People with inflammatory bowel disease (IBD) often take corticosteroids to reduce inflammation in the digestive tract. But if taken for a long period of time, these medications (which include prednisone and hydrocortisone) can interfere with bone formation. As a result, people with Crohn's disease or ulcerative colitis are 40% more likely to experience a bone fracture than the general population.

Proton pump inhibitors. Millions of people take proton pump inhibitors (see pages 18–19) to treat gastroesophageal reflux disease (GERD). These medications are very effective, but they may also interfere with the body's ability to absorb calcium. A December 2006 study in the *Journal of the American Medical Association* found that people who took a proton pump inhibitor for more than one year were 44% more likely to break a hip than people who didn't take the medication.

Keeping Your Bones Strong

Having a digestive disorder does not mean that your bones are doomed. You can fight back with a combination of calcium, vitamin D, and exercise. In fact, most of the bone-health recommendations for people without a digestive problem will work for you as well.

Calcium. After age 50, you need 1,200 mg of calcium a day to maintain bone mass and prevent osteoporosis. Eating foods rich in calcium, such as milk, yogurt, and cheese, will help you reach this goal, but don't forget to choose the low-fat versions.You can also try nondairy sources of calcium, for example, calcium-fortified orange juice as well as canned salmon and sardines with the bones.

If you can't meet your calcium requirements with food, you may want to take a calcium supplement. Two types of calcium are available: calcium carbonate, which is found in Tums, Caltrate, Os-Cal, and Viactiv; and calcium citrate, which is found in Citracal.

Whether you're getting your calcium from food or a supplement, avoid taking all of your calcium at once. Calcium is best absorbed when consumed several times a day in amounts of 500 mg or less.

Vitamin D. Vitamin D helps to maintain calcium stores in your body. Without this vitamin, dietary calcium is poorly absorbed from the intestine. The Recommended Daily Allowance (RDA) for vitamin D is 400 IU for people ages 51–70 and 600 IU for those over age 70. The latest Dietary Guidelines recommend 1,000 IU for older adults.

Fortified foods, such as milk, soymilk, and margarine, are good sources of vitamin D. The vitamin also occurs naturally in a few foods, including fish, liver, and egg yolks. Getting 10–15 minutes of sunlight without sunscreen several times a week is another way to meet the RDA for vitamin D (and shouldn't increase your risk of skin cancer).

Ask your physician if taking a multivitamin-mineral supplement plus some sun exposure will provide all the vitamin D you need.

Exercise. Round out your bone-health regimen with 30 minutes of daily exercise. The best regimen is a combination of strength training (using weights) and weight-bearing exercises (such as walking, stair climbing, and aerobics). Strength training helps muscles in the upper

Calcium and Vitamin D in Common Foods

Food	Calcium Content	Vitamin D Content
Yogurt, plain, low-fat, 1 cup	450 mg	0 IU
Milk, reduced-fat, 1 cup	285 mg	105 IU
Swiss cheese, 1 oz	225 mg	10 IU
Soymilk, fortified, 1 cup	200–300 mg	120 IU
Cottage cheese, low-fat, 1 cup	155 mg	0 IU
Orange juice, fortified, 1 cup	350 mg	100 IU
Sardines, canned in oil, with edible bones, 3 oz	325 mg	230 IU
Salmon, canned, with edible bones, 3 oz	190 mg	650 IU

Source: U.S. Department of Agriculture National Nutrient Database.

body support your bones, and weight-bearing activities strengthen bones in the lower body.

Special Instructions

Depending on your digestive disorder or the medications you are taking to manage the disorder, your bones may need some extra care.

Lactose intolerance. Most cases of lactose intolerance are mild, and you might not have to avoid dairy products altogether. For example, you may be able to eat yogurt and aged cheese, since they contain lactase-producing bacteria that lower the lactose content. You may also be able to tolerate a cup of milk a day when it is consumed with other foods.

In addition, various digestive aids may help you handle lactose better. Adding lactase-containing drops to milk can convert 75–90% of the lactose to glucose and galactose after overnight refrigeration. Specialty milks are also available that have lactase added during the manufacturing process. And lactase tablets can be taken with dairy products, although these vary in their effectiveness.

If you still have problems with dairy foods, try foods that provide calcium without the high lactose content: soymilk, calcium-fortified orange juice, and canned sardines and salmon with edible bones. In the end, you may need to take a calcium and vitamin D supplement.

Celiac disease. Make sure your diet is strictly gluten free. Most people with celiac disease who successfully eradicate gluten from their diets regain normal nutrient absorption within a few months. Once this happens, bone mass will begin to improve.

The greatest improvement (an average bone mass increase of 5%) occurs in the first year after going gluten free, but bone mineral density levels usually remain lower than in people without celiac disease. Therefore, you may need more frequent bone mineral density tests, and your doctor may recommend medication to prevent or treat osteoporosis.

Users of corticosteroids or proton pump inhibitors. Talk to your doctor about taking your corticosteroid or proton pump inhibitor at the lowest effective dose for the shortest possible time.

In general, people taking corticosteroids for longer than six months should get a bone mineral density test when beginning therapy and periodically thereafter.

They should also consider taking an osteoporosis medication (alendronate [Fosamax] and risedronate [Actonel] are approved for corticosteroid-induced osteoporosis); consume extra calcium and vitamin D (1,500 mg calcium and 800 IU vitamin D daily); and ask their doctor about topical corticosteroids, which are less likely than pills to cause bone loss. ■

constipation. The pain typically occurs in the lower abdomen, most often on the left side. This area of the abdomen may feel full or tender when touched.

Between 15% and 40% of people with diverticulosis experience mild, painless bleeding from the rectum. Excessive bleeding occurs in only about 5% of people. Bleeding occurs when a small blood vessel adjacent to the diverticulum ruptures. The bleeding usually stops on its own. If it persists or recurs, surgery to remove the portion of the colon containing the bleeding diverticulum may be necessary.

Attacks of diverticulitis can occur suddenly and without warning. The most common symptom is pain in the lower left side of the abdomen. Other possible symptoms include fever, nausea, vomiting, chills, constipation, diarrhea, painful or difficult urination, and increased frequency of urination. The severity of the symptoms depends on whether the infection has spread beyond the colon and whether any complications such as a perforation have occurred.

Diagnosis of diverticulosis and diverticulitis

Diverticulosis is often discovered by accident during a diagnostic exam (such as a barium enema, sigmoidoscopy, or colonoscopy) for another gastrointestinal ailment. If you have symptoms, and your medical history and examination suggest diverticular disease, your physician will perform one or more tests. The most common is a barium enema. A CT scan also is frequently used to diagnose diverticular disease and its complications. Your doctor may also recommend a colonoscopy to check whether cancer is causing the symptoms.

Treatment of diverticulosis and diverticulitis

For most people with diverticulosis, eating a high-fiber diet will relieve symptoms and prevent the development of diverticulitis (see the "Ask the Doctor" column on page 47). Diverticulitis is usually treated at home with bed rest, a liquid diet to rest the colon, and oral antibiotics. People with severe diverticulitis may be hospitalized and treated with intravenous antibiotics. About 80% of people with severe diverticulitis can be treated successfully without surgery.

If antibiotics do not eradicate the infection associated with diverticulitis, an abscess (a collection of pus surrounded by inflamed tissue) may form in the abdominal cavity adjacent to the colon. The abscess can be treated with more antibiotics or it may need to be drained by inserting a needle into the abscess through the skin and draining the infected fluid through a catheter. Surgical treatment is necessary in some people with a resistant infection.

Rarely, the infection may leak out of an abscess and spread into the abdominal cavity, causing a condition called peritonitis. In such cases, surgery is required immediately to clean the abdominal cavity and remove the damaged region of the colon.

A fistula (an abnormal connection between two organs) can form when an abscess erodes, creating a passage between the colon and an adjacent organ such as the bladder, small intestine, vagina, or skin. The most common type of fistula connects the colon and the bladder. This abnormality, which occurs far more often in men than in women, can lead to severe, persistent urinary tract infections. Surgery to remove the fistula and the affected part of the colon is needed to correct the problem.

Diarrhea

Diarrhea is a common problem that causes loose, watery stools. Acute diarrhea lasts no more than two weeks; diarrhea that lasts longer than two months is considered chronic.

Causes of diarrhea

Acute diarrhea is usually caused by an infectious agent. Most organisms causing diarrhea originate in feces and enter the mouth via the hands or contaminated food or water. Acute infectious diarrhea can be caused by a wide variety of bacteria, viruses, and parasites. Bacteria implicated in acute diarrhea include Salmonella, Shigella, *Campylobacter jejuni, Escherichia coli* O157:H7, and *Clostridium difficile.* Viral causes include adenoviruses, rotaviruses, and the Norwalk-like viruses known as the Noroviruses; parasites include *Entamoeba histolytica, Giardia lamblia,* and Cryptosporidium species.

Chronic diarrhea can be classified into three types: osmotic, secretory, and inflammatory. People with osmotic diarrhea usually have large amounts of undigested fat in the stool (steatorrhea). This condition is caused by ingestion of poorly absorbed substances (such as magnesium or aluminum salts in oral laxatives) or by incomplete digestion and malabsorption of food components such as lactose and sorbitol.

Secretory diarrhea usually results in large amounts of watery stools, which may contain blood. This type of diarrhea is caused by production and secretion of excessive fluid by the small intestine, usually the result of a rare, cancerous neuroendocrine tumor occurring in the digestive tract. The tumors release hormones into the bloodstream that stimulate the small intestine to secrete excessive amounts of fluid and electrolytes such as sodium and potassium.

Inflammatory diarrhea produces bloody, watery stools. It occurs when inflammation in the lining of the colon increases stool volume by decreasing the absorption of water from the stool. This type of diarrhea is common in people with Crohn's disease and ulcerative colitis, the two main types of inflammatory bowel disease discussed on pages 57–64. Diarrhea, as well as constipation, is also a hallmark of irritable bowel syndrome (see pages 64–67).

Symptoms of diarrhea

The main symptom of diarrhea is an increased number of bowel movements along with a decreased consistency of the stools, which may be semisolid or watery. Other symptoms of diarrhea include feelings of urgency and abdominal discomfort and pain.

Diagnosis of diarrhea

Most cases of acute diarrhea do not require a call to your doctor. But if diarrhea persists for more than 48 hours, is severe (more than six stools a day), or is accompanied by fever, severe abdominal pain, or blood in the stool, you should see your doctor. You may be asked to give a stool sample, which will be analyzed to identify the infectious agent causing the diarrhea.

Diagnosing chronic diarrhea is more involved. It requires a detailed evaluation that includes an upper endoscopy and/or a colonoscopy with a biopsy to rule out infections or inflammation.

Treatment of diarrhea

Most of the time, a bout of acute diarrhea requires no treatment beyond rest and drinking plenty of fluids to prevent dehydration until the symptoms subside on their own. Medications to control acute diarrhea are not recommended; you should allow the illness to run its course. However, if the diarrhea is causing you much inconvenience, you can take an antidiarrhea product such as bismuth subsalicylate (Pepto-Bismol and other brands), attapulgite (Kaopectate), or kaolin/pectin (Kao-Spen, Kapectolin) to solidify the stool. Other antidiarrhea medications, such as loperamide (Imodium A-D) or diphenoxylate/atropine (Lomotil), also are helpful because they slow the movement of feces.

Intravenous fluid administration in a hospital is required in some cases of severe diarrhea. Certain cases of infectious diarrhea, particularly those caused by bacteria like *Salmonella typhi* and *E. coli* O157:H7, can be serious. Antibiotics to eradicate the organism are usually recommended if your symptoms have not improved after 48 hours of treatment with fluids and an antidiarrhea product. The antibiotics most frequently used to treat diarrhea caused by bacteria are ciprofloxacin (Cipro) and trimethoprim plus sulfamethoxazole (Bactrim). Cases of acute diarrhea caused by a parasite are often treated with metronidazole (Flagyl). Antibiotics are most effective when started in the first three days of the illness.

Treatment of osmotic diarrhea involves avoiding foods, drinks, or medications that cause the condition. For example, stimulant laxatives such as Correctol or Dulcolax should not be used, and people should limit their use of chewing gum and foods that contain the artificial sweetener sorbitol. If the pancreas produces insufficient digestive enzymes to break down fats, supplemental digestive enzymes can be taken with meals. Treatment of secretory diarrhea caused by a neuroendocrine tumor requires locating and removing the tumor. Treatment of inflammatory diarrhea involves treating the underlying inflammatory bowel disease.

Celiac Disease

People with celiac disease are sensitive to gluten, a component of wheat and other grains. The disorder was once thought to be rare in the United States, but research now shows that about one in 100 Americans has the disease. Many people don't know they have celiac disease, either because they or their doctor have attributed the symptoms to another illness or because they have no symptoms.

Causes and symptoms of celiac disease

Celiac disease is an autoimmune disorder (the body's immune system attacks itself) and a malabsorption disorder (nutrients from foods are not absorbed). Gluten, which is found in wheat and other grains, contains a protein called gliadin. In people with celiac disease, consuming gliadin produces an immune reaction that causes the villi (finger-like projections in the intestines) to flatten or disappear. This negatively affects the ability of the villi to absorb nutrients from food. As a result, diarrhea, bloating, weight loss, anemia, and vitamin deficiencies are common and are some of the first signs of the disorder. Eventually, long-term damage to the small intestine may result.

Osteoporosis is common in people with celiac disease because of poor absorption of vitamin D and calcium. (See "Osteoporosis and Digestive Disorders" on pages 48–49.) Other possible symptoms related to poor nutrient absorption include fatigue and muscle or bone pain. Long-term malabsorption of nutrients can even damage nerves, bones, teeth, the pancreas, and the liver. In addition, a type

Immunizations You Need If You Have IBD

Your medication may increase your risk of certain illnesses

If you have an inflammatory bowel disease (IBD), the most common of which are Crohn's disease and ulcerative colitis, it's likely that you will be treated with immunosuppressive drugs such as mercaptopurine (Purinethol), azathioprine (Imuran), or infliximab (Remicade). Lowering your body's immune response can prevent flare-ups and keep your disease under control, but it can also make you more vulnerable to infections. Even if you don't take immunosuppressant drugs, a chronic medical condition like IBD puts your body under stress and can make you more likely to contract an illness.

That's why experts recommend that people with IBD should be vaccinated against the flu, pneumonia, tetanus, and other common but serious illnesses. The recommendations aren't really different from those for the general public, but they're especially important for people with IBD to follow.

Are You Protected?

Unfortunately, many people with IBD aren't getting these vaccinations. A recent study in *The American Journal of Gastroenterology* looked at the immunization status of 169 people with IBD. Eighty-six percent of the participants were taking or had taken immunosuppressive drugs, putting them at risk for contagious illnesses. Yet only 45% recalled getting a tetanus shot in the past 10 years, just 28% received regular flu vaccinations, and only 9% had received the pneumococcal vaccination. A mere 28% of the participants had received the hepatitis B vaccine, although 44% had at least one risk factor for the virus. Also, 11% of the participants couldn't remember whether they ever had chicken pox (varicella) or its vaccination.

Nearly half of the participants (49%) who didn't receive the recommended vaccinations said they weren't aware they needed to be immunized. Another 18% said they were concerned about possible side effects from the vaccinations.

But a recent study from *Inflammatory Bowel Diseases* reported that vaccines are safe, even for people currently taking immunosuppressive drugs. The only exception is live-agent vaccines, which contain a weakened rather than a completely inactivated strain of the virus. These include the measles/mumps/rubella (MMR) and varicella vaccines. The researchers also point out that people with compromised immune systems not only can tolerate other vaccinations, but also stand to benefit greatly from them.

You Should Also Be Vaccinated If...

IBD isn't the only gastrointestinal disorder that can put you at an increased risk for infections. If you have one of the following conditions, you also may need to take special precautions.

If you: have cirrhosis

You should be vaccinated against: hepatitis A and B, influenza, measles/mumps/rubella (MMR), pneumococcus, tetanus, and varicella

If you: take long-term corticosteroids for another digestive disorder besides IBD

You should be vaccinated against: Haemophilus influenzae type b (Hib), influenza, pneumococcus, and tetanus

of cancer called lymphoma is six times more likely in people with celiac disease than in those without the condition.

Risk factors for celiac disease

Celiac disease is most common in whites and people of European ancestry. Seventy percent of cases occur in women. A family history of the disease is another important risk factor. As many as 10% of

Recommended Vaccinations for People With IBD

Vaccination	How Often
Haemophilus influenzae type b (Hib)	There is no set recommended dose; follow your doctor's recommendation
Hepatitis B	Three doses: 1st: Anytime 2nd: One to two months after the first 3rd: Four to six months after the first Only recommended if you have one or more risk factors: have undergone blood transfusions or dialysis; have permanent tattoos, HIV, or nonhepatitis chronic liver disease; or have been or are an intravenous drug user or a healthcare worker
Herpes zoster (shingles)	One lifetime dose is recommended for adults age 60 and older, whether or not you have had a prior shingles episode
Influenza (flu)	One dose annually (ideally in October or November)
Pneumococcus (pneumonia)	One lifetime dose if you're age 65 or older. Two doses are recommended for those 65+ who got their first dose before age 65 if five or more years have passed since that dose. A second dose is also recommended for people with certain conditions or who are on medications like long-term steroids. Check with your doctor.
Tetanus	One dose every 10 years

Be Proactive

The American Journal of Gastroenterology study found that even though the participants with IBD saw a general practitioner at least annually and a gastroenterologist even more frequently, most of them were not offered these vaccines. If none of your physicians have mentioned vaccinations to you, each may be assuming that one of your other doctors has. You need to broach the subject with your family doctor, find out which immunizations you need, and have him or her administer them. The chart above contains a list of vaccinations recommended for people with IBD who take (or have taken) immunosuppressive drugs. ■

people with celiac disease have a close relative (a parent, child, or sibling) who also has the disease. If you have no close relatives with the disease, however, your risk of celiac disease is less than 1%.

Screening and diagnosis of celiac disease

About 20% of newly diagnosed cases of celiac disease are in people age 60 or older; some of them have had symptoms for many years.

In fact, a recent survey revealed that the average person with celiac disease has symptoms for 11 years before the condition is diagnosed. One reason is that many people with celiac disease do not have the most common symptoms—diarrhea, bloating, gas, and weight loss—and 40% have no symptoms at all. Celiac disease is especially difficult to diagnose in older adults because they are more likely to have nonspecific symptoms (for instance, pain in the joints or numbness in the legs) or nutritional deficiencies because of their age or other health problems.

If you have a close relative with celiac disease, you should be screened for the condition with a blood test. Screening should also be considered if you have thyroid disease or type 1 diabetes (which are autoimmune disorders), unexplained digestive symptoms, or weight loss. The blood test measures three specific antibodies that are present when a person with celiac disease ingests gluten. If these three antibodies are found, a biopsy of the small intestine is usually performed to look for damaged villi. The biopsy involves inserting an endoscope down the throat, through the stomach, and into the small intestine. It is important not to avoid foods that contain gluten before these tests, since avoidance could make blood test and biopsy results appear normal and prevent an accurate diagnosis.

Treatment of celiac disease

No medication or surgical procedure can cure celiac disease. The only way to treat it is to adopt a completely gluten-free diet by avoiding all food and drink containing wheat, barley, rye, and other grains. You must also look out for hidden sources of gluten, like medications, lipstick, communion wafers, and even postage stamps.

A gluten-free diet can be difficult to follow, since gluten is naturally present in many foods and is added to other products such as ice cream and salad dressings. Moreover, some labels do not indicate that a product contains gluten. Thus, you will need to ask about ingredients at restaurants, learn to substitute gluten-free ingredients in recipes, and make sure your foods don't become cross-contaminated with gluten from other foods (for example, from knives, toasters, or cutting boards).

A registered dietitian can help you recognize what foods you can and cannot eat, and the Celiac Sprue Association/USA (see page 85 for contact information) sells publications that list gluten-free foods and medicines. Joining a support group for people with celiac disease also can be helpful.

A gluten-free diet eliminates symptoms and reverses damage to the small intestine in 95% of people with celiac disease. Symptoms usually improve within a few days of eliminating gluten, although complete recovery may take anywhere from a few months to several years. To remain symptom free and avoid further damage to the small intestine, you must follow a gluten-free diet for life.

The 5% of people who do not improve on a gluten-free diet usually have severe damage to the small intestine. In these cases, medications such as the aminosalicylate anti-inflammatory compound mesalamine (Asacol, Pentasa) or the corticosteroid prednisone (see the chart on pages 60–63) may control inflammation in the small intestine and any problems from poor absorption of nutrients.

Crohn's Disease

Crohn's disease is a chronic inflammatory disorder that primarily affects the small intestine but can affect any segment of the digestive tract, including the colon, anus, mouth, and stomach. The disease can even affect the skin. About 500,000 people in the United States have Crohn's disease.

Causes of Crohn's disease

Despite extensive research, the cause of Crohn's disease is poorly understood. Three factors are believed to play a role. Genetics is one of them: Certain people inherit a susceptibility to the disease. The second factor is environmental: An unknown stimulus (perhaps a virus or a bacterium) triggers the disease by causing the body's immune system to mount an attack against the digestive tract. Once the immune system gets turned on by the trigger, it doesn't turn off properly. The third factor is race and ethnicity: Whites (particularly American Jews of European descent), followed by blacks, are more likely to get Crohn's disease than Hispanics and Asians.

Symptoms of Crohn's disease

Most often, Crohn's disease causes chronic inflammation of the small intestine. The inner lining of the small intestine becomes swollen and brittle and may develop erosions and ulcerations. These inflammatory changes usually result in abdominal pain and bloody diarrhea. The chronic inflammation can also lead to complications such as bowel perforation, peritonitis, abscesses, fistulas, and strictures.

Symptoms of Crohn's disease usually begin in the teen or young adult years. Once you have the disease you will have it for life. However, you will have symptom-free periods called remissions that can last for years. A reappearance of symptoms is called a flare-up.

Diagnosis of Crohn's disease

The tests used to diagnose Crohn's disease depend on where your doctor thinks the inflammation is occurring. An upper GI series is the best test for Crohn's disease of the small intestine. Capsule endoscopy is being investigated for diagnosis. In a 2005 study, capsule endoscopy detected more cases of Crohn's disease of the small intestine than other diagnostic techniques.

Colonoscopy is the best test for Crohn's disease of the large intestine. If a colonoscopy is not possible because of narrowing of the rectum or colon, a barium enema can be performed instead. If a fistula is suspected, the doctor may choose a more watery contrast dye called Gastrografin instead of barium.

Treatment of Crohn's disease

No drug or surgical procedure can cure Crohn's disease. Treatment is aimed at preventing and treating flare-ups and complications. Commonly prescribed drugs are listed in the chart on pages 60–63.

Because eating can irritate an inflamed bowel, severe flare-ups usually require hospital treatment with intravenous nutrition and fluids to allow the bowel to rest. You will also be given intravenous corticosteroids like methylprednisolone and mesalamine capsules (Pentasa) or tablets (Asacol) or sulfasalazine (Azulfidine) tablets to reduce inflammation. Mesalamine capsules can be used to treat disease in both the small and large intestine. If the disease is present only in the colon, mesalamine tablets or sulfasalazine tablets can be used.

If the disease responds to these treatments, you can switch from intravenous to oral corticosteroids such as prednisone or budesonide (Entocort EC). Eventually, you will be weaned off corticosteroids (but you will likely take mesalamine or sulfasalazine indefinitely). When Crohn's disease is limited to the far end of the colon and the rectum, you may receive hydrocortisone (Colocort) or mesalamine (Rowasa) enemas in addition to the treatments just mentioned.

If Crohn's disease does not improve with corticosteroids and mesalamine or sulfasalazine, immunosuppressive drugs may be tried. The most commonly used are mercaptopurine (Purinethol) and azathioprine (Imuran), both given orally. The immunosuppressant infliximab (Remicade) is especially effective when fistulas are present. It is injected about once every two months and is usually tried only when you do not respond to conventional therapy. Serious complications have been reported in people using Remicade, and in 2006, the FDA began requiring the medication's label to warn about infections and hypersensitivity reactions. Also, because Remicade can allow latent (silent) tuberculosis to develop into full-blown tuberculosis, you should receive a tuberculin skin test before beginning therapy.

In 2007, the FDA approved adalimumab (Humira) for the treatment of moderately to severely active Crohn's disease. Humira is also an immunosuppressant, but it does not require intravenous injection—the drug is packaged in an injection pen that can be self-administered once every two weeks. Humira is intended for people who cannot tolerate Remicade or who become resistant to it over time. Like Remicade, Humira carries a risk of infection, and it may increase your risk of a cancer called lymphoma.

Several other drugs to treat Crohn's disease are currently in clinical trials: abatacept (Orencia), a rheumatoid arthritis drug; natalizumab (Tysabri), a multiple sclerosis drug that was withdrawn from the market in 2005 because of a link to a rare brain infection but was then reinstated; an anti-tumor necrosis factor drug, certolizumab pegol (Cimzia); and an experimental stem-cell drug called Prochymal.

Surgical removal of a section of the bowel is required if you develop problems such as an intestinal obstruction due to serious strictures or complications like fistulas or abscesses that won't heal. In this procedure, the affected portion of the small or large intestine is removed and the two ends are reattached. This is not a cure for Crohn's disease, since the remaining bowel is still susceptible to the disease.

Ulcerative Colitis

Ulcerative colitis is a chronic inflammatory disease of the large intestine caused by an abnormal autoimmune reaction. It affects about 700,000 Americans, most of them under age 30.

The inflammation starts in the rectum and gradually progresses to the sigmoid, descending, transverse, and ascending colon and, eventually, the cecum. The inflammation does not extend beyond the colon to affect the small intestine.

Causes of ulcerative colitis

The cause of ulcerative colitis is unknown, but some people appear to have a genetic predisposition. Like Crohn's disease, ulcerative colitis is hypothesized to be activated by an environmental factor, such as an infection or food allergy, which triggers an abnormal response by the immune system. The disease is more common in whites than in nonwhites and in Jewish than in non-Jewish people.

NEW RESEARCH

Life-Threatening Colitis on the Rise in Hospital Patients

Hospitalized people are often susceptible to infection, and one that appears to be increasingly more common and deadly is *Clostridium difficile (C. difficile)* colitis, a type of colon inflammation.

C. difficile is a bacterium that lives in the intestines of 1–3% of healthy adults and about 20% of people taking antibiotics. If the normal balance of bacteria in the colon is disturbed, *C. difficile* can take over and cause symptoms such as severe diarrhea that can even lead to death. Life-threatening colitis is treated with colectomy—the removal of all or part of the colon—which carries high complication and mortality rates.

Researchers analyzed statistics from a database of hospital discharges in the United States from 1993–2003—approximately 7 million hospital stays per year. During that time period, the rate of *C. difficile* colitis cases more than doubled: from 261 cases per 100,000 discharged patients in 1993 to 546 cases per 100,000 discharged patients in 2003 (a 109% increase). Colectomy rates increased 183%, and the mortality rate for all infected patients increased 147%.

The researchers theorize that new bacterial strains, their rising antibiotic resistance, and the increasing severity of illness and ensuing susceptibility to infection among hospitalized patients may be to blame.

ARCHIVES OF SURGERY
Volume 142, page 624
July 2007

Drug Therapy for Crohn's Disease and Ulcerative Colitis 2008

Drug type: Brand (generic)	Typical daily dosages*	How to take†	Monthly cost‡: Brand (generic)
Aminosalicylate anti-inflammatory compounds			
Oral			
Asacol (mesalamine, delayed-release)	1,600–2,400 mg	One 400-mg tablet 4x/day, two 400-mg tablets 2x/day, or two 400-mg tablets 3x/day. Swallow whole (do not crush, chew, or break). Take with or without food.	$146–216
Lialda (mesalamine, delayed-release)	2.4–4.8 g	Two to four 1.2-g tablets taken once daily with a meal. Swallow whole.	$258–516
Pentasa (mesalamine, controlled-release)	4,000 mg	Four 250-mg capsules 4x/day or two 500-mg capsules 4x/day with or without food. Swallow whole.	$348–363
Azulfidine, Azulfidine-EN (sulfasalazine)	2,000–4,000 mg	One or two 500-mg tablets 4x/day with food or after meals with a glass of water.	$51–135 ($23–46)
Colazal (balsalazide)	6,750 mg	Three 750-mg capsules 3x/day with or without food.	$388
Dipentum (olsalazine)	1,000 mg	Two 250-mg capsules 2x/day with food or after meals.	$195
Rectal			
Canasa (mesalamine suppositories)	1,000 mg	Insert one 500-mg suppository into your rectum 2x/day or one 1,000-mg suppository at bedtime. For best results, have a bowel movement before using and keep in your rectum for at least 2 hours.	$300
Rowasa (mesalamine enema)	4,000 mg	At bedtime, insert the tip of one bottle into your rectum and empty the bottle's contents. For best results, use after a bowel movement and hold the medicine in your rectum overnight.	$669 ($340)
Corticosteroids			
Oral			
(prednisone)	40–60 mg	A combination of 1-, 2.5-, 5-, 10-, 20-, or 50-mg tablets 1x/day in the morning with food to prevent stomach upset.	($15–24)
Entocort EC (budesonide)	6–9 mg	Two or three 3-mg capsules 1x/day in the morning. Swallow whole (do not chew or break).	$280–392
Intravenous			
(methylprednisolone)	32–60 mg	Requires administration by a health professional who will infuse the medication into your body through a needle placed in a vein in your arm.	Not available
Rectal			
Colocort (hydrocortisone enema)	100 mg	At bedtime, insert the tip of one bottle into your rectum and empty the bottle's contents. For best results, use after a bowel movement and hold the medicine in your rectum for at least 1 hour (and preferably overnight).	$284

Precautions	Most common side effects	Call your doctor if...
Do not take if you are allergic to aspirin. Avoid alcohol to reduce the risk of dizziness and stomach bleeding. *Azulfidine only:* You'll need regular blood and urine tests to monitor the health of your blood, liver, and kidneys. *Canasa only:* Handle as little as possible, because heat from your hands can melt the suppository. *Canasa and Rowasa only:* May stain surfaces such as your clothing, floors, or countertops.	Headache, upset stomach, nausea, abdominal pain, diarrhea, gas. *Azulfidine only:* May cause skin or urine to turn orange-yellow. This is harmless and goes away when the medication is stopped.	You experience worsening stomach pain or cramping, worsening bloody diarrhea, rash, itching, yellowing eyes or skin, dark urine, fever, fatigue, headache. *Asacol and Azulfidine only:* You notice intact or partially intact tablets in your stool.
Avoid consumption of grapefruit and grapefruit juice; these foods can increase the amount of corticosteroids in your blood. Avoid exposure to people with chicken pox or measles and get your doctor's permission before having any vaccinations. If you have diabetes, monitor your blood glucose levels more closely; corticosteroids can cause your blood glucose levels to rise. Do not stop taking abruptly; to go off the drug, you need to slowly decrease the dose over time to prevent extreme fatigue, weakness, stomach upset, or dizziness. Corticosteroids can increase your risk of osteoporosis; be sure to get 1,200–1,500 mg of calcium and 400–800 IU of vitamin D a day, and have your bone density measured on a regular basis.	Headache, nausea, stomach upset, dizziness, trouble sleeping, weight gain.	You exhibit signs of high steroid levels in your body: swelling of your face and neck, acne, bruising. You have signs of infection: fever, fatigue, cough, flu-like symptoms.

* These dosages represent the usual daily dosages (unless indicated otherwise) for the treatment of Crohn's disease or ulcerative colitis. The precise effective dosage varies from person to person and depends on many factors. Do not make any changes to your medication without consulting your doctor.

† These instructions represent the typical way to take the medication. Your doctor's instructions may differ. Always follow your doctor's recommendations.

‡ Prices per drugstore.com.

continued on the next page

Drug Therapy for Crohn's Disease and Ulcerative Colitis 2008 (continued)

Drug type: Brand (generic)	Typical daily dosages*	How to take†	Monthly cost‡: Brand (generic)
Immunomodulators			
Oral			
Imuran (azathioprine)	75–150 mg	One or more 50-mg tablets 1–2x/day. Take with food to reduce stomach upset.	$142–258 ($42–71)
Purinethol (mercaptopurine)	50–100 mg	One to two 50-mg tablets 1x/day.	$156–271 ($93–186)
Intramuscular injection			
(methotrexate)	15–25 mg/week	Visit your doctor 1x/week for an injection.	Not available
Antibiotics			
Cipro (ciprofloxacin)	1,000 mg	One 500-mg tablet with or without food in the morning and evening.	$354 ($244)
Flagyl (metronidazole)	1,000–2,000 mg	One or two 500-mg tablets 2x/day in the morning and evening with food or a glass of water or milk to reduce stomach upset.	$251–502 ($19–37)
Monoclonal antibody			
Remicade (infliximab)	250–500 mg every 8 weeks	You will go to your doctor every 8 weeks to receive the medication through a needle in a vein in your arm. This takes about 2 hours.	$778–1,525
Humira (adalimumab)	40 mg every 2 weeks	You inject the medication under your skin via a single-use injection pen once every 2 weeks.	$1,400

* These dosages represent the usual daily dosages (unless indicated otherwise) for the treatment of Crohn's disease or ulcerative colitis. The precise effective dosage varies from person to person and depends on many factors. Do not make any changes to your medication without consulting your doctor.

† These instructions represent the typical way to take the medication. Your doctor's instructions may differ. Always follow your doctor's recommendations.

‡ Prices per drugstore.com.

Symptoms of ulcerative colitis

Active ulcerative colitis usually causes abdominal pain and bloody, mucusy diarrhea. Severe attacks may also produce nausea, vomiting, and fever. Like Crohn's disease, ulcerative colitis cycles between flare-ups and remissions.

Diagnosis of ulcerative colitis

The best diagnostic tests for ulcerative colitis are sigmoidoscopy and colonoscopy. The disease is diagnosed when the inner lining of the

Precautions	Most common side effects	Call your doctor if...
You should have a blood test called a complete blood count at least once a month to check for bone marrow suppression. *Methotrexate only:* Avoid alcohol, because it can cause dizziness. You will also be more sensitive to the sun, so wear sunscreen and avoid excessive sun exposure and sun lamps.	Nausea, vomiting, diarrhea, loss of appetite, stomach pain, drowsiness, dizziness.	You experience unusual bleeding or bruising or signs of infection: fever, fatigue, cough, flu-like symptoms.
Drink plenty of liquids. Consumption of dairy products (milk, yogurt, or calcium-fortified juice) greatly reduces absorption. Can cause sun sensitivity; use sunscreen and avoid excessive sunlight or sun lamps.	Stomach upset, loss of appetite, diarrhea, nausea, headache, vision changes, dizziness.	You experience a rash or signs of peripheral neuropathy: pain, burning, tingling, numbness, weakness in your hands or feet.
Alcohol should be avoided for at least 1 day afterward; the drug slows the breakdown of alcohol, which can lead to nausea and vomiting. Can cause sun sensitivity; use sunscreen and avoid excessive sunlight or sun lamps.	Diarrhea, nausea, metallic taste in the mouth, darkened urine (which is harmless).	You experience unsteadiness, seizures, mental or mood changes, numbness or tingling of your hands or feet, painful urination.
Before receiving, your doctor will do a skin test to see if you have been exposed to tuberculosis (TB). If the test is positive, you will receive treatment for TB, because Remicade and Humira can activate a latent (silent) TB infection.	Headache; nausea, vomiting, or stomach pain; redness, itching, pain, or swelling at the injection site.	You experience signs of an infection: fever, fatigue, cough, flu-like symptoms. Signs of new or worsening heart failure: shortness of breath, swelling of the ankles or feet. Signs of a blood disorder: persistent fever, bruising, bleeding, paleness. Humira only: Signs of lymphoma (unusual lumps or growths, swollen glands).

colon appears swollen, red, and brittle and contains erosions and ulcerations. Biopsies of the affected areas may be done to distinguish ulcerative colitis from other conditions affecting the colon, for example, cancer, infections, ischemia (reduced blood flow), or Crohn's disease.

Treatment of ulcerative colitis

The medications used to treat ulcerative colitis are similar to those for Crohn's disease (see the chart on pages 60–63). If you have mild disease limited to the rectum and sigmoid colon, corticosteroid- or mesalamine-containing enemas may help to control flare-ups. If this therapy fails, you may need to take oral drugs such as mesalamine (Asacol, Pentasa), olsalazine (Dipentum), sulfasalazine (Azulfidine), or balsalazide (Colazal).

If you have extensive ulcerative colitis—meaning it affects most of the colon—you may need intravenous or oral corticosteroids and oral mesalamine to treat a flare-up, followed by maintenance therapy with mesalamine to prevent future flare-ups. Severe cases may also require immunosuppressive drugs such as mercaptopurine (Purinethol) or azathioprine (Imuran) to keep the disease under control.

Surgical removal of the entire colon (called a colectomy) may be necessary if you have severe flare-ups that do not respond to corticosteroids and mesalamine, complications such as a perforation, colon cancer, or symptoms that significantly impair your quality of life.

After a colectomy, an opening called an ileostomy is made in the skin to allow fecal material to pass directly from the small intestine into an external plastic bag. Most people with an ileostomy lead normal, active lives and engage in the same job and recreational activities they did before the surgery.

Irritable Bowel Syndrome

Irritable bowel syndrome (IBS) is one of the most common—and frequently misunderstood—digestive disorders. One in five adults in the United States has symptoms of IBS, yet only a small number of people with symptoms seek treatment. In a recent poll of 201 women who had not been diagnosed with IBS but had symptoms of the disorder, 88% had heard of IBS but 21% had not talked to a doctor about their symptoms because they didn't think it was a real medical condition. And 14% didn't think there was any treatment for IBS.

The good news is that: 1) IBS can often be effectively managed once an accurate diagnosis is made—although you will require a number of tests to rule out other diseases; and 2) it appears that the disorder does not cause long-term damage to the digestive tract or lead to serious complications.

Causes of irritable bowel syndrome

The cause of IBS is not well understood. Some researchers have proposed that IBS may result from malfunctions in the rhythmic muscle contractions that propel food through the small and large intestines. Contractions that are too strong can push food contents through the intestines too quickly, causing diarrhea and bloating; weak contractions can lead to constipation.

Because women are diagnosed with IBS about three times more often than men, some experts hypothesize that symptoms may be related to hormone levels. Other proposed causes include hypersensitivity to pressure in the small and large intestines, an imbalance in neurotransmitters (chemicals found in both the brain and digestive tract), and infection.

Psychological factors may also play a role. IBS and mental stress appear to be closely related, and people with depression or anxiety tend to be more susceptible to IBS. (For more, see "Please Remain Calm" on pages 68–69.) Studies also show an increased risk of IBS in women who have been physically or sexually abused.

Symptoms of irritable bowel syndrome

The symptoms of IBS usually first appear during the teenage years or young adulthood, although the condition can develop at any time, even in older adults. One of the most common symptoms is abdominal discomfort or pain, accompanied by diarrhea, constipation, or alternating bouts of constipation and diarrhea. Other symptoms include abdominal bloating, a feeling of incomplete emptying of the bowels after passing stool, and mucus in the stool.

If you have IBS, you may find the symptoms distressing and disruptive to your life. The severity of symptoms varies: About 70% of people experience mild symptoms, although they can become more severe and even disabling at times. Some women report that IBS symptoms are worse before and during their menstrual periods. The symptoms may even awaken some people in the middle of the night.

Diagnosis of irritable bowel syndrome

IBS is difficult to diagnose because the disease causes no known physical abnormalities that doctors can identify through physical exams, imaging studies, or laboratory testing. As a result, doctors make a diagnosis only after ruling out other conditions. If you have symptoms suggestive of IBS, your doctor will take a medical history, perform a physical exam, and order blood tests. A barium enema, sigmoidoscopy, or colonoscopy may be needed to view the rectum and colon.

Once your doctor determines that your abdominal pain is not due to a physical abnormality, two of the following three criteria

NEW RESEARCH

Bolus of Steroids Still Best for Severe Ulcerative Colitis

Acute attacks of ulcerative colitis are usually treated with a bolus (high quantity) infusion of intravenous steroids, though continuous infusions—anecdotally thought to be more effective with fewer side effects—may be used. A new study, however, suggests that continuous infusion offers no greater benefit for ulcerative colitis than bolus administration.

Researchers randomly assigned 66 people having a severe attack of ulcerative colitis to receive methylprednisolone for seven days, either through a continuous I.V. infusion or two bolus I.V. injections per day. So the participants wouldn't know which treatment they were receiving, all were provided with an I.V. catheter that administered saline via an infusion pump, and the continuous-infusion group received two sham bolus injections of saline (instead of steroids) per day.

After seven days, 50% of each treatment group had complete remission of their symptoms. Steroid-related side effects—such as acne, insomnia, and muscle weakness—occurred in 28% of the participants overall but did not differ significantly between the two groups.

Since continuous infusion does not appear to offer any advantage, bolus injections should remain the preferred treatment for people experiencing severe attacks of ulcerative colitis because of the relative ease of administration.

THE AMERICAN JOURNAL OF GASTROENTEROLOGY
Volume 102, page 601
April 2007

must be met to make a diagnosis of IBS:
- Bowel movements alleviate the pain.
- The pain is accompanied by constipation or diarrhea.
- The pain is associated with a change in the form of the stool (watery, loose, or pellet-like).

These symptoms must be present, all of the time or occasionally, for at least three months.

Because the symptoms of IBS overlap with so many other digestive disorders, people with IBS are sometimes misdiagnosed. IBS can easily be confused with diverticulitis, colon cancer, intestinal obstruction, ulcerative colitis, Crohn's disease, gastrointestinal infection, celiac disease, and lactose intolerance. In fact, a study from the Netherlands found that about 25% of people diagnosed with IBS actually had lactose intolerance (an inability to properly digest lactose, a sugar found in most dairy products). When these individuals switched to a lactose-restricted diet, their symptoms improved significantly. Another study found that at least 39% of adults with unexplained, nonspecific gastrointestinal symptoms tested positive for intolerance to the sugar fructose, suggesting that many people with fructose intolerance may be mistakenly diagnosed with IBS.

Treatment of irritable bowel syndrome

Treatment of IBS focuses on relieving the most bothersome symptoms. If your main complaint is abdominal pain, anticholinergic drugs such as dicyclomine (Bentyl and other brands) and hyoscyamine (Levbid and other brands) may be used to reduce the intestinal spasms that are causing the pain. Sometimes, abdominal pain responds to a low dose of an antidepressant medication.

Constipation-predominant IBS. When constipation is your main complaint, adding fiber to your diet and increasing your fluid intake can be helpful. You may also benefit from the use of laxatives, although these medications should be used for only a week at a time unless your doctor recommends a longer period.

A drug called Zelnorm, used by many women with constipation-predominant IBS, was withdrawn from the market in April 2007 because it was suspected to increase the risk of chest pain, heart attacks, and strokes.

Diarrhea-predominant IBS. For mild to moderate diarrhea, increasing the amount of fiber in your diet or using an antidiarrhea product such as loperamide (Imodium A-D), diphenoxylate/atropine (Lomotil), or cholestyramine (Questran) may be helpful.

If you are suffering from severe diarrhea-predominant IBS and you're a woman, a drug called alosetron (Lotronex) may be considered. Lotronex has serious risks, however. It was withdrawn from the market in 2000 after reports arose of dangerous gastrointestinal side effects, including two deaths. Lotronex is now back on the market, but with strong restrictions. Only doctors registered with the drug's manufacturer can prescribe it. These doctors must agree to educate patients about Lotronex's risks and provide a written pamphlet describing these risks to their patients. Also, patients must sign an agreement, indicating that they understand the risks associated with Lotronex, prior to obtaining their first prescription.

Cilansetron (Calmactin), another drug in the same class as Lotronex, is currently in clinical trials. In a three-month study, Calmactin effectively relieved abdominal pain and discomfort and normalized bowel habits in half of the patients with diarrhea-predominant IBS who received it. The most common side effect was constipation, which affected 19% of the patients.

General advice. Keeping a diary of food intake and symptoms can help you identify foods that trigger symptoms. You may find that your symptoms are caused or worsened by fatty foods, certain vegetables (such as broccoli and cabbage), caffeine, alcohol, fructose, or sorbitol (a sweetener often used in diet candy and sugar-free gum). Certain drugs, such as antibiotics and magnesium-containing antacids or laxatives, also can be triggers.

Many people with IBS find that their symptoms improve when they exercise regularly and eat at the same times each day. If stress is a trigger for IBS, psychotherapy, hypnosis, or relaxation techniques may be beneficial. Several complementary therapies, including peppermint oil and probiotics, also show some promise.

Finally, try to talk with others who have IBS. It can be helpful to know that other people are dealing with the same challenges that you are and to share coping strategies. The website for the IBS Self Help and Support Group is www.ibsgroup.org.

Hemorrhoids

Hemorrhoids—clusters of swollen veins in and around the anus and rectum—are a common condition. More than half of all Americans develop hemorrhoids by age 50, and men and women are at equal risk. In fact, the condition is so ubiquitous that hemorrhoid sufferers have their own patron saint, St. Fiacre. Although the exact cause of hemorrhoids is not fully understood, they are thought to result from increased pressure on the veins in the anus or rectum. Hemorrhoids usually can be managed with lifestyle and self-care measures,

NEW RESEARCH

Psychological Therapies May Improve IBS Symptoms

Even with medication and dietary changes, many people with irritable bowel syndrome (IBS) do not experience relief from their symptoms. One possible reason is that IBS may have a strong psychological component, and a new review article finds that treatments directed at the mind can help.

After analyzing randomized controlled trials, meta-analyses, and journal reviews of several psychological treatments, researchers found that certain therapies were well suited for particular symptoms.

Gut-directed hypnotherapy, which focuses on imagery and techniques to normalize gastrointestinal function, appears to help some with severe IBS. Tricyclic antidepressants seem promising for people with pain and diarrhea, while selective serotonin reuptake inhibitors (SSRIs) may benefit those with constipation and pain or bloating. Cognitive behavioral therapy, which demonstrates a link between the mind and the body, may be as helpful as antidepressants but with a longer-lasting benefit. The authors suggest that a combination of talk therapy and medication may be the most beneficial.

People with IBS should not conclude that using a psychological treatment means that the condition is "all in their head," but rather it is a complex reaction to both biological and psychological factors—so they should keep an open mind to exploring psychological treatments as a potentially effective approach.

BMJ
Volume 334, page 1105
May 26, 2007

Please Remain Calm

Stress may make your digestive disorder worse

Although digestive disorders such as ulcerative colitis and irritable bowel syndrome are physical conditions, they do have an emotional aspect as well. This is not the erroneous and outdated notion that these conditions are "all in your head," but rather the idea that your mental and emotional state may affect your physical one.

Although digestive disorders aren't caused by emotional or mental stress, they do appear to be closely related. For example, people with depression or anxiety tend to be more susceptible to irritable bowel syndrome (IBS), and several studies suggest that major life events and chronic stress may worsen or cause a relapse in IBS symptoms.

The situation is similar for ulcerative colitis. A 2006 study in the journal *Gastroenterology* reported that an experimental stress test caused physical changes that may exacerbate ulcerative colitis symptoms. Heart rate and blood pressure increased, as did other inflammatory responses that can trigger an outbreak of symptoms.

The Benefits of Relaxation

Relaxing is easier said than done, but some techniques may help you cope with the stresses that can worsen digestive disorders.

Some of the most common relaxation techniques are progressive muscle relaxation, autogenic training, meditation, and guided imagery (see the inset box on the opposite page). These techniques most likely promote relaxation by reducing the activity of the sympathetic nervous system, which in turn leads to decreases in blood pressure, heart rate, respiratory rate, and muscle tension.

Relaxation techniques seem like a logical choice for the treatment of stress-related digestive disorders, and some small studies show promising results. However, until large, randomized, controlled trials confirm its effectiveness, relaxation should be used only in combination with proven treatments and not as a substitute for medication.

For ulcerative colitis. A recent German study found that individuals with ulcerative colitis who attended a 60-hour training program (which included stress management training, moderate exercise, the Mediterranean diet, behavioral techniques, and self-care strategies) reported that their quality of life was significantly improved, compared with people who received standard care for their ulcerative colitis.

Another study found that 20 people with ulcerative colitis who attended six progressive-relaxation classes had less intense and less frequent pain and a reduced need for drugs than a control group.

For IBS. A study on IBS found similar results: 16 people with IBS who were taught meditation techniques and performed two 15-minute daily sessions had significant improvements in flatulence, bloating, belching, and diarrhea two weeks later, relative to a control group. One year later, the meditation group reported even greater reductions in their symptoms. However, a more recent study found that neither cognitive behavior therapy nor relaxation training offered any benefit over standard care for individuals with IBS.

but surgical removal is required in some cases.

There are two types of hemorrhoids: internal and external. Internal hemorrhoids are located in the lower portion of the rectum and cannot be seen from outside the rectum. External hemorrhoids are visible beneath the skin around the anus.

Causes of hemorrhoids

A number of factors increase the risk of hemorrhoids or can make them worse. For example, they are more common with age, peaking at around age 65. Hemorrhoids are also associated with obesity, pregnancy and childbirth, liver disease, prostate enlargement, chronic cough, and diarrhea—all of which can increase

Four Ways To Relax

• **Progressive muscle relaxation.** Progressive muscle relaxation involves tensing and relaxing the major muscle groups of the body while breathing slowly and deeply. Starting with the muscles in the face and moving down to those in the feet, each major muscle group is tensed one at a time and then slowly relaxed. The relaxation technique can also start with the foot muscles and move up the body. Progressive muscle relaxation focuses attention on feelings of relaxation and the differences between tense and relaxed muscles.

• **Autogenic training.** Like progressive muscle relaxation, autogenic training involves focusing on different parts of the body while breathing deeply and slowly. But instead of tensing and relaxing muscles, it involves imagining that certain body parts are becoming warm and heavy one at a time. The way autogenic training works isn't completely understood, but one theory is that as you relax the body, you also relax the autonomic nervous system, which controls involuntary functions like heartbeat, blood pressure, and digestion.

• **Meditation.** Meditation is a relaxation technique that originated in India 3,000 years ago. There are many types, but the most common are transcendental meditation, breath meditation, and mindfulness meditation. Each involves sitting in a comfortable position in a quiet environment and focusing attention on something specific. In transcendental meditation, attention is focused on a simple word or sound; in breath meditation, the focus is on breathing in and out; and in mindfulness meditation, attention centers on thoughts that enter the mind.

• **Guided imagery.** In guided imagery, people use their imagination to create relaxing images. The images should involve as many of the five senses as possible. For example, you may imagine yourself lying on a beach, smelling the salt air, hearing the roar of the surf, and feeling the warmth of the sun. Picturing these images supposedly has the same relaxing effect on the brain as actually experiencing them. With practice, people are able to conjure up these relaxing images anytime they feel stressed.

How To Keep Your Cool

Mastering relaxation techniques such as those in the inset box above requires practice, and some training from a professional can be helpful. You can also find relaxation instruction on cassette or compact disc. If your primary care physician does not teach these techniques, he or she may be able to refer you to someone who does. Also, the American Holistic Medical Association website (www.holisticmedicine.org) has a directory of licensed medical doctors and doctors of osteopathic medicine who also follow holistic principles. (Click on the "Doctor Finder," and choose "Mind/Body Medicine" or "Stress Management.") ■

pressure on veins in the anus and rectum.

Contrary to popular belief, heavy lifting, long periods of sitting, and chronic constipation do not lead to hemorrhoids, although these factors can irritate existing hemorrhoids. Excessive rubbing or cleaning of the anal area also can irritate an existing condition.

Symptoms of hemorrhoids

The most common symptom of internal hemorrhoids is bleeding during a bowel movement. Such bleeding ranges in severity from blood on the toilet paper or on the outside of stools to blood in the toilet bowl. Because the membranes inside the rectum lack pain-sensitive nerves, internal hemorrhoids typically cause no pain or discomfort. However, you may experience a sensation of fullness in the rectum after a bowel movement. Internal hemorrhoids may also prolapse—meaning that the hemorrhoid protrudes outside of the anus. Prolapse can occur after straining during a bowel movement.

Unlike internal hemorrhoids, external hemorrhoids frequently cause irritation and pain, usually lasting no more than 10 days. Acute pain and inflammation can occur when a blood clot in an external hemorrhoid forms a hard lump near the anus. Mucus draining from an external hemorrhoid can cause mild itching.

See your doctor if you suspect that you have hemorrhoids and if the condition causes pain or frequent rectal bleeding.

Diagnosis of hemorrhoids

Doctors diagnose hemorrhoids by first asking about any changes in your bowel patterns and about any symptoms of pain, bleeding, or itching. The doctor may then perform an external inspection of the anus, a digital rectal exam (placing a gloved finger into the rectum to feel for hemorrhoids), and an anoscopy (an examination of the anus and lower rectum using a device called an anoscope, a short, rigid, hollow tube with a light source). Sigmoidoscopy (to view the rectum and lower colon) or colonoscopy (to view the entire colon) may be performed to see if the bleeding is originating from a source other than the hemorrhoids.

Treatment of hemorrhoids

If you have mild symptoms, lifestyle and self-care measures are frequently effective. To treat constipation that can exacerbate symptoms, you should increase your fiber and fluid intake to make stools bulkier, softer, and easier to pass. Also, you should not ignore the urge to have a bowel movement and should try not to strain when passing stool. Regular physical activity also may be helpful.

To avoid irritation of hemorrhoids, do not rub your anus too much with toilet paper after a bowel movement. Instead, try wiping gently with wet toilet paper or moist towelettes. Also, avoid sitting on the toilet for long periods.

Although research has not shown that over-the-counter suppositories, ointments, or hydrocortisone creams are effective in the treatment of hemorrhoids, many people report that they are beneficial. You may also get relief from pads containing witch hazel or a numbing agent.

To reduce irritation, try to keep the anal area clean. Avoid using soap, because it can be an irritant. Soaking in a warm bath or using a sitz water bath (a plastic basin of warm water that fits over the toilet) three to four times a day may be helpful. Afterwards, dry the anal area with a hair dryer to reduce moisture that can cause irritation. Applying cold compresses or ice packs to the anal area up to four times a day can reduce swelling.

If these conservative measures do not provide sufficient relief of symptoms, there are additional treatments for hemorrhoids. Rubber band ligation is the most common treatment for internal hemorrhoids. A small rubber band is placed at the base of the hemorrhoid to cut off its blood supply. After about a week, the hemorrhoid withers and falls off. This technique works about three quarters of the time. Sometimes, a chemical solution is injected into the hemorrhoid to shrink it—a procedure called sclerotherapy. Other options for internal hemorrhoids use laser heat or infrared light to destroy hemorrhoids. Most internal hemorrhoids can be treated effectively with one or more of these techniques.

A small percentage of people with internal hemorrhoids are not helped by the above therapies and require surgery to remove the hemorrhoids. This procedure, called a hemorrhoidectomy, requires a one- to two-day hospital stay and is the best way to ensure permanent removal of internal hemorrhoids.

For external hemorrhoids, oral pain relievers such as acetaminophen (Tylenol) or aspirin can provide some relief. However, if a hemorrhoid forms into a hard lump due to a blood clot and severe pain lasts longer than seven to 10 days, surgical removal of the clotted hemorrhoid often provides relief from symptoms.

Anal Fissure

An anal fissure is a tear in the skin that lines the anal canal, the part of the rectum closest to the anus. Most experts believe that anal fissures are caused by passing hard stool, which can tear the skin of the anal canal and cause pain and bleeding. Anal fissures are a common problem that affects most people at some point in their life. Many anal fissures heal on their own, but medication or surgery is needed if they become a chronic problem.

Causes of anal fissure

Although constipation is a common cause of anal fissures, other causes include diarrhea, childbirth, colonoscopy or sigmoidoscopy, and surgery. A high resting anal pressure (tight anus) also appears to be a factor. Tightness, or spasm, within the anus also interferes with blood supply to the anal canal, which may prevent healing of a tear. Furthermore, an anal fissure may be a sign of a more serious condition, such as syphilis, herpes, gonorrhea, chlamydia, HIV infection or AIDS, Crohn's disease, ulcerative colitis, tuberculosis, or a tumor.

Symptoms of anal fissure

The hallmark of anal fissures is pain, sometimes severe, during or after a bowel movement. The pain may be brief or continue for hours afterwards. Bleeding frequently accompanies the bowel movement, and the blood appears on the outside of the stool. About half of individuals with anal fissures also experience anal itching.

Anal fissures are frequently confused with hemorrhoids, but hemorrhoids usually do not cause pain while passing stool. Nonetheless, you can have both hemorrhoids and an anal fissure.

Diagnosis of anal fissure

To diagnose anal fissures, the doctor spreads apart your buttocks to view the anus. The fissure appears as a tear, most often in the middle of the anus toward the back of the body. While an anal fissure is usually easy to see, your doctor may use an instrument called an anoscope to view the inside of the anal canal.

Treatment of anal fissure

Between 50% and 90% of anal fissures heal on their own or with simple treatments such as eating a high-fiber diet, increasing your intake of water and other fluids, using stool-softening laxatives, and taking warm sitz baths for 10–15 minutes after each bowel movement. Topical corticosteroids and anesthetics are not effective.

If an anal fissure does not heal after six weeks of the simple treatments described above, you have a chronic anal fissure. This usually requires additional treatment, the most common of which is nitroglycerin ointment. A pea-sized amount of the ointment is placed on the fissure two to three times a day for up to eight weeks. This treatment heals between 70% and 80% of chronic anal fissures. The most common side effect of the ointment is headaches, which can be severe, though pain relievers such as acetaminophen (Tylenol) and aspirin may relieve the pain.

Other medicines used for anal fissures are calcium channel blockers—medications commonly used to treat high blood pressure and chest pain. The oral calcium channel blocker nifedipine (Procardia and other brands) heals 60% of chronic anal fissures when used for eight weeks. Nifedipine may work by decreasing anal pressure. Another calcium channel blocker, diltiazem (Cardizem), which is available in oral and cream forms, also appears to be beneficial for the treatment of chronic anal fissures. Common side effects include headache and swelling of the feet and ankles.

Low doses of botulinum toxin A (Botox), a paralyzing agent, also can be used to treat anal fissures. Studies show that a single injection can heal more than 80% of chronic anal fissures, possibly by lowering anal pressure. Although it has a high success rate, some people find the injections painful. Rare complications include bleeding, blood clots under the skin around the anus, loss of bowel control, and sepsis (a bacterial infection of the blood). (For more information, see "Botox: Not Just a Wrinkle Eraser" on pages 76–77.)

If a chronic anal fissure does not heal with medications, surgery may be necessary. Sphincterotomy, which involves cutting part of the muscle in the anal canal, is the surgery of choice. It helps heal about 98% of anal fissures. Sphincterotomy decreases the spasms and pressure in the anal canal and is a good option for people with chronic anal fissures and a high resting anal pressure. Another surgical treatment, anal dilation or a four-fingered anal stretch, heals 40–90% of chronic anal fissures. In this procedure, the physician uses four fingers to hold the anus open for four minutes to reduce spasms and pressure in the anal canal. However, almost 40% of people who undergo anal dilation have difficulty controlling flatulence or soil themselves occasionally; some 16% experience loss of bowel control.

Fecal Incontinence

Fecal incontinence (the involuntary loss of bowel control) affects more than 6.5 million Americans. Although it is a relatively common problem in older adults, it is not a normal part of aging. The inability to control your bowels can lead to embarrassment and cause you to avoid social situations, but fecal incontinence is often treatable with medication, lifestyle measures, or surgical repair of the damaged sphincter muscles. In addition, some people can benefit from an implanted device called an artificial sphincter.

Causes of fecal incontinence

Fecal incontinence is not a disease but a symptom of another gastrointestinal problem. The most common causes of fecal incontinence are:

- Damage to the sphincter muscles in the anus (usually due to hemorrhoid surgery or childbirth). These muscles normally contract to prevent stool from leaving the rectum.

• Damage to nerves in the anal sphincter muscles or rectum (due to chronic constipation, stroke, diabetes, multiple sclerosis, or childbirth). Nerve damage in the sphincter muscles leads to a loss of proper functioning of the muscles, while nerve damage in the rectum leads to loss of sensation in that area, so that you no longer recognize that stool is present.
• Loss of storage capacity in the rectum (due to rectal surgery, radiation therapy for cancer, or inflammatory bowel disease). Normally, the rectum stretches to hold stool until you reach the toilet; with loss of elasticity, an accident is much more likely.
• Diarrhea. Loose, watery stools are much harder to control than solid stools.
• Pelvic floor dysfunction (such as rectal prolapse, in which the rectum sags). By supporting the organs in the pelvis and lower abdomen, the muscles of the pelvic floor play a role in preventing fecal incontinence.

Symptoms of fecal incontinence
The symptoms of fecal incontinence are easily recognizable, ranging from the occasional leakage of liquid or solid stool and gas to the inability to hold a bowel movement until you reach the toilet. Other possible symptoms include diarrhea and constipation.

Diagnosis of fecal incontinence
Because self-treatment of fecal incontinence is rarely successful, you should see your doctor if you experience any of the symptoms above. The doctor will take a medical history, do a thorough physical examination, and may order one or more diagnostic tests. These tests could include anal manometry to measure the tightness of the anal sphincter, anorectal ultrasonography to examine the structure of the anal sphincter, proctography/defecography to determine how well the rectum holds and eliminates stool, procto-sigmoidoscopy to detect signs of diseases or other problems inside the rectum and sigmoid colon, and anal electromyography to test for nerve damage.

You should bring to your doctor's appointment a list of all the medications that you take. Some medications, such as sedatives, antacids, and muscle relaxants, can cause or increase the frequency of fecal incontinence, especially in older adults.

Treatment of fecal incontinence
Treatment depends on the cause and severity of fecal incontinence and may include changes in diet, bowel training, medication, or

surgery. Treatment helps control fecal incontinence in about 50% of patients.

Dietary changes. Because it is difficult for the anal sphincter to handle large amounts of waste material, changes in your diet may be necessary to make the stool firmer and more compact. Foods that thicken the stool include rice, bananas, yogurt, and cheese. Increasing fiber intake—to 21 g daily if you're a woman over age 50 and to 30 g daily if you're a man over age 50—by consuming more whole grains, fruits, and vegetables also may help.

Alcohol and caffeine may cause diarrhea and should be eliminated. Some people are unable to digest lactose (a sugar found in dairy products) or food additives and flavorings like sorbitol and nutmeg. Because improper digestion of these substances could contribute to diarrhea and fecal incontinence, they should be avoided as well.

Bowel training. Some people with fecal incontinence need to relearn how to control their bowels. One way to retrain the bowels is through biofeedback, which uses a computer to monitor muscle contractions as you learn exercises to strengthen the rectum and pelvic muscles. Stronger muscles can help retain stool. If fecal incontinence is caused by constipation, your doctor may recommend starting a routine of having a bowel movement at the same time every day.

Medication. Drugs may be used if fecal incontinence is caused by diarrhea. Loperamide (Imodium A-D) is an antidiarrhea medication that thickens the stool and also increases the strength of the rectal muscles. Other medications help treat fecal incontinence in other ways, for example, by decreasing intestinal secretions, contracting the muscle that closes the rectum, or slowing the movement of stool through the bowel.

External incontinence devices. If you're unable to regain fecal continence, you can wear an external device to collect any leaking stool. These prescription devices, available at medical supply stores and some pharmacies, typically consist of a drainable pouch attached to an adhesive wafer. The hole in the center of the wafer is placed over the rectum to allow stool to pass through. These devices can remain in place for 24 hours, but they must be changed if any stool leakage occurs.

Surgical repair. If fecal incontinence is caused by injury to the pelvic floor, anal canal, or anal sphincter, surgery may be performed to repair the problem. For example, damaged muscles in the anus may be replaced with muscle from the leg or arm.

Artificial sphincter. If your anal sphincter muscles are not capable of holding in stool, an artificial anal sphincter can be surgically

Botox: Not Just a Wrinkle Eraser

The popular cosmetic drug may help relieve digestive symptoms as well

Botox is best known for its ability to ease facial lines and make a person appear younger. But before the drug went Hollywood, it was originally developed for a less glamorous purpose: treating strabismus (crossed eyes) and blepharospasm (abnormal blinking).

Today, Botox is approved to treat cervical dystonia (a contraction of the neck muscles that causes abnormal movements and postures of the neck and head) and hyperhidrosis (excessive sweating). The drug is also used off-label to treat many other conditions, including some digestive disorders.

From Harmful to Helpful

Botulinum toxin A, from which Botox is derived, is a highly poisonous bacterial toxin that attacks the nerves and causes muscle paralysis. It is one of the world's most dangerous substances. But the same properties that make this toxin deadly in large doses also help relieve muscle spasms when used carefully in very small amounts.

When injected into the affected muscle, Botox prevents release of a neurotransmitter called acetylcholine from the nerve fibers controlling the muscle. As a result, the muscle loses nervous stimulation and relaxes—faces stop frowning or eyes stop crossing.

Botox offers several advantages over other treatments: Unlike oral drugs, it doesn't enter the bloodstream and typically remains in the affected muscle only, so side effects are rare. Unlike surgery, it is noninvasive, painless, and quick. Its effects typically fade after a few months, but repeat treatments appear to offer the same benefits as the first injection.

Botox for the Digestive Tract

Several digestive disorders caused by muscle spasms are candidates for Botox treatment. Achalasia was the first to benefit from Botox; now it's used for anal fissures, gastroparesis, constipation, and dysphagia. Although the U.S. Food and Drug Administration (FDA) has not approved Botox for any of these conditions, some insurance companies will cover its use.

Achalasia. This swallowing disorder occurs when the lower esophageal sphincter fails to relax and allow food to enter the stomach. Injecting Botox into the lower esophageal sphincter paralyzes and relaxes it. Several studies indicate that Botox may be helpful, but it may not be right for everyone.

A recent study in *Gastroenterology* showed that 40 people treated surgically with laparoscopic myotomy had greater symptom improvement than 40 people treated with Botox (82% vs. 66%). Two years after treatment, almost 88% of the surgical group was symptom free, compared with only 34% of the Botox group.

Another recent study in *Endoscopy* found that Botox was most successful long term in people over age 55 who had only a mild increase in pressure around the lower esophageal sphincter. Younger people with more severely increased pressure may have better results with dilation or myotomy. One theory is that older adults' nerves do not regenerate as quickly, so the paralyzing effects of Botox may last longer in this group.

Anal fissures. The internal anal sphincter, one of two muscles that control the anus, is always under tension (known as resting pressure). If the muscle contracts too often and the tension is too high, spasms and reductions in blood flow can cause tears known as fissures in the skin near the anus.

Botox injections have become a first-line therapy for anal fissures in many hospitals in the United States. In a February 2007 study in the *British Journal of Surgery*, 100 participants with anal fissures were treated with either Botox or nitroglycerin ointment (a common treatment). After two months, the fissures were completely healed in 92% of the Botox group but only 70% of the nitroglycerin group, with fewer complications with Botox. The researchers concluded that although both treatments were effective alternatives to surgery, Botox had a higher success rate with fewer complications.

Gastroparesis. This autonomic nervous system disorder, often seen in people with type 1 diabetes, involves a delay in the passage of digested food out of the stomach. The result can be an uncomfortable sense of fullness after even a small meal, nausea, vomiting, and bloating. The problem often is that the pyloric sphincter (which opens to allow food to move into the small intestine) doesn't relax properly. This cause, combined with the lack of effective medications for gastroparesis, makes Botox a viable treatment.

A recent study in *Gastrointestinal Endoscopy* showed that out of 63 people with gastroparesis who were treated with Botox, 43% had an improvement in their symptoms lasting about five months. Another small study in the same journal showed that six people treated with Botox for gastroparesis had a 55% improvement in their symptoms and a 52% increase in the time it took their stomachs to empty.

The benefits of Botox are temporary, and large-scale, randomized, controlled trials have not yet been published on the topic, but some doctors are already using Botox to help their patients reduce gastroparesis symptoms. Keep in mind that Botox is still an experimental therapy for gastroparesis and cannot be recommended to everyone until more definitive studies have been published.

Constipation. One of the common causes of constipation is when the pelvic floor muscles contract too much or don't relax enough during a bowel movement.

A November 2006 study in *The American Journal of Gastroenterology* found that Botox may help correct these muscle problems. Italian researchers injected Botox into two sites on either side of the puborectalis muscle in 24 people with chronic constipation. Two months later, 19 participants had significant improvement, and the other five experienced symptom relief after a second set of injections.

None of the participants experienced any significant side effects, and after an average of three years, all of them remained constipation free. These results are surprising, given that the effects of Botox injections usually wear off after a few months.

Although the study did not include a control group, the results suggest that Botox is a promising treatment that warrants more research. When compared with biofeedback—which is often used to treat chronic constipation—Botox is longer lasting, requires less effort, and is less expensive. However, Botox is still rarely used in the United States to treat constipation, and it is only considered after traditional therapies do not work.

Dysphagia. Dysphagia, or difficulty swallowing, is often caused by a neurological condition such as a stroke, Parkinson's disease, multiple sclerosis, or diabetes-related nerve damage.

In a December 2006 study in *Diabetes Care*, 12 people with type 2 diabetes who had severe swallowing problems received Botox injections in the upper esophageal sphincter. Ten of them experienced complete symptom relief after one injection, while the other two had significant improvement. The injection's benefits appeared within one week and lasted up to 12 weeks.

Six months after the initial treatment, symptoms reappeared in all participants, but repeat injections produced good results. The participants were then treated every three to four months, and none reported any significant side effects.

Because it is effective and noninvasive, the researchers suggest that Botox may be a first-line treatment for diabetes-related dysphagia, for which there is currently no medical treatment. Surgery is used sometimes to cut the overactive muscle causing the dysphagia, but improvements in swallowing don't always occur. Botox may be a less invasive alternative to surgery or a way to tell who would benefit from surgery. However, it is still considered an experimental therapy for dysphagia, and large, randomized, controlled trials are needed before it can be recommended.

What To Expect From Botox

Your condition will determine who administers your Botox injection—gastroenterologists typically do it for people with achalasia or gastroparesis, and surgeons usually administer it for anal fissures.

Botox is administered with a fine-gauge needle into the affected muscle. An ultrasound machine may be used to pinpoint the exact location. The injections are relatively painless, although some people experience minor discomfort. Your doctor may numb the site with a cold pack or a topical anesthetic before giving the injection.

Botox generally takes effect in a few days to a few weeks, and results last for up to six months. If you respond well, it can be repeated as needed—usually four times per year. Some people do develop a tolerance to the drug, so that it becomes less effective over time. Your doctor may try to minimize your risk of tolerance by using the lowest possible dose and the longest interval between doses.

Botox is generally considered safe, but like any drug, it has a risk of side effects. Serious reactions, such as shortness of breath, are rare. Pain and/or a pooling of blood at the injection site are slight risks. Botox may not be appropriate if you are taking aminoglycoside antibiotics or drugs that interfere with neuromuscular transmission (such as Alzheimer's drugs) or if you have an infection at the injection site. ■

implanted. This sphincter consists of a fluid-filled cuff that surrounds the anal canal, a pressure-regulating balloon in the anal canal, and a control pump located just under the skin. Normally, the cuff is full of fluid, which squeezes the anal canal closed. When you need to have a bowel movement, you squeeze the pump several times; the fluid then drains from the cuff into the balloon, and stool can pass through the open anal canal. After the bowel movement, the cuff automatically refills with fluid from the balloon. One study found that 11 of 16 patients had improved bowel control and quality of life two years after implantation of an artificial sphincter.

Colostomy. Severe fecal incontinence that does not respond to treatment may require a colostomy, a procedure in which the large intestine is connected to the abdominal wall. Instead of entering the rectum, stool goes directly from the intestine into a special bag outside the body.

Colorectal Polyps

Colorectal polyps are small, noncancerous (benign) clumps of cells that grow in the rectum and colon. Over the course of 10–15 years, some of these polyps—usually the ones that are larger than a pea—can become cancerous. Fortunately, regular screening for colorectal cancer helps to identify and remove polyps, often before they progress to cancer.

Causes of colorectal polyps

It is not known why polyps develop, but some people are more prone than others. For instance, the older you get—especially after age 50—the more likely you are to have them. You're also more likely to develop polyps if you've had them before (polyps tend to recur) or if someone in your family has had polyps or cancer of the colon. Your behavior also influences your risk: Eating a lot of fatty foods, smoking cigarettes, drinking alcohol, not exercising, and being overweight can all contribute to the formation of polyps.

Symptoms of colorectal polyps

Most polyps don't cause any symptoms. You might not know you have them until your doctor finds one or more during a physical examination or colorectal cancer screening test. However, some people notice rectal bleeding (especially after a bowel movement), constipation or diarrhea that lasts longer than a week, or blood in their stool (the stool looks black or contains red streaks). In these cases, you should see your doctor for an evaluation.

Diagnosis of colorectal polyps

Polyps can be diagnosed by a digital rectal exam, barium enema, sigmoidoscopy, or colonoscopy. The last three tests are described on pages 39–41.

Treatment of colorectal polyps

Polyps are removed during a sigmoidoscopy or colonoscopy. The removed polyps are then tested to see if they are cancerous and if any further treatment is needed.

Colorectal Cancer

In 2006, colorectal cancer—cancer of the colon or rectum—was diagnosed in about 148,500 people in the United States. It is the second most common cause of death from cancer, killing about 55,000 Americans each year. The good news is that most colorectal cancers and deaths can be prevented.

Causes of colorectal cancer

Cancer occurs when a genetic mutation causes cells in the body to reproduce in a rapid, disorderly, and dangerous manner. The precise cause of this mutation is unclear, but it appears to result from a combination of personal and environmental risk factors.

Risk factors for colorectal cancer include:

- Increasing age
- Polyps in the colon or rectum or a history of these polyps, especially an inherited condition called familial polyposis
- Breast, endometrial, or ovarian cancer
- Ulcerative colitis or Crohn's disease
- A close relative (mother, father, or sibling) diagnosed with colorectal cancer before age 60
- Dietary factors, such as red and processed meats.

Symptoms of colorectal cancer

Colorectal cancer often produces no symptoms in its early stages, which is why screening is so important. However, any of the following symptoms should prompt a visit to your doctor:

- Frequent, unexplained abdominal pain or cramps
- Blood in or on your stool or blood in the toilet or on your underwear after passing stool
- An increase or decrease in bowel movements
- Alternating between frequent bowel movements and constipation

NEW RESEARCH

High-Fruit, Low-Meat Diet May Ward Off Colorectal Cancer

Red meat has been linked in several studies with an increased risk of colorectal cancer. A new study goes one step further, suggesting that a diet high in all kinds of meat may be harmful to your colon, whereas a high-fruit diet may help protect it.

Researchers studied the dietary habits of 725 people in their 50s and 60s who underwent a colonoscopy. The test revealed adenomas (precancerous polyps) in 203 participants. Within three months of their colonoscopy, participants were asked how often they eat fruit, vegetables, and meat (including beef, pork, veal, poultry, fish, hot dogs, and luncheon meats). The researchers grouped the participants into one of three categories.

The low-meat, high-fruit eaters had the lowest occurrence of polyps: 19%. In the high-meat, low-fruit/vegetable group (with just over half the participants) 28% had a polyp. The moderate-meat, high-vegetable group, surprisingly, had the highest percentage of people with polyps: 33%.

These results don't rule out the possibility that vegetables help prevent colorectal cancer. Moderate meat consumption in the highest-risk group may have canceled out any protective effect from the vegetables. A diet low in meat and rich in fruits and vegetables is still recommended as the most promising way to protect against colorectal cancer.

THE JOURNAL OF NUTRITION
Volume 137, page 999
April 2007

- Passing narrowed stools
- Weakness and fatigue
- Unexplained weight loss.

Screening for colorectal cancer

The American College of Gastroenterology recommends regular screening for colorectal cancer in people age 50 and older. However, only one quarter of people follow this recommendation.

Colorectal cancer screening often involves a yearly fecal occult blood test beginning at age 50. The test usually involves smearing a small amount of stool on a specially designed card and bringing it to your doctor or a laboratory where it is examined for the presence of blood. If blood is found in the stool, even trace amounts, you will need to undergo a colonoscopy to find the cause of the bleeding.

If your annual fecal occult test is negative (no blood found in the stool), you will need to undergo a colonoscopy every five to 10 years starting at age 50. During a colonoscopy, the doctor can view the rectum and the entire colon and remove any polyps. In a recent report, this procedure reduced cancer risk by 76–90%. Many insurance companies now cover the cost of colonoscopy for cancer screening.

If a colonoscopy cannot be performed—perhaps because it isn't covered by your health insurance or isn't readily available in your area—the American College of Gastroenterology suggests a sigmoidoscopy once every five years in addition to a yearly fecal occult blood test, although a recent study suggested that more frequent screening may offer some benefit. The study found that, three years after sigmoidoscopy, 14% of the participants had a polyp or mass, 3% had colon cancer or adenomas (a type of polyp at high risk for becoming cancerous), and nearly 1% had advanced colon cancer or adenomas.

A third screening option, according to the American College of Gastroenterology, is a barium enema every five to 10 years. Though less expensive than a colonoscopy or sigmoidoscopy, a barium enema cannot distinguish polyps or cancer from stool, and it can produce a large number of erroneous results.

Besides regular screening, lifestyle measures may reduce the colorectal cancer risk. These include eating a diet low in animal fat and high in fruits and vegetables, exercising regularly, maintaining a healthy weight, not smoking, and not drinking alcohol excessively.

Diagnosis of colorectal cancer

Fecal occult blood testing, barium enema, sigmoidoscopy, and colonoscopy are used to diagnose colorectal cancer. Because colorectal

ASK THE DOCTOR

Q. ***I've had a colon polyp removed. What can I do to prevent colorectal cancer?***

A. One crucial step is to have a follow-up colonoscopy every three to five years, depending on the number and size of your polyps.

You also need to get moving—the American Cancer Society stresses the importance of exercise for those trying to prevent polyp recurrence. Excess body weight and inactivity are linked with shorter survival times; one study found that people who exercised regularly were about half as likely to die of colorectal cancer within four years as those who did not exercise.

No diet is guaranteed to prevent colorectal cancer recurrence, but experts suggest this recipe to help lower your risk:

- Get most of your foods from plant sources (fresh vegetables, fruits, and nuts).
- Avoid processed foods and limit those high in saturated fats (especially beef).
- Choose chicken, fish, or beans as your main protein sources.
- Avoid junk foods, including sodas and sugar-laden snacks.
- Have no more than one alcoholic drink per day.
- Get most of your nutrients from foods rather than supplements.

Finally, although some research has suggested that NSAIDs may prevent colorectal cancer, the U.S. Preventive Services Task Force recently concluded that the risks of long-term NSAID use—such as gastrointestinal bleeding, kidney problems, and hemorrhagic (bleeding) stroke—exceed the potential benefits for people at average risk for colorectal cancer.

cancer can cause intestinal bleeding, a blood test is used to check for anemia (a low red blood cell count). Imaging tests such as ultrasound, CT scans, MRI, chest x-rays, and angiography (an x-ray technique that uses an injected contrast material) may be used to visualize the intestines or to see if the cancer has spread to other sites in the body. If cancer is diagnosed, the stage of the cancer must be identified to determine the best course of treatment. The stage of the cancer is based on how large the tumor is and whether it has spread to the lymph nodes or other parts of the body.

Treatment of colorectal cancer

Surgery is the most common treatment for colorectal cancer and can eliminate the cancer in about half of all cases. It involves removal of the part of the colon or rectum that contains the cancer, some of the healthy tissue that surrounds it, and nearby lymph nodes (to determine if the cancer has spread to the lymphatic system). Common side effects of surgery include diarrhea or constipation, which usually improves on its own.

Other treatments for colorectal cancer include chemotherapy and radiation therapy, which can be used alone, in combination with each other, or with surgery. Chemotherapy delivers medication intravenously to attack cancer cells throughout the body. It can be used after surgery (to increase the odds that all cancer cells have been eliminated) or before surgery to help shrink a tumor. If colorectal cancer has spread, chemotherapy may be used to slow the progression of the cancer and relieve symptoms (without the expectation of a cure). Adverse effects may include nausea, vomiting, fatigue, diarrhea, mouth sores, hair loss, and bone marrow suppression.

Radiation therapy involves directing x-rays at the cancer cells. It is used only for rectal cancer. Unlike chemotherapy, which affects the whole body, radiation therapy specifically targets cancer cells while minimizing damage to healthy cells. As with chemotherapy, it may be used before surgery, after surgery, or for symptom relief when cancer has spread and a cure is not possible. The radiation may be delivered internally from implanted radioactive "seeds" or externally from an x-ray machine. Common adverse events include fatigue, nausea, diarrhea, appetite loss, bloody stool, and damage to the skin and other organs near the radiation site. ■

GLOSSARY

abscess—A localized accumulation of pus resulting from an infection.

achalasia—A disorder of the esophagus caused by the inability of the lower esophageal sphincter to relax and by abnormal esophageal contractions. Results in difficulty swallowing.

acute cholecystitis—Inflammation of the gallbladder producing severe pain, fever, nausea, and vomiting.

anal fissure—A tear in the skin that lines the anal canal, the part of the rectum closest to the anus.

antireflux barrier—A mechanical impediment created by the lower esophageal sphincter and the diaphragm that prevents the contents of the stomach from entering the esophagus.

anus—The opening at the end of the digestive tract through which stool is expelled. It is controlled by two sphincters and is only open during defecation.

autoimmune disease—A health problem in which the body's immune system begins to attack its own tissues.

barium x-ray—See upper GI series.

Barrett's esophagus—A disorder in which the cells that normally line the inside of the esophagus are replaced by more acid-resistant cells; associated with an increased risk of esophageal cancer.

bile—A substance synthesized by the liver, stored and concentrated in the gallbladder, and then released into the duodenum to help in the digestion and absorption of dietary fat.

bile ducts—Tubes that carry bile from the left and right lobes of the liver to the gallbladder.

biliary colic—Intermittent episodes of sharp pain in the right upper portion of the abdomen that occur when gallstones block the flow of bile from the gallbladder.

bilirubin—A component of bile made by the liver. Pigment gallstones are primarily made up of bilirubin.

bowel—The lower digestive tract, which is about 25 feet long and consists of the small and large intestines.

capsule endoscopy—A noninvasive test that allows for a full view of the small intestines, particularly the areas that are usually unreachable with an upper endoscopy or colonoscopy. You ingest a capsule that contains a video camera, which takes pictures of the digestive tract and transmits these images to a recording device.

cecum—The first part of the colon (large intestine).

celiac disease—A disorder that occurs in people who are sensitive to gluten, a component of wheat and other grains. Can cause diarrhea, bloating, weight loss, anemia, and vitamin deficiencies.

cholangitis—Infection and inflammation of the bile ducts.

cholecystectomy—Surgical removal of the gallbladder.

cirrhosis—A disease that causes the liver to slowly deteriorate and eventually malfunction as a result of the replacement of healthy tissue with scar tissue. Typically caused by alcohol abuse.

colectomy—Surgical removal of part or all of the colon.

colon—The part of the digestive tract that is connected to the small intestine. The colon absorbs water and electrolytes such as potassium from undigested foods before passing waste on to the rectum for release from the body. Also called the large intestine.

colonoscopy—A diagnostic procedure in which an endoscope is inserted through the anus and rectum to view the colon and the final portion of the small intestine (terminal ileum).

colorectal cancer—Cancer of the colon or rectum. Often preceded by the development of colorectal polyps.

common bile duct—A tube that carries bile from the liver and gallbladder to the small intestine.

constipation—A common but typically benign condition characterized by infrequent bowel movements and difficulty passing stool.

Crohn's disease—A chronic inflammatory disorder that primarily affects the small intestine but can involve any segment of the gastrointestinal tract.

cystic duct—A tube that carries bile from the gallbladder to the common bile duct.

diaphragm—The muscle that separates the chest from the abdomen; its movements play an important role in breathing.

diarrhea—An increase in the number of bowel movements and a decrease in the consistency of stools.

diffuse esophageal spasm—Prolonged and excessive contractions of the esophagus.

digital rectal exam—Insertion of a gloved finger into the rectum to feel for polyps and other abnormalities.

diverticulitis—A disorder in which small pouches in the wall of the large intestine (diverticula) become inflamed or infected.

diverticulosis—The development of small pouches (diverticula) that bulge outward through weak points in the wall of the large intestine.

duodenal bulb—The portion of the duodenum that is closest to the stomach.

duodenal ulcer—A nonhealing defect or sore that occurs in the lining of the duodenum.

duodenum—The first portion of the small intestine.

dysphagia—Difficulty swallowing food or liquids.

endoscopic dilation—An endoscopic procedure for the treatment of achalasia in which a balloon device is inserted into the esophagus to expand the lower esophageal sphincter.

endoscopic retrograde cholangiopancreatography (ERCP)—A diagnostic test that combines endoscopy with x-rays to view the pancreatic ducts and bile ducts.

endoscopy—A procedure that uses a thin, lighted viewing tube to visually examine the interior of a hollow organ, such as the esophagus, stomach, or small intestine.

esophageal manometry—A diagnostic test for esophageal disorders that measures lower esophageal sphincter pressure and evaluates esophageal contractions.

esophageal rings and webs—Thin, fragile folds in the inner lining of the esophagus that partially or completely block the esophagus.

esophageal stricture—A narrowing of the esophagus caused by chronic inflammation and scar tissue.

esophageal ulcers—Nonhealing defects in the inner lining of the esophagus.

esophagus—A muscular tube that is part of the upper digestive system. Food moves from the mouth to the throat and then to the esophagus.

fecal incontinence—The involuntary loss of bowel control; a relatively common problem in older adults.

fistula—An abnormal channel or connection in the body caused by disease. May develop between different segments of the digestive tract, or between the digestive tract and other organs, usually the bladder, vagina, or skin.

gallbladder—A pear-shaped sac located under the liver that stores bile. Plays an important role in the digestion and absorption of dietary fat.

gallstones—Small "pebbles" that form in the gallbladder and cause pain. Most gallstones are made of cholesterol, but some are made of bilirubin (a component of bile made by the liver).

gastritis—An inflammation of the inner lining of the stomach.

gastroesophageal junction—The place where the esophagus meets the stomach.

gastroesophageal reflux disease (GERD)—A backflow of the stomach's contents into the esophagus that leads to heartburn and indigestion.

Heller myotomy—A surgical procedure for the treatment of achalasia in which an incision is made through the muscle of the lower esophageal sphincter to weaken it.

hemorrhoids—Clusters of swollen veins in and around the anus and rectum that can cause pain.

hepatobiliary scintigram—A diagnostic test for acute cholecystitis in which a small amount of radioactive material is injected into a vein to visualize the bile duct system. Also called a hepato-iminodiacetic acid (HIDA) scan.

hiatal hernia—A protrusion of the gastroesophageal junction and a portion of the stomach into the chest cavity. These parts of the gastrointestinal tract are normally located in the abdominal cavity.

H_2-blockers—Drugs that inhibit gastric acid secretion. Also known as histamine H_2-antagonists.

ileostomy—A surgical procedure that attaches the last part of the small intestine (ileum) to an opening in the skin of the abdomen so that fecal material can pass out of the body.

ileum—The last portion of the small intestine.

irritable bowel syndrome—A common and frequently misunderstood digestive disorder that affects more women than men and can cause diarrhea, bloating, or constipation.

ischemia—A reduced supply of oxygen to any part of the body due to the obstruction of blood flow.

jejunum—The middle section of the small intestine.

laparoscopic surgery—A minimally invasive surgery performed through small incisions in the abdomen using specialized instruments and a tiny camera.

large intestine—The part of the digestive tract that is connected to the small intestine. It absorbs water and electrolytes such as potassium from undigested foods before passing waste on to the rectum for release from the body. Also called the colon.

liver—A large organ located on the upper-right side of your torso, opposite your stomach and behind your rib cage. Its main function is to make a substance called bile that is needed to digest food in the small intestine.

lower esophageal sphincter (LES)—A ring of muscle at the lower end of the esophagus that contracts to prevent the reflux of stomach contents into the esophagus.

main pancreatic duct—A tube that carries digestive juices from the pancreas to the duodenum.

major duodenal papilla—A protuberance in the duodenum that contains openings for the common bile duct and the main pancreatic duct.

metaplasia—A change in the cells in a tissue from a normal to an abnormal state, as occurs in Barrett's esophagus.

mucosal protectants—Drugs that increase the resistance of the inner lining of the digestive tract to damaging acid from the stomach.

Nissen fundoplication—A surgical procedure for gastroesophageal reflux disease and hiatal hernia that involves lifting a portion of the stomach and tightening it around the gastroesophageal junction to increase lower esophageal sphincter pressure.

pancreas—A long, thin gland that lies horizontally behind the bottom part of the stomach and makes digestive enzymes that flow through the pancreatic duct to the small intestine. These enzymes, along with bile from the gallbladder, break down food for use as energy.

pancreatitis—Inflammation of the pancreas.

peptic ulcer—A nonhealing defect or sore in the inner lining of the stomach or duodenum.

perforation—A hole in an organ.

peristalsis—A series of wavelike muscle contractions that occur automatically to move food and fluid through the digestive tract.

peritonitis—Inflammation or infection of the lining of the abdominal cavity.

pH—A measurement of acidity or alkalinity.

polyp—A small, noncancerous (benign) clump of cells that grows in the rectum and colon. Over the course of 10–15 years, some polyps—usually those larger than a pea—may become cancerous.

promotility agents—Drugs that increase digestive tract motility, resulting in faster removal of acid from the esophagus, greater esophageal sphincter pressure, and better emptying of the stomach.

proton pump inhibitors—Drugs that strongly suppress acid production in the stomach.

pylorus—A circular muscle that connects the opening at the end of the stomach with the duodenum.

rectum—The area into which the colon pushes waste products for storage before they are released through the anus during a bowel movement.

sigmoidoscopy—A procedure in which the last 25 inches of the colon are examined with a short, flexible endoscope inserted through the anus.

small intestine—The part of the digestive tract that absorbs nutrients from foods. The stomach passes food into the small intestine where digestive juices from the liver and pancreas help break down food. Undigested food components (waste) pass from the small intestine to the large intestine.

sphincter of Oddi—The layers of muscle that control the entry of bile and pancreatic juices into the duodenum from the common bile duct and the pancreatic duct.

steatorrhea—The presence of large amounts of undigested fat in the stool.

stomach—The portion of the digestive tract that mechanically breaks down food and mixes it with digestive juices. When the food becomes a thick liquid, it passes into the small intestine.

stricture—An abnormal narrowing of hollow tubes in the body, such as the esophagus or bile ducts, due to the formation of scar tissue.

trachea—The windpipe.

ulcer—A nonhealing defect or sore in the mucosal lining of organs such as the stomach and duodenum.

ulcerative colitis—A chronic inflammatory disease of the large intestine caused by an abnormal autoimmune reaction that causes the body to attack its own bowel.

upper endoscopy—A procedure that examines the inside lining of the esophagus, stomach, and duodenum using a long, thin, flexible tube with a light and tiny video camera at its tip, to look for abnormalities such as inflammation, ulcers, and tumors.

upper esophageal sphincter—An area of muscular tissue at the upper end of the esophagus that contracts to prevent air from entering the esophagus when swallowing is not taking place.

upper GI series—X-rays of the esophagus, stomach, and duodenum that are taken after the patient swallows a solution of barium to make the organs visible on x-ray film.

virtual colonoscopy—A noninvasive test in which a CT scan of the abdomen is done to obtain two- and three-dimensional images of the colon and rectum. It has a number of drawbacks and typically is not performed unless standard colonoscopy cannot be done.

Z-line—An irregular white line seen on endoscopy that corresponds to the gastroesophageal junction, the place where the esophagus meets the stomach.

HEALTH INFORMATION ORGANIZATIONS AND SUPPORT GROUPS

About GERD
P.O. Box 170864
Milwaukee, WI 53217-8076
☎ 888-964-2001/414-964-1799
www.aboutgerd.org
Provides general information about GERD symptoms, treatments, and new research as part of the International Foundation for Functional Gastrointestinal Disorders. Also publishes a brochure.

American College of Gastroenterology
P.O. Box 342260
Bethesda, MD 20827-2260
☎ 301-263-9000
www.acg.gi.org
A professional organization that gives patients general information and health tips pertaining to gastrointestinal disorders as well as help finding a physician.

American Gastroenterological Association
4930 Del Ray Ave.
Bethesda, MD 20814
☎ 301-654-2055
www.gastro.org
A nonprofit professional organization offering a variety of publications, magazines, news, and information about digestive health. Website provides message boards and help finding a gastroenterologist.

American Society of Colon & Rectal Surgeons
85 West Algonquin Rd., Ste. 550
Arlington Heights, IL 60005
☎ 847-290-9184
www.fascrs.org
A professional society representing more than 1,000 board-certified colon and rectal surgeons. Provides brochures, a newsletter, and help finding a surgeon.

American Speech-Language-Hearing Association
10801 Rockville Pike
Rockville, MD 20852
☎ 800-638-8255
www.asha.org
Toll-free help line gives information on communication and swallowing disorders and referrals to speech-language pathologists around the country who can help with swallowing disorders.

Celiac Sprue Association/USA Inc.
P.O. Box 31700
Omaha, NE 68131-0700
☎ 877-CSA-4CSA
www.csaceliacs.org
Sponsors a network of local chapters and support groups and publishes a list of gluten-free foods (updated annually), a quarterly newsletter, and additional education materials relating to celiac disease.

Crohn's & Colitis Foundation of America
386 Park Ave. South, 17th Fl.
New York, NY 10016-8804
☎ 800-932-2423
www.ccfa.org
A nonprofit health organization dedicated to improving the quality of life of people with Crohn's disease or ulcerative colitis. Raises funds for research, provides educational programs, and offers support such as books and brochures for patients.

International Foundation for Functional Gastrointestinal Disorders
P.O. Box 170864
Milwaukee, WI 53217-8076
☎ 888-964-2001/414-964-1799
www.iffgd.org
An education and research organization dedicated to informing and supporting patients with gastrointestinal disorders. Provides information on its website and publications on many different topics.

National Digestive Diseases Information Clearinghouse
2 Information Way
Bethesda, MD 20892-3570
☎ 800-891-5389
www.digestive.niddk.nih.gov
A branch of the National Institutes of Health. Provides publications and articles on the diagnosis, treatment, and prevention of digestive diseases.

LEADING HOSPITALS
for Digestive Disorders as Ranked by *U.S. News & World Report*

1. **Mayo Clinic**
   Rochester, MN
   ☎ 507-284-2511/507-538-3270
   www.mayoclinic.org

2. **Cleveland Clinic**
   Cleveland, OH
   ☎ 800-223-2273/216-444-2200
   www.clevelandclinic.org

3. **Johns Hopkins Hospital**
   Baltimore, MD
   ☎ 410-502-4003/410-955-5464
   www.hopkinsmedicine.org

4. **Massachusetts General Hospital**
   Boston, MA
   ☎ 617-726-2000
   www.massgeneral.org

5. **University of California, Los Angeles Medical Center**
   Los Angeles, CA
   ☎ 310-825-9111
   www.healthcare.ucla.edu

6. **University of Chicago Medical Center**
   Chicago, IL
   ☎ 888-UCH-0200/773-702-1000
   www.uchospitals.edu

7. **Duke University Medical Center**
   Durham, NC
   ☎ 888-ASK-DUKE/919-684-8111
   www.dukehealth.org

8. **Cedars-Sinai Medical Center**
   Los Angeles, CA
   ☎ 310-4-CEDARS
   www.cedars-sinai.edu

9. **Mount Sinai Medical Center**
   New York, NY
   ☎ 212-241-6500
   www.mountsinai.org

10. **Brigham and Women's Hospital**
    Boston, MA
    ☎ 617-732-5500
    www.brighamandwomens.org

INDEX

ISBN 978-1-933087-63-4
1-933087-63-3

Printed in the United States of America

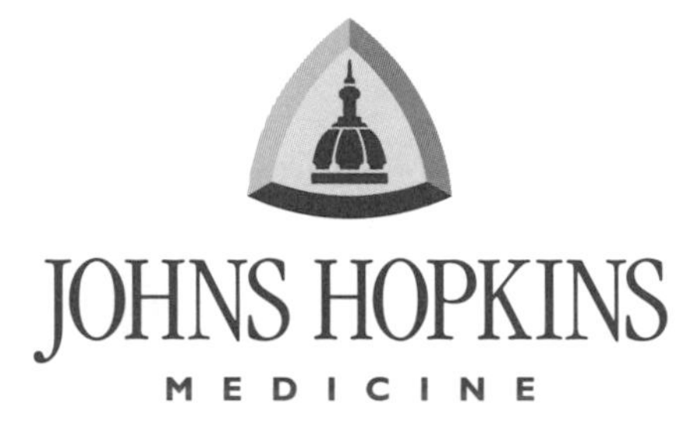

The Johns Hopkins White Papers are published yearly by Medletter Associates, LLC.

Visit our website for information on Johns Hopkins Health Publications, which include White Papers on specific disorders, home medical encyclopedias, consumer reference guides to drugs and medical tests, and our monthly newsletter *The Johns Hopkins Medical Letter: Health After 50*.
www.JohnsHopkinsHealthAlerts.com